T0227376

Neuroimaging Anatomy, Part 1: Brain and Skull

Editor

TARIK F. MASSOUD

NEUROIMAGING CLINICS OF NORTH AMERICA

www.neuroimaging.theclinics.com

Consulting Editor

SURESH K. MUKHERJI

August 2022 • Volume 32 • Number 3

ELSEVIER

1600 John F. Kennedy Boulevard • Suite 1800 • Philadelphia, Pennsylvania, 19103-2899

http://www.neuroimaging.theclinics.com

NEUROIMAGING CLINICS OF NORTH AMERICA Volume 32, Number 3
August 2022 ISSN 1052-5149, ISBN 13: 978-0-323-84997-5

Editor: John Vassallo (j.vassallo@elsevier.com)
Developmental Editor: Karen Solomon

Neuroimaging Clinics of North America (ISSN 1052-5149) is published quarterly by Elsevier Inc., 360 Park Avenue South, New York, NY 10010-1710. Months of issue are February, May, August, and November. Business and editorial offices: 1600 John F. Kennedy Blvd., Suite 1800, Philadelphia, PA 19103-2899. Business and editorial offices: 6277 Sea Harbor Drive, Orlando, FL 32887-4800. Periodicals postage paid at New York, NY, and additional mailing offices. Subscription prices are USD 401 per year for US individuals, USD 932 per year for US institutions, USD 100 per year for US students and residents, USD 469 per year for Canadian individuals, USD 946 per year for Canadian institutions, USD 546 per year for international individuals, USD 946 per year for international institutions, USD 100 per year for Canadian students and residents and USD 260 per year for foreign students and residents. To receive student/resident rate, orders must be accompanied by name of affiliated institution, date of term, and the *signature* of program/residency coordinator on institution letterhead. Orders will be billed at individual rate until proof of status is received. Foreign air speed delivery is included in all *Clinics* subscription prices. All prices are subject to change without notice. POSTMASTER: Send address changes to *Neuroimaging Clinics of North America*, Elsevier Health Sciences Division, Subscription **Customer Service, 3251 Riverport Lane, Maryland Heights, MO 63043. Telephone: 1-800-654-2452 (U.S. and Canada); 314-447-8871 (outside U.S. and Canada). Fax: 314-447-8029. E-mail: journalscustomerservice-usa@elsevier.com (for print support); journalsonlinesupport-usa@elsevier.com (for online support)**.

Reprints. For copies of 100 or more of articles in this publication, please contact the Commercial Reprints Department, Elsevier Inc., 360 Park Avenue South, New York, NY 10010-1710. Tel.: 212-633-3874; Fax: 212-633-3820; E-mail: reprints@elsevier.com.

Neuroimaging Clinics of North America is covered by *Excerpta Medical/EMBASE,* the RSNA Index of Imaging Literature, *MEDLINE/PubMed (Index Medicus),* MEDLINE/MEDLARS, SciSearch, Research Alert, and Neuroscience Citation Index.

PROGRAM OBJECTIVE

The goal of Neuroimaging Clinics of North America is to keep practicing radiologists and radiology residents up to date with current clinical practice in radiology by providing timely articles reviewing the state of the art in patient care.

TARGET AUDIENCE

Practicing radiologists, radiology residents, and other healthcare professionals who utilize neuroimaging findings to provide patient care.

LEARNING OBJECTIVES

Upon completion of this activity, participants will be able to:

1. Review the anatomy and parts of the brain, as well as its variants, to develop a better understanding of its functions.
2. Discuss the role of neuroimaging as a tool for assessing, evaluating, diagnosing, and managing structural abnormalities and dysfunction of the brain.
3. Recognize the importance of neuroimaging techniques for detecting abnormalities and dysfunction, assessing and maintaining function, and planning treatment for brain illnesses and dysfunction.

ACCREDITATION

The Elsevier Office of Continuing Medical Education (EOCME) is accredited by the Accreditation Council for Continuing Medical Education (ACCME) to provide continuing medical education for physicians.

The EOCME designates this journal-based CME activity for a maximum of 15 *AMA PRA Category 1 Credit*(s)™. Physicians should claim only the credit commensurate with the extent of their participation in the activity.

All other healthcare professionals requesting continuing education credit for this enduring material will be issued a certificate of participation.

DISCLOSURE OF CONFLICTS OF INTEREST

The EOCME assesses conflict of interest with its instructors, faculty, planners, and other individuals who are in a position to control the content of CME activities. All relevant conflicts of interest that are identified are thoroughly vetted by EOCME for fair balance, scientific objectivity, and patient care recommendations. EOCME is committed to providing its learners with CME activities that promote improvements or quality in healthcare and not a specific proprietary business or a commercial interest.

The planning committee, staff, authors, and editors listed below have identified no financial relationships or relationships to products or devices they or their spouse/life partner have with commercial interest related to the content of this CME activity:

Asthik Biswas, MBBS, DNB; Barton F. Branstetter, IV, MD; Hisham M. Dahmoush, MD; Scott E. Forseen, MD; Bruce C. Gilbert, MD; Carolina V. A. Guimaraes, MD; Lotfi Hacein-Bey, MD; Jeremy J. Heit, MD, PhD; Michael J. Hoch, MD; Susie Y. Huang, MD, PhD; Pradeep Krishnan, MBBS, MD; Michiya Kubo, MD, PhD; Pradeep Kuttysankaran; Naoya Kuwayama, MD, PhD; Tarik F. Massoud, MD, Phd, FRCR; Tomasz Matys, MD, Phd, FRCR; Adrienne M. Moraff, MD; John A. Morris, DO; Yoshiaki Ota, MD; William T. Parker, MD; Daniel J. Scoffings, MBBS, MRCP, FRCR; Gaurang Shah, MD, FACR, FASFNR; Manohar Shroff, MD, FRCPC, DABR, DMRD; Doreen Thomas-Payne, MSN, BSN, RN, PMHNP-BC; Katie Suzanne Traylor, DO; Behroze Adi Vachha, MD, PhD; Eric K. van Staalduinen, DO; Logi Vidarsson, PhD; Dylan N. Wolman, MD; Michael M. Zeineh, MD, PhD

The planning committee, staff, authors and editors listed below have identified financial relationships or relationships to products or devices they or their spouse/life partner have with commercial interest related to the content of this CME activity:

Sanjeet S. Grewal, MD: Researcher and Consultant: Boston Scientific Corp. and Medtronic, Inc.

Erik Middlebrook, MD: Researcher and Consultant: Boston Scientific Corp. and Varian Medical Systems, Inc.

Timothy M. Shepherd, MD, PhD: Ownership Interest: MICroStructure Imaging (MICSI)

UNAPPROVED/OFF-LABEL USE DISCLOSURE

The EOCME requires CME faculty to disclose to the participants:

1. When products or procedures being discussed are off-label, unlabelled, experimental, and/or investigational (not US Food and Drug Administration [FDA] approved); and
2. Any limitations on the information presented, such as data that are preliminary or that represent ongoing research, interim analyses, and/or unsupported opinions. Faculty may discuss information about pharmaceutical agents that is outside of FDA-approved labelling. This information is intended solely for CME and is not intended to promote off-label use of these medications. If you have any questions, contact the medical affairs department of the manufacturer for the most recent prescribing information.

TO ENROLL

To enroll in the *Neuroimaging Clinics of North America* Continuing Medical Education program, call customer service at 1-800-654-2452 or sign up online at http://www.theclinics.com/home/cme. The CME program is available to subscribers for an additional annual fee of USD 265.00.

METHOD OF PARTICIPATION

In order to claim credit, participants must complete the following:

1. Complete enrolment as indicated above.
2. Read the activity.
3. Complete the CME Test and Evaluation. Participants must achieve a score of 70% on the test. All CME Tests and Evaluations must be completed online.

CME INQUIRIES/SPECIAL NEEDS

For all CME inquiries or special needs, please contact elsevierCME@elsevier.com.

NEUROIMAGING CLINICS OF NORTH AMERICA

FORTHCOMING ISSUES

November 2022
Neuroimaging Anatomy, Part 2: Head, Neck, and Spine
Tarik F. Massoud, *Editor*

February 2023
Central Nervous System Infections
Tchoyoson Lim Choie Cheio, *Editor*

May 2023
MRI and Brain Trauma
Pejman Jabehdar Maralani and Sean Symons, *Editors*

RECENT ISSUES

May 2022
Mimics, Pearls, and Pitfalls of Head and Neck Imaging
Gul Moonis and Daniel T. Ginat, *Editors*

February 2022
Imaging of the Post Treatment Head and Neck
Prashant Raghavan, Robert E. Morales, and Sugoto Mukherjee, *Editors*

November 2021
Skull Base Neuroimaging
Steve E.J. Connor, *Editor*

SERIES OF RELATED INTEREST

Advances in Clinical Radiology
Available at: Advancesinclinicalradiology.com
MRI Clinics of North America
Available at: MRI.theclinics.com
PET Clinics
Available at: https://www.pet.theclinics.com/
Radiologic Clinics of North America
Available at: Radiologic.theclinics.com

THE CLINICS ARE AVAILABLE ONLINE!
Access your subscription at:
www.theclinics.com

Contributors

CONSULTING EDITOR

SURESH K. MUKHERJI, MD, MBA, FACR
Clinical Professor of Radiology and Radiation Oncology, University of Illinois, Peoria, Illinois, USA; Robert Wood Johnson Medical School, Rutgers University, New Brunswick, New Jersey, USA; Faculty, Otolaryngology Head Neck Surgery, Michigan State University, Farmington Hills, Michigan, USA; National Director of Head and Neck Radiology, ProScan Imaging, Carmel, Indiana, USA

EDITOR

TARIK F. MASSOUD, MD, PhD, FRCR
Professor of Radiology and Neuroradiology, Division of Neuroimaging and Neurointervention, Department of Radiology, Stanford University School of Medicine, Attending Diagnostic Neuroradiologist, Stanford Health Care, Director, Stanford Initiative for Multimodality Neuro-Imaging in Translational Anatomy Research (SIMITAR), Center for Academic Medicine, Palo Alto, California, USA

AUTHORS

ASTHIK BISWAS, MBBS, DNB
Department of Diagnostic Imaging, The Hospital for Sick Children, Department of Medical Imaging, University of Toronto, Toronto, Ontario, Canada; Department of Radiology, Great Ormond Street Hospital for Children NHS Trust, London, United Kingdom

BARTON F. BRANSTETTER IV, MD
Professor of Radiology, Neuroradiology Division, University of Pittsburgh School of Medicine, Pittsburgh, Pennsylvania, USA

HISHAM M. DAHMOUSH, MD
Clinical Assistant Professor of Radiology, Stanford University School of Medicine, Department of Radiology, Stanford University, Stanford, California, USA

SCOTT E. FORSEEN, MD
Department of Radiology and Imaging, Medical College of Georgia at Augusta University, Augusta, Georgia, USA

BRUCE C. GILBERT, MD
Neuroradiology, Neuroradiology Section, Department of Radiology and Imaging, Medical

College of Georgia at Augusta University, Augusta, Georgia, USA

SANJEET S. GREWAL, MD
Assistant Professor, Department of Neurosurgery, Mayo Clinic, Jacksonville, Florida, USA

CAROLINA V.A. GUIMARAES, MD
Clinical Professor of Radiology, Division Chief of Pediatric Radiology, University of North Carolina, School of Medicine, Department of Radiology, Chapel Hill, North Carolina, USA

LOTFI HACEIN-BEY, MD
Division of Neuroradiology, Radiology Department, University of California, Davis School of Medicine, Sacramento, California, USA

JEREMY J. HEIT, MD PhD
Department of Radiology, Department of Neuroimaging and Neurointervention, Stanford University School of Medicine, Stanford, California, USA; Assistant Professor of Radiology and Neurosurgery Stanford University School of Medicine, Center for Academic Medicine, Palo Alto, California, USA

MICHAEL J. HOCH, MD
Department of Radiology, University of Pennsylvania, Philadelphia, Pennsylvania, USA

SUSIE Y. HUANG, MD, PhD
Director of Translational Neuro MR Imaging, Associate Professor of Radiology, Division of Neuroradiology and Athinoula A. Martinos Center for Biomedical Imaging, Department of Radiology, Massachusetts General Hospital, Harvard Medical School, Charlestown, Massachusetts, USA

PRADEEP KRISHNAN, MBBS, MD
Department of Diagnostic Imaging, The Hospital for Sick Children, Department of Medical Imaging, University of Toronto, Toronto, Ontario, Canada

MICHIYA KUBO, MD, PhD
Department of Neurosurgery, Stroke Center, Saiseikai Toyama Hospital, Department of Neurosurgery, University of Toyama, Toyama, Japan

NAOYA KUWAYAMA, MD, PhD
Toyama Red Cross Hospital, Department of Neurosurgery, University of Toyama, Toyama, Japan

TARIK F. MASSOUD, MD, PhD, FRCR
Professor of Radiology and Neuroradiology, Division of Neuroimaging and Neurointervention, Department of Radiology, Stanford University School of Medicine, Attending Diagnostic Neuroradiologist, Stanford Health Care, Director, Stanford Initiative for Multimodality Neuro-Imaging in Translational Anatomy Research (SIMITAR), Center for Academic Medicine, Palo Alto, California, USA

TOMASZ MATYS, MD, PhD, FRCR
Associate Professor and Honorary Consultant Neuroradiologist, Department of Radiology, University of Cambridge, Cambridge Biomedical Campus, Department of Radiology, Cambridge University Hospitals NHS Foundation Trust, Addenbrooke's Hospital, Cambridge Biomedical Campus, Cambridge, United Kingdom

ERIK H. MIDDLEBROOKS, MD
Professor of Radiology, Consultant Departments of Radiology and Neurosurgery, Mayo Clinic, Jacksonville, Florida, USA

ADRIENNE M. MORAFF, MD
Assistant Professor, Division of Neurosurgery, Howard University, Howard University School of Medicine, Washington, DC, USA

JOHN A. MORRIS, DO
Department of Radiology and Imaging, Medical College of Georgia at Augusta University, Augusta, Georgia, USA

YOSHIAKI OTA, MD
Division of Neuroradiology, Department of Radiology, University of Michigan, Ann Arbor, Michigan, USA

WILLIAM T. PARKER, MD
Neuroradiology, Neuroradiology Section, Department of Radiology and Imaging, Medical College of Georgia at Augusta University, Augusta, Georgia, USA

DANIEL J. SCOFFINGS, MBBS, MRCP, FRCR
Consultant Neuroradiologist, Department of Radiology, Cambridge University Hospitals NHS Foundation Trust, Addenbrooke's Hospital, Cambridge Biomedical Campus, Cambridge, United Kingdom

GAURANG SHAH, MD, FACR, FASFNR
Professor of Radiology, Division of Neuroradiology, Department of Radiology, University of Michigan, Ann Arbor, Michigan, USA

TIMOTHY M. SHEPHERD, MD, PhD
Department of Radiology, NYU Langone School of Medicine, New York, New York, USA

MANOHAR SHROFF, MD, FRCPC, DABR, DMRD
Department of Diagnostic Imaging, The Hospital for Sick Children, Department of Medical Imaging, University of Toronto, Toronto, Ontario, Canada

KATIE SUZANNE TRAYLOR, DO
Assistant Professor of Radiology, Neuroradiology Division, Director of Head and Neck Imaging, University of Pittsburgh School of Medicine, Pittsburgh, Pennsylvania, USA

BEHROZE ADI VACHHA, MD, PhD
Associate Attending, Neuroradiology, Department of Radiology, Brain Tumor Center, Memorial Sloan Kettering Cancer Center, New York, New York, USA

ERIC K. VAN STAALDUINEN, DO
Department of Radiology, Stanford University, Stanford, California, USA

LOGI VIDARSSON, PhD
Department of Diagnostic Imaging, The Hospital for Sick Children, Department of Medical Imaging, University of Toronto, Toronto, Ontario, Canada

DYLAN N. WOLMAN, MD
Department of Radiology, Department of Neuroimaging and Neurointervention, Stanford University School of Medicine, Center for Academic Medicine, Palo Alto, California, USA

MICHAEL M. ZEINEH, MD, PhD
Associate Professor, Department of Radiology, Stanford University, Stanford, California, USA

Contents

Foreword: Neuroimaging Anatomy, Part 1: Brain and Skull xv

Suresh K. Mukherji

Preface: Neuroimaging Anatomy, Part 1: Brain and Skull xvii

Tarik F. Massoud

Anatomy of the Calvaria and Skull Base 447

Tomasz Matys, Daniel J. Scoffings, and Tarik F. Massoud

A thorough understanding of the skull anatomy is of key importance to radiologists as well as specialist physicians and surgeons. We describe the anatomy of the neurocranium comprising calvaria (the skull vault) and the skull base and discuss the most common and clinically relevant anatomic variants.

Anatomy of the Cerebral Cortex, Lobes, and Cerebellum 463

Behroze Adi Vachha, Tarik F. Massoud, and Susie Y. Huang

Strong foundational knowledge of the anatomy of the cerebral cortex, lobes, and cerebellum is key to guide the search for potential lesions based on clinical presentation and known focal neurologic deficits. This article provides an introduction and overview of cerebral cortical anatomy, including the key sulci that divide the 4 lobes of the cerebral cortex, as well as the major gyral and sulcal landmarks within each lobe. The organization of the cerebellum and its major anatomic constituents are also described. Commonly encountered anatomic variants and asymmetries in cerebral cortical anatomy are presented and discussed.

Medial Temporal Lobe Anatomy 475

Eric K. van Staalduinen and Michael M. Zeineh

The medial temporal lobe (MTL) is a complex anatomic region encompassing the hippocampal formation, parahippocampal region, and amygdaloid complex. To enable the reader to understand the well-studied regional anatomic relationships and cytoarchitecture that form the basis of functional connectivity, the authors have created a detailed yet approachable anatomic reference for clinicians and scientists, with special attention to MR imaging. They have focused primarily on the hippocampal formation, discussing its gross structural features, anatomic relationships, and subfield anatomy and further discuss hippocampal terminology and development, hippocampal connectivity, normal anatomic variants, clinically relevant disease processes, and automated hippocampal segmentation software.

Brain Functional Imaging Anatomy 491

Behroze Adi Vachha and Erik H. Middlebrooks

Human brain function is an increasingly complex framework that has important implications in clinical medicine. In this review, the anatomy of the most commonly assessed brain functions in clinical neuroradiology, including motor, language, and vision, is discussed. The anatomy and function of the primary and secondary sensorimotor areas are discussed with clinical case examples. Next, the dual stream of language processing is reviewed, as well as its implications in clinical medicine

and surgical planning. Last, the authors discuss the striate and extrastriate visual cortex and review the dual stream model of visual processing.

Cerebral White Matter Tract Anatomy 507

Asthik Biswas, Pradeep Krishnan, Logi Vidarsson, and Manohar Shroff

Advances in MR imaging techniques have allowed for detailed in vivo depiction of white matter tracts. The study of white matter structure and connectivity is of paramount importance in leukodystrophies, demyelinating disorders, neoplasms, and various cognitive, neuropsychiatric, and developmental disorders. The advent of advanced "function-preserving" surgical techniques also makes it imperative to understand white matter anatomy and connectivity, to provide accurate road maps for tumor and epilepsy surgery. In this review, we will describe cerebral white matter anatomy with the help of conventional MRI and diffusion tensor imaging.

MRI-Visible Anatomy of the Basal Ganglia and Thalamus 529

Michael J. Hoch and Timothy M. Shepherd

Conventional MR imaging does not discriminate basal ganglia and thalamic internal anatomy well. Radiology reports describe anatomic locations but not specific functional structures. Functional neurosurgery uses indirect targeting based on commissural coordinates or atlases that do not fully account for individual variability. We describe innovative MR imaging sequences that improve the visualization of normal anatomy in this complex brain region and may increase our understanding of basal ganglia and thalamic function. Better visualization also may improve treatments for movement disorders and other emerging functional neurosurgery targets. We aim to provide an accessible review of the most clinically relevant neuroanatomy within the thalamus and basal ganglia.

Brain Connectomics 543

Erik H. Middlebrooks and Sanjeet S. Grewal

A central tenet of modern neuroscience is the conceptualization of the brain as a collection of complex networks or circuits with a shift away from traditional "localizationist" theories. Connectomics seeks to unravel these brain networks and their role in the pathophysiology of neurologic diseases. This article discusses the science of connectomics with the examples of its potential role in clinical medicine and neuromodulation in multiple disorders, such as essential tremor, Parkinson's disease, obsessive-compulsive disorder, and epilepsy.

MRI-Visible Anatomy of the Brainstem 553

Timothy M. Shepherd and Michael J. Hoch

Human brainstem internal anatomy is intricate, complex, and essential to normal brain function. The brainstem is affected by stroke, multiple sclerosis, and most neurodegenerative diseases—a 1-mm focus of pathologic condition can have profound clinical consequences. Unfortunately, detailed internal brainstem anatomy is difficult to see with conventional MRI sequences. We review normal brainstem anatomy visualized on widely available clinical 3-T MRI scanners using fast gray matter acquisition T1 inversion recovery, probabilistic diffusion tractography, neuromelanin, and susceptibility-weighted imaging. Better anatomic localization using these recent innovations improves our ability to diagnose, localize, and treat brainstem diseases. We aim to provide an accessible review of the most clinically relevant brainstem neuroanatomy.

Fetal Brain Anatomy 663

Carolina V.A. Guimaraes and Hisham M. Dahmoush

Fetal brain development has been well studied, allowing for an ample knowledge of the normal changes that occur during gestation. Imaging modalities used to evaluate the fetal central nervous system (CNS) include ultrasound and MRI. MRI is the most accurate imaging modality for parenchymal evaluation and depiction of developmental CNS anomalies. The depiction of CNS abnormalities in a fetus can only be accurately made when there is an understanding of its normal development. This article reviews the expected normal fetal brain anatomy and development during gestation. Additional anatomic structures seen on brain imaging sequences are also reviewed.

Imaging of Normal Brain Aging 683

Yoshiaki Ota and Gaurang Shah

Understanding normal brain aging physiology is essential to improving healthy human longevity, differentiation, and early detection of diseases, such as neurodegenerative diseases, which are an enormous social and economic burden. Functional decline, such as reduced physical activity and cognitive abilities, is typically associated with brain aging. The authors summarize the aging brain mechanism and effects of aging on the brain observed by brain structural MR imaging and advanced neuroimaging techniques, such as diffusion tensor imaging and functional MR imaging.

Foreword
Neuroimaging Anatomy, Part 1: Brain and Skull

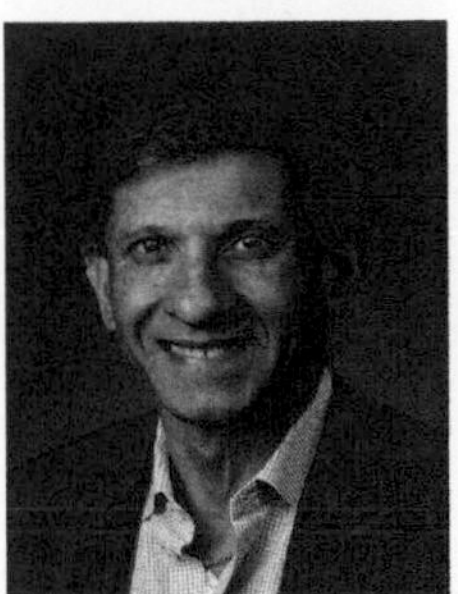

Suresh K. Mukherji, MD, MBA, FACR
Consulting Editor

I recently shared a long cab ride with the editor of one the major radiology journals, and they asked me what I did in my academic "spare" time. My spontaneous response was that I like to review old anatomic textbooks and papers. I was taken aback after "listening" to my own answer since I have built my academic career on applications of evolving technologies for diagnosis and management of Head & Neck Cancer. However, then I read Dr Tarik Massoud's preface of this issue of *Neuroimaging Clinics*, which states "[a] natomy should rightly be regarded as the firm foundation of the whole art of medicine and its essential preliminary" (Andreas Vesalius, De Humani Corporis Fabrica [1543]) and "[a]t least half of learning neuroradiology is understanding neuroanatomy" (Dr Anne G. Osborn), and I was relieved!

We have entered the era of physiologic imaging, and every trainee is exposed to advanced techniques that assess various biologic pathways, which has been enhanced by applications of artificial intelligence. However, we should always remember that the role of imaging is to directly visualize anatomy, and we will never be able to identify pathologic conditions and add fundamental value to patient care if we do not have a strong foundation in normal anatomy.

I am often asked what the most comprehensive book is for reviewing neuroanatomy, and I could not think of anything recent. So, to rectify this educational gap, I asked Dr Massoud to guest edit a 2-part issue of *Neuroimaging Clinics* devoted to Neuroimaging Anatomy. This topic is dedicated to the brain and skull base anatomy and contains fifteen articles that review both structural and functional neuroanatomy. The authors are recognized experts in their fields, and the articles are outstanding.

I would like to personally thank the article authors for their outstanding contributions. I would especially like to thank Dr Massoud for agreeing to edit this wonderful contribution. I remember discussing this opportunity when I was a Visiting Professor at Stanford a few years ago. Tarik not only accepted the invitation but also took this project to a new level. This issue has reached and exceeded Dr Massoud's stated goal of presenting anatomic facts of practical value to clinical neuroradiologists, other clinical neuroscientists, and their trainees and will be a wonderful reference for years to come! Thank you to all who contributed and especially to Tarik!

Suresh K. Mukherji, MD, MBA, FACR
Marian University
Head and Neck Radiology
ProScan Imaging
Carmel, IN 46032, USA

E-mail address:
sureshmukherji@hotmail.com

Neuroimag Clin N Am 32 (2022) xv
https://doi.org/10.1016/j.nic.2022.05.005
1052-5149/22/© 2022 Published by Elsevier Inc.

Preface
Neuroimaging Anatomy, Part 1: Brain and Skull

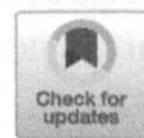

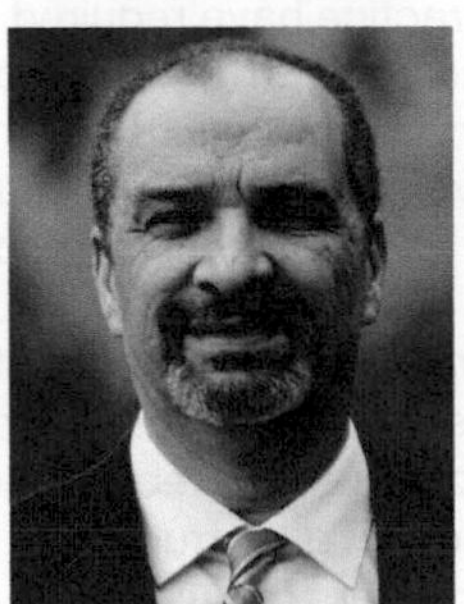

Tarik F. Massoud, MD, PhD, FRCR
Editor

Two wonderful quotations capture the intended essence and objective for compiling this and the next issue of *Neuroimaging Clinics* on the subject of neuroimaging anatomy: "[a]natomy should rightly be regarded as the firm foundation of the whole art of medicine and its essential preliminary" (Andreas Vesalius, De Humani Corporis Fabrica [1543]), and "[a]t least half of learning neuroradiology is understanding neuroanatomy" (Dr Anne G. Osborn).

This issue of *Neuroimaging Clinics* on neuroimaging anatomy of the brain and skull appears after an unusually long interval since this topic was last reviewed in this series (8:1, February 1998; guest editor, Lindell Gentry), in part dictated by the need to await the steady evolution of neuroimaging techniques we have witnessed over the last two decades that would help us better depict the stunning neuroanatomy we encounter in our daily neuroradiological practice. We believe this *Neuroimaging Clinics* issue covering brain and skull anatomy will help clinical neuroradiologists and specialists in allied fields appreciate the exquisitely detailed anatomy that underlies neuroimaging. We aim to update the reader about the role of current and new advances in imaging techniques that help us visualize and understand this complex anatomy. As such, this issue is not intended to be a formal or exhaustive treatise on anatomy (classical textbooks and atlases are intended for that purpose) but aims to give an updated anatomic background, which would assist clinical practitioners in the diagnosis and treatment of disorders of the brain and skull.

The importance of anatomy in imaging cannot be overstated. As radiologists, we are exceedingly privileged to be able to indirectly see the internal anatomy of our patients. There are many reasons neuroanatomy is the underpinning of our neuroradiology practice. This is not only because we noninvasively review intricate neuroanatomic structures on images but also, in practice, because we clinically and educationally disseminate the anatomic knowledge we have gained to others. The reasons for the importance of neuroimaging anatomy include the fact that its knowledge is highly relevant to the daily work of neuroradiologists in distinguishing normal and variant anatomy from pathologic signs of disease.

Neuroimag Clin N Am 32 (2022) xvii–xix
https://doi.org/10.1016/j.nic.2022.05.004
1052-5149/22/

Thus, to correlate structural and functional neuroimaging findings with the clinical information of patients, to issue radiologic reports, and to communicate meaningfully and on par with referring physicians all require a deep understanding of neuroanatomy and the language used to describe it. The central role of these neuroimaging interpretations rooted in knowledge of neuroanatomy has never been stronger for clinical decision making within contemporary clinical care.

As neuroradiology becomes ever more fundamental to clinical pathways and as a hub for decision making in the clinical neurosciences, an understanding of neuroimaging anatomy is essential to the neuroradiologists of tomorrow. The aim of including anatomy in radiology curricula for residents and fellows in training is not to produce anatomists, but rather, to produce radiologists who will be able to apply anatomic scientific principles, methods, and knowledge to the clinical practice of radiology. I often tell radiology trainees that "radiologists are but applied anatomists." As neuroradiology educators, we must convey to our trainees a sound core knowledge of neuroimaging anatomy. This will form a cornerstone of their future practice and will instill confidence during training by lessening the occurrence of anatomic misinterpretations, defined as errors in identifying the correct anatomic locations of brain pathologic conditions.

The symbiosis of anatomy and radiology is crucial to the practice of medicine, and it is also an important element of doctors as scholars and scientists. We therefore also hope that the fine collection of up-to-date reviews contained within this issue will represent a useful foundation of knowledge for neuroradiologists as scientists and physician-investigators aiming to effectively contribute to advancements in the clinical neurosciences. This may entail performance of "reverse translational" neuroimaging anatomy research, where clinical problems can be identified and addressed with studies of anatomy and morphometry as depicted on neuroimages. For example, in a manner that answers hypothesis-driven questions, anatomy pertinent to improving safety and efficacy of interventional neuroendovascular or intracranial neuroendoscopic procedures can be studied using morphometric measurements and statistical analyses of brain anatomic information seen on neuro-MRI images, all to the ultimate benefit of our patients.

Until now, no succinct book has been available as a comprehensive updated source of information and knowledge on neuroimaging anatomy of the brain and skull. While the actual neuroanatomy has not changed since the previous *Neuroimaging Clinics* issue on this subject, more recent advances in neuroradiology have enabled new imaging techniques for diagnostic neuroimaging and therapeutic neurointerventions that have rendered some of the older techniques obsolete. These changes as well as advances in clinical neuroscientific knowledge and practice have required revision of all previous articles, with the addition of several new ones and many more illustrations of modern, more informative structural and functional ways to visualize brain anatomy using neuroimaging.

This issue of *Neuroimaging Clinics* consists of 15 articles providing reference material on the latest methods to visualize craniocerebral neuroimaging anatomy, including structural and functional imaging, brain connectomics, and age-related changes in brain anatomy spanning fetal development to changes in the aging brain. This issue is organized to provide a broad core knowledge related to imaging anatomy of the brain and skull, extending from the outer cranium, through the organization of the brain lobes and cortex, then deeper and downward into the central brain and the hindbrain. The contents of this issue are presented as separate review articles, any one of which is complete in itself. Each article is beautifully illustrated with many high-resolution images that present the relevant anatomy in multiple planes.

Of note, we tried to conform as much as possible to standard anatomic English terminology shown in the *Terminologia Anatomica* and *Terminologia Neuroanatomica* (two of the international standards for human anatomic terminology developed by the International Federation of Associations of Anatomists [IFAA]), with sporadic Latin usage. In the future, neuroradiologists will inevitably need to adhere to the recommendations of these two international standards to uniformly adopt more accurate terminology for craniocerebral anatomy. As for eponyms, we have for now continued the use of standard, well-known eponyms. However, the use of eponyms is counter to the recommendation of the IFAA to omit all eponyms in the description of anatomic structures (with the exception of a few terms; curiously, those relevant to neuroimaging being Schwann for Schwann cells, and Ammon Ra for Ammon's horn of the hippocampus). The slow replacement of eponyms in our neuroimaging anatomic language will be uncomfortable for older generations of neuroradiologists, but for future generations, it will be a relief. On the other hand, we did not shy away from presenting common neuroimaging anatomic variants. These may be defined as slight deviations from the accepted standard human neuroanatomy without causing a demonstrable impairment in function. However, an in-depth description of anatomic variations is a vast topic in its own right and beyond the scope of this issue, as there exists an extremely wide range of "normal" in the body.

Finally, we compiled this issue with the goal of presenting anatomic facts of practical value to clinical neuroradiologists, other clinical neuroscientists, and their trainees. We are immensely grateful to each one of the team of expert contributors to this issue who have provided readers with the most up-to-date knowledge on neuroimaging anatomy of the brain and skull. The success of this issue is largely a result of their time, effort, and expertise in preparing their articles.

It has been a privilege and a pleasure for me to guest edit this issue. I wish to express my sincere thanks to Dr Suresh Mukherji, consulting editor, for his invitation, and to Elsevier for their excellent support throughout the process leading to completion of this issue.

Tarik F. Massoud, MD, PhD, FRCR
Division of Neuroimaging and Neurointervention
Department of Radiology
Stanford University School of Medicine
Stanford Health Care
Stanford Initiative for Multimodality Neuro–Imaging in Translational Anatomy Research (SIMITAR)
Center for Academic Medicine
Radiology MC: 5659
453 Quarry Road
Palo Alto, CA 94304, USA

E-mail address:
tmassoud@stanford.edu

Anatomy of the Calvaria and Skull Base

Tomasz Matys, MD, PhD, FRCR[a,c,*], Daniel J. Scoffings, MBBS, MRCP, FRCR[c], Tarik F. Massoud, MD, PhD, FRCR[b]

KEYWORDS

- Anatomy • Skull • Calvaria • Skull vault • Skull base • Radiological anatomy

KEY POINTS

- The neurocranium includes the calvaria (skull vault) and skull base.
- The complex development of the calvaria and the skull base leads to anatomic variations, most of which are of no clinical significance but can potentially lead to interpretative errors, or can be of importance in the planning of surgical procedures.
- A thorough understanding of skull anatomy and common normal variants is of key importance to radiologists and specialist physicians and surgeons.

INTRODUCTION

We describe the anatomy of the calvaria (skull vault) and the skull base, which jointly form the neurocranium – the part of the skull that encases and protects the brain. We exclude the facial skeleton (viscerocranium) and the anatomy of the petrous pyramids of the temporal bones. Discussion of anatomic variants and abnormal findings is limited to those that are most common or can be potential sources of diagnostic errors.

ANATOMY OF THE CALVARIA

The calvaria (the skull vault) is composed of the frontal, parietal, temporal, and occipital bones (**Fig. 1**A, B), which develop in a membrane (desmocranium) through the condensation of mesenchyme derived from occipital somatomeres around the developing brain (**Table 1**).[1,2] The bones continue to grow during fetal development and early childhood following the growth of the cerebrum, their final size determined by brain volume.[1] Ossification starts around the 10th week in utero and by the time of birth is almost complete, with the exception of sutures and fontanelles that remain open to enable bone overlapping during delivery (**Fig. 1**C, D). Sutures can widen in the first two months of life before starting to progressively ossify.[1,3] With the exception of the metopic suture, which usually closes in early childhood, the major sutures remain open until adulthood (**Table 2**).

Premature suture fusion (craniosynostosis) leads to reduced skull growth perpendicular to the affected suture (craniostenosis), elongation of the skull parallel to the affected suture, and may cause asymmetric head shape (plagiocephaly). Premature closure can be owing to the absence of normal stretch forces across the suture following arrested brain growth, or to mechanical constraints on the head in utero.[2] Craniosynostosis can also happen postpartum but premature fusion after 3 to 5 years of life does not result in skull deformity, as by this age the brain approaches its adult size.[1] Most cases of craniosynostosis are sporadic although it can also be syndromic.[2]

[a] Department of Radiology, University of Cambridge, Cambridge Biomedical Campus, Hills Road, Cambridge CB2 0QQ, UK; [b] Division of Neuroimaging and Neurointervention, Department of Radiology, Stanford University School of Medicine, Stanford Health Centre, Palo Alto, CA, USA; [c] Department of Radiology, Cambridge University Hospitals NHS Foundation Trust, Addenbrooke's Hospital, Cambridge Biomedical Campus, Hills Road, Cambridge CB2 0QQ, UK
* Corresponding author.
E-mail address: tm418@cam.ac.uk
Twitter: @neuroradtom (T.M.); @brainscandan (D.J.S.)

Neuroimag Clin N Am 32 (2022) 447–462
https://doi.org/10.1016/j.nic.2022.04.011
1052-5149/22/

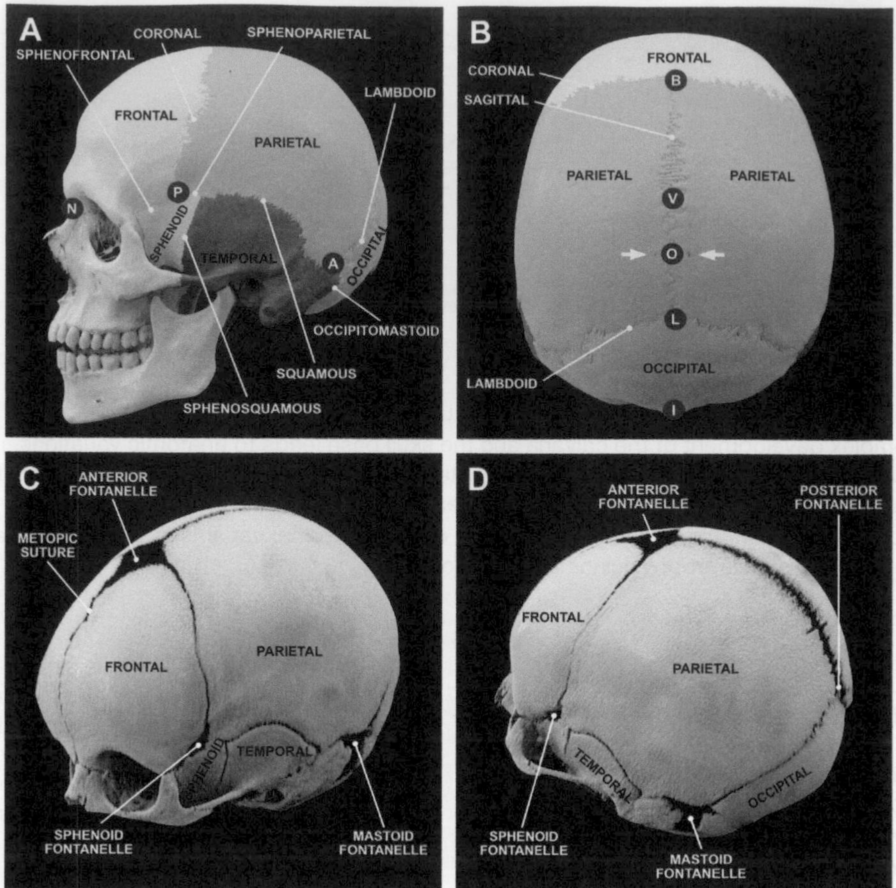

Fig. 1. Cinematic CT volume rendering demonstrating bones (*black*), sutures (*white*), and fontanelles of the cranial vault in adult (*A, B*) and infant skull (*C, D*). Anatomic landmarks: N-nasion, P-pterion, A-asterion, B-bregma, V-vertex, O-obelion, L-lambda, I-inion. Arrows point to parietal foramina.

There are 17 named sutures, that is, synarthroses, unique to the skull. The major sutures of the adult skull and landmarks found at their junctions are shown in **Fig. 1**A, B. Pterion is an important neurosurgical landmark that approximates the intracranial location of the sphenoid ridge and the anterior branch of the middle meningeal artery.[4] The vertex, is the most superior aspect of the calvaria, near the midpoint of the sagittal suture. Other important skull landmarks are whereby there are palpable bony protuberances or depressions: nasion, is the midline depression between the orbits whereby the frontal and 2 nasal bones meet; glabella, is just superior to the nasion as a slight depression joining the 2 brow ridges; and inion, is the tip of the external occipital protuberance.

Table 1
Development of the bones of neurocranium

Membranous (Desmocranium)	Cartilaginous (Chondrocranium)
• Frontal	• Ethmoid
• Parietal	• Sphenoid
• Occipital	• Occipital
○ Interparietal	○ Supraoccipital, exoccipital and basioccipital
• Temporal	• Temporal
○ Squamous	○ Petrous
○ Tympanic	○ Mastoid
	○ Styloid process

Diverse atypical patterns of calvarial ossification can result in ectopic sutures, accessory bones, and unusual foramina in the skull. Appreciation of these fracture mimics is important when interpreting trauma on head CT, and in children when imaging nonaccidental injury. The metopic suture may persist in 10% of adults[1,5] On account of complex embryology of the occipital bone, unfused sutural variants may persist, for example, midline fissures, transverse occipital sutures (including Mendosal sutures), and superior median fissures. Mendosal

Table 2
Characteristics of normal sutures and fontanelles

Normal width of the sutures	
At birth	up to 17 mm (sagittal suture)
2 mo – 12 mo	≤ 3 mm
> 3 years	≤ 2 mm
Age of closure of skull vault sutures	
Metopic suture	childhood (<2 y)
Sagittal suture	20–30 y
Coronal suture	30–40 y
Lambdoid suture	40–50 y
Age of closure of skull base synchondroses	
Anterior intraoccipital	8–10 y
Posterior intraoccipital	4–7 y
Occipitomastoidal	12–15 y
Petrooccipital	16–18 y
Spheno-occipital	16–18 y
Age of closure of the fontanelles	
Anterior	1.5–24 mo
Posterior	2–6 mo
Sphenoidal	3–6 mo
Mastoid	6–24 mo

sutures can persist in 2.5% of skulls, with partial persistence in 16%,[6] extending horizontally through the occipital bone and separating an interparietal bone (Inca bone or Goethe's ossicle) from the supraoccipital part (Fig. 2A, B).[1,5]

Wormian (sutural) bones (Olaus Worm, 1643) are small ossicles within the sutures or fontanelles occurring in 40% of skulls, most commonly in the lambdoid and coronal sutures (see Fig. 2A,D).[7,8] Their etiology is related to increased intracranial pressure leading to sutural opening and defective ossification,[2] with a larger number of Wormian bones associated with higher cranial volumes.[9] Wormian bones are also characteristically seen in osteogenesis imperfecta and other causes of defective mineralization, whereby their number depends on the severity of the disease.[2,7]

Enlarged parietal foramina (fenestrae parietalis, foramina parietalia permagna, or Catlin marks) are usually symmetric, bilateral defects in the parietal bones,[1,10] which, in contrast to the normal 1 to 2 mm parietal foramina (see Fig. 2B), can reach 3 to 5 cm in diameter (see Fig. 2C). Enlarged and nonenlarged parietal foramina can coexist and occur owing to disrupted parietal bone ossification rather than around emissary venous channels.[10] Enlarged parietal foramina are rare (1:15,000–1:50,000) and hereditary.[10] In infants they may initially present as a midline defect termed cranium bifidum (see Fig. 2D), subsequently bridged by bone. Enlarged parietal foramina are usually asymptomatic but may be associated with cephaloceles, abnormal cortical development, and vascular malformations.[10] Enlarged parietal foramina should be differentiated from biparietal osteodystrophy (senile biparietal atrophy), a gradual thinning of parietal bones most often seen in elderly women, and usually of no clinical significance (see Fig. 2E, F).

The skull diploic veins (and venous lacunae or lakes, when enlarged) are a relatively consistent network connecting cerebral veins and dural sinuses to the extracranial veins,[11] most often seen in parasagittal frontal and parietal bones (Fig. 3A). Four common major pathways for these veins have been demonstrated: the pteriofrontoparietal, fronto-orbital, occipitoparietal, and occipitocervical routes,[12] and these may conform to fixed spatial patterns as well.[13] Arachnoid granulations may protrude into the skull vault usually causing small focal defects (see Fig. 3B), or, on occasion, larger defects owing to giant arachnoid granulations. Both diploic veins and arachnoid granulations are usually of no clinical significance, although they can be mistaken for lytic lesions, and brain herniation into arachnoid granulations has been linked to headaches and epilepsy.[14,15]

Cranial emissary veins are valveless and transmit bidirectional blood flow usually from extracranial veins to intracranial venous sinuses, and often communicate with skull diploic veins. They serve to equalize intracranial pressure and cool the brain. They are often seen on MR imaging, CT, and angiography. Those relevant clinically include the (retro)mastoid, posterior condylar, occipital, ophthalmic, sphenoidal ovale, and Vesalian veins, as well as the petrosquamosal sinus.

Copperbeaten skull refers to the appearance of prominent gyral impressions on the inner skull table in conditions with chronically raised intracranial pressure in children such as craniosynostosis or obstructive hydrocephalus (see Fig. 3C).[16] Lückenschädel (lacunar skull) is an abnormality of membranous bone development associated with Chiari II malformation leading to well defined lucent areas bounded by normally ossified bone (see Fig. 3D).[17]

Hyperostosis frontalis interna is an overgrowth of the inner frontal table, usually symmetric and bilateral (see Fig. 3E, F), affecting 18% of women above 65 years of age and usually of no clinical significance.[18] More rarely, the overgrowth may be more widespread as hyperostosis frontoparietalis or hyperostosis calvariae diffusa.

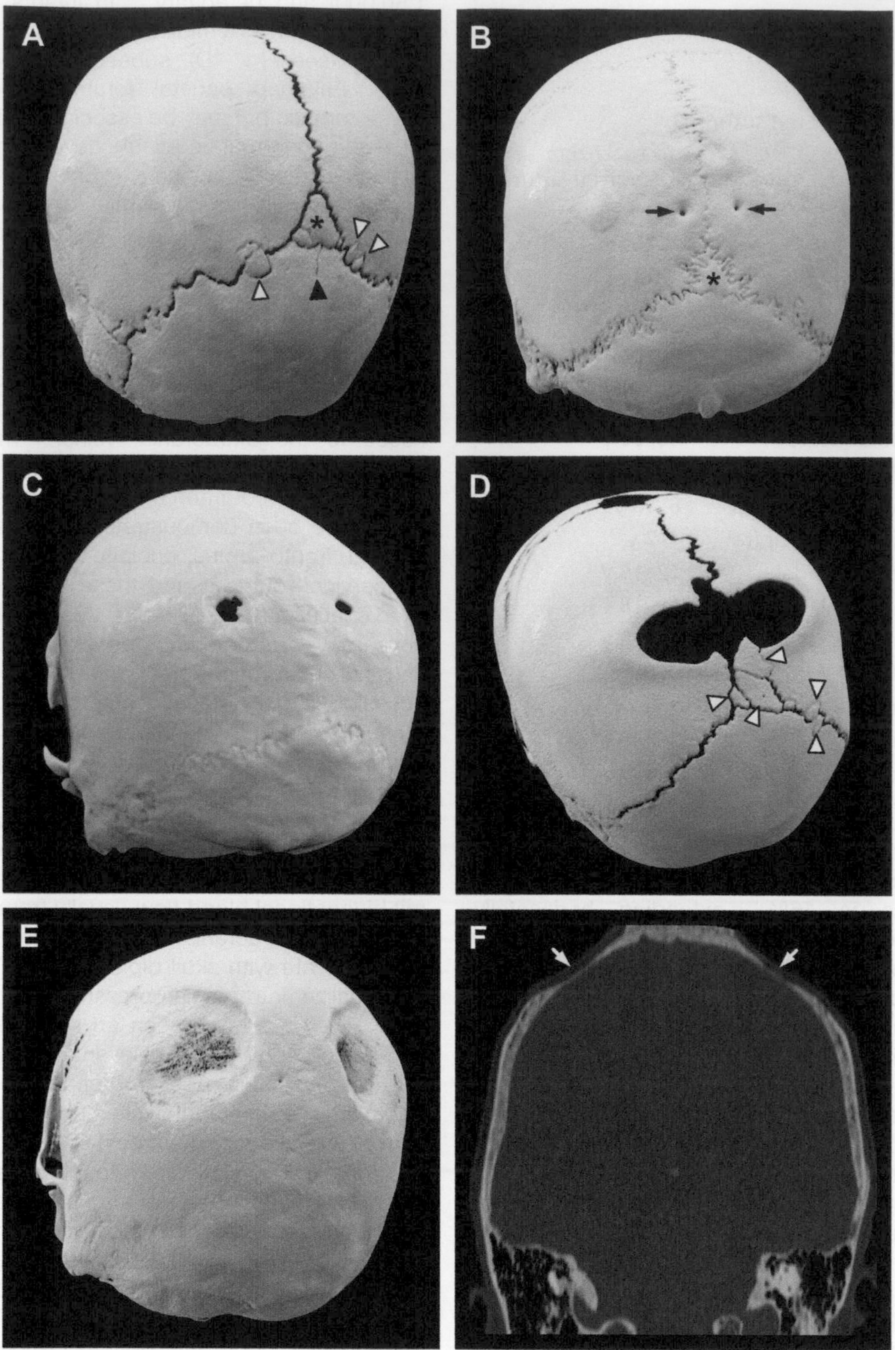

Fig. 2. Anatomic variants and abnormalities of the skull vault. (*A*) Inca bone (*asterisk*), and Wormian bones (white *arrowheads*) in a child; accessory suture in the midline (*black arrow*). (*B*) Inca bone (*asterisk*) in an adult; short arrows–normal parietal foramina. (*C*) Enlarged parietal foramina. (*D*) Cranium bifidum defect and multiple Wormian bones (*white arrowheads*). (*E*, *F*) Biparietal osteodystrophy on (*E*) volume rendered and (*F*) coronal CT reformats.

ANATOMY OF THE SKULL BASE

The bones of the skull base include the frontal, ethmoid, sphenoid, temporal, and occipital bones. Most of the skull base is formed in cartilage (see **Table 1**) around existing nerves and blood vessels, resulting in variable anatomy of the resulting foramina.[1,18] The interior surface of the skull base is divided into anterior, middle, and posterior cranial fossae (**Fig. 4**A).

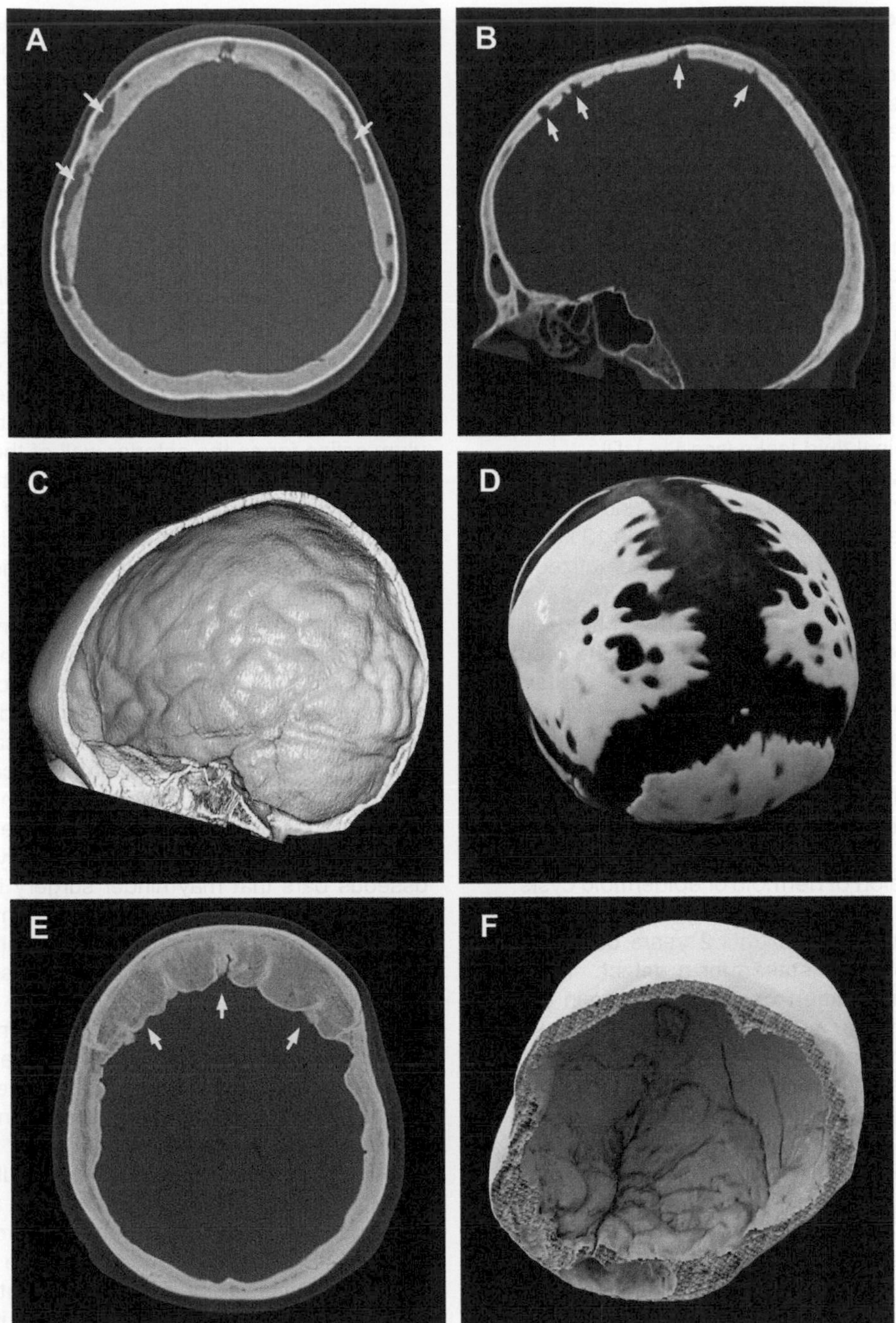

Fig. 3. Anatomic variants and abnormalities of the skull vault. (*A*) Venous lacunae (venous lakes) and (*B*) Arachnoid granulations, which can be mistaken for lytic lesions. (*C*) Prominent gyral impressions resulting in copper-beaten appearance. (*D*) Lückenschädel skull in Chiari type II malformation. (*E*) Axial CT and (*F*) volume renderings demonstrating hyperostosis frontalis interna.

Anterior Cranial Fossa

Anterior cranial fossa extends from the inner surface of the frontal bones to the sphenoid ridge and anterior clinoid processes (see **Fig. 4**B). Its floor is formed by horizontal orbital plates of the frontal bone that join the ethmoid bone and lesser wings of the sphenoid bone.[19] The central part of the ethmoid bone is formed by the lamina cribrosa (cribriform plate) on each side of the perpendicular plate, which protrudes intracranially as the crista galli. The cribriform plate itself is made of two medial and lateral lamellae.[19] Perforations in lamina cribrosa transmit olfactory fibers from the olfactory recesses of the nasal cavity to the olfactory bulbs. The olfactory bulbs and tracts lie in the olfactory grooves, which are the most inferior parts of the olfactory fossae (see Fig. 4C).[19] Beyond the lateral margins of the cribriform plate, bilateral fovea ethmoidalis form the roofs of the ethmoid air cells. The variable depth of the olfactory fossa is of importance in sinonasal surgery and is graded according to the Keros classification.[19] Defects in the cribriform plate can be a site of congenital or acquired cephaloceles and cerebrospinal fluid leaks (see Fig. 4D).[20,21]

The crista galli forms an anterior attachment of the cerebral falx. Its bone marrow undergoes fatty replacement by 14 years of age.[22] In 13% to 14% of adults the crista galli is pneumatized (see Fig. 4E),[18] usually by extension of frontal sinus pneumatization.[23] Anterior to the crista galli lies the foramen cecum – a remnant of the prenasal space, which during development contains a dural diverticulum extending to the skin of the nose.[22] Failure of its involution may result in the formation of dermoid or epidermoid cysts, nasal gliomas or encephaloceles. Widening of the foramen cecum and bifid or dystrophic crista galli are important imaging findings suggesting intracranial extension of dermoid or epidermoid cysts.[2,22] The skull base around the foramen cecum can remain cartilaginous until 2 years of life, which should not be mistaken for a defect.[1] In 1% of adults the foramen cecum may remain patent, transmitting a vein connecting the superior sagittal sinus and nasal vein (see Fig. 4F).[24] A patent foramen cecum is usually of no clinical significance although it has been reported as a site of cerebrospinal fluid rhinorrhea.[25]

Posterior to the ethmoid bone lies the planum sphenoidale (jugum sphenoidale), the superior surface of the sphenoid bone terminating posteriorly as the limbus sphenoidale.[26] The latter consists of two parts. The superior limbus is continuous anteriorly with the planum sphenoidale, and laterally, it joins the lesser wings of the sphenoid. The inferior limbus is continuous anteriorly with the tuberculum sellae, and laterally it joins the anterior clinoid processes.

Middle Cranial Fossa

The middle cranial fossa extends from the limbus sphenoidale, anterior clinoid processes, and sphenoid ridges anteriorly to the dorsum sellae and the petrous ridges posteriorly.[4] Bones forming the middle cranial fossa include the sphenoid bone anteriorly, squamous part of the temporal bone anterolaterally, and petrous temporal bone posteromedially.

The central portion of the middle cranial fossa (Fig. 5A) includes the prechiasmatic sulcus containing the optic chiasm, and sella turcica containing the pituitary gland. The prechiasmatic sulcus lies immediately posterior to the limbus sphenoidale, limited laterally by the anterior clinoid processes.[4,26] At its lateral aspects, the optic foramina form the cranial openings of the optic canals, limited inferiorly by optic struts extending from the anterior clinoid process to the body of the sphenoid. Inferior to the optic struts the tuberculum sellae forms the anterior wall of the pituitary fossa and small lateral projections form the middle clinoid processes. The posterior wall of the pituitary fossa is formed by the dorsum sellae, which extends superolaterally as the posterior clinoid processes.[4,27]

The clinoid processes provide attachment sites for the tentorium, diaphragm sellae, and smaller dural folds and ligaments.[4] Mineralization of ligaments between the anterior and middle clinoid processes results in the formation of a caroticoclinoid canal traversed by the internal carotid artery.[28] Interclinoid ligaments between the anterior and posterior (see Fig. 5B) or the middle and posterior clinoid process can also ossify forming osseous bars that may hinder surgery in this region.[27,28] Other surgically relevant variants include the pneumatization of optic struts and anterior clinoid processes posing a risk of cerebrospinal fluid leaks.[4]

The body of the sphenoid bone contains the sphenoid sinus, which varies in volume from 0.5 to 30 mL averaging 7.5 mL.[18] The degree of pneumatization is of importance in transsphenoidal and skull base surgery (see Fig. 5C).[4]

Multiple foramina connect the middle cranial fossa to the orbit, pterygopalatine fossa and infratemporal fossa, transmitting nerves, arteries, and veins (Table 3). The optic canal (see Fig. 5A; Fig. 6A) courses from the prechiasmatic sulcus to the orbital apex tapering toward its orbital end.[4] In 2.7% of skulls it can be duplicated with a smaller inferior canal transmitting the ophthalmic artery.[29] The metoptic canal is a small channel traversing the optic strut inferolateral to the optic canal in 8% of skulls, and duplication is a subtype of this variant.[29] The inferior wall of the optic canal can be grooved which is known as a "key-hole anomaly."[29]

Lateral to the sella, the anterior wall and floor of the middle cranial fossa are traversed by several openings positioned along an arc-shaped curve

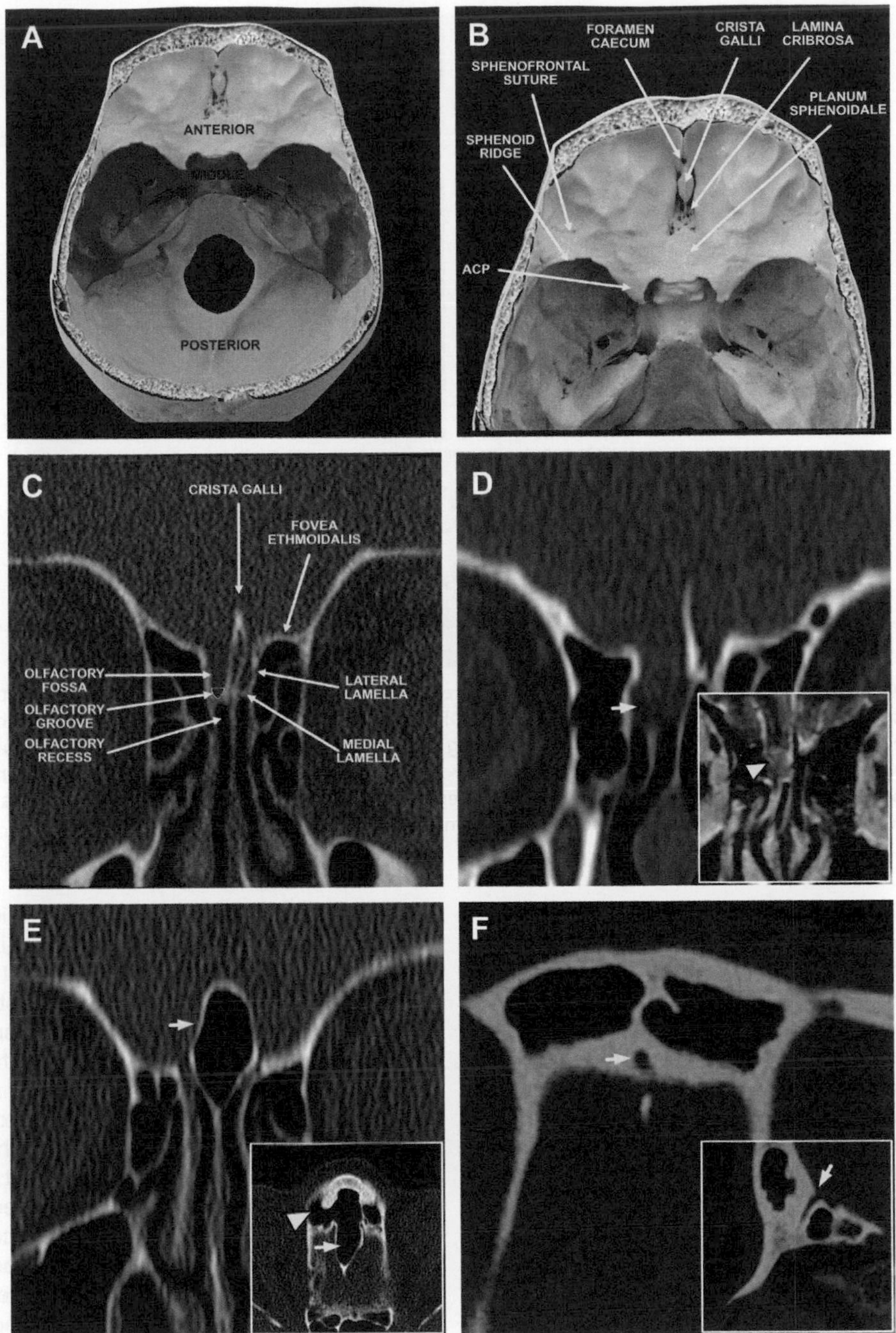

Fig. 4. (*A*) Overview of the anterior, middle, and posterior cranial fossa. (*B*) The main anatomic structures of the anterior cranial fossa on volume rendered CT; ACP–anterior clinoid process. (*C*) Coronal CT showing detail of the anterior skull base; the olfactory groove is the most inferior aspect of the olfactory fossa (*orange*) limited by the medial and lateral lamellae of lamina cribrosa, and crista galli medially. The olfactory recess is the most superior aspect of the nasal cavity below lamina cribrosa. (*D*) Lamina cribrosa defect with soft tissue (*arrow*) protruding into the nasal cavity. Coronal T2W MR imaging (inset) confirms a cephalocele with brain herniation through the defect (*white arrowhead*). (*E*) Pneumatized crista galli (*arrow*) formed by extension of frontal sinus pneumatization (inset–*arrowhead* on axial image)). (*F*) Axial and sagittal (inset) CT reformats showing patent foramen cecum in an adult.

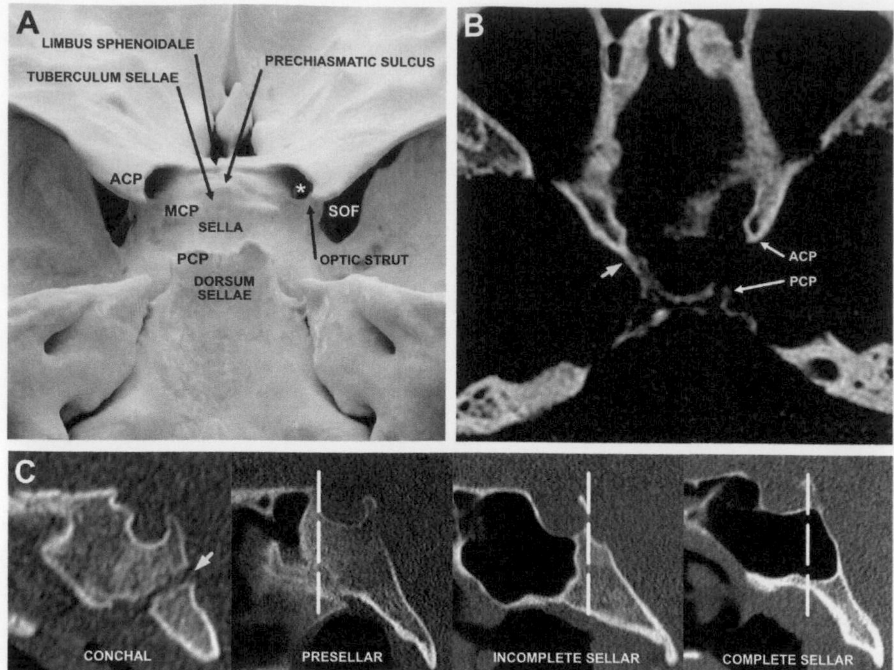

Fig. 5. (*A*) Anatomic features of the central aspect of the middle cranial fossa; ACP, MCP, and PCP–anterior, middle and posterior clinoid process, asterisk–optic canal, SOF–superior orbital fissure. (*B*) Variant interclinoid bar (*arrow*) between ACP and PCP may be of importance during neurosurgical procedures. (*C*) Classification of sphenoid sinus pneumatization–conchal type is almost exclusively seen in children below 12; arrow–open sphenooccipital synchondrosis. Pneumatization extending up to the anterior sellar wall (presellar) is seen in 26%. Sellar pneumatization (incomplete–up to posterior sellar wall and complete–postsellar) account for 74%.

described as the "sphenoidal crescent of foramina" (Fig. 6A–C).

The superior orbital fissure is limited by the lesser sphenoid wing superiorly and the greater wing inferiorly and opens into the orbit. Its profile is variable, encompassing a spectrum between racket-shaped and egg-shaped varieties,[29] or between type A or B (with or without discrete narrowing).[30] In less than 1% skulls, the inferior aspect of the superior orbital fissure can be separated by a bridge forming a Warwick's foramen.[29] Inferomedial to the superior orbital fissure lies the foramen rotundum leading into the pterygopalatine fossa. Both openings arise from the developmental foramen lacerum anterius between the orbitosphenoid and alisphenoid (precursors of the lesser and greater sphenoid wings), which rarely persist in humans.[5]

The Vidian canal (pterygoid canal) courses from the region of the foramen lacerum to the pterygopalatine fossa through the junction of the sphenoid body and pterygoid processes (see Fig. 6D).[4,27] On its course it is usually embedded in bone but in a third of individuals it may protrude into the sphenoid sinus; in 3% the nerve travels entirely within sinus often on an osseous stalk, and can be dehiscent in 6% (see Fig. 6E).[18] An intrasphenoid course of the nerve poses a risk of injury during sinus surgery but can be of benefit in Vidian neurectomy performed to treat vasomotor rhinitis or gustatory lacrimation, enabling transsphenoidal transection as an alternative to a transnasal approach.[31]

The foramen ovale lies posterolateral to the foramen rotundum and anterolateral to the cranial opening of the carotid canal (Fig. 7A). It develops from the foramen lacerum medius between the alisphenoid, basisphenoid, and periotic capsule of the petrous bone, which becomes separated into foramen ovale and foramen lacerum. Persistence of foramen lacerum medius resulting in the absence of foramen ovale is rare.[32] The anterior venous aspect of the foramen ovale transmitting an emissary vein between the cavernous sinus and the pterygoid plexus is sometimes separated by a thin spur. The shape and size of the foramen ovale depend on the diameter of the transmitted veins and are highly variable.[1,18,32] The foramen ovale provides a route of access to the trigeminal (Gasserian) ganglion for percutaneous rhizotomy for the treatment of trigeminal neuralgia. Needle access to the foramen can be obstructed by

Table 3
Skull base openings and transmitted structures

Optic Canal	Optic Nerve Ophtalmic Artery
Superior orbital fissure – lateral part	Lacrimal nerve (from Va) Frontal nerve (from Va) Superior ophthalmic vein Trochlear nerve (IV)
Superior orbital fissure – middle part	Oculomotor nerve (III) – superior division Nasociliary nerve (from Va) Oculomotor nerve (III) – inferior division Abducens nerve (VI)
Superior orbital fissure – medial part	Inferior ophthalmic vein
Foramen rotundum	Maxillary nerve (Vb) Emissary veins Artery of foramen rotundum
Vidian canal	Vidian nerve (greater superficial and deep petrosal)
Inferior rotundal canal (10%–16%)	*Emissary vein (pterygoid plexus – cavernous sinus)*
Foramen of Vesalius (80%) Foramen ovale *Canaliculus innominatus (12%–16%)*	Emissary vein (pterygoid plexus – cavernous sinus) Mandibular nerve (Vc) Lesser superficial petrosal verve
Foramen spinosum	Middle meningeal artery and vein, nervus spinosus
Orbitomeningeal foramen of Hyrtl (42%–44%)	*Anastomoses of meningo-lacrimal artery or recurrent meningeal branch of lacrimal artery*
Jugular foramen – pars nervosa	Glossopharyngeal nerve (IX)
Jugular foramen – pars vasculosa	Vagus nerve (X), accessory nerve (XI) Jugular bulb
Foramen magnum	Medulla oblongata Vertebral and spinal arteries and veins Accessory nerve (XI, spinal root)
Hypoglossal canal	Hypoglossal nerve (XII)
Condylar foramen (31%–50%)	*Emissary vein*
Mastoid foramen (>80%)	*Emissary vein*
Foramen magnum	Medulla oblongata Vertebral and spinal arteries and veins Spinal root of the accessory nerve (XI)

(inconstant features shown in italics)

ligamentous ossification in the infratemporal fossa, in particular, pterygoalar and pterygospinous bars (see **Fig.** 7B).[28,33]

The foramen spinosum lies posterolateral to the foramen ovale (see **Fig.** 7A); it may lack its medial or posterior wall appearing as a groove or notch (see **Fig.** 7C). Its anterior wall can be absent, leading to fusion with foramen ovale. In the absence of foramen spinosum (see **Fig.** 7D) the middle meningeal artery enters the skull via the foramen ovale or can be replaced by an ophthalmic artery branch entering the skull through the superior orbital fissure or through the orbito-meningeal foramen.[18] Absence of the foramen spinosum is also associated with a persistent stapedial artery.[34]

The foramen lacerum is a remnant of foramen lacerum medius between the sphenoid body and petrous apex at the anterior aspect of the spheno-petrosal and petro-occipital fissures (see **Fig.** 7A).[32] The anteromedial aspect of the horizontal segment of the carotid artery passes superior to foramen lacerum turning upwards to enter the cavernous sinus.[32] The foramen lacerum does

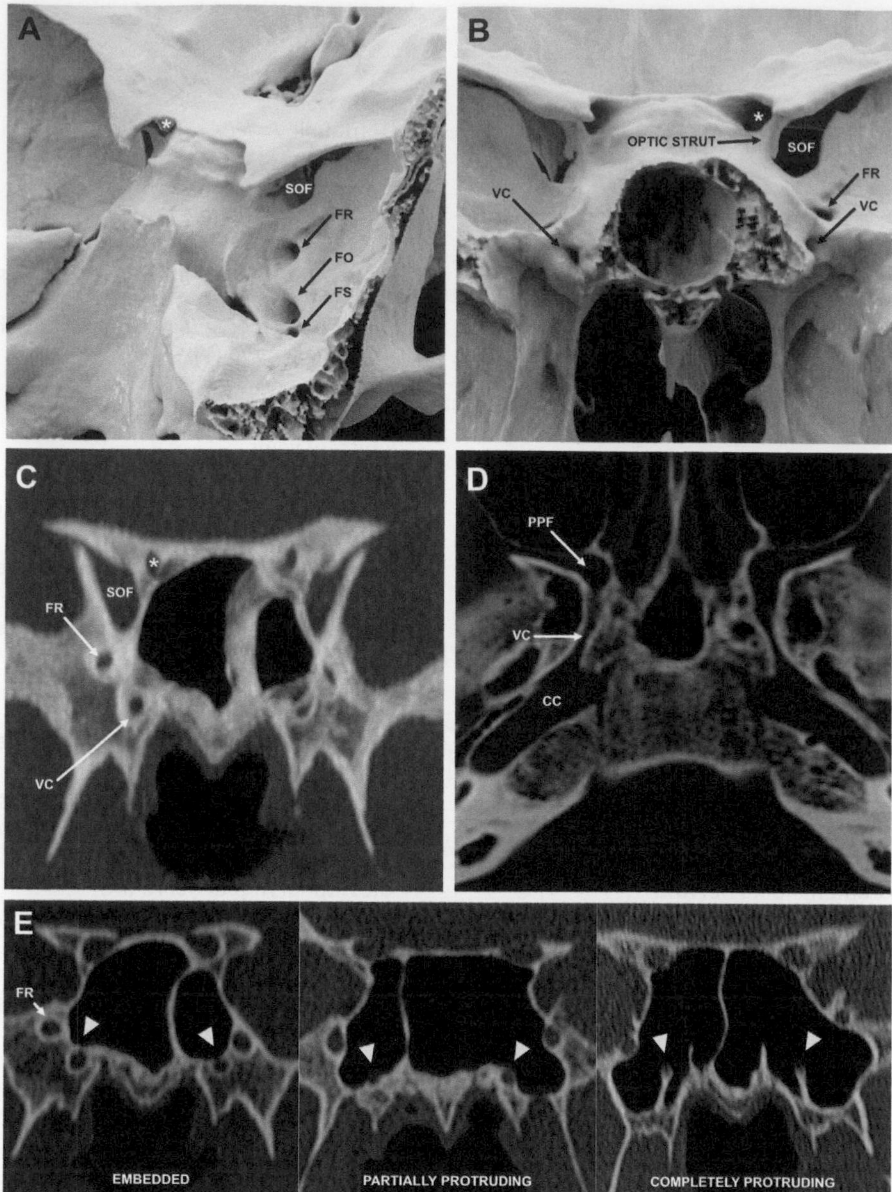

Fig. 6. (*A, B*) Anatomic features of the lateral aspect of the middle cranial fossa with "crescent of foramina" – SOF–superior orbital fissure, FR–foramen rotundum, VC–Vidian canal, FO–foramen ovale, and FS–foramen spinosum; asterisk–optic canal. (*C*) Owing to their complex spatial arrangements, the foramina of the anterior wall of the middle cranial fossa are difficult to demonstrate on a single CT image but can be seen on 5 mm oblique maximum intensity projections. (*D*) Axial CT image showing anatomic relationships of the Vidian canal, which courses from the anterior aspect of the carotid canal (CC) to the pterygopalatine fossa (PPF). (*E*) Variations in course of the Vidian canal (arrowheads) through the sphenoid bone.

not transmit any major neural or vascular structures but its significance stems from it providing a route for intracranial spread of infection from the nasopharynx.[1,32]

The foramen of Vesalius (sphenoid emissary foramen, canaliculus sphenoidalis, foramen venosum) lies anteromedial to foramen ovale, providing an alternative route for the emissary vein (see Fig. 7E, F). Its inferior opening lies in the scaphoid fossa between the two legs of the attachment of the medial pterygoid plate.[1,5,32] A similar venous channel termed the inferior rotundal canal occurs more anteriorly with its cranial opening near the foramen rotundum, and exocranial opening in the pterygoid fossa between the lateral and medial pterygoid plates (see Fig. 7F).[32] Both

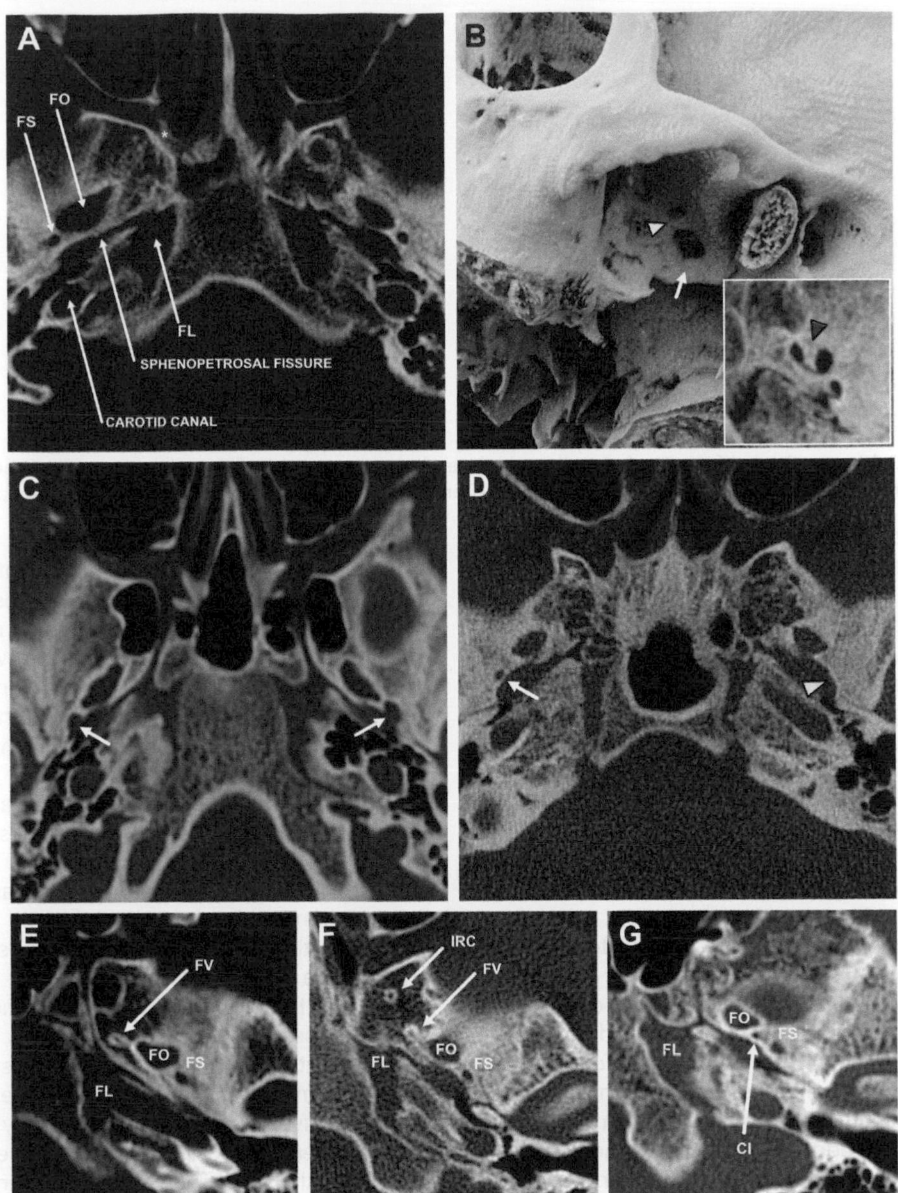

Fig. 7. (*A*) Axial CT image showing foramen ovale (FO) and spinosum (FS) with no inconstant foramina. Note asymmetry of FO, which is a common finding. Sphenopetrosal fissure courses medially to the foramina joining foramen lacerum (FL). (*B*) Volume rendering showing pterygoalar (*white arrowhead*) and pterygospinous bars (*white arrow*) obstructing access to FO from the infratemporal fossa; (inset) on axial maximum intensity projection the pterygospinous bar (*red arrowhead*) traverses the lumen of FO. (*C*) Variant incomplete FS seen as a notch on the medial surface of the sphenoid bone. (*D*) Absence of the left FS (*white arrowhead*) with normal contralateral foramen (*arrow*). (*E*) Inconstant foramen of Vesalius (FV) at the anteromedial aspect of FO. (*F*) Inferior rotundal canal (IRC) located anterior to FV. (*G*) Canaliculus innominatus (CI) located between FO and FS.

foramina may provide a way of spread of extracranial infections to the cavernous sinus.[18] The foramen of Vesalius may also pose a risk of bleeding if engaged by a misplaced needle during percutaneous trigeminal rhizotomy.[35]

The canaliculus innominatus (foramen petrosum, foramen of Arnold) occurs between the foramen ovale and foramen spinosum (see Fig. 7G) and transmits the lesser petrosal nerve, which in its absence travels via the foramen ovale.[32]

The orbitomeningeal foramen (of Hyrtl) (Fig. 8A) transmits connections between the internal and external carotid circulation, usually an

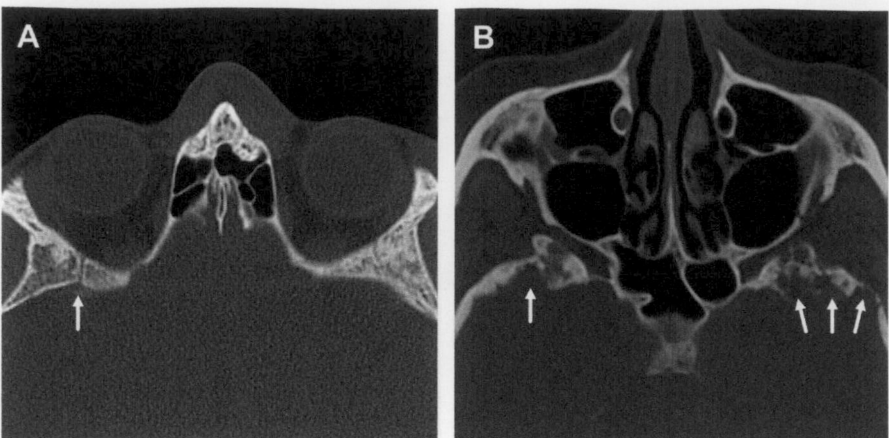

Fig. 8. (A) Orbitomeningeal foramen (arrows) at the lateral superior aspect of the posterior wall of the orbit can be mistaken for a fracture. (B) Arachnoid pits (arrows) in the anterior wall of the middle cranial fossa.

anastomosis of the meningo-lacrimal artery (an orbital branch of the middle meningeal artery) and the recurrent meningeal branch of the ophthalmic artery. Alternatively, a recurrent meningeal branch of the lacrimal artery (from the ophthalmic artery) may anastomose with the middle meningeal artery. The foramen can be single or multiple and usually occurs in the frontosphenoidal suture superolaterally to the superior orbital fissure or within the adjacent frontal bone opening in the middle cranial fossa (M-type) or anterior cranial fossa (A-type). Large anastomotic arteries can represent a surgical hazard, and the foramen can be mistaken for a fracture.[29,36,37]

The middle cranial fossa is a characteristic location of arachnoid pits – small defects of the inner table resulting from the presence of aberrant arachnoid granulations outside of the dural venous sinuses (see Fig. 8B). Arachnoid pits can be incidental but can also be associated with altered cerebrospinal fluid hydrodynamics in idiopathic intracranial hypertension.[38] In this setting, they can undergo progressive enlargement and lead to the formation of cephaloceles; in particular lateral sphenoid cephaloceles.[20,38]

Posterior Cranial Fossa

The posterior cranial fossa is formed by the occipital bone, with the body of sphenoid bone contributing to the anterosuperior aspect of the clivus, and petrous pyramids forming its anterolateral walls.

The occipital bone develops both in cartilage and membrane (see Table 1) from six ossification centers.[39] The cartilaginous part develops from four segments around the foramen magnum separated by intraoccipital synchondroses (Fig. 9A, B), which start to close at 1 to 2 years of age and become seamlessly incorporated into the bone by 10 years of age (Table 3).[40] The interparietal bone develops in membrane from two ossification centers above the Mendosal suture as described earlier (see Fig. 2A, B). Whereas knowledge of this arrangement helps differentiate synchondroses from fractures, variant ossification patterns may lead to atypical sutures which can be mistaken for pathology.[41,42]

The central part of the posterior cranial fossa includes the clivus extending from the dorsum sellae to the anterior margin of the foramen magnum, formed by the basisphenoid and the basiocciput. The sphenooccipital synchondrosis remains open until the teenage years to allow skull base growth (see Fig. 9A).[1,40]

Laterally the clivus articulates with the petrous apices across the petrooccipital fissure, which on the ossification of the sphenooccipital synchondrosis becomes a petroclival fissure (see Fig. 9B). The petroclival fissure extends anteriorly to the foramen lacerum and posteriorly to the anterior aspect of the jugular foramen and contains the inferior petrosal sinus joining the jugular bulb. The jugular foramen lies between the petrous temporal bone and jugular notch of the occipital bone.[1] Its anterior part (pars nervosa) can be separated from the posterior part (pars vasculosa) by an osseous strut (jugular spine, see Fig. 9B). Posterior to the jugular foramen the bone surface contains a deep groove for sigmoid sinus (see Fig. 9B) that continues posteriorly as a groove for transverse sinus joining its contralateral counterpart at the internal occipital prominence in the posterior aspect of the occipital bone (see Fig. 9C).[1] Together with a vertical groove for superior sagittal sinus and the internal occipital crest between the internal occipital prominence and the foramen magnum (see Fig. 9C), these osseous markings

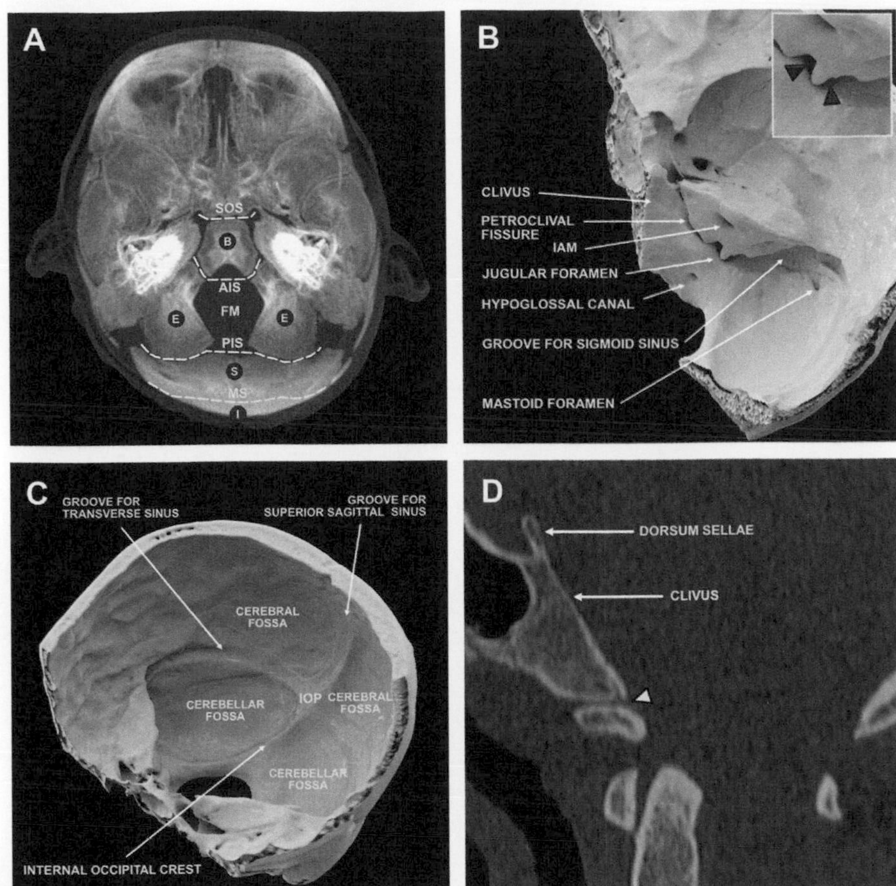

Fig. 9. (*A*) Thick slab average intensity projection of an infant head CT demonstrating developmental parts of the occipital bone–basioccipital (*B*), exoccipital (E), supraoccipital (S) and interparietal (I) bone separated by anterior (AIS) and posterior (PIS) intraoccipital synchondroses and the metopic suture (MS); SOS–spheno-occipital synchondrosis. (*B, C*) Volume renderings showing anatomic structures of the posterior cranial fossa. Jugular foramen (inset in *B*) is separated by the jugular spine into anterior pars nervosa (*blue arrowhead*) and posterior pars vascularis (*read arrowhead*). (*D*) Inferior type of canalis basilaris medianus (*arrowhead*).

form a cruciform (or cruciate) eminence dividing the internal surface of the occipital bone into paired cerebral fossae (containing the occipital lobes) and cerebellar fossae (containing the cerebellar hemispheres).

The canalis basilaris medianus is a midline clival canal seen in 4% to 5% of adults.[43] It is considered to be a notochondral remnant but can also contain a venous channel. Several variants are described depending on the completeness of the canal (patent or blind-ending) and location of its openings.[43] The inferior complete variant traverses the basiocciput opening on the anterior pharyngeal aspect of the clivus (see Fig. 9D). An incomplete canal can present as a long channel ending blindly near the dorsum sellae. An Incomplete canal can also present as a recess on the ventral surface of the basioccipiut (foveola pharyngica) which can mimic a lytic lesion. Complete variants are a potential site of meningocele and can predispose to meningitis.[43]

The foramen magnum is of variable shape and may demonstrate a notch (keyhole-shaped foramen)[18] or a projection at its anterior margin (basion tubercle).[44] The basion is the midsagittal point of the anterior margin of foramen magnum. Posteriorly there may be a small cleft, or a projection (Kerckring's ossicle) which is a remnant of an independent ossification center.[39] The size of the foramen magnum can be reduced in achondroplasia, whereas Arnold–Chiari malformation results in its enlargement.[2,18]

The hypoglossal canal opens inferomedially to the jugular foramen at the anterolateral margin of the foramen magnum and courses inferolaterally opening at the anterior margin of the occipital

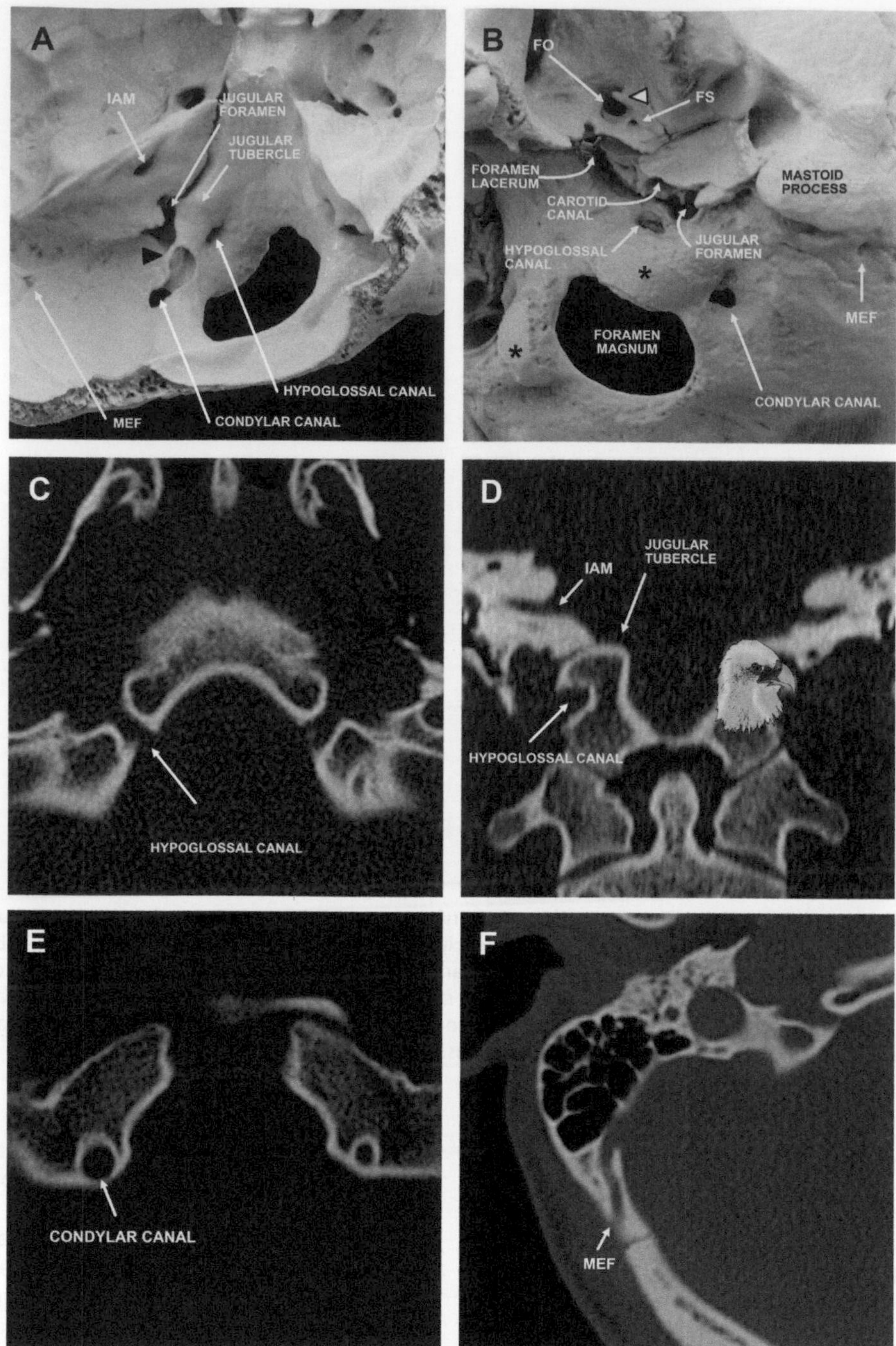

Fig. 10. (*A*) Volume rendering showing foramina of the posterior cranial fossa. Example of a condylar canal that grooves the floor and enters the jugular foramen under a thin osseous strut (*black arrowhead*). IAM–internal acoustic meatus. MEF–mastoid emissary foramen. (*B*) External surface of the posterior skull base and associated foramina. The hypoglossal canal opens anterolaterally to the occipital condyle (*asterisk*), whereas the condylar canal opens posterior to the condyle. Note a partial pterygoalar bar (*white arrowhead*) narrowing the foramen ovale. (*C, D*) Hypoglossal canal demonstrated on axial (*C*) and coronal (*D*) images, the latter demonstrating an "eagle sign." (*E*) Condylar canal and (*F*) mastoid emissary foramen on axial CT images.

condyle (Fig. 10A–C). It can demonstrate osseous spurs and bridging involving different parts of the canal, and sometimes its entire length, resulting in its duplication.[5] Coronal CT through the skull base can demonstrate the typical appearance of the occipital condyle and jugular tubercle, mimicking an eagle in profile (eagle sign, see Fig. 10D), with the hypoglossal canal running under the neck and beak of the bird. The condylar canal traverses the occipital bone opening posteriorly to the occipital condyle and transmits an emissary vein connecting the jugular bulb or the sigmoid sinus to the suboccipital venous plexus (see Fig. 10A, B and E).[32,45] The (retro)mastoid foramen occurs at the posterior margin of the mastoid process, usually within or near the temporo-occipital suture, transmitting a mastoid emissary vein between the sigmoid sinus and posterior auricular or occipital veins (see Fig. 10A, B and F). If large, it may cause tinnitus of venous origin,[46] and injury to an emissary vein during mastoidectomy may pose a risk of hemorrhage, venous sinus thrombosis, or air embolism.[47]

SUMMARY

Anatomy of the calvaria, and especially of the skull base, demonstrates a high degree of variability. Knowledge of the imaging anatomy and common anatomic normal variants presented here is of key importance to neuroradiologists and other clinical neuroscientists.

CLINICS CARE POINTS

- Appreciation of ectopic sutures and accessory bones is important when interpreting trauma head CT – using 3D volume-rendered reformats allows easier evaluation of their spatial configuration and differentiation from fractures.
- Diploic veins (venous lacunae) and arachnoid granulations should not be mistaken for lytic lesions.
- Arachnoid pits of the middle cranial fossa can be associated with altered cerebrospinal fluid dynamics in idiopathic intracranial hypertension.
- Anatomic variants of potential significance in planning surgical procedures include endosinal course of the Vidian canals, the type of sphenoid sinus pneumatization, and ossification of skull base ligaments.

DISCLOSURE

This work was supported by the NIHR Cambridge Biomedical Research Centre (BRC-1215-20014). The views expressed are those of the author(s) and not necessarily those of the NIHR or the Department of Health and Social Care.

REFERENCES

1. Belden CJ. The skull base and calvaria. Adult and pediatric. Neuroimaging Clin N Am 1998;8:1–20.
2. Sanchez P, Graham JM. Congenital Anomalies of the Skull. In: Swaiman KF, Ashwal S, Ferriero DM, et al, editors. Swaiman's pediatric neurology. Elsevier; 2017. p. 233–41.
3. Schuenke M, Schulte E, Schumacher U. Head, neck, and neuroanatomy (Thieme Atlas of Anatomy). Thieme; 2015.
4. Rhoton AL. The sellar region. Neurosurgery 2002;51: S335–74.
5. Keskil S, Gözil R, Calgüner E. Common surgical pitfalls in the skull. Surg Neurol 2003;59:228–31 [discussion: 231].
6. Tubbs RS, Salter EG, Oakes WJ. Does the mendosal suture exist in the adult. Clin Anat 2007;20:124–5.
7. Bellary SS, Steinberg A, Mirzayan N, et al. Wormian bones: a review. Clin Anat 2013;26:922–7.
8. Cirpan S, Aksu F, Mas N. The Incidence and Topographic Distribution of Sutures Including Wormian Bones in Human Skulls. J Craniofac Surg 2015;26: 1687–90.
9. Hanninger SE, Schwabegger AH. A case of an extremely large accessory bone with unusual sutures and foramina parietalia permagna in multiple premature craniosynostoses. J Craniomaxillofac Surg 2012;40:555–8.
10. Griessenauer CJ, Veith P, Mortazavi MM, et al. Enlarged parietal foramina: a review of genetics, prognosis, radiology, and treatment. Childs Nerv Syst 2013;29:543–7.
11. Ugga L, Cuocolo R, Cocozza S, et al. Spectrum of lytic lesions of the skull: a pictorial essay. Insights Imaging 2018;9:845–56.
12. Tsutsumi S, Nakamura M, Tabuchi T, et al. Calvarial diploic venous channels: an anatomic study using high-resolution magnetic resonance imaging. Surg Radiol Anat 2013;35:935–41.
13. Hershkovitz I, Greenwald C, Rothschild BM, et al. The elusive diploic veins: anthropological and anatomical perspective. Am J Phys Anthropol 1999;108:345–58.
14. Ciochon UM, Sehested PC, Skejø HPB, et al. The controversial entity of brain herniations into arachnoid granulations: A report of three cases with literature review. Radiol Case Rep 2021;16: 2768–73.

15. Rodrigues JR, Santos GR. Brain herniation into giant arachnoid granulation: an unusual case. Case Rep Radiol 2017;2017:8532074.
16. Ittyachen AM, Anand R. Copper beaten skull. BMJ Case Rep 2019;12:e230916.
17. Glass RB, Fernbach SK, Norton KI, et al. The infant skull: a vault of information. Radiographics 2004;24: 507–22.
18. Tunali S. Skull. In: Tubbs RS, Shoja MM, Loukas M, editors. Bergman's comprehensive encyclopedia of human anatomic variation. Hoboken, New Jersey: John Wiley & Sons; 2016. p. 1–21.
19. Bates NS, Massoud TF. Ambiguous "olfactory" terms for anatomic spaces adjacent to the cribriform plate: A publication database analysis and quest for uniformity. Clin Anat 2021;34:1186–95.
20. Connor SE. Imaging of skull-base cephalocoeles and cerebrospinal fluid leaks. Clin Radiol 2010;65: 832–41.
21. Scoffings DJ. Imaging of Acquired Skull Base Cerebrospinal Fluid Leaks. Neuroimaging Clin N Am 2021;31:509–22.
22. Lowe LH, Booth TN, Joglar JM, et al. Midface anomalies in children. Radiographics 2000;20:907–22. quiz 1106.
23. Som PM, Park EE, Naidich TP, et al. Crista galli pneumatization is an extension of the adjacent frontal sinuses. AJNR Am J Neuroradiol 2009;30:31–3.
24. Lang J. Skull base and related structures. Schattauer Verlag; 2001.
25. Gaffey MM, Friedel ME, Fatterpekar GM, et al. Spontaneous cerebrospinal fluid rhinorrhea of the foramen cecum in adulthood. Arch Otolaryngol Head Neck Surg 2012;138:79–82.
26. Guthikonda B, Tobler WD, Froelich SC, et al. Anatomic study of the prechiasmatic sulcus and its surgical implications. Clin Anat 2010;23:622–8.
27. Rhoton AL. The cavernous sinus, the cavernous venous plexus, and the carotid collar. Neurosurgery 2002;51:S375–410.
28. Touska P, Hasso S, Oztek A, et al. Skull base ligamentous mineralisation: evaluation using computed tomography and a review of the clinical relevance. Insights Imaging 2019;10:55.
29. Regoli M, Bertelli E. The revised anatomy of the canals connecting the orbit with the cranial cavity. Orbit 2017;36:110–7.
30. Caldarelli C, Benech R, Iaquinta C. Superior Orbital Fissure Syndrome in Lateral Orbital Wall Fracture: Management and Classification Update. Craniomaxillofac Trauma Reconstr 2016;9:277–83.
31. Liu SC, Wang HW, Su WF. Endoscopic vidian neurectomy: the value of preoperative computed tomographic guidance. Arch Otolaryngol Head Neck Surg 2010;136:595–602.
32. Ginsberg LE, Pruett SW, Chen MY, et al. Skull-base foramina of the middle cranial fossa: reassessment of normal variation with high-resolution CT. AJNR Am J Neuroradiol 1994;15:283–91.
33. Matys T, Ali T, Zaccagna F, et al. Ossification of the pterygoalar and pterygospinous ligaments: a computed tomography analysis of infratemporal fossa anatomical variants relevant to percutaneous trigeminal rhizotomy. J Neurosurg 2019;132:1942–51.
34. Silbergleit R, Quint DJ, Mehta BA, et al. The persistent stapedial artery. AJNR Am J Neuroradiol 2000; 21:572–7.
35. Elnashar A, Patel SK, Kurbanov A, et al. Comprehensive anatomy of the foramen ovale critical to percutaneous stereotactic radiofrequency rhizotomy: cadaveric study of dry skulls. J Neurosurg 2019;132:1414–22.
36. Georgiou C, Cassell MD. The foramen meningo-orbitale and its relationship to the development of the ophthalmic artery. J Anat 1992;180:119–25.
37. Macchi V, Regoli M, Bracco S, et al. Clinical anatomy of the orbitomeningeal foramina: variational anatomy of the canals connecting the orbit with the cranial cavity. Surg Radiol Anat 2016;38:165–77.
38. Settecase F, Harnsberger HR, Michel MA, et al. Spontaneous lateral sphenoid cephaloceles: anatomic factors contributing to pathogenesis and proposed classification. AJNR Am J Neuroradiol 2014;35:784–9.
39. Bernard S, Loukas M, Rizk E, et al. The human occipital bone: review and update on its embryology and molecular development. Childs Nerv Syst 2015;31:2217–23.
40. Madeline LA, Elster AD. Suture closure in the human chondrocranium: CT assessment. Radiology 1995; 196:747–56.
41. Choudhary AK, Jha B, Boal DK, et al. Occipital sutures and its variations: the value of 3D-CT and how to differentiate it from fractures using 3D-CT. Surg Radiol Anat 2010;32:807–16.
42. Sanchez T, Stewart D, Walvick M, et al. Skull fracture vs. accessory sutures: how can we tell the difference. Emerg Radiol 2010;17:413–8.
43. Currarino G. Canalis basilaris medianus and related defects of the basiocciput. AJNR Am J Neuroradiol 1988;9:208–11.
44. Zdilla MJ, Russell ML, Bliss KN, et al. The size and shape of the foramen magnum in man. J Craniovertebr Junction Spine 2017;8:205–21.
45. Matsushima K, Kawashima M, Matsushima T, et al. Posterior condylar canals and posterior condylar emissary veins-a microsurgical and CT anatomical study. Neurosurg Rev 2014;37:115–26.
46. Lee SH, Kim SS, Sung KY, et al. Pulsatile tinnitus caused by a dilated mastoid emissary vein. J Korean Med Sci 2013;28:628–30.
47. Kim LK, Ahn CS, Fernandes AE. Mastoid emissary vein: anatomy and clinical relevance in plastic & reconstructive surgery. J Plast Reconstr Aesthet Surg 2014;67:775–80.

Anatomy of the Cerebral Cortex, Lobes, and Cerebellum

Behroze Adi Vachha, MD, PhD[a,b], Tarik F. Massoud, MD, PhD[c], Susie Y. Huang, MD, PhD[d,*]

KEYWORDS

- Cerebral cortex • Cerebellum • Central sulcus • Parieto-occipital sulcus • Sylvian fissure
- Cingulate gyrus • Precentral gyrus • Inferior frontal gyrus

KEY POINTS

- Each cerebral hemisphere is divided into 4 lobes based on key fissures and sulci: the Sylvian fissure (lateral sulcus), central sulcus, parieto-occipital sulcus, and cingulate sulcus.
- The central sulcus is an important anatomic landmark separating the frontal and parietal lobes.
- The Sylvian fissure is a key landmark that separates the insula medially and the frontal lobe superiorly from the temporal lobe.
- The frontal lobe is the largest lobe within the cerebral hemisphere and is composed of 4 major gyri: the superior, middle, and inferior frontal gyri and the precentral gyrus.
- The parietal lobe is located posterior to the central sulcus and is divided into 4 regions: the postcentral gyrus anteriorly, the superior and inferior parietal lobules posteriorly, and the precuneus medially.

INTRODUCTION

A strong grasp of cerebral cortical, lobar, and cerebellar anatomy is essential for any practitioner of neuroimaging. Neuroanatomy provides the map to identify and communicate the locations of lesions and understand their functional implications. This understanding is especially relevant to the localization of lesions before biopsy or neurosurgical intervention. Detailed knowledge of neuroanatomy is also necessary for clinical correlation with neurologic symptoms in patients presenting with suspected neurologic diseases. Neuroanatomical knowledge provides an essential foundation to help guide the search for potential lesions based on the clinical presentation and known focal neurologic deficits.

Advances in neuroimaging techniques over the past few decades have enabled the detailed visualization of brain structures at unprecedented spatial and contrast resolution. High-resolution 3-dimensional cross-sectional imaging is now acquired routinely, leveraging the latest computed tomography (CT) and MRI technology to enable the precise localization of small lesions in the cerebrum and cerebellum. Therefore, the ability to identify the location of key gyri and sulci within the cerebral cortex has become an essential skill for the practiced clinical neuroimager and will be of paramount importance as noninvasive techniques for imaging the brain continue to evolve and become more sophisticated.

The cerebral cortex of each cerebral hemisphere is part of the telencephalon that covers

[a] Department of Radiology, Memorial Sloan Kettering Cancer Center, 1275 York Avenue, New York, NY 10065, USA; [b] Brain Tumor Center, Memorial Sloan Kettering Cancer Center, 1275 York Avenue, New York, NY 10065, USA; [c] Division of Neuroimaging and Neurointervention, Department of Radiology, Stanford University School of Medicine, Center for Academic Medicine, 453 Quarry Road, Palo Alto, CA 94304, USA; [d] Division of Neuroradiology and Athinoula A. Martinos Center for Biomedical Imaging, Department of Radiology, Massachusetts General Hospital, Harvard Medical School, 149 13th Street, Room 2301, Charlestown, MA 02129, USA
* Corresponding author.
E-mail address: susie.huang@mgh.harvard.edu

Neuroimag Clin N Am 32 (2022) 463–473
https://doi.org/10.1016/j.nic.2022.04.008
1052-5149/22/

neuroimaging.theclinics.com

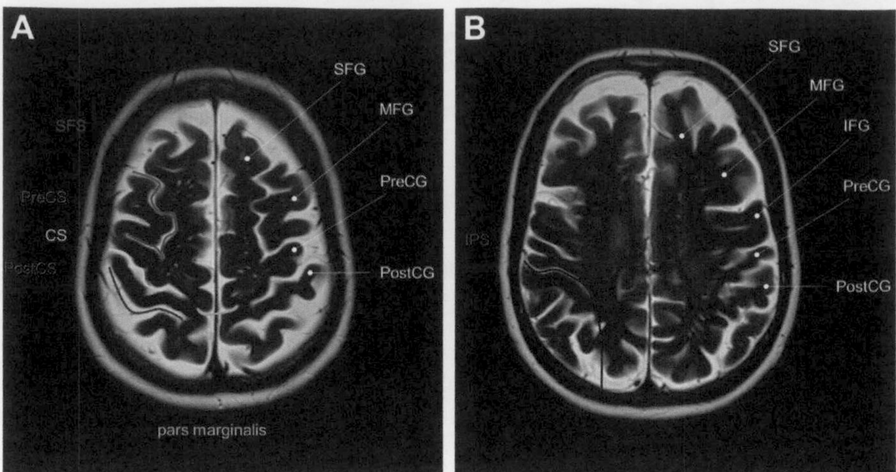

Fig. 1. Axial T2-weighted spin-echo images at the level of the (*A*) central sulcus and (*B*) intraparietal sulcus. Labeled gyri include the superior frontal gyrus (SFG), middle frontal gyrus (MFG), precentral gyrus (PreCG), and postcentral gyrus (PostCG). Labeled sulci include the superior frontal sulcus (SFS, *blue*), precentral sulcus (PreCS, *orange*), central sulcus (CS, *yellow*), postcentral sulcus (PostCS, *red*), pars marginalis of the cingulate sulcus (*green*), and intraparietal sulcus (IPS, *purple*).

the deeper diencephalic structures of the forebrain (the prosencephalon). Each hemispheric cortex is divided into 4 lobes based on key fissures and sulci, namely, the Sylvian fissure (lateral sulcus), central sulcus (CS), parieto-occipital sulcus, and cingulate sulcus. These fissures and sulci are large and readily identifiable between individuals based on their well-defined and characteristic configurations, locations, and depths along the cerebral hemispheres. The 4 major lobes are divided into smaller sulci and gyri that also exhibit defined patterns that can be recognized and learned through systematic review and practice in identifying these landmarks on routine neuroimaging studies.

The normal brain is almost but not quite perfectly symmetric across the interhemispheric fissure, and subtle inherent structural asymmetries may be apparent on neuroimaging, as reviewed recently by Kuo and Massoud.[1] Brain structural asymmetries can be rotational or pure right-left asymmetries. Yakovlevian torque results from the right hemisphere rotating slightly forward relative to the left, which may make the right frontal lobe bigger and wider, and the left occipital lobe wider and extend rightward. This torque also makes the left Sylvian fissure longer and flatter, resulting in a larger planum temporale. There are also right-left asymmetries in the cortex, white matter structures, deep gray nuclei, lateral ventricles, and hindbrain.[1] Brain asymmetries are not entirely random but result from distinct patterns in evolutionary structural design that confer functional advantages.

Frontal Lobe

The frontal lobe is the largest lobe within the cerebral hemisphere and is located anterior to the CS and above the Sylvian fissure. The frontal pole represents the most anterior portion of the frontal lobe. The prefrontal cortex corresponds to the anterior part of the frontal lobe. The prefrontal cortex plays a key role in the regulation of higher-order cognitive, emotional, and behavioral functioning. The frontal lobe is composed of 4 major gyri: the superior, middle, and inferior frontal gyri and the precentral gyrus. On axial images, the superior frontal gyrus is a vertically oriented gyrus along the superiormost margin of the frontal lobe (Fig. 1, SFG). The middle frontal gyrus (see Fig. 1, MFG) is a wide bar of tissue that parallels and is separated from the superior frontal gyrus by the superior frontal sulcus (see Fig. 1). The precentral gyrus crosses the superior frontal gyrus along the superior frontal convexity, which is well seen on axial images (see Fig. 1, PreCG). The precentral gyrus delineates the most posterior portion of the frontal lobe and extends inferiorly to the Sylvian fissure.

The inferior frontal gyrus is part of the lateral and inferior surface of the frontal lobe that overlies the insula anteriorly and is separated from the middle frontal gyrus by the inferior frontal sulcus.[2,3] The Sylvian fissure lies along its inferior edge; the anterior and ascending rami arising from the Sylvian fissure divide the inferior frontal gyrus into 3 parts, giving it the shape of the letter "M," known as the

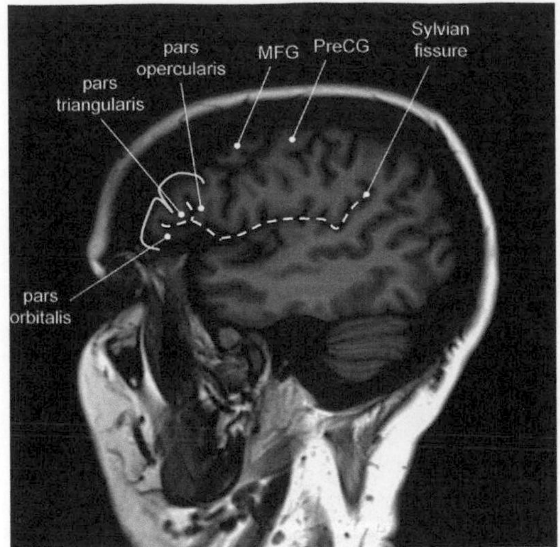

Fig. 2. Far lateral sagittal T1-weighted image at the level of the Sylvian fissure and frontal operculum. Labeled gyri include the yellow M-shaped inferior frontal gyrus, consisting of the pars orbitalis, pars triangularis, and pars opercularis; middle frontal gyrus (MFG), and precentral gyrus (PreCG). The Sylvian fissure courses horizontally across the image as denoted by the dashed line, with its anterior and ascending rami separating the pars orbitalis, pars triangularis, and pars opercularis of the inferior frontal gyrus, respectively.

"M sign" (Fig. 2, yellow line).[2] From anterior to posterior, the 3 parts of the "M" shape are the pars orbitalis, the pars triangularis, and the pars opercularis (see Fig. 2). Traditionally, the pars opercularis and pars triangularis are considered to form the Broca area (Brodmann areas 44 and 45) in the left hemisphere.[4] The functions of the traditional Broca and Wernicke areas are discussed in detail in the article "Brain Functional Imaging Anatomy" in this issue. The pars opercularis overlies the anterior insula and abuts the orbitofrontal cortex, which runs parallel to the gyrus rectus along the inferior surface of the frontal lobe (Fig. 3). The orbitofrontal cortex rests upon the orbital portion of the frontal bone and is composed of 4 gyri delineated by a distinctive H-shaped sulcus on axial views: the anterior, medial, posterior, and lateral orbital gyri (see Fig. 3B). The medial orbital gyrus abuts the vertically oriented olfactory sulcus, which is bordered superiorly by the olfactory tract and divides the orbital gyri from the gyrus rectus (see Fig. 3A).

Central Sulcus

The CS of Rolando separates the frontal and parietal lobes and is an important anatomic landmark when interpreting structural neuroimaging.[2,5,6] The CS is flanked by the precentral gyrus, which houses the primary motor cortex anteriorly, and the postcentral gyrus, which houses the primary somatosensory cortex posteriorly.[2,7] Along the medial surface of the brain, near the interhemispheric fissure at the apex of the CS, the precentral and postcentral gyri fuse to form the paracentral lobule, whereas inferolaterally these gyri fuse to form the subcentral gyrus.[2,3,8,9] This continuous loop of tissue surrounding the CS has been proposed as a separate lobe referred to as

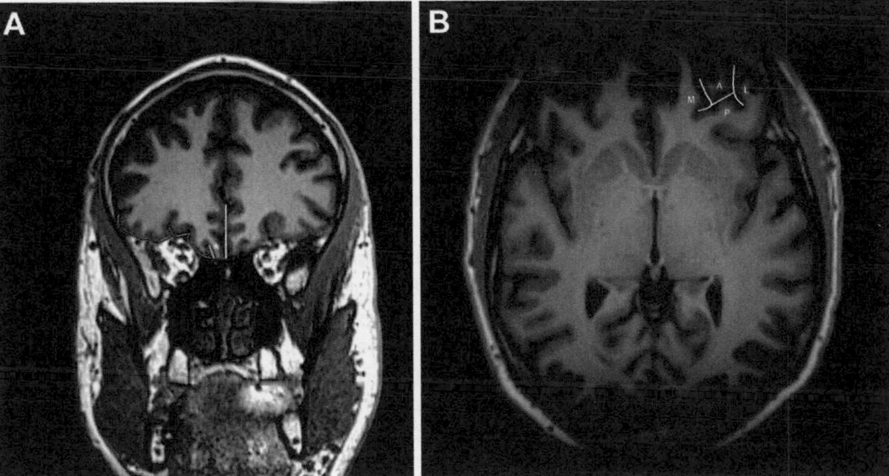

Fig. 3. Coronal and axial T1-weighted magnetization-prepared gradient echo (MPRAGE) images through the level of the orbitofrontal cortex. (*A*) Far anterior coronal image shows the orbitofrontal cortex (*red outline*), which is separated from the gyrus rectus (*asterisk*) by the vertically oriented olfactory sulcus (*orange line*). The interhemispheric fissure is delineated as a yellow line dividing the cerebral hemispheres. (*B*) Axial image shows the H-shaped orbital sulcus separating the anterior (*A*), lateral (*L*), posterior (*P*), and medial (*M*) orbital gyri.

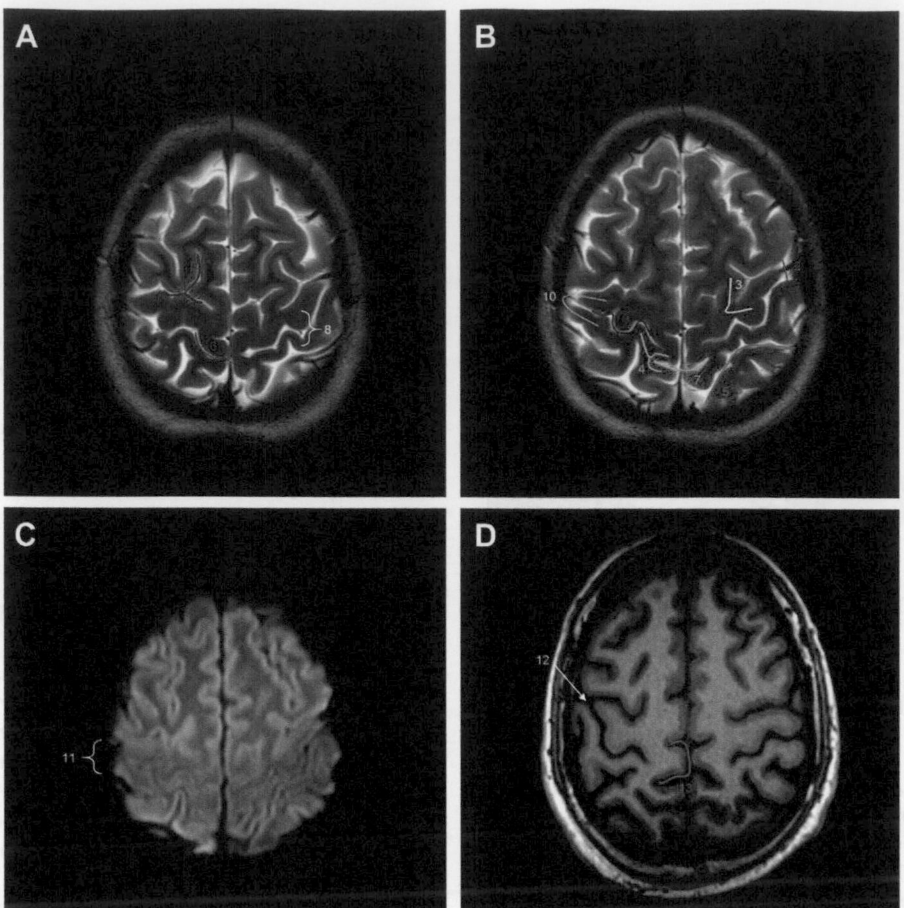

Fig. 4. Montage of signs indicating the location of the central sulcus on (*A, B*) axial T2-weighted images, (*C*) axial diffusion-weighted image, and (*D*) axial T1-weighted MPRAGE image along the superior convexity. 1, Superior frontal sulcus-precentral sulcus sign (upper T sign); 2, inferior frontal sulcus-precentral sulcus sign (lower T sign); 3, L sign; 4, bifid postcentral gyrus sign; 5, intraparietal sulcus sign; 6, midline sulcus sign; 7, pars bracket sign; 8, thin postcentral gyrus sign; 9, handknob or reverse-omega sign; 10, U sign; 11, invisible cortex sign; 12, white gray sign; 13, white paracentral lobule sign.

the central lobe, although the term has yet to gain wide acceptance.[2]

Several signs and landmarks have been described on structural imaging using CT and MRI to identify the CS, most of which rely on relationships and patterns between sulci and gyri (Fig. 4). Although most of these signs are 85% to 98% reliable in localizing the CS, morphologic variations or changes owing to adjacent cerebral lesions (Fig. 5) can be limiting factors, suggesting the need to combine several signs in concert to increase confidence in localization.[2] **Table 1** lists the most commonly described signs for identification of the CS, which are also illustrated in Fig. 4.

Cingulate Gyrus

Along the medial surface of the cerebral hemisphere, the cingulate gyrus parallels the corpus callosum, separated from it by the callosal sulcus, as best seen on sagittal imaging (Fig. 6). The cingulate gyrus is bordered superiorly by the superior frontal gyrus and paracentral lobule. The cingulate gyrus is separated from the superior frontal gyrus and paracentral lobule by the cingulate sulcus (see Fig. 6),[2] which runs parallel to the corpus callosum along its anterior portion and bends superiorly to form the pars marginalis.

The cingulate gyrus is a major limbic area and part of the Papez circuit (the medial or hippocampal limbic circuit), which begins at the hippocampus, continues as the fimbria and fornix, and ends in the mammillary body. From the mammillary body, the mammillothalamic tract reaches the anterior nuclear group of the thalamus and then the cingulum (the white matter core of the cingulate gyrus), which turns around the splenium of the corpus callosum to end as the radiation of

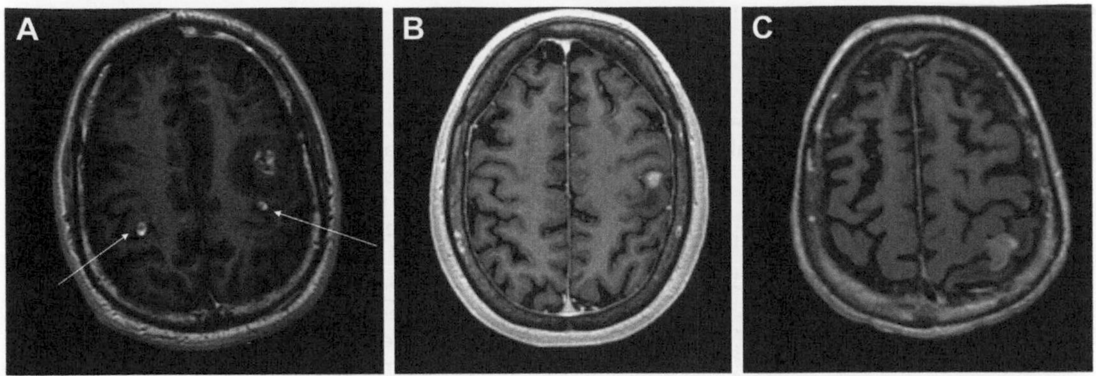

Fig. 5. Postcontrast axial T1-weighted fast spoiled gradient echo images demonstrating metastatic lesions involving the precentral and postcentral gyri. (*A*) Small enhancing metastases (*white arrows*) in the bilateral precentral gyri. A larger enhancing lesion in the posterior aspect of the middle frontal gyrus is associated with marked surrounding edema that extends into the precentral gyrus. (*B*) Enhancing metastasis involving the left postcentral gyrus with adjacent edema. (*C*) Lobulated enhancing lesion centered in the left postcentral gyrus extends into the central sulcus.

the cingulum into the hippocampus and uncus of the temporal lobe, thus completing the circuit[10]; this is in contradistinction to the basolateral or amygdaloid limbic circuit.[10,11]

Parietal Lobe

The parietal lobe is located posterior to the CS and can be divided into 4 regions: the postcentral gyrus anteriorly, the superior and inferior parietal lobules posteriorly, and the precuneus medially. The postcentral gyrus is located immediately posterior to and runs parallel to the CS (see Fig. 1). The postcentral gyrus is bordered posteriorly by the postcentral sulcus. The superior and inferior parietal lobules are located posterior to the postcentral sulcus and are divided by the intraparietal sulcus (see Fig. 1). The precuneus is located posterior to the postcentral sulcus and can be readily identified on the medial surface of the hemisphere on sagittal images (see Fig. 6). The precuneus is contiguous with the superior parietal lobule along the superior aspect of the parietal lobe. The parieto-occipital sulcus is posterior to the precuneus and divides the parietal lobe from the occipital lobe (see Fig. 6). The parieto-occipital sulcus is readily identified on sagittal images as a diagonally oriented sulcus that parallels and is located posterior to the ascending ramus of the cingulate sulcus Between the pars marginalis of the cingulate sulcus and the parieto-occipital sulcus lies a sulcus known as the subparietal sulcus (see Fig. 6), which separates the precuneus from the posterior portion of the cingulate gyrus.

On the lateral surface of the brain, the posterior part of the Sylvian fissure angles superiorly to form the ascending ramus, which terminates in an inverted U-shaped gyrus known as the supramarginal gyrus (Fig. 7). The angular gyrus is usually located immediately posterior to the supramarginal gyrus. This relationship may vary anatomically even within an individual (see Fig. 7), with the interposition of accessory gyri between the supramarginal and angular gyri (see Fig. 7B).[12] Taken together, the supramarginal and angular gyri form the inferior parietal lobule. The inferior parietal lobule is separated from the superior parietal lobule by the intraparietal sulcus. The primary intermediate sulcus descends from the intraparietal sulcus to divide the supramarginal gyrus from the angular gyrus.

Temporal Lobe

The Sylvian fissure (also known as the lateral sulcus or lateral fissure) is a key landmark that separates the insula medially and the frontal lobe superiorly from the temporal lobe. The lateral aspect of the Sylvian fissure separates the frontal and parietal opercula from the temporal operculum. The temporal pole lies under the Sylvian fissure at the anterior margin of the temporal lobe, along the most rostral portion of the middle cranial fossa. The circular sulcus outlines the insular cortex and is best visualized on sagittal planes medial to the Sylvian fissure. The circular sulcus consists of anterior, superior, and inferior segments that separate the insula from the frontal, temporal, and parietal opercula.[13] The posterior segment of the Sylvian fissure is contiguous with the superior and inferior segments of the circular sulcus of the insula. The limen insula is located at the junction of the anterior and posterior segments of the Sylvian fissure and delineates the

Table 1
Central sulcus signs

Signs	Description
Superior frontal sulcus-precentral sulcus sign (upper T sign)	The easily identifiable superior frontal sulcus joins the precentral sulcus; this intersection has the shape of an upper case T (see Fig. 1) and is considered 85% specific.[2,9,19] The precentral sulcus lies at the posterior end of the superior frontal sulcus, the precentral gyrus is found posterior to the precentral sulcus; and the CS is the next posterior sulcus[2,9]
L sign	The intersection between the superior frontal gyrus and the precentral gyrus resembles the capital letter "L" with the CS immediately posterior to the precentral gyrus[9,20]
Bifid postcentral gyrus sign	The pars marginalis of the cingulate sulcus splits the postcentral gyrus into a bifid configuration near the interhemispheric fissure[9,19,]
Intraparietal sulcus sign	The intraparietal sulcus intersects the postcentral sulcus and can be used to identify the central sulcus.[2]
Midline sulcus sign	The CS is identified as the longest sulcus running horizontally and closely approaching the interhemispheric fissure[9]
Pars bracket sign	The bihemispheric pars marginalis formed by the posterior-superior extension of the cingulate sulcus takes the shape of an anteriorly shaped bracket. The CS passes anterior to the pars marginalis on each side and medial to the lateral edge of the pars bracket.[2]
Thin postcentral gyrus sign	The precentral gyrus is thicker than the postcentral gyrus in anteroposterior diameter.[2] In addition, the thickness of the cortical gray matter within the precentral gyrus is thicker than that of the postcentral gyrus.[2]
Handknob or reverse-omega sign	The motor hand knob area refers to the posterior convex bulge of the precentral gyrus resulting in a symmetric or asymmetrical reverse-omega or epsilon shape in the axial plane.[2,20,21,22] In the sagittal plane, the hand motor area resembles a backward-oriented hook known as the sigmoidal hook sign[2,20,21]
U sign	The inferolateral aspect of the CS is enclosed by the U-shaped subcentral gyrus[9]
Invisible cortex sign	The cortices abutting the CS appears isointense relative to adjacent white matter on diffusion-weighted MRI sequences.[6] This observation is highly accurate in identifying the inferolateral aspect of the CS[6]
White gray sign	Increased T1 signal of the anterior and posterior cortices along the CS; the reduced gray-white contrast around the central sulcus was noted to be a reliable sign for identification of the CS on T1-weighted 3D inversion recovery fast-spoiled gradient echo images[23]
White paracentral lobule sign	The high signal intensity of the paracentral lobule cortex on T1-weighted imaging compared with that in the superior frontal cortex is useful for CS identification.[5]
Disappearing central sulcus sign	On double inversion recovery sequences, the CS cortex signal intensity is lower than that of the adjacent sulci, and this characteristic can be used to identify the CS[24]

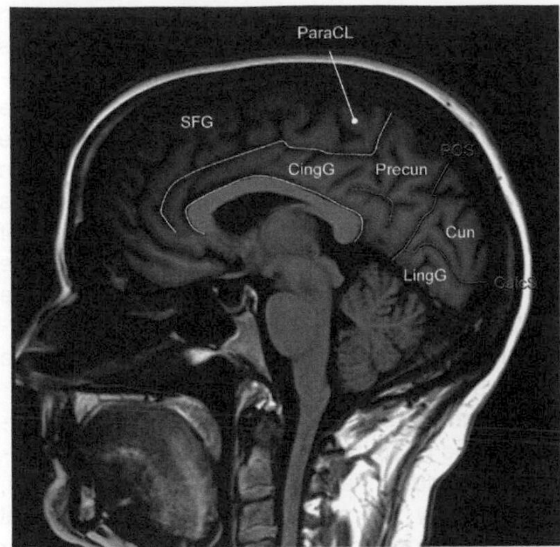

Fig. 6. Sagittal T1-weighted image demonstrating key gyri and sulci identifiable along the midline. Labeled gyri include the superior frontal gyrus (SFG), paracentral lobule (ParaCL), cingulate gyrus (CingG), precuneus (Precun), cuneus (Cun), and lingual gyrus (LingG). Outlined sulci include the cingulate sulcus (*white line*), callosal sulcus (*yellow line*), subparietal sulcus (*blue line*), parieto-occipital sulcus (*red line*, POS), and calcarine sulcus (*orange line*, CalcS).

point at which the insular cortex meets the amygdala and superior temporal gyrus.

The temporal lobe consists of 3 gyri: the superior, middle, and inferior temporal gyri (Fig. 8). The superior temporal sulcus separates the superior and middle temporal gyri, and the inferior temporal sulcus separates the middle and inferior temporal gyri. The traditional Wernicke area (Brodmann Area 22) is considered to lie in the posterior part of the superior temporal gyrus in the dominant hemisphere.[8] The inferior temporal gyrus is separated by the lateral occipito-temporal sulcus from the lateral occipito-temporal gyrus (see Fig. 8). The lateral occipito-temporal gyrus is separated from the parahippocampal gyrus by the collateral sulcus (see Fig. 8). The hippocampal fissure separates the parahippocampal gyrus from the hippocampus (see Fig. 8). The temporal stem connects the temporal and frontal lobes and lies in close proximity to the insula. The temporal stem is a key landmark that may be affected in several disorders, including seizures, tumors, and infection.

The demarcation between the insula and temporal lobes is readily identified on axial and sagittal views (Fig. 9). The insula is generally divided into 5 gyri. The anterior, middle, and posterior short insular gyri are separated from the anterior and posterior long insular gyri by the CS of the insula, which divides the insula into larger anterior and smaller posterior lobules.[14] On axial views, the posterior long insular gyrus is separated from the transverse temporal gyrus or Heschl gyrus (see Fig. 9), which is the location of primary auditory cortex. Heschl sulcus is posterior to Heschl gyrus and represents the anterior boundary of the planum temporale, an auditory association area.

Occipital Lobe

Along the medial surface of the cerebral hemisphere, the parieto-occipital sulcus separates the

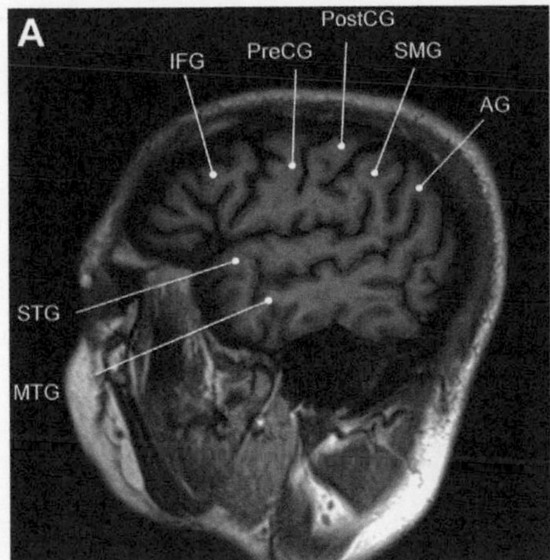

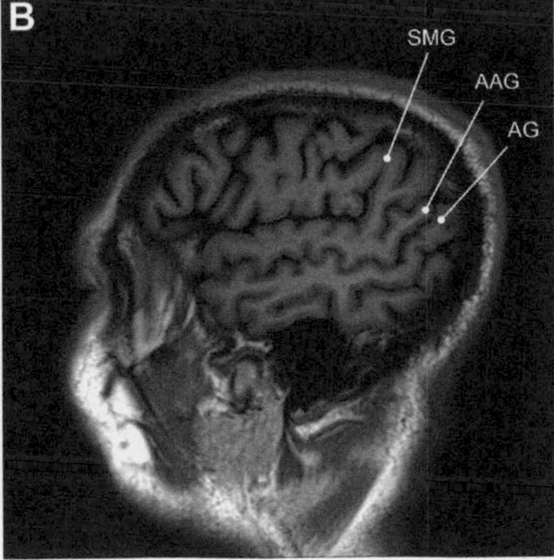

Fig. 7. Sagittal T1-weighted images along the lateral aspects of the cerebral convexities at the level of the Sylvian fissure illustrating variations in parietal lobe anatomy within an individual. (*A*) Right lateral view of the frontal, temporal, and parietal lobes. Labeled gyri include the inferior frontal gyrus (IFG), precentral gyrus (PreCG), postcentral gyrus (PostCG), supramarginal gyrus (SMG), angular gyrus (AG), superior temporal gyrus (STG), and middle temporal gyrus (MTG). (*B*) Sagittal image of the contralateral hemisphere demonstrates the presence of an accessory preangular gyrus (AAG) interposed between the supramarginal gyrus (SMG) and angular gyrus proper (AG).

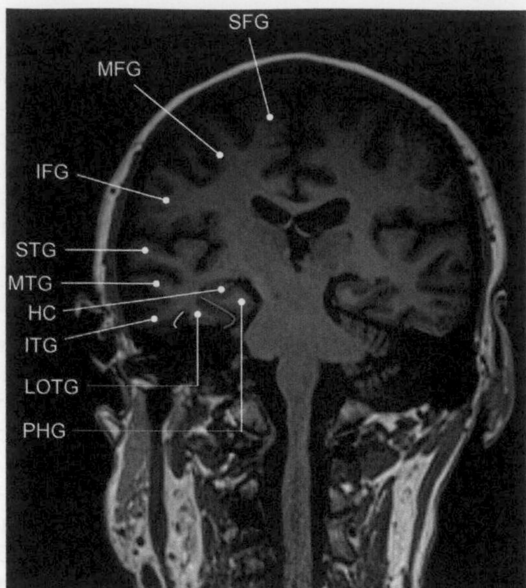

Fig. 8. Coronal image at the level of the foramina of Monro of the lateral ventricles demonstrating the major gyri and sulci of the frontal and temporal lobes. Labeled gyri include the superior frontal gyrus (SFG), middle frontal gyrus (MFG), inferior frontal gyrus (IFG), superior temporal gyrus (STG), middle temporal gyrus (MTG), hippocampus (HC), inferior temporal gyrus (ITG), lateral occipito-temporal gyrus (LOTG) and parahippocampal gyrus (PHG). Outlined sulci include the lateral occipitotemporal sulcus (*yellow line*) separating the inferior temporal gyrus and lateral occipitotemporal gyrus and the collateral sulcus (*blue line*) dividing the lateral occipitotemporal gyrus from the parahippocampal gyrus.

precuneus in the parietal lobe from the cuneus in the occipital lobe (see Fig. 6). The calcarine sulcus runs nearly orthogonal to the parietooccipital sulcus and divides the occipital lobe into the triangular-shaped cuneus superiorly and the tongue-shaped lingual gyrus inferiorly as seen on sagittal imaging (see Fig. 6). The calcarine sulcus separates the superior and inferior portions of the primary visual cortex. The anterior calcarine sulcus extends anteriorly and inferiorly from the junction of the parieto-occipital sulcus and calcarine sulcus to separate the lingual gyrus from the continuation of the cingulate sulcus.

Along the lateral surface of the cerebral hemisphere, the occipital lobe is composed of the superior, middle, and inferior occipital gyri, separated by the superior and inferior occipital sulci.[2] The superior occipital gyrus drapes over the convexity onto the medial surface to form the cuneus. The superior occipital sulcus or intraoccipital sulcus is contiguous with the intraparietal sulcus and parallels the interhemispheric fissure on axial views. The intraoccipital sulcus runs perpendicular to the parieto-occipital sulcus, which is readily identified on axial images as a bifid, barbell-shaped sulcus crossing midline. On axial views, the precuneus sits anterior to the parieto-occipital sulcus, and the cuneus is located posterior to the parieto-occipital sulcus.

The inferior occipital sulcus extends posteriorly from the inferior temporal sulcus. The middle occipital gyrus lies just posterior to the junction of the temporal and parietal lobes and abuts the

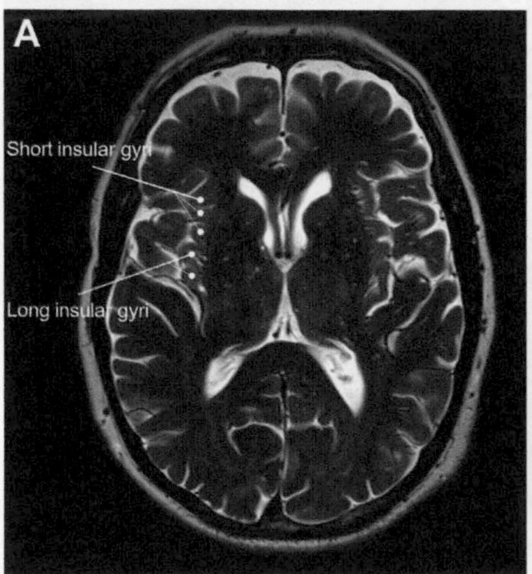

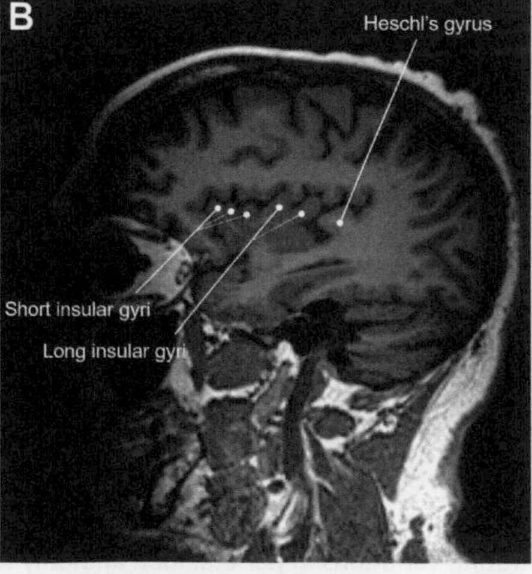

Fig. 9. Axial and sagittal images of the insula. (*A*) Axial T2-weighted spin-echo image demonstrating the division of the insula into the anterior, middle, and posterior short insular gyri anteriorly and the anterior and posterior long insular gyri posteriorly. (*B*) Sagittal T1-weighted image shows the short and long insular gyri separated by the central sulcus of the insula, and Heschl gyrus posteriorly.

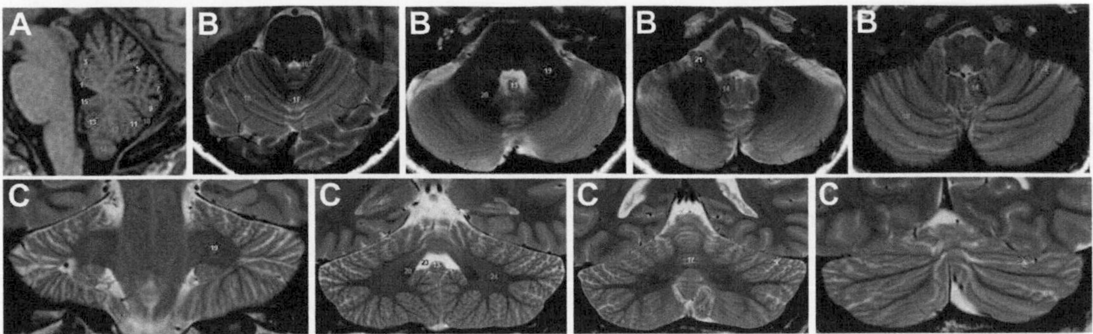

Fig. 10. (*A*) Sagittal, (*B*) axial, and (*C*) coronal images of the cerebellum. 1, Superior medullary velum; 2, lingula; 3, central lobule; 4, culmen; 5, tentorial fissure; 6, declive; 7, folium; 8, horizontal fissure; 9, tuber; 10, suboccipital fissure; 11, pyramid; 12, uvula; 13, nodulus; 14, tonsil; 15, inferior medullary velum; 16, superior cerebellar peduncle; 17, vermis; 18, cerebellar hemisphere; 19, middle cerebellar peduncle; 20, dentate nucleus; 21, flocculus; 22, cerebellar folia; 23, fourth ventricle; 24, cerebellar white matter (arbor vitae).

supramarginal gyrus, the angular gyrus, the superior temporal gyrus, and the middle temporal gyrus. The middle occipital gyrus occupies the most area along the lateral aspect of the occipital lobe and is divided into superior and inferior portions by the horizontally oriented middle occipital sulcus.[2]

Cerebellum

The cerebellum is located in the posterior cranial fossa and is a major feature of the hindbrain (the rhombencephalon). More specifically, along with the pons, it forms the metencephalon or the upper part of the hindbrain. All cerebellar connections with other parts of the brain pass through the cerebellar peduncles. The cerebellum consists of a highly-folded layer of cerebellar gray matter cortex overlying white matter surrounding a fluid-filled fourth ventricle at its base (**Fig. 10**). Four deep cerebellar nuclei are embedded in the white matter. The first detailed descriptions of cerebellar MRI anatomy were provided by Courchesne and colleagues[15] and Press and colleagues.[16,17]

The cerebellum is divided into 2 cerebellar hemispheres, connected by a narrow midline zone termed the *vermis* (see **Fig. 10**). The vermis has been described as consisting of 9 named lobules: lingula, central lobule, culmen, clivus, folium of the vermis, tuber, pyramid, uvula, and nodule or nodulus.[18] Three lobes can be distinguished within the cerebellum: the anterior or superior lobe (above the primary or horizontal fissure), the posterior or inferior lobe (below the primary fissure), and the flocculonodular lobe (below the posterior fissure). A set of folds divides the overall structure of the cerebellum into about 10 smaller lobules (I to V in anterior lobe, VI to IX in posterior lobe, and X is considered the flocculonodular lobe). Each surface ridge or gyrus in the cortex is called a folium. Underneath the gray matter folia lies white matter (the arbor vitae, or tree of life, because of its branched appearance on cross section), made up largely of myelinated nerve fibers running to and from the cortex. Embedded within the white matter is a cluster of 4 deep cerebellar nuclei, composed of gray matter, the dentate, globose, emboliform, and fastigial nuclei. Each of these communicates with different parts of the brain and cerebellar cortex. The dentate nucleus is the largest and is a thin, convoluted layer of gray matter. The flocculus of the flocculonodular lobe is the only part of the cerebellar cortex that does not project to the deep nuclei; its output goes to the vestibular nuclei.

Connecting the cerebellum to different parts of the brain and spinal cord are 3 paired cerebellar peduncles (superior, middle, and inferior). Each superior cerebellar peduncle (brachium conjunctivum) is made of white matter that connects the cerebellum to the midbrain. The middle cerebellar peduncle (brachium pontis) only contains fibers from the pons to the cerebellum arranged in 3 fasciculi: superior, inferior, and deep. The pontine nuclei (or griseum pontis) in the ventral pons are the nuclei involved in motor activity. Corticopontine fibers carry information from the primary motor cortex to the ipsilateral pontine nucleus, and the pontocerebellar projection then carries that information to the contralateral cerebellum through the middle cerebellar peduncle. The inferior cerebellar peduncle (made of restiform and juxtarestiform bodies) is at the lower part of the fourth ventricle and connects the cerebellum to the spinal cord and medulla oblongata. The inferior cerebellar peduncle carries several input and output fibers for integration of proprioceptive sensory input and motor vestibular functions such as balance and posture maintenance.

The cerebellopontine fissure, also called the cerebellopontine angle, is a V-shaped fissure formed by the cerebellum wrapping around the pons and middle cerebellar peduncle. Inferiorly, the cerebellar tonsil is equivalent to a rounded lobule on the undersurface of each cerebellar hemisphere, continuing medially into the uvula of the vermis and superiorly into the flocculonodular lobe.

CLINICS CARE POINTS

- **Morphologic variations in the configuration of the CS or alterations in its configuration owing to adjacent cerebral lesions may require combining several imaging signs in concert to increase confidence in localizing this key anatomic landmark.**
- **The temporal stem connects the temporal and frontal lobes and is a key structure that may be affected in several disorders, including seizures, tumors, and infection.**

FUNDING INFORMATION

NIH/NCI Cancer Center Support (Grant P30 CA008748, PI: Thompson). NIH grant numbers U01-EB026996, P41-EB030006, K23-NS096056, P41-EB017183, and R01-NS118187.

DISCLOSURES

None.

REFERENCES

1. Kuo F, Massoud TF. Structural asymmetries in normal brain anatomy: a brief overview. Ann Anat 2022;241:151894.
2.. Naidich T, Tang C, Ng J, et al. Surface anatomy of the cerebrum. In: Naidich T, Castillo M, Cha S, et al, editors. Imaging of the brain. Philadelphia: Elsevier Inc; 2013. p. 127–53.
3. Ulmer S. Neuroanatomy and cortical landmarks. In: Ulmer S, Jansen O, editors. *fMRI:* Basics and clinical applications. 3rd edition ed. Switzerland: Springer Nature; 2020. p. 5–13.
4. Sibilla L. Functional anatomy of the major lobes. In: Agarwal N, Port J, editors. Neuroimaging: anatomy meets function. Switzerland: Springer International Publishing; 2018. p. 81–99.
5. Cho S, Kurokawa R, Hagiwara A, et al. Localization of the central sulcus using the distinctive high signal intensity of the paracentral lobule on T1-weighted images. Neuroradiology 2021;64(2):289–99.
6. Su S, Yang N, Gaillard F. Invisible cortex sign: a highly accurate feature to localize the inferolateral central sulcus. J Med Imaging Radiat Oncol 2019; 63(4):439–45.
7. Hill VB, Cankurtaran CZ, Liu BP, et al. A practical review of functional MRI Anatomy of the language and motor systems. AJNR Am J Neuroradiol 2019;40(7): 1084–90.
8. Naidich T, Yousry T. Functional Neuroanatomy. In: Stippich C, editor. Clinical functional MRI: Presurgical functional neuroimaging. Berlin-Heidelberg: Springer-Verlag; 2007. p. 53–86.
9. Wagner M, Jurcoane A, Hattingen E. The U sign: tenth landmark to the central region on brain surface reformatted MR imaging. AJNR Am J Neuroradiol 2013;34(2):323–6.
10. Shah A, Jhawar SS, Goel A. Analysis of the anatomy of the Papez circuit and adjoining limbic system by fiber dissection techniques. J Clin Neurosci 2012; 19(2):289–98.
11. Duprez TP, Serieh BA, Raftopoulos C. Absence of memory dysfunction after bilateral mammillary body and mammillothalamic tract electrode implantation: preliminary experience in three patients. AJNR Am J Neuroradiol 2005;26(1):195–7.
12. Naidich TP, Valavanis AG, Kubik S. Anatomic relationships along the low-middle convexity: Part I--normal specimens and magnetic resonance imaging. Neurosurgery 1995;36(3):517–32.
13. Destrieux C, Terrier LM, Andersson F, et al. A practical guide for the identification of major sulcogyral structures of the human cortex. Brain Struct Funct 2017;222(4):2001–15.
14. Naidich TP, Kang E, Fatterpekar GM, et al. The insula: anatomic study and MR imaging display at 1.5 T. AJNR Am J Neuroradiol 2004;25(2):222–32.
15. Courchesne E, Press GA, Murakami J, et al. The cerebellum in sagittal plane–anatomic-MR correlation: 1. the vermis. AJR Am J Roentgenol 1989;153(4):829–35.
16. Press GA, Murakami J, Courchesne E, et al. The cerebellum in sagittal plane–anatomic-MR correlation: 2. the cerebellar hemispheres. AJR Am J Roentgenol 1989;153(4):837–46.
17. Press GA, Murakami JW, Courchesne E, et al. The cerebellum: 3. anatomic-MR correlation in the coronal plane. AJR Am J Roentgenol 1990;154(3): 593–602.
18. Monte Bispo RF, Casado Ramalho AJ, Buarque de Gusmao LC, et al. Cerebellar vermis: topography and variations. Int J Morphol 2010;28(2):439–43.
19. Naidich T, Brightbill T. Systems for localizing frontoparietal gyri and sulci on axial CT and MRI. Int J Neuroradiol 1996;2:313–38.
20. Raabe A. The Craniotomy Atlas. Stuttgart, Germany: Thieme; 2019.

21. Yousry TA, Schmid UD, Alkadhi H, et al. Localization of the motor hand area to a knob on the precentral gyrus. A new landmark. Brain 1997;120(Pt 1): 141–57.
22. Caulo M, Briganti C, Mattei PA, et al. New morphologic variants of the hand motor cortex as seen with MR imaging in a large study population. AJNR Am J Neuroradiol 2007;28(8):1480–5.
23. Kaneko OF, Fischbein NJ, Rosenberg J, et al. The "White Gray Sign" identifies the central sulcus on 3t high-resolution t1-weighted images. AJNR Am J Neuroradiol 2017;38(2):276–80.
24. Mark IT, Luetmer PH, Rydberg CH, et al. Signal intensity of peri-rolandic cortex identifies the central sulcus on double inversion recovery MRI. J Neurosurg Sci 2019;66(1):1–8.

Medial Temporal Lobe Anatomy

Eric K. van Staalduinen, DO[a], Michael M. Zeineh, MD, PhD[b,*]

KEYWORDS

• Medial temporal lobe anatomy • Mesial temporal lobe • Hippocampal formation • Hippocampus
• Cornu ammonis • CA fields • Dentate gyrus

KEY POINTS

- Knowledge of normal hippocampal anatomy and development improves recognition of hippocampal pathology.
- Deciphering hippocampal subfield anatomy on routine clinical imaging is now possible, with greater confidence owing to improved imaging techniques and higher field strength MR scanners.

INTRODUCTION

The medial temporal lobe (MTL) is a complex anatomic region in the ventromedial aspect of the temporal lobe. It consists of the hippocampal formation, the parahippocampal region, and the amygdaloid complex and plays a key role in numerous cognitive processes, including the creation, retrieval, and consolidation of new memories, spatial navigation, emotion, and social behavior.[1,2] Although much work has been done to elucidate the complex anatomic relationships, cytoarchitecture, and functional connectivity within the MTL, the authors' goal is to create an anatomic reference for clinicians and scientists that highlights and summarizes this region, with special attention to MR imaging. They have therefore focused primarily on the hippocampal formation, discussing its gross structural features and anatomic relationships, relevant subfield anatomy, and hippocampal connectivity. They detail how this complex anatomy appears on MR imaging and also discuss hippocampal terminology and development, normal anatomic variants, clinically relevant disease processes, and automated segmentation software common to hippocampal analysis. **Table 1** lists important anatomic terms in this review.

HIPPOCAMPAL TERMINOLOGY AND DEVELOPMENT

The classic gross appearance of the human hippocampal formation is that of a prominent, bulging eminence in the floor of the temporal horn of the lateral ventricle (**Fig. 1**).[2] The term "hippocampus" (or sea horse) was first used by the Italian anatomist and surgeon Giulio Cesare Aranzio (Arantius) in 1587, although it is unclear which aspect of the hippocampus reminded him of a sea horse, as he also likened the hippocampus to a silkworm.[2] Centuries later, Winslow (1732) likened the appearance to a ram's horn, and de Garengoet (1742) named the hippocampus "Ammon's horn" after the Egyptian deity Amun, who has the head of a ram.[3] Lorente de Nó (1934) appropriated the term "Cornu Ammonis" (CA) for the hippocampus proper, a term that remains synonymous with the hippocampus today.[4]

Although much of the cerebral cortex consists of a 6-cell-layer neocortex, the mesial temporal structures are formed of more primitive allocortex (which consists of 3, 4, or 5 cell layers), which begins in early fetal life as a flat cortical plate along the medial wall and floor of the temporal horn.[5] Unequal growth and thickening of the dentate gyrus

[a] Department of Radiology, Stanford University, 453 Quarry Road, Stanford, CA 94304, USA; [b] Department of Radiology, Stanford University, 1201 Welch Road, Room P271, Stanford, CA 94305, USA
* Corresponding author.
E-mail address: mzeineh@stanford.edu

Neuroimag Clin N Am 32 (2022) 475–489
https://doi.org/10.1016/j.nic.2022.04.012

Table 1
Anatomic terms

Ambient gyrus	The most prominent bulge in the medial temporal lobe; composed of entorhinal cortex and categorized as medial extension of parahippocampal gyrus; part of the anterior uncus
Band of Giacomini	The most superficial part of the dentate gyrus in the hippocampal head, present along the inferior and medial uncal surfaces; continues caudally in the hippocampal body as the margo denticulatus
Collateral sulcus	Runs in an anteroposterior course along the inferior temporal and occipital lobes; anteriorly separates the parahippocampal gyrus medially from the fusiform (or lateral occipitotemporal) gyrus laterally; posteriorly separates the lingual gyrus medially from the lateral occipitotemporal gyrus laterally
Endorhinal sulcus	Separates the anterior perforated substance from the uncus; used as a landmark to identify the piriform cortex; seen on coronal MR at the level of the limen insulae
Fasciola cinerea	The superficial continuation of the margo denticulatus along the hippocampal tail; situated between the gyrus fasciolaris and the gyrus Andreas Retzius
Gyrus of Andreas Retzius	The superficial continuation of the CA1 field along the hippocampal tail; demonstrates characteristic small, rounded bulges on its surface
Gyrus fasciolaris	The superficial continuation of the CA3 field along the hippocampal tail; covered by alveus
Gyrus intralimbicus	Also known as the uncal apex; is a small, rounded medial protrusion posterior to the band of Giacomini in the posterior uncus; is composed of CA4 and CA3; and is covered by alveus; fimbria attaches to its caudal extremity; demarcates the caudal aspect of the hippocampal head
Intrarhinal sulcus	Shallow sulcus within the entorhinal cortex
Limen insulae	Also known as the frontotemporal junction, formed at the junction between the frontal and temporal lobes; forms the lateral limit of the anterior perforated substance and represents the level at which the middle cerebral artery bifurcates; marks the reference level for the piriform cortex, amygdala, and entorhinal cortex
Margo denticulatus	The most superficial part of the dentate gyrus along the hippocampal body
Piriform lobe	Consists of cortical amygdala, anterior segment of uncus, and anterior parahippocampal gyrus
Rhinal sulcus	Rostral continuation of the collateral sulcus; separates the temporal pole from the parahippocampal gyrus
Semiannular sulcus	Also known as sulcus semiannularis; along the medial surface of the anterior uncus; separates the semilunar gyrus (amygdala) above from the ambient gyrus (parahippocampal gyrus) below
Semilunar gyrus	Covers the corticomedial nuclei of the amygdala in the anterior uncus
Superficial hippocampal sulcus	Present along the inferior border of the hippocampal body, separating the margo denticulatus from the subiculum
Uncal sulcus	Along the medial surface of the posterior uncus, separates the hippocampus above from the parahippocampal gyrus below
Uncinate gyrus	Forms part of the posterior uncus; is continuous rostrally with the ambient gyrus; composed of CA1 and subiculum

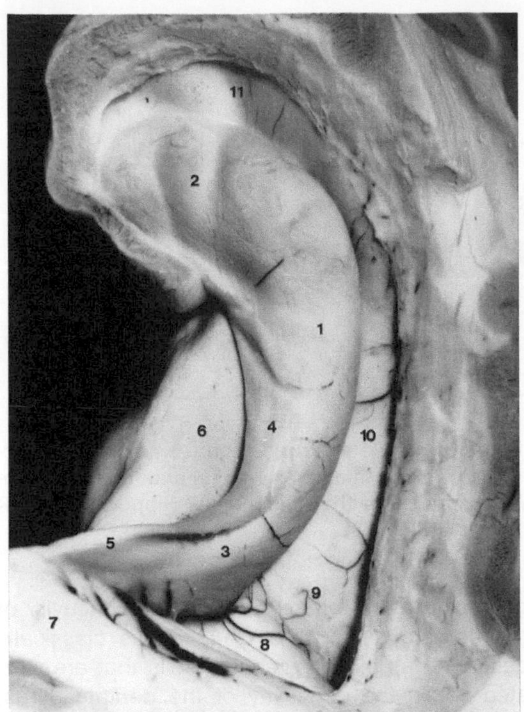

Fig. 1. Intraventricular aspect of the hippocampus, viewed from above. The temporal horn has been opened and choroid plexus removed. 1, hippocampal body; 2, hippocampal head and internal digitations; 3, hippocampal tail; 4, fimbria; 5, crus of fornix; 6, subiculum; 7, splenium of corpus callosum; 8, calcar avis; 9, collateral trigone; 10, collateral eminence; 11, uncal recess of the temporal horn. (*From* Duvernoy HM. *The Human Hippocampus: Functional Anatomy, Vascularization and Serial Sections with MRI*. Springer Berlin Heidelberg; 2005.)

initiates the process of hippocampal infolding, whereby the hippocampal sulcus deepens and shifts from a location between the dentate gyrus and cornu ammonis to a location between the dentate gyrus and subiculum (Fig. 2); this results in the characteristic interlocking C-shape configuration of the adult hippocampus, with the external surfaces of the dentate gyrus and CA1/subiculum in contact around a diminutive hippocampal sulcus.[6]

SURFACE AND SUBFIELD ANATOMY OF THE MEDIAL TEMPORAL LOBE

The term "hippocampal formation" refers to a collection of cytoarchitectonically distinct components that are linked by predominantly unidirectional internal connections and organized as a functional unit. These components consist of the dentate gyrus (or gyrus dentatus/DG), hippocampus proper (or cornu ammonis/CA fields), subicular complex, and some include the entorhinal cortex as part of the formation. Although the term "hippocampus" consists of the dentate gyrus and CA fields in an anatomic sense of the word, some definitions have also included the subicular complex, as the subiculum is not easily distinguished from the CA fields on MR images.

Hippocampus

The hippocampus is an arched bilaminar gray and white matter structure located in the MTL that demonstrates an enlarged anterior extremity and a posterior extremity that narrows as a comma (see Fig. 1; Fig. 3).[7] It has a length of approximately 4.5 cm along the rostrocaudal axis[2] and is commonly divided into 3 parts: (1) an anterior part or head; (2) a middle part or body; (3) a posterior part or tail. The CA fields and dentate gyrus are gray matter structures that form 2 interlocking U-shaped laminae, which are partially separated by the vestigial hippocampal sulcus (Fig. 4).[7] The alveus and fimbria are white matter structures that together constitute the fornix. Several fissures surround the hippocampus, including the lateral extension of the ambient cistern, termed the transverse fissure of Bichat, which separates the thalamus above from the parahippocampal gyrus below (see Fig. 14). The superolateral extension of the transverse fissure is the choroidal fissure, whereas the inferolateral extension is the hippocampal fissure, which is often obliterated but separates the dentate gyrus from the subiculum and CA fields. In general, the gray matter structures of the hippocampus appear as other gray matter structures on MR imaging, with signal intensity matching that of cortex and deep gray nuclei elsewhere throughout the brain, except for the stratum lacunosum moleculare, which contains myelinated white matter of the perforant pathway.

Although a comprehensive discussion of internal hippocampal architecture is beyond the scope of this chapter, a concise review is provided for completeness. The hippocampus proper consists of 6 layers, from the ventricular cavity to the vestigial hippocampal sulcus: alveus (1, see Fig. 4), stratum oriens (2), stratum pyramidale (3), stratum radiatum (4), stratum lacunosum (5), and stratum moleculare (6). As allocortex typically shows only 3 layers, the 6 layers of the CA listed above are grouped into 3 layers: stratum oriens (2), stratum pyramidale (3), and the molecular zone (4–6, a layer that combines the strata *r*adiatum, *l*acunosum, and *m*oleculare, commonly termed the SRLM).[4,7] Along the other side of the hippocampal sulcus is the dentate gyrus, a trilaminate cortical region consisting of a molecular layer (8), a

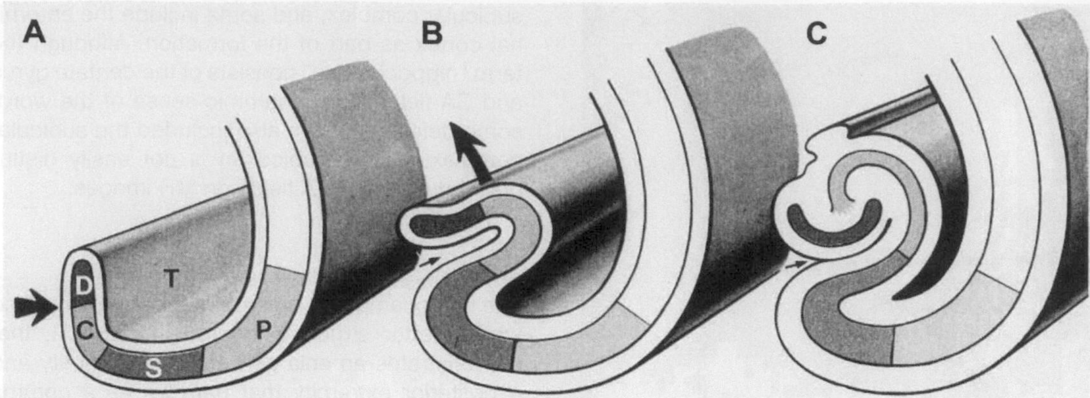

Fig. 2. Coronal plane illustration of hippocampal infolding stages. D, dentate gyrus; C, cornu ammonis; S, subiculum; P, parahippocampal gyrus; T, temporal horn. Large arrow in (*A*) and small arrows in (*B*) and (*C*), hippocampal sulcus. (*From* Kier EL, Kim JH, Fulbright RK, Bronen RA. Embryology of the Human Fetal Hippocampus: MR Imaging, Anatomy, and Histology. *AJNR Am J Neuroradiol*. 1997;18:525-532.)

granular layer (9), and a polymorphic layer (arrowhead).[8,9]

Lorente de Nó (1934) described 4 distinct hippocampal fields based on cytoarchitectural analysis, termed CA1–4 (see **Fig. 4**).[2,4] The CA1 field borders the subiculum medially and continues along the inferior aspect of the hippocampus laterally, curving upward along the temporal horn of the lateral ventricle; this coincides with an expanded pyramidal cell layer, and the CA1/CA2 border is denoted by a marked transition to the dense, narrow pyramidal cell layer of CA2.[2] The CA2/3 border roughly corresponds to an expansion of the CA3 pyramidal layer. The CA3 field is thought to correspond to the superomedial curve, or genu of the CA, where it enters the concavity of the dentate gyrus. The CA4 field is classically described as those pyramidal cells that are situated within the concavity of the dentate gyrus, enclosed by the granule cell layer. Some suggest grouping the CA3 and CA4 fields together, as there is no cytoarchitectonic or connectional reason to distinguish CA4 from CA3,[2] with commonality present of the incoming mossy fibers and colocalization of the outgoing endfolial pathway joining the Schaffer collaterals. Yet, there is not a laminate structure to CA4.[8] The CA1 field has a specific sensitivity to anoxia and has thus been termed the vulnerable sector (or Sommer sector), whereas CA3 is known as the resistant sector (or

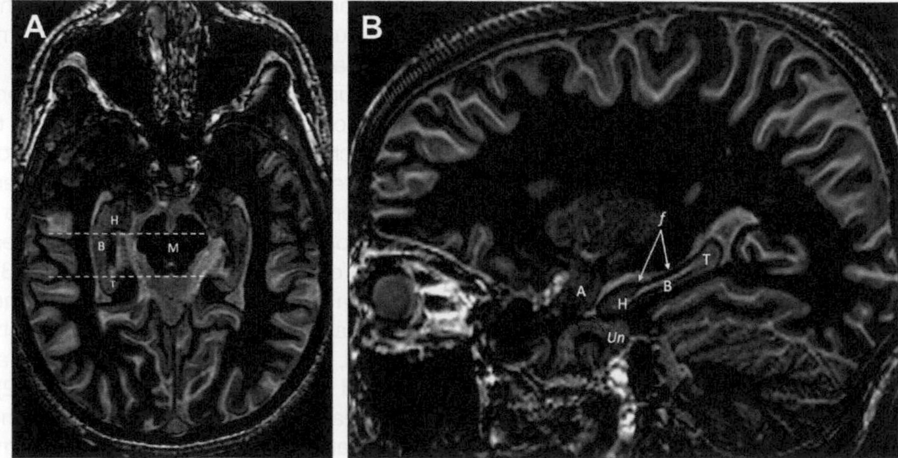

Fig. 3. (*A*) Axial and (*B*) sagittal fGATIR 3T images. The hippocampal head (H) is located anterior to the plane of the interpeduncular cistern, whereas the tail (T) is posterior to the midbrain (M) and the body (B) is in between. The amygdala (A) is separated from the hippocampal head by the uncal recess of the temporal horn (Un). Fimbria (*f*), uncal apex (*yellow arrow*).

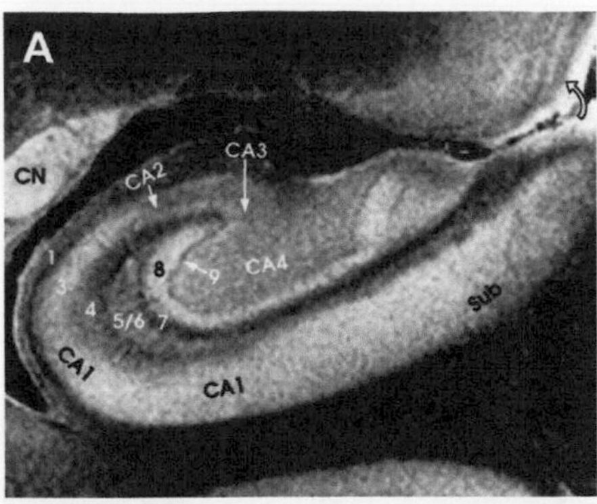

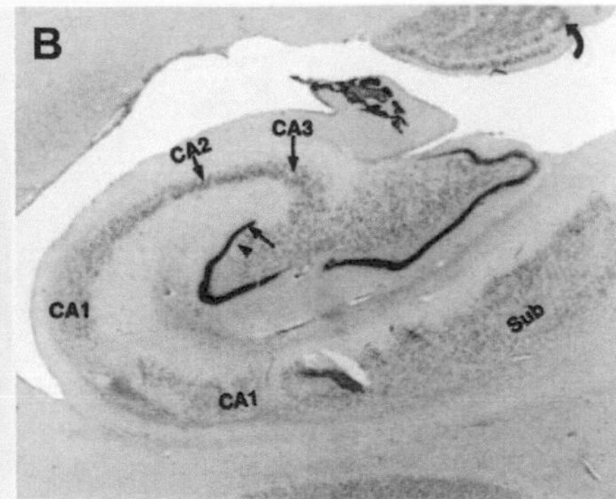

Fig. 4. (*A*) Magnetic resonance microscopy (MRM) of the hippocampal body coronally at 9.4 T. (*B*) Nissl stain specimen corresponding to A. From lateral to medial, the MRM displays the following: 1, alveus; 2, stratum oriens (between 1 and 3); 3, stratum pyramidale; 4, stratum radiatum; 5, stratum lacunosum; 6, stratum moleculare; 7, hippocampal sulcus; 8, stratum moleculare; 9, dentate granule cell layer (*straight arrow* in *B*); and 10, polymorphic layer (*arrowhead* in *B*). Also seen are cornu ammonis, CA1 to CA4, caudate nucleus tail (CN), subiculum (Sub), and the lamellar retinotopic organization of the lateral geniculate body (*curved arrow*). (*From* Fatterpekar GM, Naidich TP, Delman BN, et al. Cytoarchitecture of the Human Cerebral Cortex: MR Microscopy of Excised Specimens at 9.4 Tesla. *AJNR Am J Neuroradiol*. 2002;23:1313-1321.)

Spielmeyer sector).[7] CA2 is thought to be involved with Lewy body disease.[10]

MR imaging of these strata and subfields has been challenging before the advent of high-field, high-resolution MR imaging, with prior studies showing that these structures cannot be precisely or reliably predicted as macroscopic, anatomic landmarks.[11] However, more recent studies using higher field strengths (≥3T) and improved imaging techniques suggest that some of these boundaries and strata can be visualized *in vivo* with reproducibility.[9,12–14]

The authors now review the hippocampal head, body, and tail with greater detail, emphasizing the structural anatomy that can be readily appreciated on MR imaging, beginning with the body, where the laminate architecture is more tractable. Intraventricular components refer to visibility along the floor of the temporal horn of the lateral ventricle during dissection, whereas extraventricular (or cisternal) parts refer to visibility along the surface of the ambient cistern.

Hippocampal body

The intraventricular hippocampal body (see Figs. 1 and 3) is an element in the floor of the temporal horn of the lateral ventricle that is hidden by choroid plexus and has ependyma covering the protruding alveus. Its medial border is defined by the fimbria, whereas the lateral border consists of the collateral eminence (which is the intraventricular protrusion of cortex covering the collateral sulcus).[7] The extraventricular part is visible medially (Fig. 5).

On coronal MR images (Fig. 6; see Fig. 11), the hippocampal body has the traditional C within a C architecture, with the slightly hyperintense hilus (including the dentate gyrus and CA4) present centrally; CA3, CA2, and CA1 wrapping around the hypointense SRLM; the hippocampal sulcus and SRLM separating the remainder of CA1 from the DG; and contiguity with the subicular complex. Notably, the subicular complex often shows some hypointensity, likely related to multiple myelinated perforant pathway bundles that shorten T2 relaxation.

Hippocampal head The hippocampal head (Fig. 7; see Fig. 11F, G) represents the anterior component of the hippocampal arc. It features 2 to 4 internal digitations consisting of transverse folds of CA around a central extension of the DG.[7] The DG is present more posteriorly within the hippocampal head, whereas CA fields and subiculum predominate more anteriorly. The extraventricular part of the hippocampal head forms the posterior segment of the uncus, with the uncinate gyrus and uncal apex (also known as the gyrus intralimbicus) representing prominent bulges in the MTL at the mid- and caudal aspects. The uncinate gyrus is continuous with the ambient gyrus rostrally and has been described as a strip of CA1 and subiculum,[5] whereas the uncal apex is present as a small round protuberance medial to the usual profile of the hippocampus, is composed of CA4 and CA3 fields, and is firmly attached to the fimbria at its extremity; this is an important anatomic landmark for MR imaging, as it is used to demarcate the posterior margin of the hippocampal head and approximate the caudal limits of the entorhinal and perirhinal cortices.[14] A useful method for confidently identifying the uncal apex/GIL is to look

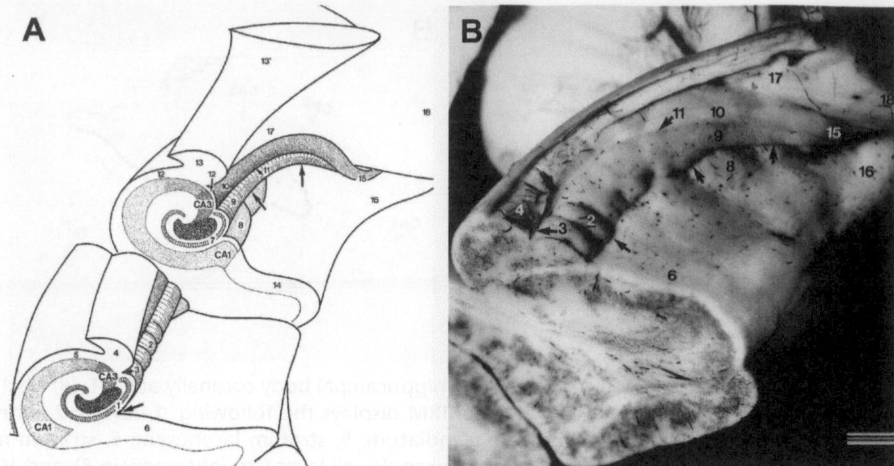

Fig. 5. Schematic (*A*)/specimen (*B*) images of the hippocampal body/tail. The most superficial part of the dentate (1 and 7) along the hippocampal body is termed *margo denticulatus* (2). Rounded surface protrusions termed *dentes* represent a superficial manifestation of dentate gyrus folding (2). White matter fibers from the alveus (5 and 12) continue caudally along the superomedial surface as fimbria (4 and 13). The fimbriodentate sulcus (3) separates the margo denticulatus from the fimbria, whereas the superficial hippocampal sulcus (*arrows*) separates the margo denticulatus from the subjacent subiculum (6 and 14).[5] As the body transitions to tail, the fimbria (4 and 13) begins to separate from the margo denticulatus (2) as it ascends to join the crus of the fornix (13′). Concomitant widening of the fimbriodentate sulcus (3) exposes the superficial continuation of CA3 covered by alveus, termed *gyrus fasciolaris* (10). The CA1 field appears progressively at the surface, often producing small, rounded bulges, termed the *gyri of Andreas Retzius* (8). As the margo denticulatus continues caudally, it becomes smooth and narrow, forming the *fasciola cinerea* (9).[5] The terminal segment covers the subsplenial surface, thus termed subsplenial gyrus (15). Although controversial, it is favored to consist of CA without dentate gyrus, with CA3 along the medial edge and CA1 constituting its majority.[5] The subiculum (14) is continuous caudally as the isthmus of the cingulate cortex (16). The sulcus dentatofasciolaris (11), splenium of the corpus callosum (18), and subcallosal trigone (17) are labeled for completeness. (*From* Duvernoy HM. The Human Hippocampus: Functional Anatomy, Vascularization and Serial Sections with MRI. Springer Berlin Heidelberg; 2005.)

for the fimbria, as it can often be seen attaching to its caudal extremity (see **Figs. 3**, **7**D, **9**, **11**G). Although the anterior part of the uncus is also visualized at the level of the hippocampal head, it is important to note that the ambient gyrus (see **Figs. 7**B and **11**E), the most prominent bulge in the MTL, is actually entorhinal cortex, which is categorized as medial extension of the parahippocampal gyrus.[15]

Hippocampal tail The hippocampal tail represents the posterior part of the hippocampal arc. It also appears as a transverse bulge in the floor of the lateral ventricle without surface digitations. The internal architecture is composed of CA, centered by digital extensions of DG, with CA fields extending beyond the DG in the caudal-most aspect, as in the head. The intraventricular part is thickly covered by alveus and subependymal veins, whereas its medial border is flanked by fimbria, and its lateral border is the collateral trigone.[7] The extraventricular part demonstrates continuation of the hippocampal formation, with similar surface features (see **Fig. 5**).

On coronal MR images (**Fig. 8**), the tail seems to widen because of its superomedial curvature (see **Figs. 1** and **3**, posteriorly), and the division between body and tail often coincides with the appearance of the wing of the ambient cistern. Typical hippocampal architecture is observed, with CA fields surrounding the SRLM and central dentate gyrus.

A few practical points are highlighted before continuing the discussion later. First, the structure of the hippocampus is the same throughout its different segments, consisting of the U-shaped dentate gyrus and surrounding CA. Second, the segment of dentate gyrus visible from within the ventricle and along its medial surface is known by 3 terms depending on location: the band of Giacomini in the head/uncus, margo denticulatus in the body, and fasciola cinerea in the tail.

Parahippocampal region

The parahippocampal gyrus forms the medial edge of the brain, extending from the rhinal sulcus (6, **Fig. 9**) anteriorly to the splenium posteriorly.[16] It encompasses the perirhinal, entorhinal, and

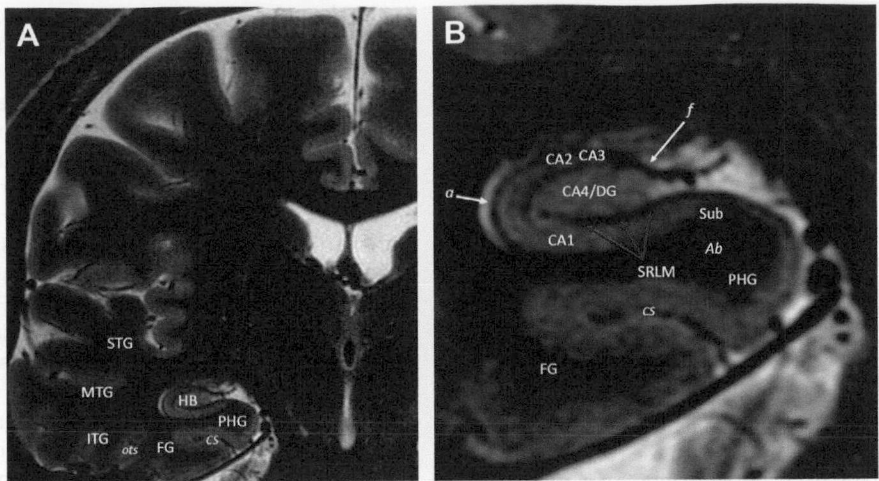

Fig. 6. (*A*) Large and (*B*) small field-of-view coronal 3T of the hippocampal body. (*A*) Regional anatomy: hippocampal body (HB), parahippocampal gyrus (PHG), fusiform gyrus (FG), inferior temporal gyrus (ITG), middle temporal gyrus (MTG), superior temporal gyrus (STG), collateral sulcus (*cs*), and occipitotemporal sulcus (ots). (*B*) Hippocampal subfield anatomy: CA1–4, hilus (CA4/DG), subiculum (Sub), SRLM (stratum radiatum, lacunosum, and moleculare; *red arrows*), angular bundle (*Ab*), alveus (*a*), and fimbria (*f*).

parahippocampal cortices and subiculum along its rostrocaudal extent and is continuous along its longitudinal axis, although it can be divided into anterior and posterior segments. The anterior segment, also known as the piriform lobe, consists of the uncus and the entorhinal area, whereas the posterior segment is separated from the hippocampus by the uncal sulcus, consists of subiculum superomedially and parahippocampal cortex inferiorly, and continues caudally to join the isthmus of the cingulate gyrus below the splenium of the corpus callosum (see Fig. 9).

The subiculum (or "bed" of the hippocampus) is a trilaminate cortex composed of a superficial molecular layer, a central pyramidal cell layer, and a deep polymorphic layer. It borders the CA1 field of the hippocampus and is subdivided into several segments, from lateral to medial: prosubiculum

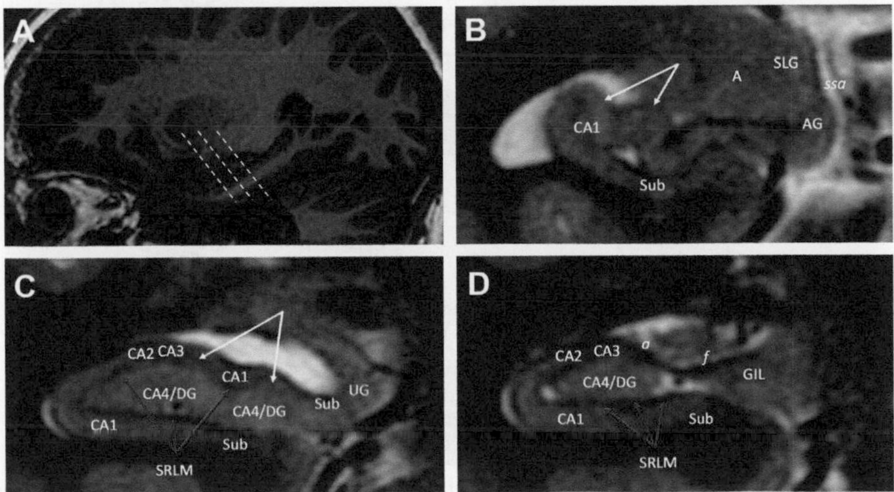

Fig. 7. The hippocampal head at 3T, with a sagittal cross-reference image (*A*) and zoomed-in coronal images at the rostral, mid, and caudal aspects (*B–D*). The hippocampal head is widened owing to anteromedial wrapping (as seen in Figs. 1 and 3, anteriorly) and demonstrates an undulated appearance due to interdigitations (images *B* and *C*, *white arrows*). Approximate boundaries of CA1–4, subiculum (Sub), amygdala (A), semilunar gyrus (SLG), ambient gyrus (AG), sulcus semiannularis (*ssa*), SRLM (stratum radiatum, lacunosum, and moleculare; *red arrows*), uncinate gyrus (UG), gyrus intralimbicus (GIL), fimbria (*f*), alveus (*a*).

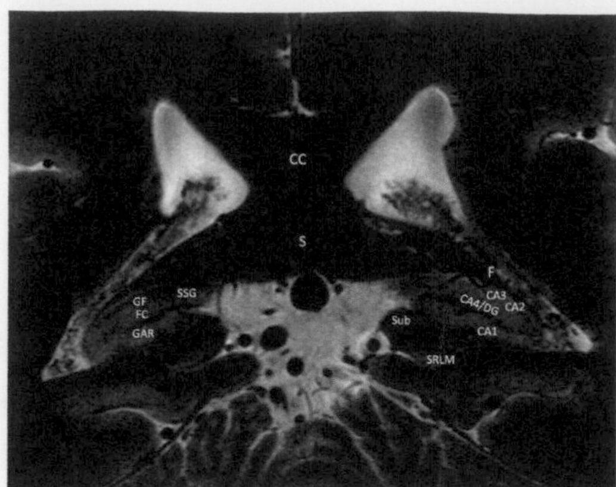

Fig. 8. Coronal T2W-FSE MR image of the hippocampal tail at 7T. Surface anatomy on the radiologic right: gyrus fasciolaris (GF), fasciola cinerea (FC), gyrus of Andreas Retzius (GAR), subsplenial gyrus (SSG). Subfield anatomy on the left: CA1-4, SRLM (stratum radiatum, lacunosum, and moleculare, *red arrow*), subiculum (Sub). Splenium (S), corpus callosum (CC), crus of the fornix (F).

(continuous with CA1 but not universally agreed on as a separate region), subiculum, presubiculum, and parasubiculum.[17,18] The parasubiculum passes around the medial margin of the parahippocampal gyrus and is contiguous with the entorhinal area. The subiculum contains anteroposterior projecting myelinated fibers from the perforant pathway[8] and thus has lower signal on T2-weighted fast spin-echo MR images (see Fig. 6).

The entorhinal cortex (Figs. 10 and 11) is composed of periallocortex that is obliquely oriented and contiguous with the parasubiculum. It is the most rostrally situated component of the hippocampal formation, with its rostral extreme identified just behind the limen insulae and its caudal-most portion defined as one slice caudal to the gyrus intralimbicus on coronal MR images.[19] Its medial portion forms the ambient gyrus, extending to the sulcus semiannularis (small arrow, see Fig. 10).[15] Its lateral border extends to the medial bank of the collateral sulcus, where it borders the perirhinal cortex.[19] It demonstrates a 6-layer pattern, with characteristic islands of large pyramidal cells in layer II (see Fig. 10). Macroscopically, this shows small, raised mounds on the surface termed "verrucae hippocampi."[2] Despite its small size, it is the principal input to the hippocampus, with the origin of the perforant/alvear pathways arising from its layer II/III neurons.[7] In addition, it is one of the hallmark locations of tau deposition and neurodegeneration in Alzheimer disease (AD), closely following transentorhinal/perirhinal tau.[20]

The white matter of the parahippocampal gyrus situated deep to the subicular complex is called the angular bundle. Within this region, fibers of the perforant path system travel to caudal levels

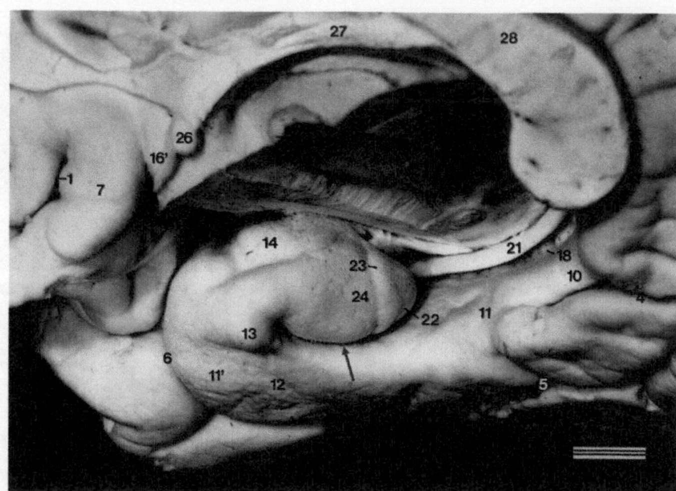

Fig. 9. Sagittal dissection of the right hemisphere. Surface anatomy demonstrates the parahippocampal gyrus (11′ and 11), semilunar gyrus (14), ambient gyrus (13), entorhinal area with islands (12), isthmus of the cingulate cortex (10), rhinal sulcus (6), uncal sulcus (*red arrow*), uncinate gyrus (24), band of Giacomini (23), uncal apex (22), fimbria (21), fornix (27), subcallosal gyrus (7) and sulcus (1), paraterminal gyrus (16′), anterior commissure (26), corpus callosum (28), dentate gyrus (18), anterior calcarine sulcus (4), collateral sulcus (5). (*Adapted from* Duvernoy HM. *The Human Hippocampus: Functional Anatomy, Vascularization and Serial Sections with MRI*. Springer Berlin Heidelberg; 2005.)

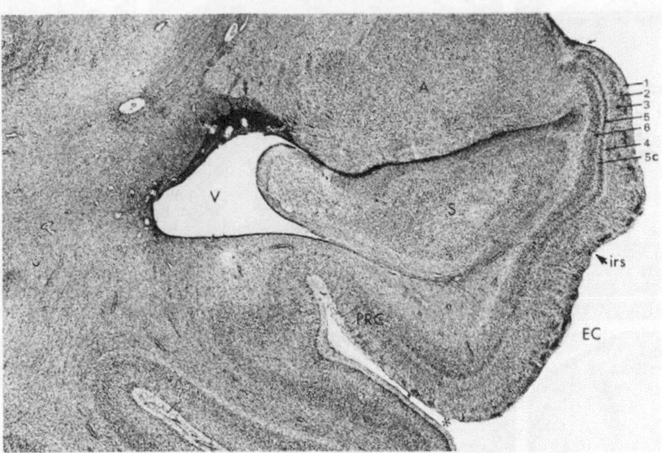

Fig. 10. Coronal, thionin-stained section of the human hippocampus and entorhinal cortex (EC). The numbers at the top right of the image indicate the layers of the EC. Note the shallow intrarhinal sulcus (irs) located in the EC. Amygdala (A), subiculum (S), temporal horn of the lateral ventricle (V), and perirhinal cortex (PRC). An asterisk marks the collateral sulcus, whereas small arrows demarcate the dorsomedial and ventrolateral extents of EC layer II. (*From* Insausti R, Amaral DG. Hippocampal Formation. In: *The Human Nervous System*. Elsevier; 2012:896-942.)

of the hippocampal formation, perforate through the subiculum and hippocampus, and terminate in CA1 and the outer two-thirds of the molecular layer of the dentate gyrus.[2,8] It is well defined and partially myelinated at birth.

Amygdaloid complex

The amygdala is an almond-shaped, gray matter structure consisting of many nuclei (see Fig. 11). Its rostral portion approximates that of the entorhinal cortex (where it can be identified by the limen insula), and it is bounded medially by the piriform and periamygdaloid cortices, together termed the piriform cortex-cortical amygdaloid (PCA) region.[21] Except at its rostral-most level, the amygdala reaches the medial surface of the temporal lobe throughout its rostrocaudal extent, forming the semilunar gyrus.[22] Three main regions constitute the amygdala body, including a group of deep nuclei called the basolateral nuclear group, a superficial laminated region in the anterior part of the uncus termed the corticomedial group, and a central group.[22] The corticomedial nuclei are olfactory centers, whereas the basolateral and central nuclei have limbic functions.[7] The amygdala is separated from the hippocampus by the anterior aspect of the temporal horn (see Fig. 3B), and a well-defined hippocampal-amygdaloid transitional area, which is approximately coincident with the choroidal fissure.[23]

Hippocampal Connectivity

Hippocampal connectivity consists of many intrinsic and extrinsic pathways, with a predominantly forward loop of excitatory connections and inhibitory neurons between the entorhinal cortex and the rest of the hippocampal formation. A detailed discussion of hippocampal circuitry is beyond the scope of this chapter; however, a comprehensive schematic is provided in Fig. 12.

Subcortical output from the hippocampal formation largely originates in the CA3 field and subiculum and extends into the alveus and fimbria to the fornix. A smaller precommissural projection, arising mainly from the cells of the hippocampus proper, extends to the septal region, primarily innervating the lateral septal nucleus, whereas a much larger postcommissural bundle, arising primarily from the subicular complex, provides input to the mammillary bodies. Impulses then reach the anterior thalamic nucleus, either directly or via the mammillary bodies from the mammillothalamic tract, before finally reaching the posterior cingulate, retrosplenial, and anterior cingulate cortices.[7]

Hippocampal Vascularization

The hippocampus is supplied by the anterior, middle, and posterior hippocampal arteries, which are variably derived from the posterior cerebral artery and its branches as well as the anterior choroidal artery. The hippocampal head and uncus are supplied by the anterior hippocampal artery, whereas the body and tail are vascularized by the middle and posterior hippocampal arteries (Fig. 13). The anterior hippocampal artery courses through the

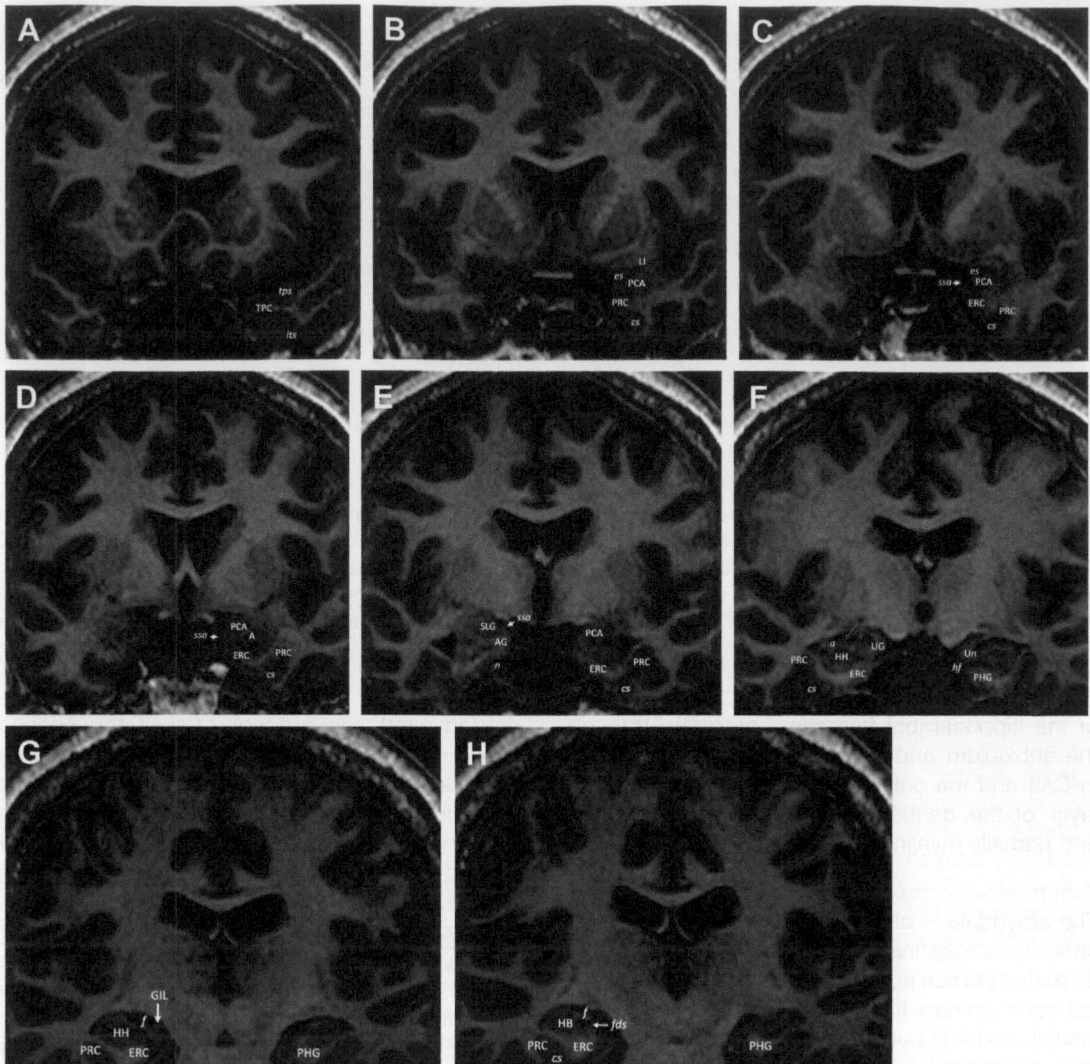

Fig. 11. Coronal T1W 3T MR images of the anteromedial temporal lobe (*A–H*, rostral to caudal). Anatomic landmarks used to identify the hippocampal formation, parahippocampal region, and amygdaloid complex are delineated. (*A*) The lateral edge of the temporopolar sulcus (*tps*) demarcates the dorsal limit of the temporopolar cortex (TPC), whereas the medial edge of the inferotemporal sulcus (*its*) delineates its ventrolateral extent. (*B*) The limen insulae (LI), also known as the frontotemporal junction, approximates the rostral extremes of the piriform cortex-cortical amygdaloid region (PCA) and the perirhinal cortex (PRC). At this level, the PCA extends from the fundus of the endorhinal sulcus (*es*) one-third of the distance to the most convex point of the medial temporal lobe. The perirhinal cortex is the caudal continuation of the temporopolar cortex. It represents the most rostral aspect of the parahippocampal gyrus (PHG) and extends to the lateral bank of the collateral sulcus (cs). (*C*) The entorhinal cortex (ERC) begins just caudal to the limen insulae, extending medially to the sulcus semiannularis (*ssa*) and laterally to the medial bank of the collateral sulcus. The PRC extends from there to the lateral bank of the collateral sulcus. At this level, the PCA extends from the fundus of the endorhinal sulcus to the sulcus semiannularis. (*D*) The amygdala (A) is just caudal to the limen insulae. The PCA, ERC, and PRC are all visible at this level. (*E*) The semilunar gyrus (SLG) is separated from the ambient gyrus (AG) by the sulcus semiannularis. The uncal notch (N) is visualized along the inferior surface of the AG. (*F*) The hippocampal head (HH) demonstrates internal digitations (*red arrows*) with a thin overlying strip of alveus (A). The uncinate gyrus (UG) is visualized. Note flattening and loss of internal digitations in the left hippocampal head. The hippocampal fissure (*hf*) separates the uncus (Un) from the PHG. (*G*) The caudal aspect of the right hippocampal head is demarcated by the gyrus intralimbicus (GIL), which is the most caudal of the uncal bulges and is seen as a small, round superomedial protrusion. The fimbria (*F*) is firmly adhered to its caudal extremity. (*H*) One slice caudal to the GIL, demarcating the first slice of hippocampal body (HB). Note the fimbria (*F*) and fimbriodentate sulcus (fds); this is the last slice that contains the ERC, whereas the PRC extends an additional slice and wraps medially behind the ERC. Beyond that, the parahippocampal cortex continues along the medial aspect of the temporal lobe.

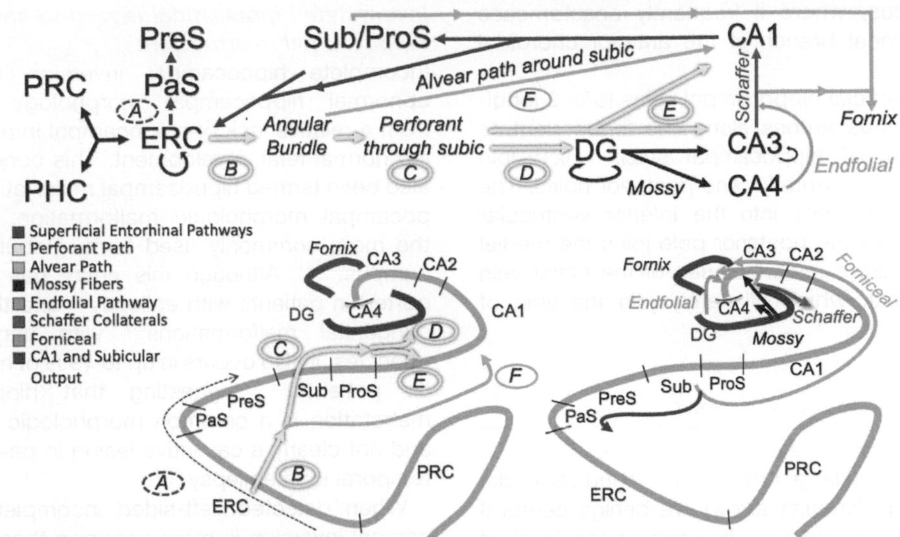

Fig. 12. Hippocampal circuitry. (*Top*) (A–F) The components of the perforant path system largely identified in animal studies. Major pathways are represented by solid lines, whereas minor pathways are represented by dotted lines. (A) = "sublamina supratangentialis" (*dotted red*), a minor superficial entorhinal bundle projecting to the parasubiculum and presubiculum. (B) = entorhinal projection to the angular bundle (*yellow*). (C) = angular bundle fibers (*yellow*) perforating through the subiculum. D + E = these same fibers projecting superiorly (D) into the dentate gyrus or inferiorly (E) into the hippocampal CA fields (*yellow*). F = angular bundle fibers subjacent to the subiculum projecting into the CA fields (alvear path, *light blue*). The remaining hippocampal circuitry includes mossy fibers projecting from the dentate gyrus to CA3 and CA4 (*dark blue*), the endfolial pathway projecting from CA4 toward and through CA3 (*light brown*), CA3 projecting to the fornix (*green*) and to CA1 (Schaffer collaterals, *orange*), followed by CA1 and subiculum output to ERC and subicular output to the fornix (*green*). CA, cornu ammonis; DG, dentate gyrus; ERC, entorhinal cortex; PaS, parasubiculum; PHC, parahippocampal cortex; PRC, perirhinal cortex; PreS, presubiculum; ProS, prosubiculum; Sub, subiculum. (*From* Zeineh MM, Palomero-Gallagher N, Axer M, et al. Direct Visualization and Mapping of the Spatial Course of Fiber Tracts at Microscopic Resolution in the Human Hippocampus. *Cereb Cortex*. Published online February 13, 2016:bhw010.)

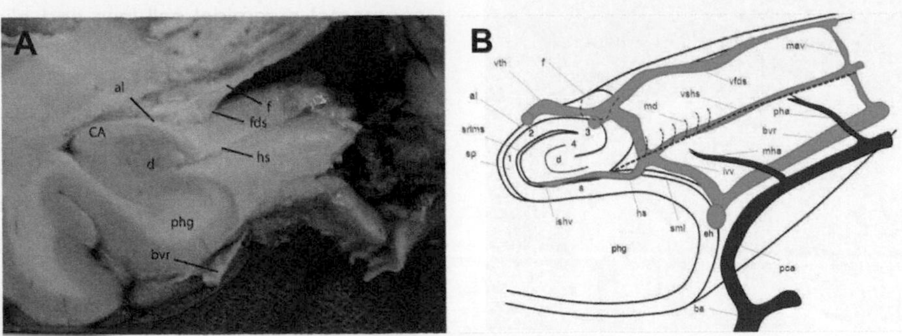

Fig. 13. Gross (*A*) and schematic (*B*) images depicting the superficial arteries and veins of the hippocampal body. Cornu ammonis (CA) and CA1–4 subfields, dentate gyrus (D), alveus (aL), fimbria (F), fimbriodentate sulcus (fds), superficial hippocampal sulcus (hs), parahippocampal gyrus (phg), basal vein of Rosenthal (bvr), middle and posterior hippocampal arteries (mha and pha), posterior cerebral artery (pca), basilar artery (ba), vein of the fimbriodentate sulcus (vfds), vein of the superficial hippocampal sulcus (vshs), vein of the temporal horn (vth), intrasulcal hippocampal vein (ishv), inferior ventricular vein (ivv), medial atrial vein (mav), stratum pyramidale (sp), compilation of strata radiatum, lacunosum, and moleculare (srlms), subiculum (*S*), superficial medullary lamina (sml), entorhinal area (eh), margo denticulatus (md). (*From* Thomas BP, Welch EB, Niederhauser BD, et al. High-resolution 7T MRI of the human hippocampus in vivo. *J Magn Reson Imaging*. 2008;28(5):1266-1272.)

uncal sulcus, where it frequently anastomoses with the uncal branch of the anterior choroidal artery.[7]

The superficial hippocampal veins form 2 longitudinal venous arches along the fimbriodentate and superficial hippocampal sulci, which join together at their anterior and posterior poles. The anterior pole flows into the inferior ventricular vein, whereas the posterior pole joins the medial atrial vein. Both are tributaries of the basal vein of Rosenthal, which ultimately join the vein of Galen.[7]

Normal Hippocampal Variants

Sulcal remnant and choroidal fissure cysts

Sulcal remnant (large arrow, Fig. 14) and choroidal fissure cysts (smaller arrow) are benign cerebral cysts that are occasionally seen at the level of the vestigial hippocampal sulcus and the choroidal fissure. Sulcal remnant cysts result from lack of obliteration of the hippocampal sulcus, thus they are most commonly located between the CA and dentate gyrus in the lateral aspect of the hippocampal apex. The cause of choroidal fissure cysts is less clear, although developmental variation may occur along the choroidal fissure at the time of primitive choroid plexus formation. On MR imaging, both types of cysts demonstrate signal intensity that follows cerebrospinal fluid on all sequences without demonstrating contrast enhancement or restricted diffusion. Both are asymptomatic and incidentally discovered.[5]

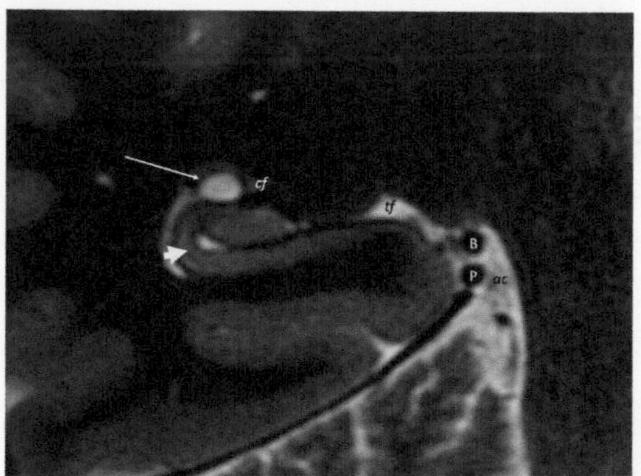

Fig. 14. Coronal T2W-FSE MR image at 3T demonstrates a small choroidal fissure cyst (*long, thin arrow*) and a smaller sulcal remnant cyst in the vestigial hippocampal sulcus (*short, wide arrow*). The fissures surrounding the hippocampus are delineated, including the ambient cistern (*ac*), transverse fissure (*tf*), and choroidal fissure (*cf*). The hippocampal fissure is largely obliterated. The basal vein of Rosenthal (B) and posterior cerebral artery (P) are also labeled.

Incomplete hippocampal inversion and hippocampal malrotation

Incomplete hippocampal inversion refers to abnormal hippocampal morphology resulting from a relative lack of hippocampal infolding during normal fetal development. This condition has also been termed hippocampal malrotation or hippocampal morphologic malformation, including the more commonly used term, globular hippocampus.[24,25] Although this entity has been reported in patients with epilepsy[25] and those with congenital malformations[26] with varying frequencies, it also occurs in up to 19% of nonepileptic patients,[27] suggesting that hippocampal malrotation is a common morphologic variation, and not clearly a causative lesion in patients with temporal lobe epilepsy.[28,29]

When detected, left-sided incomplete hippocampal inversion is more common than bilateral, and isolated right-sided hippocampal malrotation is rare.[27] It is assessed in the coronal plane at the level of the red nucleus and hippocampal body, classically demonstrating a round or pyramidal hippocampal shape, a deep collateral sulcus with increased vertical orientation, and a lateralized, somewhat prominent temporal horn. Hippocampal signal intensity is normal (Fig. 15). This entity is a lesser form along the spectrum of a vertical hippocampus (a more complete and severe form of hippocampal malrotation), which occurs in developmental malformations such as holoprosencephaly.

Clinical Relevance

Temporal lobe epilepsy and hippocampal sclerosis

Hippocampal sclerosis is characterized by segmental pyramidal cell loss and gliosis and is the most common histopathologic abnormality found in adults with drug-resistant temporal lobe

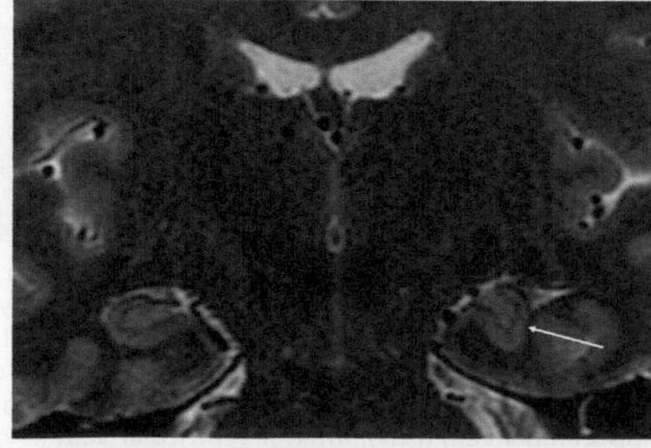

Fig. 15. Coronal T2W-FSE MR image at 3T through the hippocampal body demonstrates incomplete left hippocampal inversion (*arrow*).

epilepsy.[30] Classic imaging features on MR include noticeable hippocampal atrophy and increased signal intensity on T2-weighted images, particularly involving the hilus (DG and CA4). Another key imaging feature is altered architecture, specifically the loss of internal digitations anteriorly, and blurring of the gray-white matter junction, such that the SRLM is less conspicuous. Secondary signs with less specificity are ipsilateral mammillary body and forniceal column volume loss, ipsilateral temporal horn dilation, and choroidal fissure widening. Hippocampal volumetry is an adjunct to visual inspection, and the degree of hippocampal subfield neuronal loss has been shown to correlate with degree of atrophy.[30] Three main patterns of subfield neuronal loss and gliosis are described by the International League Against Epilepsy, including type 1 (affecting CA1, CA4, and DG regions), type 2 (CA1-predominant), and type 3 (CA4-predominant).[30] An important adjunct to MR imaging findings is hypometabolism on interictal PET, which characteristically extends to involve the temporal pole (Fig. 16).

Alzheimer disease

AD is a common progressive, ultimately fatal, neurodegenerative disorder and the most common cause of dementia. Histopathologically, there is extracellular β-amyloid plaques and neurofibrillary tangles with progressive neuron and synapse loss. Imaging has shown MTL volume loss with disproportionate atrophy in the CA1 region, subiculum, and entorhinal cortex compared with normal controls (Fig. 17), although these findings lack specificity and can be challenging to distinguish from senescent volume loss or atrophy associated with other neurodegenerative disorders (e.g., PART or hippocampal sclerosis of aging).[14,31–33] One qualitative imaging assessment is the MTL atrophy score,[34] whereas a more recently described qualitative assessment is the entorhinal cortical atrophy score.[35] Reduced clarity of the SRLM is another imaging feature described in those with amnestic AD.[31,32] A significant challenge in the strict use of volumetry is the wide distribution of volume among healthy populations, and it is important to judge if the hippocampal volume loss is reflective of global volume loss or specific to the hippocampus. In addition, there are hippocampal sparing forms of AD.[36]

Image Segmentation Software

Image segmentation software has become increasingly useful for quantification in neuroimaging. Hippocampal subfield segmentation software, such as FreeSurfer and Automatic Segmentation of Hippocampal Subfields, is currently more research oriented, whereas several other automated segmentation software packages are Food and Drug Administration approved for clinical use, including IcoMetrix and NeuroQuant. These latter packages provide fully automated volumes of numerous brain structures, including cerebral white and gray matter, hippocampus, amygdala, and basal ganglia nuclei, which is clinically relevant, as volumetric changes have been implicated in neurodegenerative diseases, such as AD, and can be helpful in discriminating volume loss in mesial temporal sclerosis.

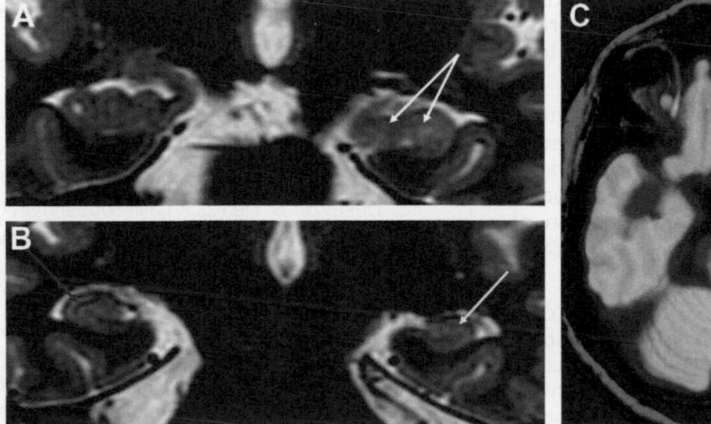

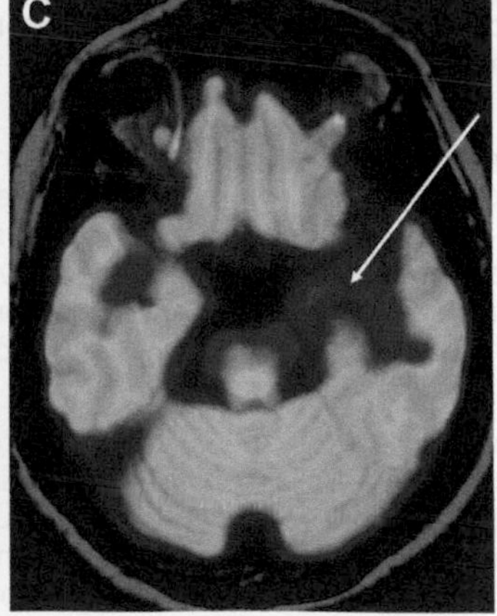

Fig. 16. Coronal T2W-FSE MR images at 3T through the hippocampal head (*A*) and body (*B*) demonstrate ILAE-type 1 hippocampal sclerosis. There is loss of internal digitations with increased T2 signal and blurring of internal architecture in the left hippocampal head (*white arrows* in (*A*). There is also atrophy of the left hippocampal body with reduced clarity of the SRLM (*yellow arrow* in (*B*), compared with a normal SRLM on the right (*red arrow*). Fused axial FDG-PET/MR image (*C*) demonstrates markedly decreased interictal metabolic activity in the left medial temporal lobe.

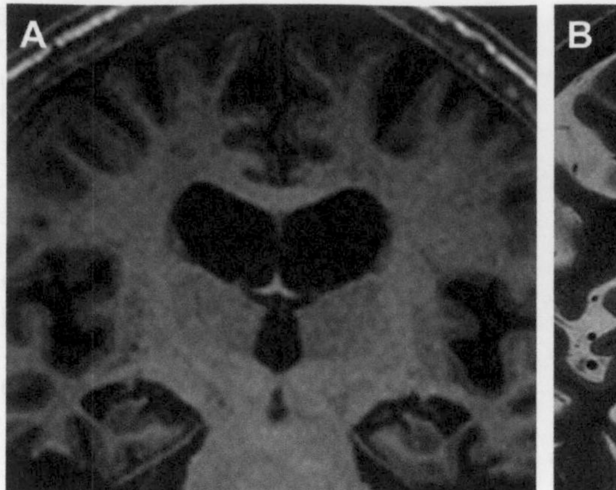

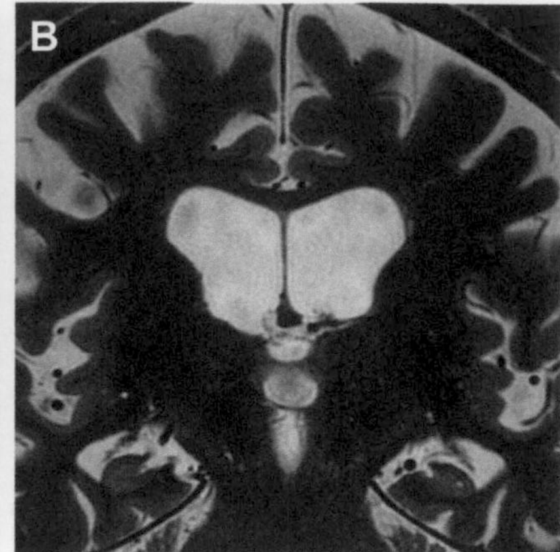

Fig. 17. Coronal (*A*) T1- and (*B*) T2-weighted MR images through the hippocampal body at 3T in a patient with early onset Alzheimer disease, showing global and hippocampal volume loss.

SUMMARY

The anatomic relationships of the MTL are fascinating and complex, including structural and functional anatomy of the hippocampal formation, the parahippocampal region, and the amygdaloid complex. As neuroimaging techniques continue to improve, an understanding of hippocampal subfield anatomy is requisite, as these structures will be more clearly visualized, with clinical relevance given their unique contributions to cognition and sensitivities to pathology.

CLINICS CARE POINTS

- Important anatomic landmarks for evaluating the MTL include the hippocampal head/body/tail boundaries, the collateral sulcus, limen insulae, uncal apex (gyrus intralimbicus), and SRLM.
- Hippocampal malrotation refers to abnormal hippocampal morphology, characterized by a round or pyramidal hippocampal shape, a deep collateral sulcus with increased vertical orientation, and a lateralized position of a nondilated temporal horn. Hippocampal signal intensity is normal.
- Hippocampal sclerosis is characterized by neuronal cell loss and gliosis, with specific types described by the International League Against Epilepsy based on CA field involvement. MR imaging depicts hippocampal volume loss, increased signal on T2-weighted images, loss of internal digitations, blurring of the gray-white matter, ipsilateral mammillary body and forniceal column volume loss, ipsilateral temporal horn dilation, and choroidal fissure widening.
- AD demonstrates disproportionate atrophy in the CA1 region, subiculum, and entorhinal cortex as well as reduced clarity of the SRLM, although it can be challenging to distinguish these changes from overall brain volume loss and senescent changes.

DISCLOSURE

There are no relevant disclosures.

REFERENCES

1. Andersen P. The hippocampus book. New York: Oxford University Press; 2007.
2. Insausti R, Amaral DG. Hippocampal formation. In: The human nervous system. Elsevier; 2012. p. 896–942. https://doi.org/10.1016/B978-0-12-374236-0.10024-0.
3. Lewis F. The significance of the term hippocampus. J Comp Neurol 1923;35:213–30.
4. Lorente de Nó R. Studies on the structure of the cerebral cortex. II. continuation of the study of the ammonic system. J Psychol Neurol 1934;46:113–77.
5. Dekeyzer S, De Kock I, Nikoubashman O, et al. Unforgettable" – a pictorial essay on anatomy and pathology of the hippocampus. Insights Imaging 2017; 8(2):199–212.
6. Kier EL, Kim JH, Fulbright RK, et al. Embryology of the human fetal hippocampus: mr imaging, anatomy, and histology. AJNR Am J Neuroradiol 1997;18:525–32.
7. Duvernoy HM. The human hippocampus: functional anatomy, vascularization and serial sections with MRI. Springer Berlin Heidelberg; 2005. https://doi.org/10.1007/b138576.
8. Zeineh MM, Palomero-Gallagher N, Axer M, et al. Direct visualization and mapping of the spatial course of fiber tracts at microscopic resolution in

the human hippocampus. Cereb Cortex. Published online February 13, 2016:bhw010. doi:10.1093/cercor/bhw010

9. Fatterpekar GM, Naidich TP, Delman BN, et al. Cytoarchitecture of the human cerebral cortex: MR microscopy of excised specimens at 9.4 tesla. AJNR Am J Neuroradiol 2002;23:1313–21.
10. Dickson DW, Ruan D, Crystal H, et al. Hippocampal degeneration differentiates diffuse Lewy body disease (DLBD) from Alzheimer's disease. Neurology 1991;41(9):1402.
11. Amunts K, Kedo O, Kindler M, et al. Cytoarchitectonic mapping of the human amygdala, hippocampal region and entorhinal cortex: intersubject variability and probability maps. Anat Embryol (Berl) 2005;210(5):343–52.
12. Thomas BP, Welch EB, Niederhauser BD, et al. High-resolution 7T MRI of the human hippocampus in vivo. J Magn Reson Imaging 2008;28(5):1266–72.
13. Coras R, Milesi G, Zucca I, et al. 7T MRI features in control human hippocampus and hippocampal sclerosis: an ex vivo study with histologic correlations. Epilepsia 2014;55(12):2003–16.
14. Mueller SG, Stables L, Du AT, et al. Measurement of hippocampal subfields and age-related changes with high resolution MRI at 4T. Neurobiol Aging 2007;28(5):719–26.
15. Insausti R, Córcoles-Parada M, Ubero MM, et al. Cytoarchitectonic areas of the gyrus ambiens in the human brain. Front Neuroanat 2019;13:21.
16. Naidich TP, Castillo M, Cha S, et al. Surface anatomy of the cerebrum. In: Imaging of the brain. Saunders; 2012. p. 127–53.
17. Ding SL. Comparative anatomy of the prosubiculum, subiculum, presubiculum, postsubiculum, and parasubiculum in human, monkey, and rodent: comparative neuroanatomy of the subicular cortices. J Comp Neurol 2013;521(18):4145–62.
18. Bienkowski MS, Sepehrband F, Kurniawan ND, et al. Homologous laminar organization of the mouse and human subiculum. Sci Rep 2021;11(1):3729.
19. Insausti R, Juottonen K, Soininen H, et al. MR Volumetric analysis of the human entorhinal, perirhinal, and temporopolar cortices. AJNR Am J Neuroradiol 1998;19:659–71.
20. Braak H, Braak E. Neuropathological stageing of Alzheimer-related changes. Acta Neuropathol 1991;82(4):239–59.
21. Pereira PMG, Insausti R, Artacho-Perula E, et al. MR Volumetric analysis of the piriform cortex and cortical amygdala in drug-refractory temporal lobe epilepsy. AJNR Am J Neuroradiol 2005;26:319–32.
22. Yilmazer-Hanke DM. Amygdala. In: The human nervous system. Elsevier; 2012. p. 759–834. https://doi.org/10.1016/B978-0-12-374236-0.10022-7.
23. Frankó E, Insausti AM, Artacho-Pérula E, et al. Identification of the human medial temporal lobe regions on magnetic resonance images: human medial temporal lobe landmarks. Hum Brain Mapp 2014;35(1):248–56.
24. Barsi P, Kenez J, Solymosi D, et al. Hippocampal malrotation with normal corpus callosum: a new entity? Neuroradiology 2000;42:339–45.
25. Bernasconi N, Kinay D, Anderman F, et al. Analysis of shape and positioning of the hippocampal formation: an MRI study in patients with partial epilepsy and healthy controls. Brain 2005;128:2442–52.
26. Sato N, Hatakeyama S, Shimizu N, et al. MR evaluation of the hippocampus in patients with congenital malformations of the brain. AJNR Am J Neuroradiol 2001;22:387–93.
27. Bajic D, Wang C, Kumlien E, et al. Incomplete inversion of the hippocampus—a common developmental anomaly. Eur Radiol 2008;18(1):138–42.
28. Bajic D, Kumlien E, Mattsson P, et al. Incomplete hippocampal inversion—is there a relation to epilepsy? Eur Radiol 2009;19(10):2544–50.
29. Tsai MH, Vaughan DN, Perchyonok Y, et al. Hippocampal malrotation is an anatomic variant and has no clinical significance in MRI-negative temporal lobe epilepsy. Epilepsia 2016;57(10):1719–28.
30. Blümcke I, Thom M, Aronica E, et al. International consensus classification of hippocampal sclerosis in temporal lobe epilepsy: a task force report from the ILAE commission on diagnostic methods. Epilepsia 2013;54(7):1315–29.
31. Firbank MJ, Blamire AM, Teodorczuk A, et al. High resolution imaging of the medial temporal lobe in alzheimer's disease and dementia with lewy bodies. J Alzheimers Dis 2010;21(4):1129–40.
32. Su L, Hayes L, Soteriades S, et al. Hippocampal stratum radiatum, lacunosum, and moleculare sparing in mild cognitive impairment. In: Hornberger M, editor. J Alzheimers Dis 2017;61(1):415–24.
33. Yushkevich PA, Pluta JB, Wang H, et al. Automated volumetry and regional thickness analysis of hippocampal subfields and medial temporal cortical structures in mild cognitive impairment: Automatic Morphometry of MTL Subfields in MCI. Hum Brain Mapp 2015;36(1):258–87.
34. Scheltens P, Leys D, Barkhof F, et al. Atrophy of medial temporal lobes on MRI in "probable" Alzheimer's disease and normal ageing: diagnostic value and neuropsychological correlates. J Neurol Neurosurg Psychiatry 1992;55(10):967–72.
35. Enkirch SJ, Traschütz A, Müller A, et al. The ERICA score: an MR imaging–based visual scoring system for the assessment of entorhinal cortex atrophy in alzheimer disease. Radiology 2018;288(1):226–333.
36. Whitwell JL, Dickson DW, Murray ME, et al. Neuroimaging correlates of pathologically defined subtypes of Alzheimer's disease: a case-control study. Lancet Neurol 2012;11(10):868–77.

Brain Functional Imaging Anatomy

Behroze Adi Vachha, MD, PhD[a,b,*], Erik H. Middlebrooks, MD[c,d]

KEYWORDS

• Functional imaging • fMRI • Functional anatomy • Diffusion tractography • Dual stream model

KEY POINTS

- The primary sensorimotor cortex and corticospinal tracts are critical motor and sensory areas, which generally show limited plasticity.
- The dual stream model of language is the most widely accepted model of language function, subserved by a dorsal phonologic stream and ventral semantic stream.
- The traditional Broca area has been proved to relate to prearticulatory planning rather than the "speech production" center, and damage to this cortical area does not typically result in long-term speech disorders.
- Retinotopic mapping with fMRI can be used to assess and predict visual field deficits.

INTRODUCTION

Neuroimaging techniques, such as functional MR imaging (fMRI) and diffusion tractography, have played a vital role in the modern conception of brain function. At the same time, the clinical use of these tools requires an in-depth knowledge of brain functional anatomy. In this review, the anatomy of the most commonly assessed brain functions in clinical neuroradiology, including motor, language, and vision, is discussed. The anatomy and function of the primary and secondary sensorimotor areas are discussed with clinical case examples. Next, the dual stream of language processing is reviewed, as well as its implications in clinical medicine and surgical planning. Last, the authors discuss the striate and extrastriate visual cortex and review the dual stream model of visual processing.

SENSORIMOTOR CORTICES

The sensorimotor strip follows a medial-posterior-superior to lateral-anterior-inferior course from the apex to the Sylvian fissure.[1] The primary motor cortex and the somatosensory cortex are contained within the precentral and postcentral gyri, respectively, separated by the central sulcus.[2–4] At the apex of the central sulcus, the precentral and postcentral gyri fuse to form the paracentral lobule.[1,3] Inferiorly the precentral and postcentral gyri fuse to form the U-shaped subcentral gyrus, which appears as a distinct anatomic structure enclosing the Sylvian end of the central sulcus.[5]

Several anatomic landmarks and signs have been described as being variably useful in identifying the precentral gyrus, postcentral gyrus, and central sulcus in normal brains. These landmarks are described in greater detail in the article detailing

Funding Information: NIH/NCI Cancer Center Support (Grant P30 CA008748, PI: Thompson).

[a] Department of Radiology, Neuroradiology Section, Memorial Sloan Kettering Cancer Center, 1275 York Avenue, New York, NY 10065, USA; [b] Brain Tumor Center, Memorial Sloan Kettering Cancer Center, 1275 York Avenue, New York, NY 10065, USA; [c] Department of Radiology, Mayo Clinic, 4500 San Pablo Road, Jacksonville, FL 32224, USA; [d] Department of Neurosurgery, Mayo Clinic, 4500 San Pablo Road, Jacksonville, FL 32224, USA

* Corresponding author. Department of Radiology, Neuroradiology Section, Memorial Sloan Kettering Cancer Center, 1275 York Avenue, New York, NY 10065.

E-mail address: vachhab@mskcc.org

Neuroimag Clin N Am 32 (2022) 491–505
https://doi.org/10.1016/j.nic.2022.04.001
1052-5149/22/

the anatomy of the cerebral cortex, lobes, and the cerebellum. For example, Kido and colleagues[6] demonstrated that the junction between the superior frontal sulcus and precentral sulcus marks the anterior border of the precentral gyrus, also known as the "inverted T sign." Another typical landmark of the precentral gyrus is the region responsible for hand motor function seen as a "reverse omega"-shaped or epsilon-shaped structure known as the "motor hand knob" on axial imaging and depicted as a hook in the sagittal plane.[4,7,8] The postcentral gyrus follows the contour of the precentral gyrus with a similar omega-shaped structure in the postcentral gyrus containing the somatosensory functions for the hand area. However, the radiologist can differentiate these 2 gyri by remembering that the precentral gyrus is thicker than the postcentral gyrus in anteroposterior dimension.[1,3,4]

Primary Motor Cortex

Anatomy: The primary motor cortex (PMC) corresponds to Brodmann area 4 (BA 4) and is designated as M1. It is important for the radiologist to note that the PMC does not encompass the entire thickness of the precentral gyrus but rather occupies the posterior margin of the precentral gyrus, anterior bank of the central sulcus, and anterior part of the paracentral lobule.[2,9,10] This fact is reflected in fMRI, as is illustrated in **Fig. 1**A that demonstrates hand motor activation along the posteriormost aspect of the hand motor knob of the precentral gyrus.

Connections and functions: Axonal fibers from the pyramidal cells in the PMC descend through the pyramidal tract to synapse on neurons in the spinal cord (corticospinal tract; **Fig. 2**) and brainstem (corticobulbar tract; see **Fig. 2**). The PMC initiates voluntary movements of the trunk, as well as the upper and lower extremities through the corticospinal tract, which also receives fibers from the premotor, supplementary, and somatosensory cortices.[2,9] Most fibers cross to the contralateral side at the pyramidal decussation descending within the lateral corticospinal tract to synapse directly or indirectly on lower motor neurons in the spinal cord supplying distal muscles.[11,12] Nondecussating fibers continue on the same side within the spinal cord as the anterior corticospinal tract innervating the proximal muscles, as well as the trunk.[12] Fibers of the corticobulbar tract arise mainly from the lateral aspect of the PMC and descend similarly to the corticospinal tract, but exit to synapse with neurons within the brainstem motor cranial nerve nuclei (except to the facial nucleus of the lower face) and are involved in the movement of the face, head, and neck.[11,12]

Somatotopic organization: Several studies have demonstrated a somatotopic organization to the PMC representation of movement, such that each part of the body is reliably mapped to a specific region of the PMC with a progression through foot, legs, trunk, arm, hands, face, and tongue from superomedial to inferolateral portions of the frontal lobe.[13,14] In addition, the area of PMC representing a part of the body is not proportional to the size of the part, but rather to the intricacy of movements in the region resulting in a distorted homunculus in which the face, lips, fingers, and hands have greater representation than the remaining parts of the body.[9,15,16]

Eloquent Motor Regions in Presurgical Mapping

Motor fMRI paradigms for presurgical mapping are selected based on the individual patient's clinical presentation and the proximity of the lesion to eloquent motor regions, such as the hand motor area, foot motor area, and the tongue and lips. These 3 areas are discussed in more detail in the following subsections. **Fig. 1** illustrates the normal fMRI activation of these regions, whereas **Fig. 3** demonstrates example fMRI clinical cases affecting the motor network.

Hand motor area

Traditionally, the part of the brain that controls hand motor function is believed to reside in the "hand knob" or reverse omega shape in the precentral gyrus on axial images (see **Figs.** 1A and 3).[7,17,18] However, several studies indicate that the structural "hot spot" corresponding to functional hand motor activation region is located adjacent to but not within the hand knob of the precentral gyrus for all patients.[19–21] For example, studies using fMRI and electrocorticography demonstrated a topographic layout for the little finger to the thumb proceeding from medial to lateral, suggesting that specific finger-oriented activation is not controlled by the hand knob.[20–22] Hamidian and colleagues[23] showed that the maximum bilateral functional and structural connectivity was achieved when a region of interest (ROI) was placed near the thumb representation in the precentral gyrus lateral to the hand motor knob compared with an ROI in the traditional hand knob region.

Foot motor area

The foot motor area is represented within the most medial aspect of the precentral gyrus adjacent to the interhemispheric fissure at the high frontal convexity (see **Figs.** 1B and 3). Although the medial termination of the central sulcus in

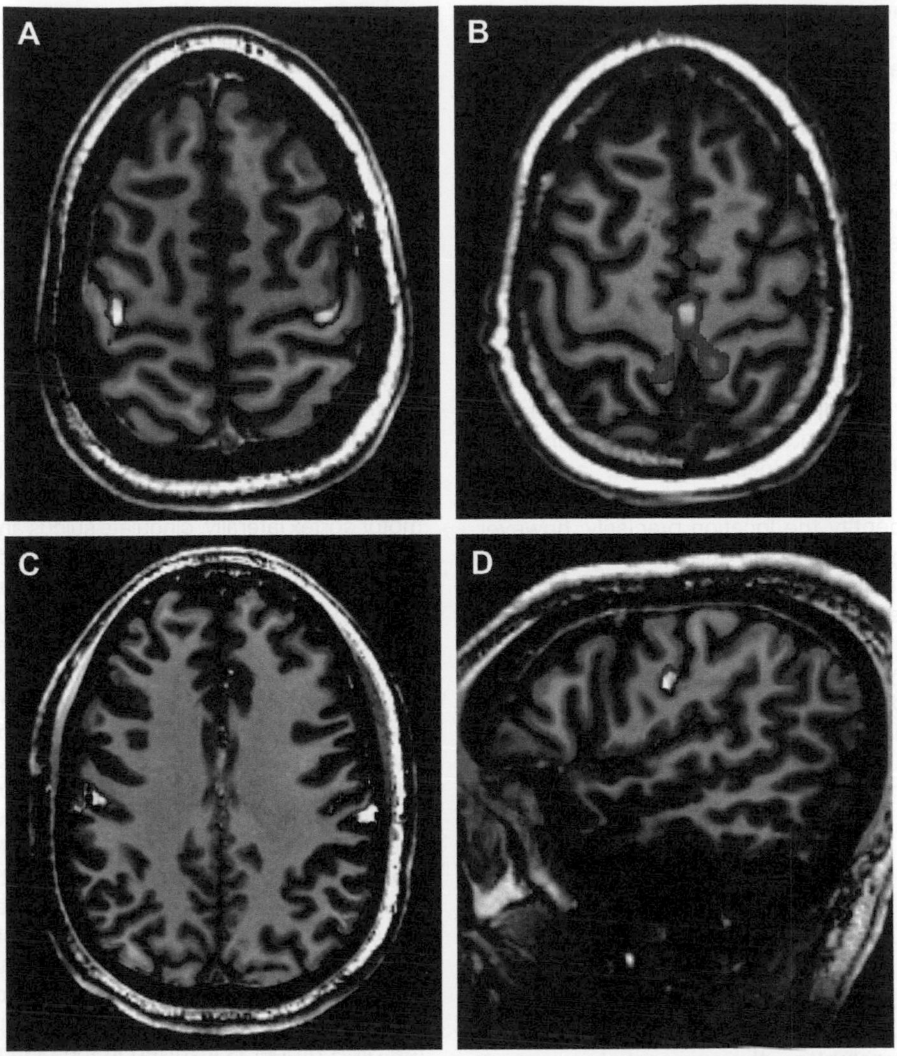

Fig. 1. Functional brain MR images showing the normal activation patterns for (*A*) motor hand, (*B*) motor foot, and (*C,D*) motor tongue.

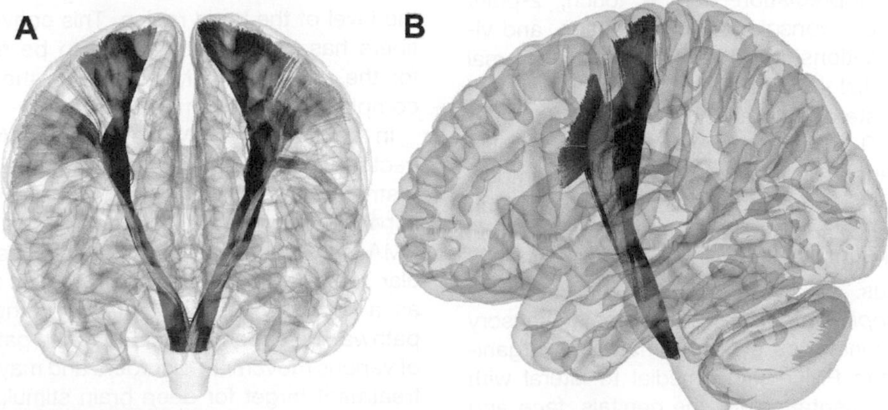

Fig. 2. (*A*) Coronal and (*B*) sagittal diffusion tractography images highlighting the course of the corticospinal (*blue*) and corticobulbar (*orange*) tracts.

normal hemispheres is used as a guide to localize the foot motor region, precise location of the foot motor area is limited owing to lack of definite anatomic landmarks on structural MR imaging.[24] In addition, the border between the more caudally placed primary foot motor area and the more rostrally placed supplementary area is not clearly defined by a sulcus making the distinction between these 2 regions difficult on routine MR imaging.

Facial motor area

The PMC of lip representation and tongue movements is located at the lateral aspect of the precentral gyrus adjacent to the Sylvian fissure (see **Fig. 1**C,D).[1] In axial sections, this portion of the precentral gyrus does not have a specific anatomic feature to serve as an anatomic landmark to identify the location precisely; however, in the sagittal plane, lip and tongue movements result in functional activation in the region formed by the fusion of the precentral and postcentral gyri at the base of the sensorimotor cortex bound dorsally by the posterior subcentral sulcus.[1] Specifically, during task-based fMRI, tongue movements will result in activation about the lateral aspect of the precentral gyrus lower than and overlapping with that produced by lip puckering.[25]

Somatosensory Areas

Anatomy: The primary somatosensory cortex (S1) corresponds to BA 3a, 3b, 1, and 2.[10,26] The primary somatosensory cortex is located behind the central sulcus in the postcentral gyrus, which closely resembles the precentral gyrus in configuration.[1]

Connections and function: The primary somatosensory area receives sensory input regarding conscious appreciation of fine touch, 2-point discrimination, conscious proprioception, and vibration sensations from the body, from the dorsal column medial lemniscus pathway mainly via the ventral posterorolateral nucleus of the thalamus.[10,16] The primary somatosensory area also receives sensory input regarding pain and temperature (lateral spinothalamic tract), as well as crude touch (anterior spinothalamic tract) via projection fibers from the ventral posterorolateral nucleus of the thalamus.[10,16]

Somatotopic organization: The somatosensory cortex demonstrates similar somatotopic organization as the PMC going medial to lateral with greater representation for the genitals, face and lips, as well as fingers and hands than the remaining parts of the body.[13,27]

SUPPLEMENTARY MOTOR AREA

Traditionally, the supplementary motor area (SMA) is divided into the posterior or caudal SMA proper (referred to as SMA in this article) and the more anterior or rostral pre-SMA. Both areas are separated by indistinct borders and have overlapping functions suggesting they probably represent a continuum rather than discrete anatomic regions.[2,28] However, they are discussed separately with the SMA discussed in this section and the pre-SMA discussed in the secondary language areas section.

Anatomy: The SMA proper is located in the dorsomedial superior frontal gyrus anterior to the foot motor representation of the PMC and corresponds to medial BA 6 or area 6aα of Vogt.[3,29] The SMA is bounded by the interhemispheric falx medially, premotor cortex laterally, cingulate sulcus and gyri inferiorly, foot motor area posteriorly, and pre-SMA anteriorly.[2,3] The precentral sulcus separates the lateral posterior border of the SMA from the leg area of the PMC; however, the border between the medial posterior SMA and the foot motor area is not distinct.[24,30] Anteriorly, the anatomic border line between the SMA proper and the pre-SMA is accepted as a vertical imaginary line traversing the anterior commissure and perpendicular to a line joining the anterior and posterior commissures.[30,31]

Connections and function: The SMA is an eloquent region with connections to the motor, premotor, and cingulate cortex, as well as with the superior parietal lobule, insula, basal ganglia, thalamus, cerebellum, and contralateral SMA.[2,30] The SMA proper sends fibers to join the corticospinal tract[32,33]; through this corticospinal projection, the SMA proper is involved in the planning, initiation, and execution of movements.[34] Additionally Vergani and colleagues[34] demonstrated the presence of short U-fibers directly connecting the SMA with the PMC with convergence of fibers at the level of the hand region. This convergence of fibers has been hypothesized to be responsible for the role of the SMA proper in the control of complex hand movements.[34,35]

In addition, the SMA and pre-SMA are connected to the caudate and putamen via the frontostriatal tract, which functions in different aspects of motor and speech control.[29,34,36] The SMA is also connected to the thalamus, in particular the ventralis oralis nucleus, and may serve as a relay from pallidothalamic pathways. This pathway has been implicated in the pathogenesis of various movement disorders and may serve as a treatment target for deep brain stimulation, such as dystonic tremor[37] and tremor related to multiple sclerosis.[38] Recent studies also demonstrated

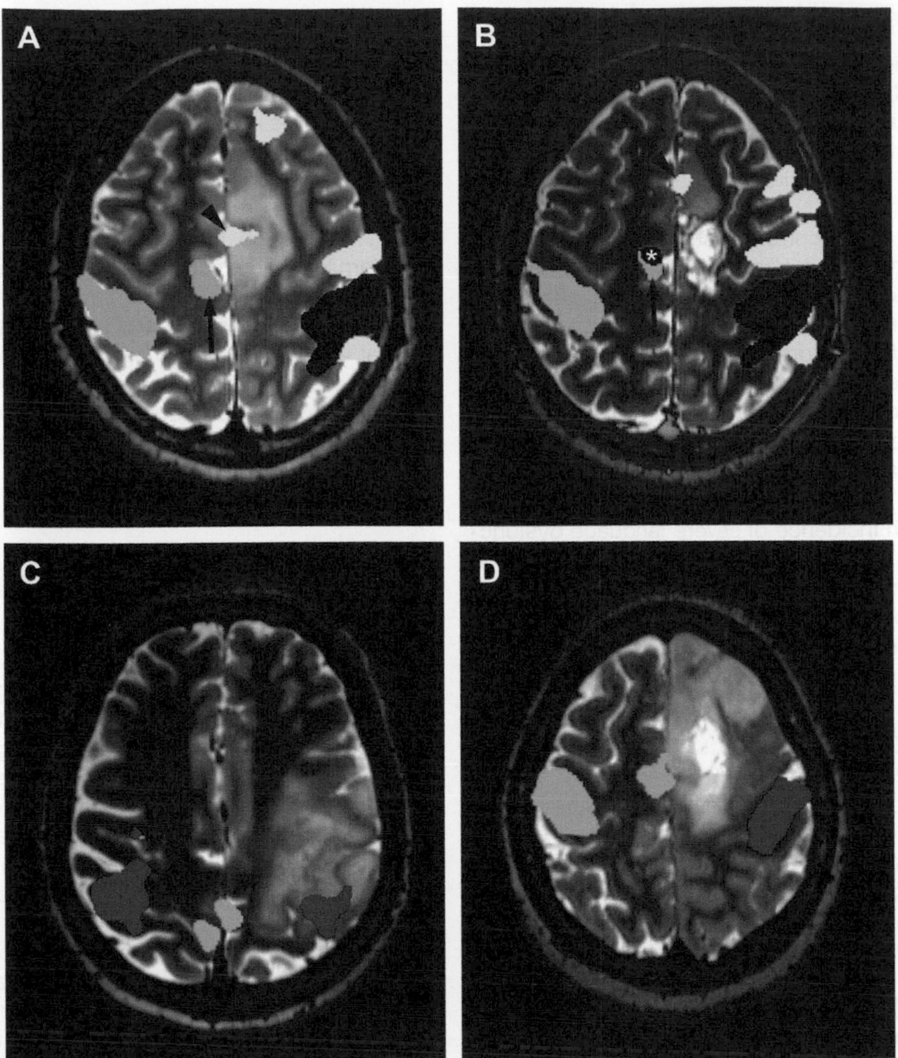

Fig. 3. Examples of fMRI clinical cases affecting the motor network. (*A*) Patient 1 has a left frontal glioma. Right hand motor task (*blue*) shows normal activation in primary motor hand cortex, but no supplementary motor area (SMA) activation with right hand motor movement. There is normal activation from left hand motor movement (*green*), in the right hemisphere primary motor cortex, and in the supplementary motor area (SMA; *arrow*). Sentence completion language task (*yellow*) shows left hemisphere language dominance with activation in the left pre-SMA (*arrowhead*) adjacent to the left frontal glioma. (*B*) Postoperatively, the patient had a transient SMA syndrome. Repeat fMRI shows right hand SMA now in the left SMA (*blue*; *asterisk*), colocalized with the left hand SMA (*green*). This case highlights neurovascular uncoupling on the preoperative fMRI leading to a false-negative of left hemisphere SMA function, which underwent reorganization postoperatively. There is also reorganization of the pre-SMA more anteriorly (*arrow*). (*C*) Patient 2 has a left frontoparietal glioma with preserved motor hand (*red*) and foot (*green*) function in the area of tumor infiltration. (*D*) Patient 3 has a left frontal glioma with no SMA activation with right hand motor task (*red*) and normal left hand motor function (*green*). Patient also had a postoperative SMA syndrome suggesting neurovascular uncoupling and false-negative fMRI.

that the SMA is connected with the pars opercularis of the inferior frontal gyrus through the frontal aslant tract[35] and is thought to facilitate speech initiation owing to this connection. Last, the SMA is connected with the precuneus and anterior cingulate cortex through the most medial portion of the superior longitudinal fasciculus (SLF I) and may function in initiation of motor activity and higher-order control of body-centered action.[29]

Somatotopic organization: The SMA demonstrates a crude somatotopic map of the body with the head, trunk, upper extremity, and lower extremity represented anteroposteriorly within the SMA.[3,39,40]

SPEECH AND LANGUAGE AREAS

The traditional "localizationist" models of language pioneered by Paul Broca and Carl Wernicke were revolutionary concepts in understanding brain functional anatomy. However, decades of subsequent research have entirely dispelled this simplistic model, and the "connectomic" model is widely accepted as the current best model of human language. This "dual stream" model highlights that speech and language are complex functions spread across wide areas of the brain, but generally subserved by a dorsal "phonologic" stream and a ventral "semantic" stream.[41] No discrete areas of language comprehension and language production exist, as posited in the early theories of language. Although language function is widespread, it seems that these regions can largely be divided into those with a high incidence of severe language dysfunction when damaged versus less critical areas that may be more easily compensated for by other network pathways. This section primarily focuses on those regions thought to be most critical for language mapping and preservation.

Traditional Speech Areas

Frontal speech areas (Broca area)

The inferior frontal gyrus lies between the inferior frontal sulcus dorsally and the anterior part of the lateral fissure ventrally and is divided into 3 parts, which from anterior to posterior are the pars orbitalis, pars triangularis, and pars opercularis.[1,4,42] The anterior ramus of the lateral fissure separates the pars orbitalis from the pars triangularis, whereas the ascending ramus separates the pars triangularis from the pars opercularis (Fig. 4).[4,43] Although there is disagreement on the anatomic definition,[44] Broca area (BA 44 and 45) is most commonly considered as the pars opercularis and pars triangularis (Fig. 5).[45] Nevertheless, this lack of precision in anatomic definitions highlights the need for more precise terminology in place of older eponyms.[44]

The classical model of language suggests that Broca area in the left hemisphere is involved in speech production and language processing, whereas Broca area homolog in the nondominant right hemisphere has been implicated in linguistic prosody.[45,46] However, the traditional theory has been largely disproven and shows that the pars opercularis is more involved in prearticulatory planning and lexical retrieval, with onset of activation preceding the onset of speech motor function.[47] The pars opercularis can be considered as a gateway to releasing phonetic codes to the ventral premotor cortex (vPMC) before the initiation of speech.

Temporal Language Areas (Wernicke Area)

The anatomic definition of the traditional Wernicke area is even less clear,[44] but often considered as BA 22 and lies in the posterior portion of the superior temporal gyrus in the dominant hemisphere (see Fig. 4).[3] Historically, this area is considered to be involved in language comprehension; however, this notion has also been disproven with modern language research. After initial phonologic perception through the middle superior temporal gyrus and superior temporal sulcus (audio) or the visual word form area (vWFA) (written), the phonemes are retrieved through the posterior superior temporal gyrus.[48] Damage to this area can result in impaired word retrieval or phonemic paraphasias that may be interpreted as anomia in awake mapping.[49]

DUAL STREAM MODEL OF LANGUAGE FUNCTION

First proposed by Hickok and Poeppel,[41] the dual stream neurocognitive model of language function suggests that distinct neuroanatomical networks subserve lexical-semantic processing (ventral stream) and motor-phonological processing (dorsal stream) of speech and language. The investigators proposed that the dorsal stream is left lateralized, whereas the ventral stream is bilaterally organized with some differences between the hemispheres.[41]

The ventral stream involves a ventrolateral pathway along the extreme capsule that involves the middle and inferior temporal gyri and the ventrolateral prefrontal cortex.[50] The major white matter tracts of the ventral stream include: (1) the inferior fronto-occipital fasciculus (IFOF), which extends from the middle occipital gyrus, inferior occipital gyrus, and precuneus to the dorsolateral prefrontal cortex (BA 46), pars orbitalis (BA 47), and pars triangularis (BA 45); (2) inferior longitudinal fasciculus (ILF) extending from the dorsolateral occipital cortex to the temporal pole; and (3) uncinate fasciculus that consists of an anterolateral portion connecting the temporal polar region with the dorsolateral frontal lobe and the ventromedial region connecting the amygdala and parahippocampal gyrus with the medial orbitofrontal cortex, septal region, and nucleus accumbens.[51] Fig. 6A,B illustrate the white matter tracts of the ventral stream.

The dorsal stream of language originates within the superior temporal gyrus (STG) and superior temporal sulcus and projects dorsoposteriorly through the supramarginal gyrus to the inferior frontal gyrus and premotor cortex.[41,50,52] The

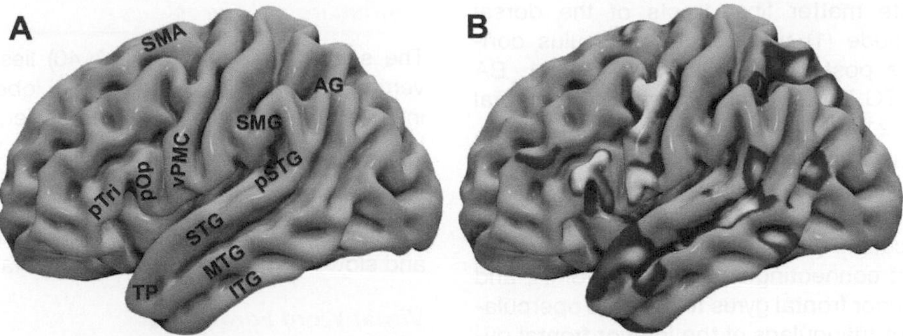

Fig. 4. (*A*) Surface and (*B*) fMRI anatomy of language function showing common areas of activation related to the ventral stream semantic processing in the angular gyrus (AG), middle (MTG) and inferior temporal gyrus (ITG), and temporal pole. Areas of the dorsal stream, including the posterior superior temporal gyrus (pSTG; classic Wernicke area), supramarginal gyrus (SMG), ventral premotor cortex (vPMC), pars opercularis (pOp; classic Broca area), pars triangularis (pTri), and supplemental motor area (SMA).

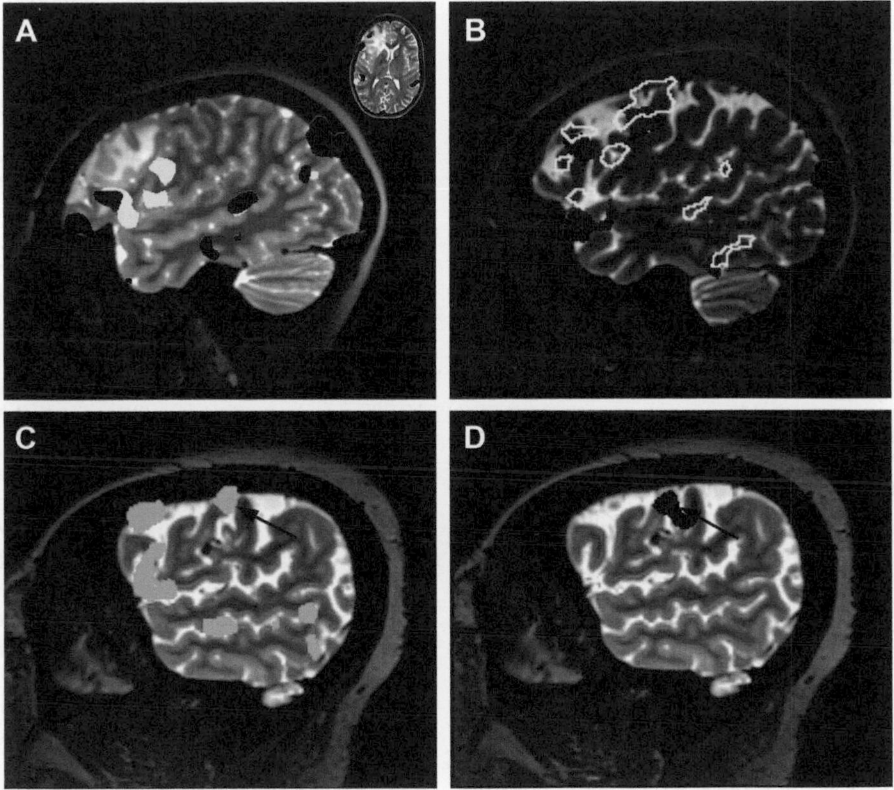

Fig. 5. Example clinical fMRI cases. (*A*) Patient 1 is a right-handed patient who had previous surgery in the right frontal lobe for low grade glioma and experienced an unexpected postoperative decline in language after surgery. Subsequent fMRI shows right hemisphere language dominance. The semantic decision task (*blue*) shows greater activation in areas of semantic processing, such as the angular gyrus, middle temporal gyrus, and pars orbitalis. The phonologic-heavy rhyming task (*yellow*) produces greater activation in areas of phonologic processing, such as the pars opercularis and ventral premotor cortex. (*B*) Patient 2 has a left temporal cavernous venous malformation. Phonologic task (*rhyming*; *yellow*) versus semantic decision (*blue*) language tasks again show difference in activation patterns between the 2 tasks. (*C*) Patient 3 has a left inferior frontal gyrus cavernous venous malformation. The language activation using a sentence completion task (*green*) reveals activation in the superior portion of the ventral premotor cortex (*arrow*) likely reflecting "mirror neuron" activation in the tongue premotor region that is shown in (*D*) with motor tongue task (*blue*).

major white matter fiber tracts of the dorsal stream include (1) the arcuate fasciculus connecting the posterior STG (BA 22, BA 41, BA 42), mid STG BA 22), and mid middle temporal gyrus (BA 21) to the pars opercularis (BA 44), pars triangularis (BA 45) in 40% of cases, and vPMC (BA 6)[51,53]; (2) the SLF part III, which connects the supramarginal gyrus (BA 40) to the pars opercularis (BA 44)[51,53]; and (3) the frontal aslant tract connecting the pre-SMA, SMA, and lateral superior frontal gyrus to the pars opercularis and pars triangularis of the inferior frontal gyrus.[54] **Fig. 6**C,D illustrate the white matter tracts of the dorsal stream.

SECONDARY LANGUAGE AREAS

Research continues to support a complex and nuanced interaction between cortical and subcortical regions of the brain that support the multiple facets of language. The subsequent subsections briefly discuss the anatomic localization and function of some of these "secondary" cortical language areas that are often activated in conjunction with the historically "primary" Broca and Wernicke language areas.

Pre-SMA: The pre-SMA is located in the dorsomedial superior frontal gyrus anterior to the SMA proper and corresponds to medial BA 6 or area 6aβ of Vogt (**Fig. 3**).[3,28,31,55] The pre-SMA is bounded by the interhemispheric falx medially, premotor cortex laterally, SMA proper posteriorly, and anterior cingulate motor area ventrally (inferiorly).[2,24,56]

The pre-SMA is heavily connected with the prefrontal cortex and caudate nucleus, whereas the SMA is more heavily connected with the motor cortex and putamen, suggesting functional differences between the SMA and pre-SMA with the SMA involved in motor control, whereas the pre-SMA involved in higher-order function in language production.[29]

Angular gyrus: The angular gyrus (BA 39) is a horseshoe-shaped gyrus in the inferior parietal lobule that surrounds the posterior termination of the superior temporal sulcus.[51,57] Although the exact function of the angular gyrus is not known, the extensive structural and functional connections with several brain regions[58] substantiate this region as a hub of several networks involved in complex language functions, including lexical-semantic processing and syllable discrimination and identification.[57] In addition, lesions affecting the left parietal lobe, specifically angular gyrus, result in the characteristic tetrad of finger agnosia, left-right disorientation, acalculia, and agraphia known as Gerstmann syndrome.[59]

Supramarginal Gyrus

The supramarginal gyrus (BA 40) lies along the ventrolateral aspect of the parietal lobe within the inferior parietal lobule. As stated earlier, this region is connected with the pars opercularis via the SLF III and plays a role in phonologic working memory.[53,60] Direct cortical stimulation of the supramarginal gyrus has resulted in slurring, stutters, and slowed speech, as well as anomia.[61,62]

Visual Word Form Area

The vWFA (BA 37) is localized to the ventral occipitotemporal cortex of the dominant hemisphere (**Fig. 7**).[63] There is structural and functional connectivity between the vWFA and the superior temporal, inferior parietal, and lateral prefrontal regions implicated in language-related functions. This region plays a role in decoding written forms of words with lesions in this region or resection resulting in pure alexia.[64]

Ventral Premotor Cortex

The vPMC lies posterior superior to the pars opercularis and at the foot of the precentral gyrus.[51] The inferior half of the vPMC region plays a role in phonologic processing and the bridge to motor representation of articulatory gestures (tongue, lip, and pharynx control). Direct cortical stimulation of the vPMC typically results in dysarthria/anarthria.[65] It is likely that many cases of speech arrest in awake mapping are attributable to the vPMC rather than the pars opercularis, and this area has been shown to have little plasticity. Owing to its role in phonologic processing, it is likely that more heavily phonologic tasks elicit greater activation of vPMC, even in the absence of overt speech. Overt speech tasks, however, may produce greater activation compared with silent language tasks.[66]

The more superior part of the vPMC region contains an execution-observation matching system known as the "mirror neuron" system,[67] so called because these neurons mirror the actions and behaviors of other neurons. The mirror neuron system is not fully understood in humans, but it has been shown that speech perception can produce activation in the vPMC, including overlap with the same region as speech motor, such as the tongue (see **Fig. 5**C,D).

VISUAL AREAS

Primary Visual Cortex

The primary visual cortex (V1), also known as the striate cortex (BA 17), is located in and around the calcarine fissure in the occipital lobe. V1

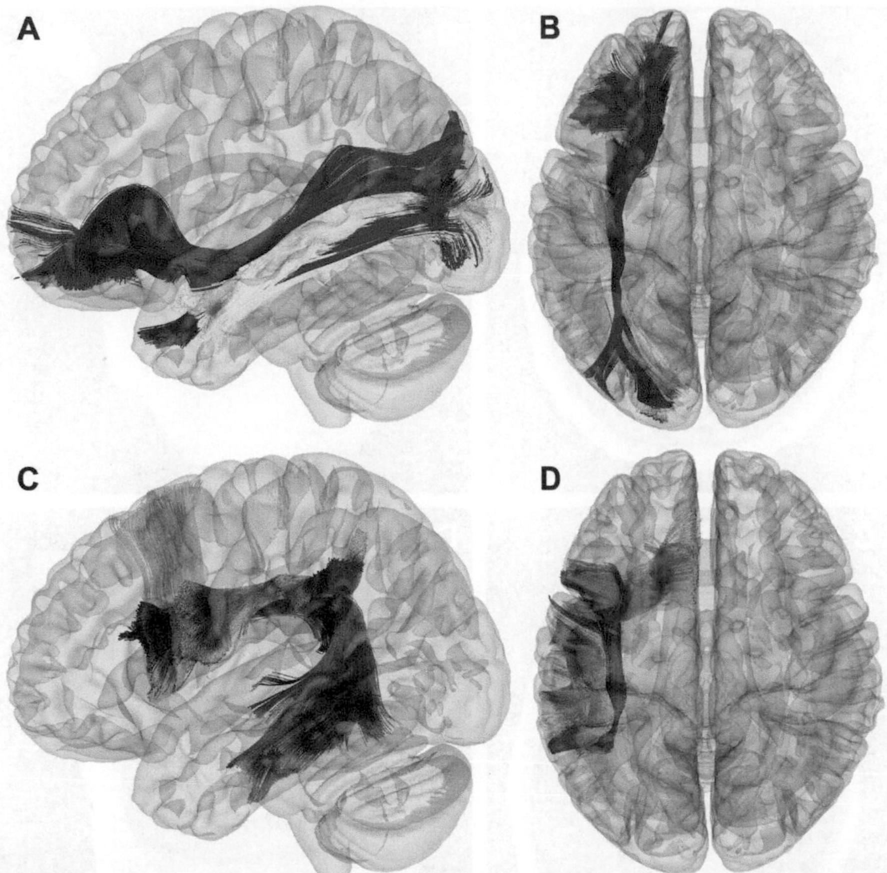

Fig. 6. (*A*) Sagittal and (*B*) axial images of the tracts of the ventral semantic stream including the inferior fronto-occipital fasciculus (*red*), inferior longitudinal fasciculus (*yellow*), and uncinate fasciculus (blue). (*C*) Sagittal and (*D*) axial images of the tracts of the dorsal phonologic stream including the arcuate fasciculus (*purple*), superior longitudinal fasciculus 3 (*orange*), and frontal aslant tract (*green*).

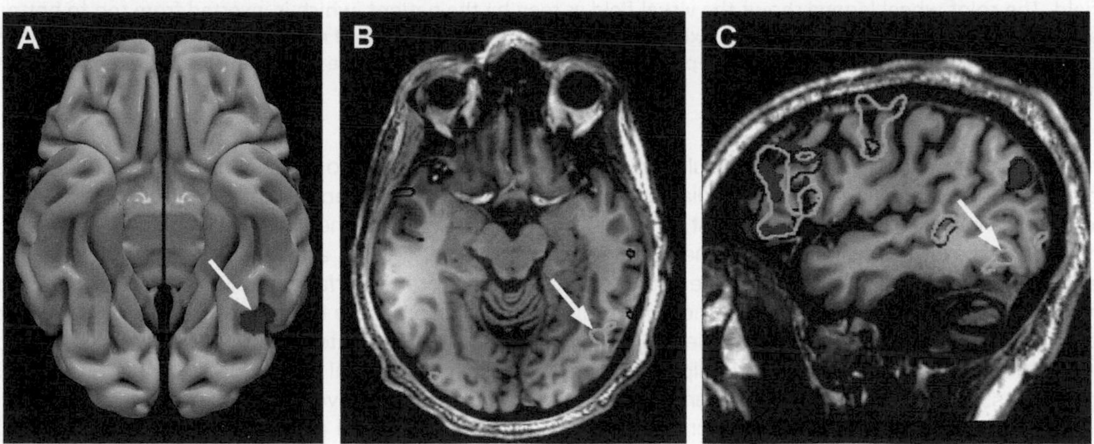

Fig. 7. (*A*) Inferior view of the brain showing the location of the visual word form area (*arrow*) along the lateral occipitotemporal sulcus and mid fusiform gyrus. Axial (*B*) and sagittal (*C*) language fMRI in a patient with epilepsy. Visual sentence completion task (*green*) elicits activation in the visual word form area (*arrow*), whereas audio semantic decision (*red*) and audio story comprehension task (*blue*) fail to elicit activation in the visual word form area.

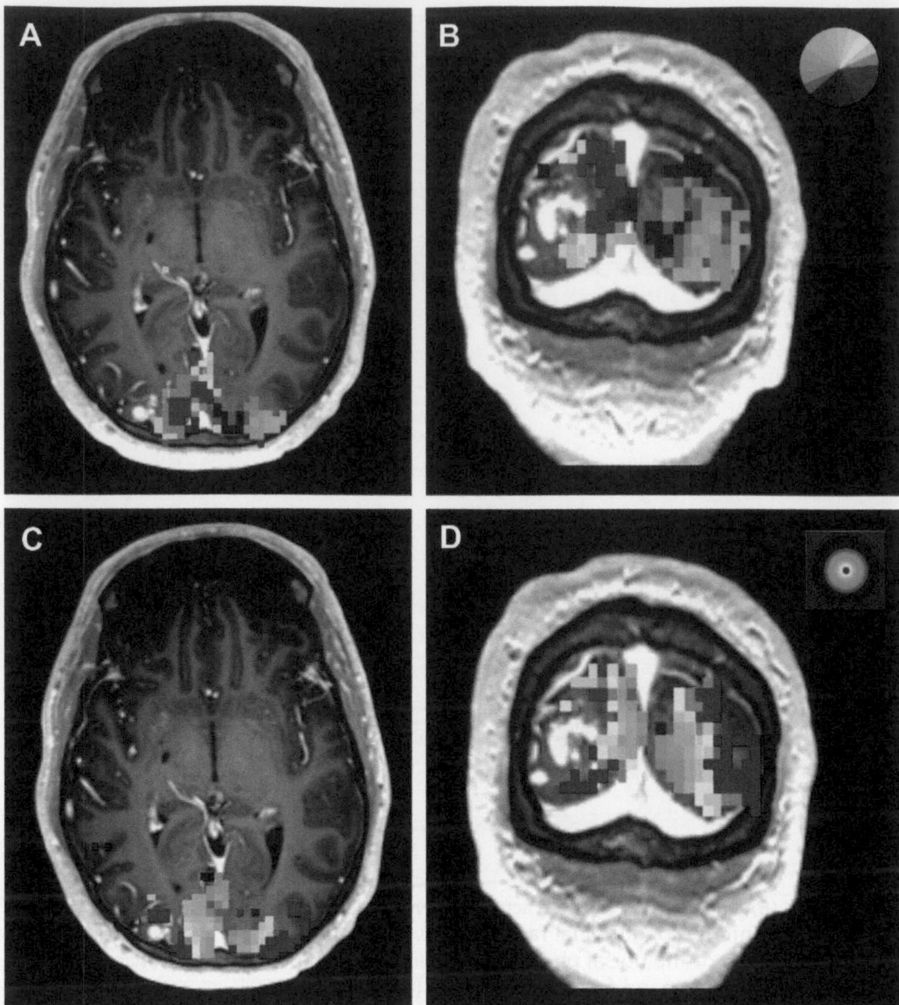

Fig. 8. Retinotopic mapping for a right occipital arteriovenous malformation (AVM). (*A*) Axial and (*B*) coronal polar angle fMRI map shows the AVM to occupy portions of both the right upper and lower quadrants of the visual field. The color wheel legend shows the visual field as seen by the patient, which is inverted from top to bottom and flipped left-right in the brain. (*C*) Axial and (*D*) coronal eccentricity fMRI map shows the AVM to lie nearest the foveal region. The legend shows the patient's visual field referenced to the color map, with the red representing the central fovea.

receives axons from the lateral geniculate nucleus of the thalamus through the optic radiations (geniculocalcarine tract) and is the first of several cortical maps of the visual field.[68] The human visual cortex is organized into multiple retinotopic maps.[69] The retrolenticular fibers of the optic radiation representing the inferior visual field (superior retinal field) terminate in the superior lip of the calcarine fissure.[42] The sublenticular fibers of the optic radiation representing the superior visual field (inferior retinal field) first pass around the rostral pole of the temporal horn of the lateral ventricle within the temporal lobe as the Meyer loop before terminating in the inferior lip of the calcarine fissure.[42] The center of gaze (fovea) is represented at the caudalmost part of the occipital lobe, whereas the peripheral fields are represented more anteriorly near the junction of the parieto-occipital sulcus and the calcarine sulcus.[68] A larger cortical surface area is dedicated to the representation of the fovea relative to the cortical surface area dedicated to the peripheral visual field, known as cortical magnification, which has implications for improved visual performance including visual acuity and perception.[69,70] The primary visual cortex is the first site that segregates and then recombines the visual inputs of the retinogeniculocortical pathways, which are then sent out to different extrastriate cortical areas for further analysis.[68]

Extrastriate and Visual Association Cortices

Extrastriate and visual association cortices refer to visually responsive cortical regions other than the primary visual cortex, which receive input from the primary visual cortex, as well as from relays through other extrastriate areas.[68,69,71] These regions encompass the occipital lobe and extend to adjacent areas of the posterior parietal lobe, temporal lobe, and even into selected regions in the frontal lobe.[56,68] At present, our knowledge of the various cortical visual areas and networks connecting them is largely based either on homologous regions extrapolated in humans from studies in macaque monkey brains or through lesion-related findings of visual deficits in humans.[71] However, both stimulus-based fMRI data and functional connectivity studies are adding to our knowledge of different organizations of visual processing pathways in humans.[72]

In its most simplistic form, cortical visual processing was proposed to proceed along 2 major processing streams: a slower ventral stream involved in object recognition ("what" pathway) and a faster dorsal stream involved in spatial information and attention ("where" pathway).[73,74] Specifically, the ventral stream connects the occipital cortex to the anterior part of the inferior temporal cortex.[68,75] The fusiform gyrus, located in the middle of the ventral temporal lobe, is an important region in the ventral stream that participates in facial recognition and recognition of object features.[76] The dorsal stream projects from the striate cortex to the parietal lobe and the middle temporal visual complex.[71] In addition to mediating spatial perception, recent studies show that the dorsal stream also involves projections to the prefrontal cortex, premotor cortex, and medial temporal lobe that mediate spatial working memory, visually guided action, and navigation.[75] Finally, although beyond the scope of this review, recent studies have modified and added to the complexity of these streams that are more likely to be highly interactive and interconnected rather than separate.[71]

SUMMARY

While our understanding of human brain function continues to increase in complexity, so do the tools that allow us to explore such function. These tools, such as fMRI and diffusion tractography, have the potential to vastly improve precision medicine, and already have made an impact in patient care. To properly interpret the normal and dysfunctional brain, a thorough knowledge of brain functional anatomy is required.

CLINICS CARE POINTS

- Radiologists and clinicians managing a patient who is a potential candidate for resective surgery should be aware that task-based functional activation of hand motor regions may not always be within the hand knob and that individual variability in concert with tumor-related mass effect can result in relocation of eloquent cortices.
- The location of the foot motor area adjacent to and under the superior sagittal sinus makes it difficult to approach for intraoperative direct cortical stimulation, emphasizing the role that task-based fMRI plays in accurately localizing this region during presurgical mapping. Furthermore, small displacements in patient head position during routine imaging acquisition with or without mass effect related to tumor and/or edema can result in significant differences in the position of local anatomic landmarks. These differences can lead radiologists to misjudge the correct location of the foot motor region.[24]
- Tongue and lip movements are frequently involved in mastication, swallowing, and articulation; these functions may be compromised by lesions or injury in the frontotemporal region.[77]
- Complex motor and sensory tasks result in activation within the contralateral SMA proper, and this area is seen activated along with activation in the appropriate region of the precentral gyrus during fMRI motor tasks such as finger tapping (see **Figs. 1** and **3**).[56] Surgical resection of a unilateral SMA results in an SMA syndrome, which is characterized by temporary global akinesia that is more pronounced contralaterally, and mutism if the lesion is in the dominant hemisphere. Improvement or recovery is common in the ensuing weeks to months postsurgery,[34,78,79] and the extent of preservation of anatomic connections of the SMA can increase the likelihood of recovery.[80]
- Awake stimulation of the traditional Broca area may sometimes elicit speech disturbances, such as anomia, whereas damage to this cortical area does not typically result in long-term speech disorders.[81] It is likely that long-term speech disorders from inferior frontal gyrus damage are the result of damage to the adjacent vPMC (discussed later) or to the underlying bottleneck of eloquent white matter tracts, such as the arcuate fasciculus, frontal aslant tract, and lateral SLF (SLF

III). Likewise, during awake mapping, the traditional Broca area may be mistaken for ventral premotor area or the inappropriate use of language tasks. For example, anomia may be mistaken for speech arrest if simply asked to name an object, but can easily be discerned by the patient being asked to lead with "This is a..." before naming the object to distinguish speech arrest from anomia.

- White matter tract damage is generally considered to have less plasticity than cortical damage; therefore, we must consider several eloquent tracts in the language streams. Damage to the arcuate fasciculus may produce phonologic paraphasias, repetition disorders, or transcortical motor aphasia.[82] The lateral portion of the SLF (SLF III) is part of the phonologic working memory loop and is associated with anarthria/dysarthria with potential for severe speech output disorders when injured.[83] Injury to the frontal aslant tract can result in decline of verbal fluency with deficits in speech initiation and articulatory planning.[80] Anomia or semantic paraphasias can be seen with injury to either IFOF or the ILF.[51,84] Additionally, ILF injury may result in impaired reading or alexia.[85]
- Language paradigms in fMRI often elicit activation in both primary language areas and in secondary language areas. The neuroradiologist should pay attention to these secondary language areas and their proximity to the lesion marked for resection and convey this information to the neurosurgeon, because injury to these areas can also result in functional postoperative deficits.
- As already described, injury or resection of the SMA complex can result in the SMA syndrome. However, direct cortical stimulation of the SMA complex during surgery can fail to produce a deficit but may still result in postoperative SMA syndrome[86] suggesting the importance of identifying these regions on preoperative functional mapping to predict the risk of developing postoperative SMA syndrome (see Fig. 3).
- Although there is bilateral representation of the vPMC, this region shows limited plasticity with persistent postoperative deficits corresponding to the percentage of the vPMC resected[83] emphasizing the importance of locating the vPMC preoperatively using functional mapping.
- Although visual field deficits are expected in resections of lesions in the occipital lobe, the neuroradiologist should consider the risk of visual field deficits when resections disrupt the course of the geniculocalcarine fiber tract, including within the temporal lobe. In addition, as described in later sections, vision-related cortex extends beyond V1 in the occipital lobe and into adjoining parts of the temporal and parietal lobes, as well as into regions in the frontal lobe.[69] Insults to this extensive, interconnected visual network can result in a range of selective visual deficits. fMRI vision mapping has been used in presurgical planning in patients with pathology or potential surgical resection of central visual pathways. Fig. 8 provides an example of retinotopic mapping in clinical practice.

DISCLOSURE

B.A.V. has no disclosures. E.H.M. receives unrelated research support from Varian Medical Systems, Inc., Boston Scientific Corp., and Vigil Neuroscience, Inc. E.H.M. is a consultant for Boston Scientific Corp. and Varian Medical Systems, Inc.

REFERENCES

1. Ulmer S. Neuroanatomy and cortical landmarks. In: Ulmer S, Jansen O, editors. fMRI: basics and clinical applications. 3rd edition. Cham, Switzerland: Springer Nature; 2020. p. 5–14.
2. Hill VB, Cankurtaran CZ, Liu BP, et al. A practical review of functional MRI anatomy of the language and motor systems. AJNR Am J Neuroradiol 2019;40(7): 1084–90.
3. Naidich T, Yousry T. Functional neuroanatomy. In: Stippich C, editor. Clinical functional MRI: presurgical functional neuroimaging. Berlin-Heidelberg (Germany): Springer-Verlag; 2007. p. 53–86.
4. Naidich T, Tang C, Ng J, et al. Surface anatomy of the cerebrum. In: Naidich T, Castillo M, Cha S, et al, editors. Imaging of the brain. Philadelphia (PA): Elsevier Inc; 2013.
5. Wagner M, Jurcoane A, Hattingen E. The U sign: tenth landmark to the central region on brain surface reformatted MR imaging. AJNR Am J Neuroradiol 2013;34(2):323–6.
6. Kido DK, LeMay M, Levinson AW, et al. Computed tomographic localization of the precentral gyrus. Radiology 1980;135(2):373–7.
7. Yousry TA, Schmid UD, Alkadhi H, et al. Localization of the motor hand area to a knob on the precentral gyrus. A new landmark. Brain 1997;120(Pt 1): 141–57.
8. Raabe A. The craniotomy atlas. Stuttgart (Germany): Thieme; 2019.
9. Pressman P, Rosen H. Disorders of frontal lobe function. In: Zigmond M, Rowland L, Coyle J, editors. Neurobiology of brain disorders biological basis of

neurological and psychiatric disorders. Waltham, MA: Elsevier; 2015. p. 542–57.
10. Vanderah T, Gould D. Nolte's the human brain. an introduction to its functional anatomy. 8th edition. Philadelphia (PA): Elsevier; 2021.
11. Felten D, O'Banion M, Maida M. Motor Systems. In: Felten D, O'Banion M, Maida M, editors. Netter's atlas of neuroscience. Philadelphia, PA: Elsevier; 2016. p. 391–420.
12. Lemon RN. Descending pathways in motor control. Annu Rev Neurosci 2008;31:195–218.
13. Penfield W, Boldrey E. Somatic motor and sensory representation in the cerebral cortex of man as studied by electrical stimulation. Brain 1937;60(4):389–443.
14. Schellekens W, Petridou N, Ramsey NF. Detailed somatotopy in primary motor and somatosensory cortex revealed by Gaussian population receptive fields. Neuroimage 2018;179:337–47.
15. Overduin SA, Servos P. Distributed digit somatotopy in primary somatosensory cortex. Neuroimage 2004; 23(2):462–72.
16. Watson C, Kirkcaldie M, Paxinos G. The brain: an introduction to functional neuroanatomy. Amsterdam (the Netherlands): Elsevier; 2010.
17. Caulo M, Briganti C, Mattei PA, et al. New morphologic variants of the hand motor cortex as seen with MR imaging in a large study population. AJNR Am J Neuroradiol 2007;28(8):1480–5.
18. Vigano L, Fornia L, Rossi M, et al. Anatomo-functional characterisation of the human "hand-knob": A direct electrophysiological study. Cortex 2019;113: 239–54.
19. Ahdab R, Ayache SS, Brugieres P, et al. The hand motor hotspot is not always located in the hand knob: a neuronavigated transcranial magnetic stimulation study. Brain Topogr 2016;29(4):590–7.
20. Hlustik P, Solodkin A, Gullapalli RP, et al. Somatotopy in human primary motor and somatosensory hand representations revisited. Cereb Cortex 2001; 11(4):312–21.
21. Siero JC, Hermes D, Hoogduin H, et al. BOLD matches neuronal activity at the mm scale: a combined 7T fMRI and ECoG study in human sensorimotor cortex. Neuroimage 2014;101:177–84.
22. Dechent P, Frahm J. Functional somatotopy of finger representations in human primary motor cortex. Hum Brain Mapp 2003;18(4):272–83.
23. Hamidian S, Vachha B, Jenabi M, et al. Resting-state functional magnetic resonance imaging and probabilistic diffusion tensor imaging demonstrate that the greatest functional and structural connectivity in the hand motor homunculus occurs in the area of the thumb. Brain Connect 2018;8(6):371–9.
24. Moreno RA, Holodny AI. Functional brain anatomy. Neuroimaging Clin N Am 2021;31(1):33–51.
25. Ulmer JL, Hacein-Bey L, Mathews VP, et al. Lesion-induced pseudo-dominance at functional magnetic resonance imaging: implications for preoperative assessments. Neurosurgery 2004;55(3):569–79 [discussion: 580-561].
26. Borich MR, Brodie SM, Gray WA, et al. Understanding the role of the primary somatosensory cortex: opportunities for rehabilitation. Neuropsychologia 2015;79(Pt B):246–55.
27. Roux FE, Djidjeli I, Durand JB. Functional architecture of the somatosensory homunculus detected by electrostimulation. J Physiol 2018;596(5):941–56.
28. Nachev P, Kennard C, Husain M. Functional role of the supplementary and pre-supplementary motor areas. Nat Rev Neurosci 2008;9(11):856–69.
29. Bozkurt B, Yagmurlu K, Middlebrooks EH, et al. Microsurgical and tractographic anatomy of the supplementary motor area complex in humans. World Neurosurg 2016;95:99–107.
30. Potgieser AR, de Jong BM, Wagemakers M, et al. Insights from the supplementary motor area syndrome in balancing movement initiation and inhibition. Front Hum Neurosci 2014;8:960.
31. Picard N, Strick PL. Imaging the premotor areas. Curr Opin Neurobiol 2001;11(6):663–72.
32. He SQ, Dum RP, Strick PL. Topographic organization of corticospinal projections from the frontal lobe: motor areas on the medial surface of the hemisphere. J Neurosci 1995;15(5 Pt 1):3284–306.
33. Wise SP. Corticospinal efferents of the supplementary sensorimotor area in relation to the primary motor area. Adv Neurol 1996;70:57–69.
34. Vergani F, Lacerda L, Martino J, et al. White matter connections of the supplementary motor area in humans. J Neurol Neurosurg Psychiatry 2014;85(12): 1377–85.
35. Catani M, Dell'acqua F, Vergani F, et al. Short frontal lobe connections of the human brain. Cortex 2012; 48(2):273–91.
36. Lehericy S, Ducros M, Krainik A, et al. 3-D diffusion tensor axonal tracking shows distinct SMA and pre-SMA projections to the human striatum. Cereb Cortex 2004;14(12):1302–9.
37. Tsuboi T, Wong JK, Eisinger RS, et al. Comparative connectivity correlates of dystonic and essential tremor deep brain stimulation. Brain 2021;144(6):1774–86.
38. Foote KD, Seignourel P, Fernandez HH, et al. Dual electrode thalamic deep brain stimulation for the treatment of posttraumatic and multiple sclerosis tremor. Neurosurgery 2006;58(4 Suppl 2). ONS-280-285.
39. Chainay H, Krainik A, Tanguy ML, et al. Foot, face and hand representation in the human supplementary motor area. Neuroreport 2004;15(5):765–9.
40. Fontaine D, Capelle L, Duffau H. Somatotopy of the supplementary motor area: evidence from correlation of the extent of surgical resection with the clinical patterns of deficit. Neurosurgery 2002;50(2): 297–303 [discussion: 303-295].

41. Hickok G, Poeppel D. Dorsal and ventral streams: a framework for understanding aspects of the functional anatomy of language. Cognition 2004;92(1–2):67–99.
42. Boling W, Olivier A. Anatomy of important functioning cortex. In: Byrne R, editor. Functional mapping of the cerebral cortex. Cham, Switzerland: Springer International Publishing; 2016. p. 23–40.
43. Idowu OE, Soyemi S, Atobatele K. Morphometry, asymmetry and variations of the sylvian fissure and sulci bordering and within the pars triangularis and pars operculum: an autopsy study. J Clin Diagn Res 2014;8(11):AC11–4.
44. Tremblay P, Dick AS. Broca and Wernicke are dead, or moving past the classic model of language neurobiology. Brain Lang 2016;162:60–71.
45. Sibilla L. Functional anatomy of the major lobes. In: Agarwal N, Port J, editors. Neuroimaging: anatomy meets function. Cham, Switzerland: Springer International Publishing; 2018. p. 81–99.
46. Belyk M, Brown S. Perception of affective and linguistic prosody: an ALE meta-analysis of neuroimaging studies. Soc Cogn Affect Neurosci 2014; 9(9):1395–403.
47. Flinker A, Korzeniewska A, Shestyuk AY, et al. Redefining the role of Broca's area in speech. Proc Natl Acad Sci U S A 2015;112(9):2871–5.
48. Binder JR. The Wernicke area: modern evidence and a reinterpretation. Neurology 2015;85(24): 2170–5.
49. Quigg M, Fountain NB. Conduction aphasia elicited by stimulation of the left posterior superior temporal gyrus. J Neurol Neurosurg Psychiatry 1999;66(3): 393–6.
50. Saur D, Kreher BW, Schnell S, et al. Ventral and dorsal pathways for language. Proc Natl Acad Sci U S A 2008;105(46):18035–40.
51. Middlebrooks EH, Yagmurlu K, Szaflarski JP, et al. A contemporary framework of language processing in the human brain in the context of preoperative and intraoperative language mapping. Neuroradiology 2017;59(1):69–87.
52. Hickok G, Poeppel D. The cortical organization of speech processing. Nat Rev Neurosci 2007;8(5): 393–402.
53. Yagmurlu K, Middlebrooks EH, Tanriover N, et al. Fiber tracts of the dorsal language stream in the human brain. J Neurosurg 2016;124(5):1396–405.
54. La Corte E, Eldahaby D, Greco E, et al. The frontal aslant tract: a systematic review for neurosurgical applications. Front Neurol 2021;12:641586.
55. Picard N, Strick PL. Motor areas of the medial wall: a review of their location and functional activation. Cereb Cortex 1996;6(3):342–53.
56. Chung GH, Han YM, Jeong SH, et al. Functional heterogeneity of the supplementary motor area. AJNR Am J Neuroradiol 2005;26(7):1819–23.
57. Binder JR, Desai RH, Graves WW, et al. Where is the semantic system? A critical review and meta-analysis of 120 functional neuroimaging studies. Cereb Cortex 2009;19(12):2767–96.
58. Seghier ML. The angular gyrus: multiple functions and multiple subdivisions. Neuroscientist 2013; 19(1):43–61.
59. Ardila A. Gerstmann Syndrome. Curr Neurol Neurosci Rep 2020;20(11):48.
60. Vigneau M, Beaucousin V, Herve PY, et al. Meta-analyzing left hemisphere language areas: phonology, semantics, and sentence processing. Neuroimage 2006;30(4):1414–32.
61. Chang EF, Breshears JD, Raygor KP, et al. Stereotactic probability and variability of speech arrest and anomia sites during stimulation mapping of the language dominant hemisphere. J Neurosurg 2017;126(1):114–21.
62. Mandonnet E, Sarubbo S, Duffau H. Proposal of an optimized strategy for intraoperative testing of speech and language during awake mapping. Neurosurg Rev 2017;40(1):29–35.
63. Purcell JJ, Shea J, Rapp B. Beyond the visual word form area: the orthography-semantics interface in spelling and reading. Cogn Neuropsychol 2014; 31(5–6):482–510.
64. Sabsevitz DS, Middlebrooks EH, Tatum W, et al. Examining the function of the visual word form area with stereo EEG electrical stimulation: a case report of pure alexia. Cortex 2020;129:112–8.
65. Tate MC, Herbet G, Moritz-Gasser S, et al. Probabilistic map of critical functional regions of the human cerebral cortex: Broca's area revisited. Brain 2014; 137(Pt 10):2773–82.
66. Huang J, Carr TH, Cao Y. Comparing cortical activations for silent and overt speech using event-related fMRI. Hum Brain Mapp 2002;15(1):39–53.
67. Morin O, Grezes J. What is "mirror" in the premotor cortex? A review. Neurophysiol Clin 2008;38(3): 189–95.
68. Gill S, Ulmer J, DeYoe E. Vision and higher cortical function. In: Holodny A, editor. Functional neuroimaging a clinical approach. New York: Informa Health Care; 2008. p. 67–80.
69. DeYoe EA, Raut RV. Visual mapping using blood oxygen level dependent functional magnetic resonance imaging. Neuroimaging Clin N Am 2014; 24(4):573–84.
70. Song C, Schwarzkopf DS, Kanai R, et al. Neural population tuning links visual cortical anatomy to human visual perception. Neuron 2015;85(3): 641–56.
71. DeYoe EA, Ulmer JL, Mueller WM, et al. Imaging of the functional and dysfunctional visual system. Semin Ultrasound CT MR 2015;36(3):234–48.
72. Goelman G, Dan R, Keadan T. Characterizing directed functional pathways in the visual system

by multivariate nonlinear coherence of fMRI data. Sci Rep 2018;8(1):16362.
73. Milner AD, Goodale MA. Two visual systems reviewed. Neuropsychologia 2008;46(3):774–85.
74. Ungerleider L, Mishkin M. Two visual systems. In: Ingle D, Goodale MA, Mansfield R, editors. Analysis of visual behavior. Cambridge (MA): MIT Press; 1982.
75. Kravitz DJ, Saleem KS, Baker CI, et al. A new neural framework for visuospatial processing. Nat Rev Neurosci 2011;12(4):217–30.
76. Zhang W, Wang J, Fan L, et al. Functional organization of the fusiform gyrus revealed with connectivity profiles. Hum Brain Mapp 2016;37(8):3003–16.
77. Xiao FL, Gao PY, Qian TY, et al. Cortical representation of facial and tongue movements: a task functional magnetic resonance imaging study. Clin Physiol Funct Imaging 2017;37(3):341–5.
78. Krainik A, Lehericy S, Duffau H, et al. Postoperative speech disorder after medial frontal surgery: role of the supplementary motor area. Neurology 2003; 60(4):587–94.
79. Laplane D, Talairach J, Meininger V, et al. Clinical consequences of corticectomies involving the supplementary motor area in man. J Neurol Sci 1977; 34(3):301–14.
80. Kinoshita M, de Champfleur NM, Deverdun J, et al. Role of fronto-striatal tract and frontal aslant tract in movement and speech: an axonal mapping study. Brain Struct Funct 2015;220(6):3399–412.
81. Gajardo-Vidal A, Lorca-Puls DL, Team P, et al. Damage to Broca's area does not contribute to long-term speech production outcome after stroke. Brain 2021;144(3):817–32.
82. Chang EF, Raygor KP, Berger MS. Contemporary model of language organization: an overview for neurosurgeons. J Neurosurg 2015;122(2):250–61.
83. van Geemen K, Herbet G, Moritz-Gasser S, et al. Limited plastic potential of the left ventral premotor cortex in speech articulation: evidence from intraoperative awake mapping in glioma patients. Hum Brain Mapp 2014;35(4):1587–96.
84. Duffau H, Gatignol P, Mandonnet E, et al. New insights into the anatomo-functional connectivity of the semantic system: a study using cortico-subcortical electrostimulations. Brain 2005;128(Pt 4):797–810.
85. Herbet G, Zemmoura I, Duffau H. Functional anatomy of the inferior longitudinal fasciculus: from historical reports to current hypotheses. Front Neuroanat 2018;12:77.
86. Rosenberg K, Nossek E, Liebling R, et al. Prediction of neurological deficits and recovery after surgery in the supplementary motor area: a prospective study in 26 patients. J Neurosurg 2010;113(6):1152–63.

Cerebral White Matter Tract Anatomy

Asthik Biswas, MBBS, DNB[a,b,c,*], Pradeep Krishnan, MBBS, MD[a,b], Logi Vidarsson, PhD[a,b], Manohar Shroff, MD, FRCPC, DABR, DMRD[a,b]

KEYWORDS

• White matter • Anatomy • MRI • DTI • Neuroimaging

KEY POINTS

- Advances in MR imaging techniques have allowed for detailed in vivo depiction of white matter tracts.
- In addition to leukodystrophies, demyelinating disorders, and neoplasms, there is increasing evidence of involvement of white matter structures in various cognitive, developmental, and neuropsychiatric disorders. Identification and further assessment of these structures (eg, using volume and fractional anisotropy) will play a key role in the neuroradiological evaluation of many of these disorders.
- Knowledge of white matter anatomy and connectivity also plays a key role in preoperative surgical planning, for example, in providing a road map for tumor and epilepsy surgery, and in assessing the risk of potential neurologic deficits that may result from the resection of specific regions of interest.

> *"It is impossible to explain the movements of a machine if the contrivance of its parts is unknown"*
>
> *—Nicholas Steno (Discourse on the Anatomy of the Brain, 1665)*

INTRODUCTION

The major neurons comprising gray matter are interneurons and long projection neurons. Myelinated axons sprouting from long projection neurons arrange themselves in fibers, and subsequently, bundles of fibers, thereby forming compact structures, which in the healthy state traverse in predictable directions to reach their destination of interest. White matter (WM) tracts, therefore, form complex 3-dimensional structures within the brain and spinal cord. The directionality of WM tracts makes it possible for in vivo imaging, exploiting the concept of fractional anisotropy (ie, the preferential movement of water molecules along the long axis of WM tracts). In this article, we will review the anatomy of the cerebral WM with the help of conventional MRI and diffusion tensor imaging (DTI) techniques. WM tracts of the brainstem will be covered in detail by Shepherd and Hoch in this issue.

A BRIEF HISTORY OF THE NOMENCLATURE AND CLASSIFICATION OF WHITE MATTER TRACTS

Historically, WM anatomy was described in terms of their regional distribution (eg, centrum semiovale; corona radiata; internal, external, and extreme capsules). The centrum semiovale was named so by Vieussens on account of its semioval shape, and referred to cerebral WM that was located above the level of the lateral ventricles.[1] The corona radiata, on the other hand, was named for its radiating appearance in sagittal sections, and represents the caudal continuum of the

[a] Department of Diagnostic Imaging, The Hospital for Sick Children, 555, University Avenue, Toronto, Ontario M5G1X8, Canada; [b] Department of Medical Imaging, University of Toronto, Toronto, Ontario M5G1X8, Canada; [c] Department of Radiology, Great Ormond Street Hospital for Children NHS Trust, London WC1N3JH, United Kingdom

* Corresponding author. Department of Radiology, Great Ormond Street Hospital for Children NHS Trust, London WC1N3JH, United Kingdom.

E-mail address: asthikbiswas@gmail.com

Neuroimag Clin N Am 32 (2022) 507–528
https://doi.org/10.1016/j.nic.2022.05.001

centrum semiovale. The term *"capsule"* was used to describe WM tracts passing ("encapsulated") in between the cortex and deeper gray matter structures. Indeed, these WM structures do not conform to specific tracts, and rather, serve as *"conduits"* for various WM fibers. For instance, the corona radiata is not a single tract but is collectively formed by the corticospinal, corticopontine, corticobulbar, and the thalamocortical projections. Similarly, the internal capsule comprises a number of projection fibers including the corticospinal and thalamocortical tracts.

Individual WM tracts have been named on the basis of either their relationship to the cortical structure (eg, corticospinal tract), or their location (eg, superior longitudinal fasciculus), or their shape (eg, arcuate fasciculus), and this nomenclature continues to be the most widely used in the medical literature.[1] In this article, we will describe WM anatomy based on this most commonly accepted nomenclature. It is important to note, however, that there is ongoing debate regarding the need for a more systematic taxonomic anatomic classification as proposed in a recent review.[1] Furthermore, despite the increasing need (especially in preoperative planning), for the usage of tract specific terminologies, the utility of regional WM terminology is commonly retained in everyday radiology parlance, and will therefore be discussed in addition to tract specific WM structures.

Based on connectivity, WM tracts may be divided into 3 major types: the projection fibers, commissural fibers, and association fibers, each of which is further described later in discussion. We will then discuss the major WM conduits that constitute important landmarks in the brain. **Tables 1** and **2** summarise the major WM tracts and conduits.

PROJECTION FIBERS

Projection fibers comprise afferent and efferent tracts that interconnect the cortex with the deep gray nuclei, the brainstem, cerebellum, and spinal cord (**Fig. 1**). The major projection fibers identifiable on DTI are the corticospinal, corticobulbar, corticopontine, and the optic radiations (geniculocalcarine tracts). The internal capsules and cerebral peduncles serve as the major conduits for the projection fibers.

Corticospinal Tracts

Corticospinal tracts (CST), also known as the pyramidal tracts, are paired descending tracts that arise from the neocortical internal cell (layer 5) of the frontal and parietal lobes, connecting the motor cortex (primary, supplementary and premotor), the somatosensory cortex and the cingulate gyrus to the spinal cord.[2–5] Fibers of the CST traverse the centrum semiovale, converge into the corona radiata before forming the compact posterior limb of internal capsule (PLIC). From the PLIC, the CST fibers enter the mesencephalon via the cerebral peduncles, course along the basis pontis, and continue in the ventral medulla forming the medullary pyramids. At the level of the caudal medulla, the majority (75–90%) of the fibers cross over to the contralateral side and proceed to descend to the lateral corticospinal tracts in the spinal cord.[6] The fibers that do not cross continue ipsilaterally as the anterior CST. The lateral CST, therefore, comprise fibers originating in the contralateral cerebral hemisphere and descend in the posterior part of the lateral funiculus of the spinal cord; whereas the anterior CST comprise mainly ipsilateral fibers and descend along the anterior column of the spinal cord on either side of the midline.[2] Eventual termination of the CST fibers is in the spinal gray matter, with the lateral CST terminating ipsilateral to its side of descent, and the anterior CST terminating contralateral to its side of descent.

The trajectory and somatotopic distribution of the CST at various levels are depicted in **Figs 2** and **3**; and are detailed as follows:

a *Corona radiata:* At this level, the anterior fibers of the CST represent the face, the middle fibers represent the hand and the posterior fibers represent the lower limbs.[7]
b *Posterior limb of internal capsule:* The CST occupy the posterior aspect of the PLIC. Similar to the corona radiata, the fibers representing the hand are located anterior to those representing the feet.[2]
c *Cerebral peduncles:* The CST occupy the middle thirds of the crus cerebri, with face fibers traversing medially, hand fibers in between, and feet fibers situated laterally.[8,9]
d *Basis pontis:* The fibers representing the hand are anteromedial to the fibers representing the feet.[10]
e *Medulla:* The CST form ventral bumps on either side of the midline known as the medullary pyramids. Similar to the pons, the fibers representing the hand are located medial to those representing the feet.[11]

Normal variants and asymmetry of corticospinal tracts

- Ipsilateral lateral CST and contralateral anterior CST have been described.[2]

Table 1
White matter tracts, their connections and main functions

White Matter Tract	Connection	Function
A. Projection fibers		
1. Corticospinal tracts	Motor cortex, somatosensory cortex and the cingulate gyrus to the spinal cord.	Upper motor neuron innervation from neck to feet.
2. Corticobulbar tracts	Primary motor, premotor and supplementary motor cortex to motor nuclei of V, VII, IX, X, XI, and XII cranial nerves.	Upper motor neuron innervation of face, head and neck.
3. Corticopontine tracts	All areas of the cerebral cortex to the pontine nuclei, which then form pontocerebellar tracts that communicate with the contralateral cerebellar hemispheres.	Coordination of planned motor functions.
4. Thalamic radiations	Reciprocal connections with the cerebral cortex.	Relay of sensory information (except olfaction).
5. Optic radiations	Lateral geniculate body and pulvinar of thalamus to the primary visual cortex.	Transmission of visual input.
B. Association fibers		
1. Superior longitudinal fasciculus	Frontal lobes to the temporal, parietal and occipital lobes.	Speech and language, visuospatial cognition, attention and working memory.
2. Middle longitudinal fasciculus	Temporal lobe with the parietal and occipital lobes.	Postulated to play a role in the perception of auditory representations and the integrity of auditory and visual information.
3. Inferior longitudinal fasciculus	Anterior and medial aspects of the temporal lobes with the occipital lobes.	Ventral visual stream which is critical for face and object recognition.
4. Inferior fronto-occipital fasciculus	Inferior frontal lobe with the parietal and occipital lobes.	Semantic language processing via the ventral stream, visual recognition system, reading and writing tasks and goal oriented behaviour.
5. Uncinate fasciculus	Orbitofrontal cortex to the anterior temporal lobes.	Language processing, emotional understanding and empathy.
6. Frontal aslant tract	Superior frontal gyrus to the inferior frontal gyrus and anterior insula.	Speech, language, cognitive and executive functions.
C. Commissural fibers		
1. Corpus callosum	Homologous cortical regions of contralateral cerebral hemispheres.	Major association tract contributing to interhemispheric motor, sensory and auditory connectivity.

(continued on next page)

Table 1
(continued)

White Matter Tract	Connection	Function
2. Anterior commissure	Olfactory bulb, anterior olfactory nucleus and the anterior perforated substance; homologous structures of the temporal lobe (amygdala; inferior temporal, parahippocampal and fusiform gyri; and the inferior occipital cortex).	Olfaction, memory, instinct and emotion.
3. Posterior commissure	Midbrain, thalamus and hypothalamus.	Upward eye movements via reciprocal connections with the superior colliculus. Possibly other functions, largely unknown.
4. Hippocampal commissure	Crura of fornices	Part of limbic system.
D. Fibers of the limbic system		
1. Cingulum	Cingulate gyrus and medial aspects of the frontal, parietal and temporal lobes, and the hippocampus.	Emotion, motivation, executive function, memory.
2. Fornix	Hippocampi to the septal area, basal forebrain, mamillary bodies and anterior nuclei of the thalami.	Formation of memory.
3. Stria terminalis	Amygdala to the hypothalamus and septal nuclei.	Modulates emotional and behavioural responses to stress.

- Asymmetry within the CST is common, with the left-sided CST shown to have higher fractional anisotropy values on account of high myelin content, possibly reflective of hand dominance.[12] An increasing fractional anisotropy (FA) has also been noted with increasing age.[13]

Corticobulbar Tracts

The corticobulbar tracts provide upper motor neuron innervation to the cranial nerves that supply the face, head, and neck. Fibers originate predominantly from the primary motor cortex, the premotor area (PMA) and supplementary motor area (SMA), pass through the corona radiata and genu of the internal capsule, run medial to the CST at the level of the cerebral peduncles, and descend along the ventral aspect of the brainstem to directly innervate the motor nuclei of trigeminal, facial, glossopharyngeal, vagus, accessory, and hypoglossal nerves (see **Fig. 3**). The corticobulbar tracts also indirectly exert effects on the muscles supplied by oculomotor, trochlear, and abducens nerves via the medial longitudinal fasciculus and the paramedian part of the pontine formation.[14]

Corticopontine Tracts

The corticopontine fibers arise from all areas of the cerebral cortex (ie, frontal, temporal, parietal, and occipital cortices), with the largest contribution from the frontal lobes.[15] These fibers then traverse the internal capsule and the cerebral peduncles before terminating in the pontine nuclei. Second-order neurons from the pontine nuclei give rise to the pontocerebellar tracts, which communicate with the contralateral cerebellar hemisphere via the middle cerebellar peduncles.[2,16] This pathway serves to allow for the coordination of planned motor functions.[15]

Table 2
White matter conduits and their constituent tracts

White Matter Conduit	Types of fibers	Major Tracts
Corona radiata	Projection and commissural	Corticospinal Corticopontine Corticobulbar Corticoreticular Corticothalamic Corticostriatal Thalamocortical
Internal capsule	Projection	*Anterior limb* Anterior thalamic radiation Frontopontine *Genu* Corticobulbar Corticoreticular Superior thalamic radiation *Posterior limb* Corticospinal Corticorubral Corticopontine Superior thalamic radiation Posterior thalamic radiation *Retrolenticular* Optic radiation Parietopontine Occipitopontine *Sublenticular* Auditory radiation Temporopontine Inferior thalamic radiation
External capsule	Association	Superior longitudinal fasciculus Inferior fronto-occipital fasciculus Uncinate fasciculus
Extreme capsule	Association	Inferior fronto-occipital fasciculus Uncinate fasciculus
Temporal stem	Association and projection	Inferior fronto-occipital fasciculus Uncinate fasciculus Meyer's loop of optic radiation Posterior bundle of anterior commissure
Sagittal stratum	Association and projection	Optic radiation Middle longitudinal fasciculus Inferior frontooccipital fasciculus Inferior longitudinal fasciculus
Cerebral peduncle	Projection	*Medial* Frontopontine *Middle* Corticospinal *Lateral* Temporopontine Parietopontine

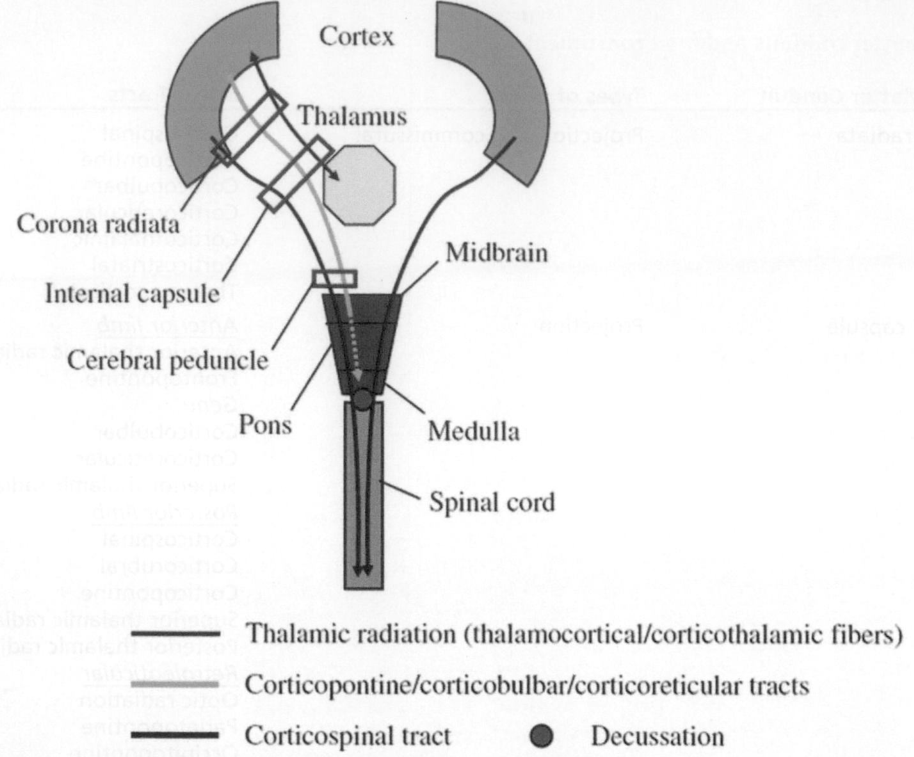

Fig. 1. Schematic representation of trajectories of the projection fibers. The decussation at the level of inferior medulla is that of the corticospinal tracts. (*From* Oishi K, Faria AV, Zijl PCM van, Mori S. MRI Atlas of Human White Matter. Academic Press; 2010].)

Thalamic Radiations

The thalamus, being the primary relay center of the brain, has widespread reciprocal connections with the cerebral cortex. These fibers form the anterior, posterior, superior and inferior thalamic radiations that course in the internal capsule and then fan out

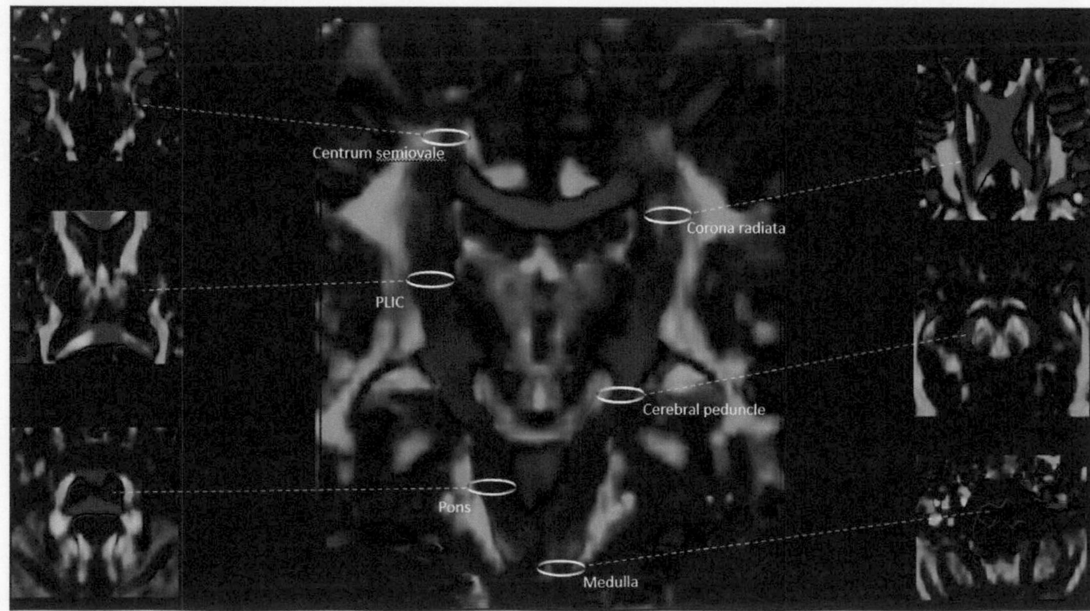

Fig. 2. Corticospinal tract trajectory and its position at various levels.

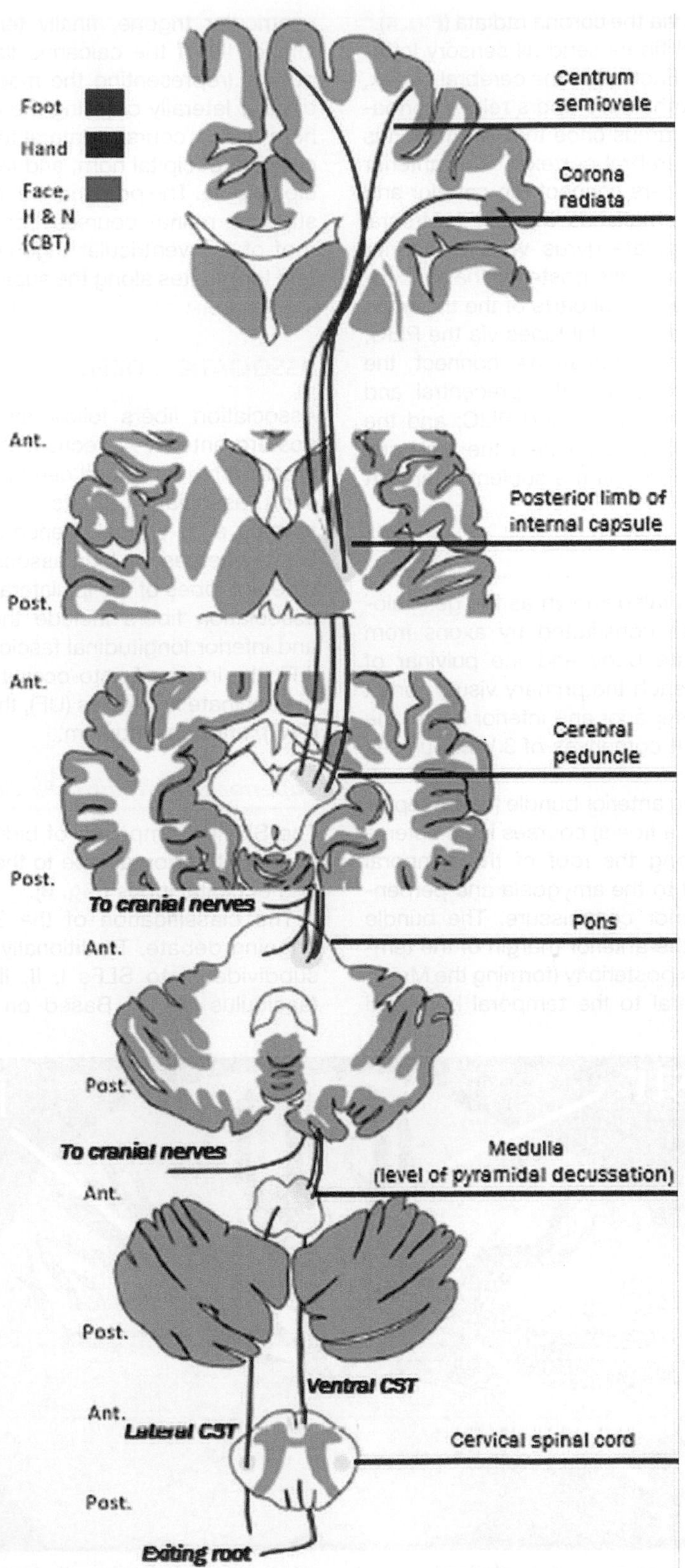

Fig. 3. Somatotopic distribution of the corticospinal tracts. (*Adapted from* Wycoco V, Shroff M, Sudhakar S, Lee W. White matter anatomy: what the radiologist needs to know. Neuroimaging Clin N Am. 2013;23(2):197 to 216.)

toward the cortices via the corona radiata (Fig. 4).[2] The thalamocortical fibers send all sensory information (except for olfaction) to the cerebral cortex, whereas the corticothalamic fibers relay information back to the thalamus once the information is processed in the cerebral cortex.[17] The anterior thalamic radiation fibers connect the anterior and medial nuclei of the thalamus with the prefrontal cortex and the cingulate gyrus via the anterior limb of internal capsule; the posterior thalamic radiations connect the caudal parts of the thalamus with the parietal and occipital lobes via the PLIC; the superior thalamic radiations connect the ventral thalamic nuclei with the precentral and postcentral gyri via the genu and PLIC; and the inferior thalamic radiations connect the thalamus with the temporal lobes via the sublenticular part of internal capsule.[17]

Optic Radiations

The optic radiations (also known as the geniculocalcarine tracts) are constituted by axons from the lateral geniculate body and the pulvinar of the thalamus that reach the primary visual cortex situated within the superior and inferior lips of the calcarine fissure.[18] It comprises of 3 WM bundles (Fig. 5).

From its origin, the anterior bundle (which represents the lower retina fibers) courses in an anterolateral direction along the roof of the temporal horn, posterolateral to the amygdala and perpendicular to the anterior commissure. The bundle then drapes along the anterior margin of the temporal horn and turns posteriorly (forming the Meyer loop), coursing lateral to the temporal horn and ventricular trigone, finally terminating along the inferior lip of the calcarine fissure.[18] The central bundle (representing the macular region) passes directly laterally crossing the roof of the temporal horn before coursing lateral to the ventricular trigone and occipital horn, and terminating at the occipital pole. The posterior bundle (representing the superior retina) courses posteriorly forming the roof of the ventricular trigone and occipital horn and terminates along the superior lip of the calcarine fissure.[2,18]

ASSOCIATION FIBERS

Association fibers follow an antero-posterior or postero-anterior direction, connecting cortical areas within ipsilateral cerebral hemispheres. The short association fibers connect adjacent gyri forming a "U-shape" (hence also known as *U-fibers*), whereas the long association fibers connect different lobes of the ipsilateral hemisphere. Major association fibers include the superior, middle, and inferior longitudinal fasciculi (SLF, MdLF, and ILF), the inferior fronto-occipital fasciculus (IFOF), the uncinate fasciculus (UF), the frontal aslant tract (FAT), and the cingulum.

Superior Longitudinal Fasciculus

The SLF is composed of bidirectional fibers that connect the frontal lobe to the temporal, parietal, and occipital lobes (Fig. 6).[19]

The classification of the SLF is a matter of ongoing debate. Traditionally, the SLF has been subdivided into SLFs I, II, III, and the arcuate fasciculus (AF).[19] Based on this classification,

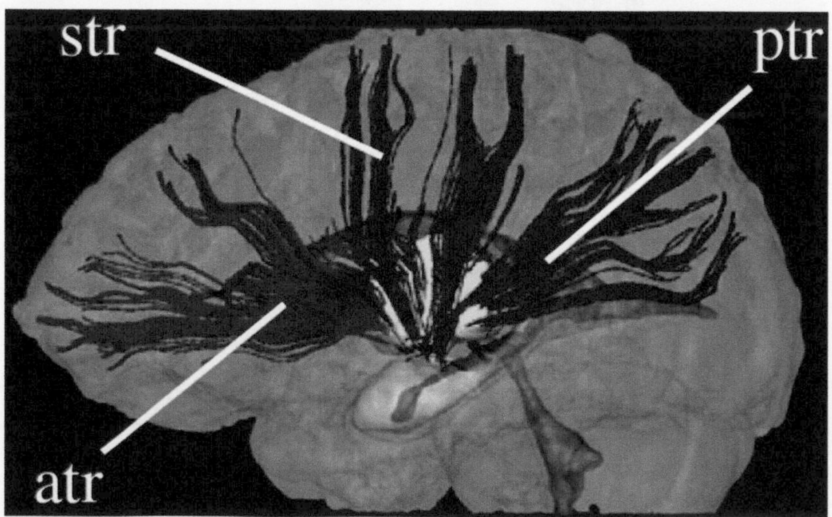

Fig. 4. DTI-based reconstruction of the thalamic radiations. atr, anterior thalamic radiation; str, superior thalamic radiation; ptr, posterior thalamic radiation. The inferior thalamic radiations are not shown in this image. (*From* Oishi K, Faria AV, Zijl PCM van, Mori S. MRI Atlas of Human White Matter. Academic Press; 2010.)

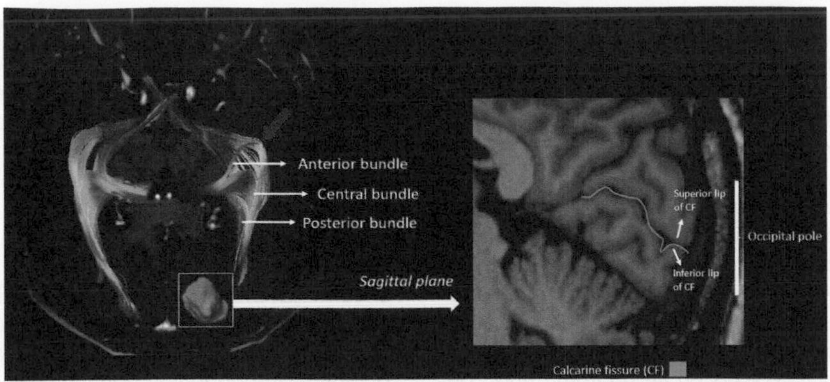

Fig. 5. DTI-based reconstruction of the optic radiations. Meyer's loop is represented by the red arrow. *(Adapted from* Bertani GA, Bertulli L, Scola E, et al. Optic Radiation Diffusion Tensor Imaging Tractography: An Alternative and Simple Technique for the Accurate Detection of Meyer's Loop. World Neurosurgery. 2018;117:e42-e56.)

the SLF I connects the dorsal and medial parts of the parietal lobe with the dorsal and medial parts of the frontal lobe; SLF II connects the angular gyrus with the caudal middle frontal gyrus and dorsal precentral gyrus; SLF III connects the supramarginal gyrus with the ventral precentral gyrus and pars opercularis; whereas the AF originates in the caudal aspect of the superior temporal gyrus and runs contiguous with the SLF II.

Recent evidence, however, challenges this conventional SLF I–III classification, which was primarily based on simian anatomy. In 2015, Wang and colleagues[20] used high angular diffusion spectrum imaging (DSI) in healthy humans and showed that only SLF II and SLF III could be identified as separate bundles, whereas SLF I could not be delineated as a separate tract and was, therefore, either part of the cingulum or very closely related to it. In addition, the study demonstrated a strong asymmetry with certain fibers of the SLF II being present only in the left hemisphere, and certain fibers of the SLF III located only in the right hemisphere. In an effort to address the ongoing debate, Nakajima and colleagues[21] reclassified the SLF into 4 components based on anatomical structure and functional segregation: the dorsal SLF, ventral SLF, posterior SLF, and AF; which correspond to traditional SLF II, SLF III, posterior AF, and long segment AF, respectively (see Fig. 6D).

The SLF can be identified readily on coronal color-coded FA images as a high anisotropic WM bundle that courses along the superior margin of the insula (see Fig. 6B). The SLF plays a major role in speech and language, visuospatial cognition, attention and working memory.[22]

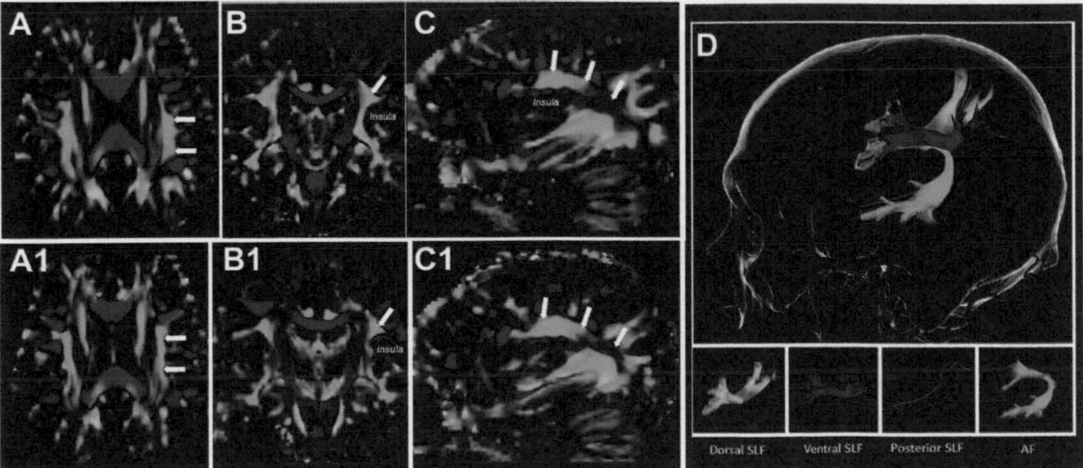

Fig. 6. Trajectory of the superior longitudinal fasciculus indicated by arrows in the axial (*A*), coronal (*B*), and sagittal (*C*) planes. DTI tractography depicting the 4 segments of the SLF (*D*). (Image D is from Nakajima R, Kinoshita M, Shinohara H, Nakada M. The superior longitudinal fascicle: reconsidering the fronto-parietal neural network based on anatomy and function. Brain Imaging and Behavior. 2020;14(6):2817 to 2830.)

Middle Longitudinal Fasciculus

The MdLF was initially described to connect the superior temporal gyrus with the inferior parietal lobule.[2,23] Recent studies, however, show more extensive connectivity between the temporal and parietal lobes, as well as the temporal and occipital lobes (**Fig. 7**).[24,25] Subsegments of the MLF remain a matter of debate, with different studies yielding various results, showing its composition as a single bundle,[26] two components,[25,27] three components,[24] and six components, respectively.[23] Similarly, the functional importance of the MdLF remains unclear. Based on its anatomy and connectivity pattern, it has been postulated to play a role in the perception of auditory representations and the integrity of auditory and visual information.[24]

Inferior Longitudinal Fasciculus

The ILF primarily connects the anterior and medial temporal lobe with the occipital lobe (**Fig. 8**).[28] It courses along the lateral wall of the temporal horn of the lateral ventricle at which point it is in direct contact with the uncinate fasciculus and the inferior fronto-occipital fasciculus.[3,28] It then forms part of the sagittal stratum before reaching the occipital lobe.[29] Recent dissection and DTI studies have shown that the ILF is composed of a least 4 layers: a fusiform branch which connects the fusiform gyrus to the anterior temporal region; a dorsolateral occipital branch which connects the occipital gyri to the anterior temporal region; a lingual branch which connects the lingual gyrus to the middle temporal gyrus, and a cuneal branch which connects the cuneus to the temporal lobe.[30,31] The ILF is

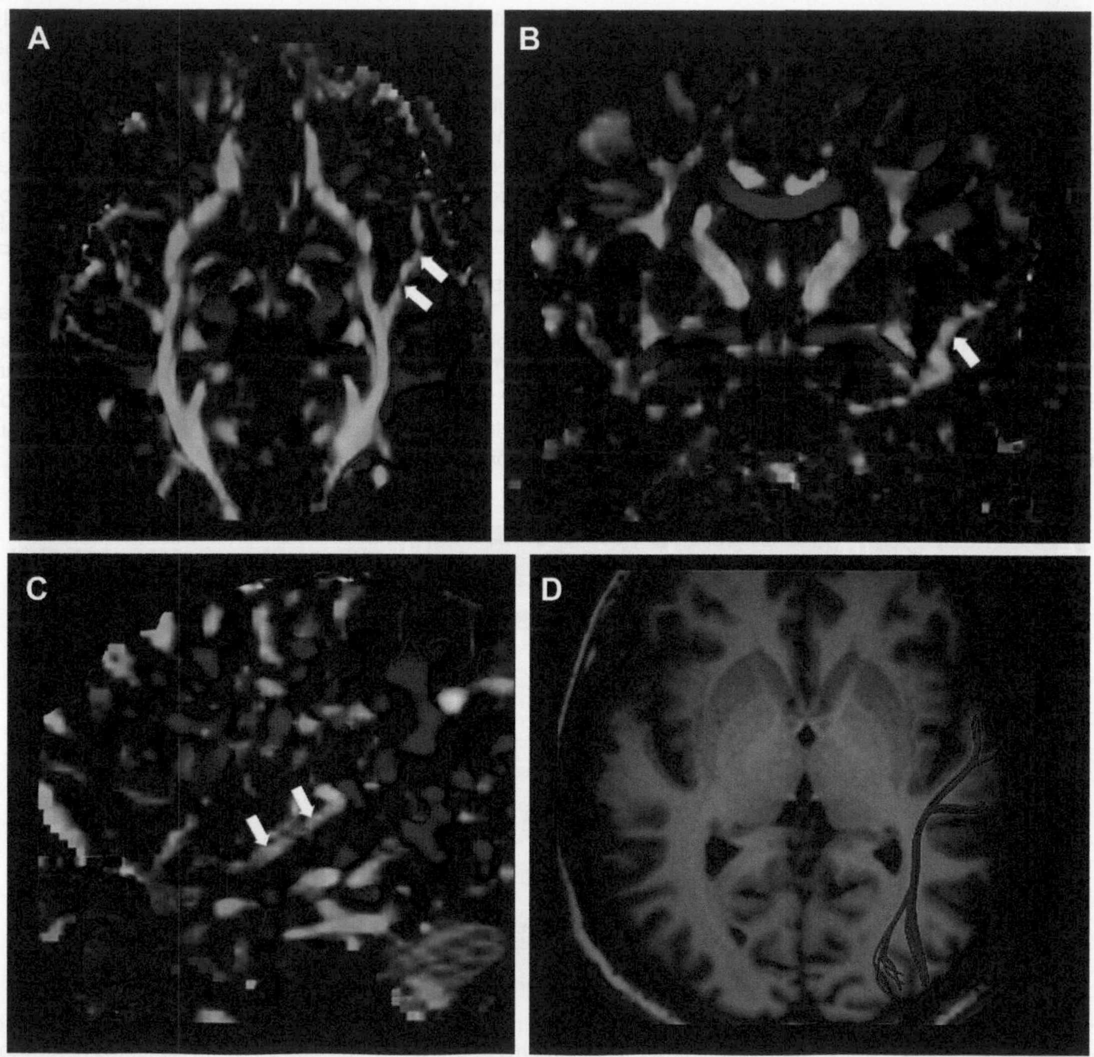

Fig. 7. Trajectory of the middle longitudinal fasciculus (MdLF) indicated by arrows in the axial (*A*), coronal (*B*), and sagittal (*C*) planes. Trajectory of the left MdLF superimposed on an axial T1 weighted image (*D*).

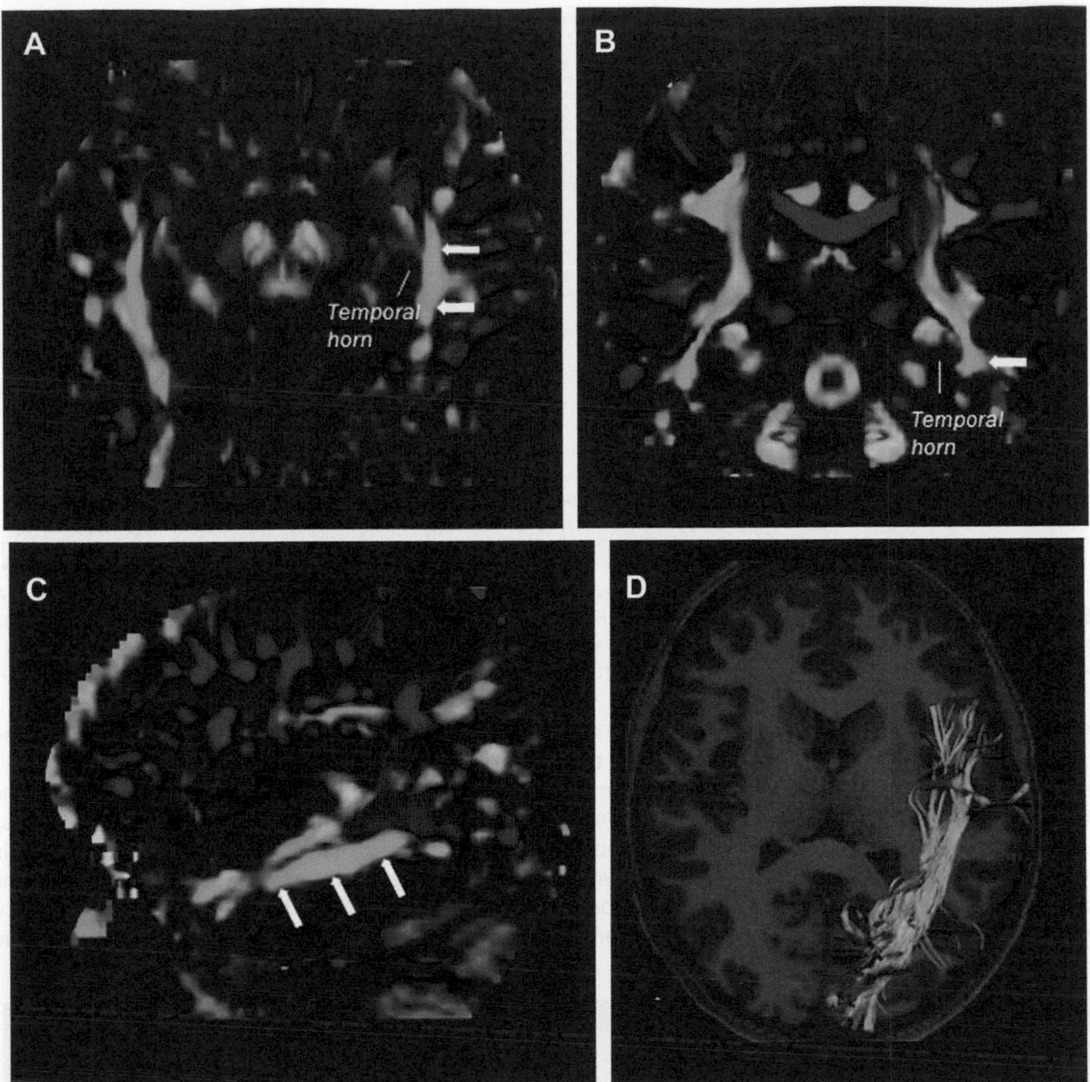

Fig. 8. Trajectory of the inferior longitudinal fasciculus (ILF) indicated by arrows in the axial (*A*), coronal (*B*), and sagittal (*C*) planes. The ILF courses just lateral to the temporal horn of the lateral ventricle (*A* and *B*). DTI tractography (*D*) depicting the left ILF overlaid on a T1 weighted image. (Image D is courtesy of A Conner, MD and C O'Neal, MD, Oklahoma City, Oklahoma.)

identifiable on color-coded FA images as a high anisotropic WM bundle that courses lateral to the temporal horn (see Figs. 8A and B).

The ILF is involved in the ventral visual stream which is critical for face and object recognition, and its disruption has been linked to visual agnosia and prosapagnosia.[32,33]

Superior Fronto-occipital Fasciculus

The SFOF is well documented to connect the frontal and occipital lobes in monkeys. Based on fiber dissection techniques, Türe and colleagues,[34] as early as 1997, proposed that the SFOF did not exist in humans. However, it was not until 2015 when Meola and colleagues confirmed that prior imaging reconstructions of the SFOF in humans were generated by false continuations between the superior and posterior thalamic peduncles and stria terminalis.[35] Similarly, Bao and colleagues were unable to localize the SFOF in fiber dissection studies.[36]

Inferior Fronto-occipital Fasciculus

The IFOF connects primarily the inferior frontal lobe with the parietal and occipital lobes. From the inferior frontal lobe at the opercular region,

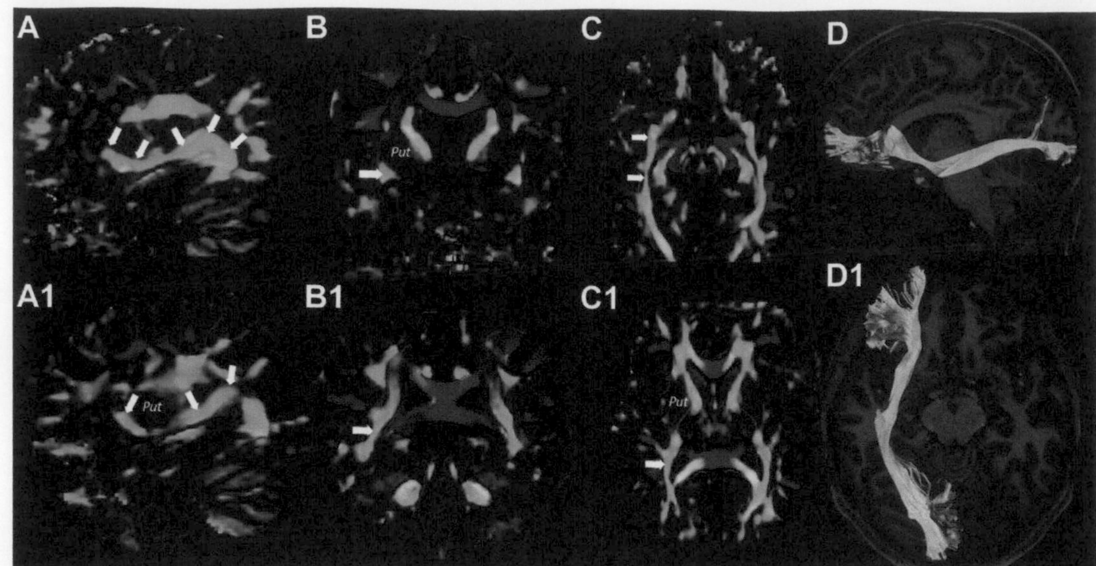

Fig. 9. Trajectory of the inferior fronto-occipital fasciculus (IFOF) indicated by arrows in the sagittal (*A*), coronal (*B*), and axial (*C*) planes. Note *"S-shape"* of the IFOF on sagittal images (*A* and *D*). The IFOF courses inferolateral to the putamen *(Put)* on the coronal plane (*B*). DTI tractography (D and D1) depicting the right IFOF overlaid on T1 weighted images. (Images D and D1 are courtesy of A Conner, MD and C O'Neal, MD, Oklahoma City, Oklahoma.)

the IFOF courses medial to the insula via the external and extreme capsules, forms part of the temporal stem and the sagittal stratum, and terminates in the parietal and occipital lobes (Fig. 9).[37] Anterior projections to the lateral and medial fronto-orbital gyri and the middle frontal gyrus have also been described; whereas posterior projections terminate in the middle and inferior occipital gyri, lingual gyrus, with some fibers also projecting in the temporal and parietal lobes.[38,39]

The IFOF can be identified in the coronal plane as a high anisotropic WM bundle that courses just inferolateral to the putamen (see Fig. 9B). In the temporal stem and the external and extreme capsules, the IFOF is located superior to the uncinate fasciculus (Fig. 10C). On sagittal color-coded

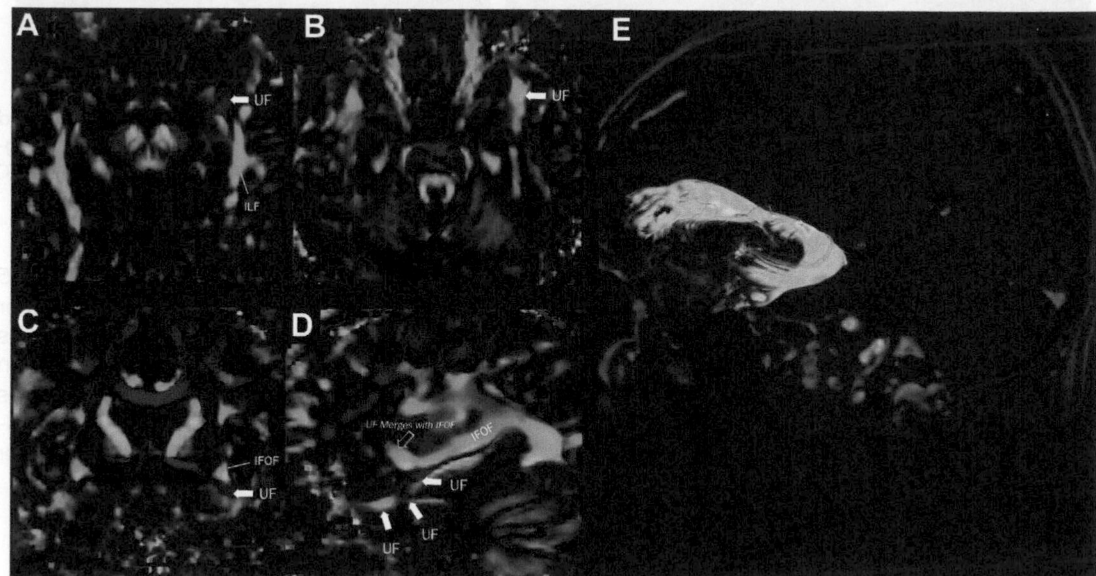

Fig. 10. Trajectory of the uncinate fasciculus (UF) indicated by arrows in the axial (*A* and *B*), coronal (*C*), and sagittal (*D*) planes. DTI tractography (*E*) depicting the right UF overlaid on contrast-enhanced T1 weighted image. (Image E is courtesy of S Kierońska, MD, Bydgoszcz, Poland.)

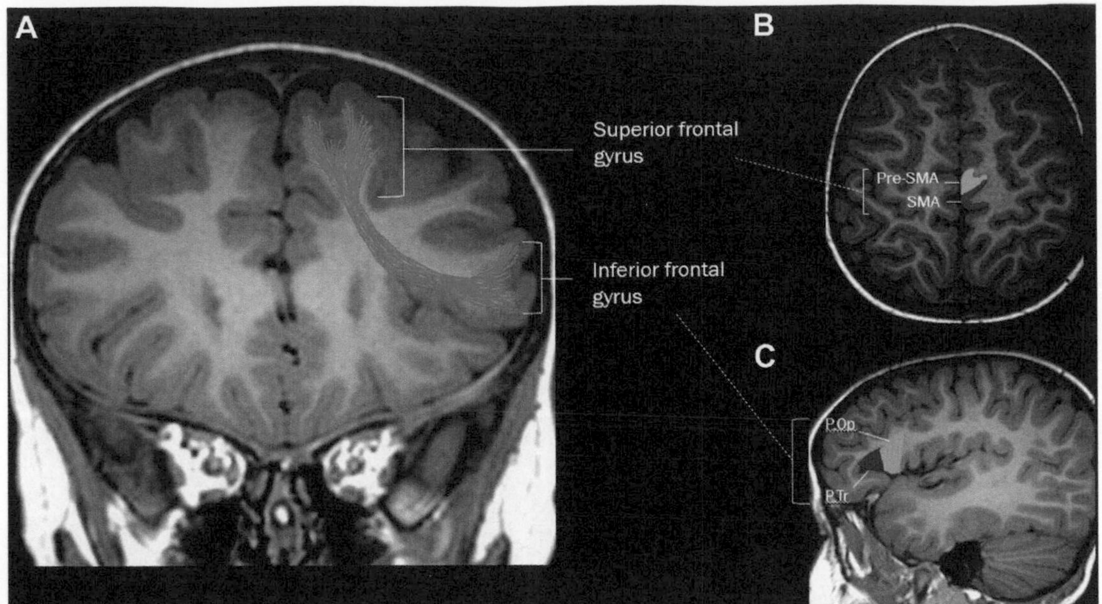

Fig. 11. Trajectory of the frontal aslant tract overlaid on coronal T1 weighted image (*A*). Presupplementary motor area (pre-SMA) and SMA overlaid on axial T1 weighted image (*B*). Pars triangularis (P.Tr) and pars opercularis (P.Op) overlaid on sagittal T1 weighted image (*C*).

DTI images, the IFOF has a characteristic *"S-shape"* (see Fig. 9A).

The IFOF plays a critical role in semantic language processing via the ventral stream, visual recognition system, reading and writing tasks, and goal-oriented behavior.[37]

Uncinate Fasciculus

The UF is a hook shaped bundle of bidirectional fibers that connects the orbitofrontal cortex to the anterior temporal lobes via the temporal stem.[2,40] From the anterior temporal lobe, it gradually curves forming a J-shape as it courses medial to the insula in the external and extreme capsules to eventually terminate in the orbitofrontal gyri (see Fig. 10).[40,41] In the temporal lobe, the UF fibers course anteromedial to the ILF fibers (see Fig. 10A), and in the temporal stem, the UF fibers course inferior to the IFOF fibers (see Fig. 10C). It has been noted to be larger in the right hemisphere where it is associated with emotional understanding and empathy.[42,43] On the left, the UF is known to play a role in language processing.[40]

Frontal Aslant Tract

The FAT (so named on account of its oblique course in the frontal WM) is a recently identified WM bundle that connects the presupplementary motor area (pre-SMA), supplementary motor area (SMA), and lateral aspects of the superior frontal gyrus (SFG) to the pars opercularis and pars triangularis of the inferior frontal gyrus (IFG), as well as the anterior insula (Fig. 11).[44,45] The FAT plays an important role in speech, language, cognitive and executive functions.[44]

COMMISSURAL FIBERS

Commissural fibers connect homologous cortical regions between the two cerebral hemispheres. The major commissural tracts include the corpus callosum, the anterior commissure, and the posterior commissure.

Corpus Callosum

The corpus callosum is the primary commissural tract connecting the cerebral hemispheres and forms the largest WM fiber bundle in the brain (Fig. 12). The anterior section of the corpus callosum is formed by the rostrum and genu, the middle section comprises the body and the posterior section is represented by the isthmus and splenium. The fibers are most dense in the genu, decrease in density toward the isthmus, and increase in density again in the splenium. Anatomic and functional topographic representation of the different cortical areas is demonstrated in the CC, and this is reflected in fiber composition. For instance, large diameter fibers traversing the posterior body, isthmus, and splenium represent sensory fibers carrying information at high speed, whereas small fibers that connect association

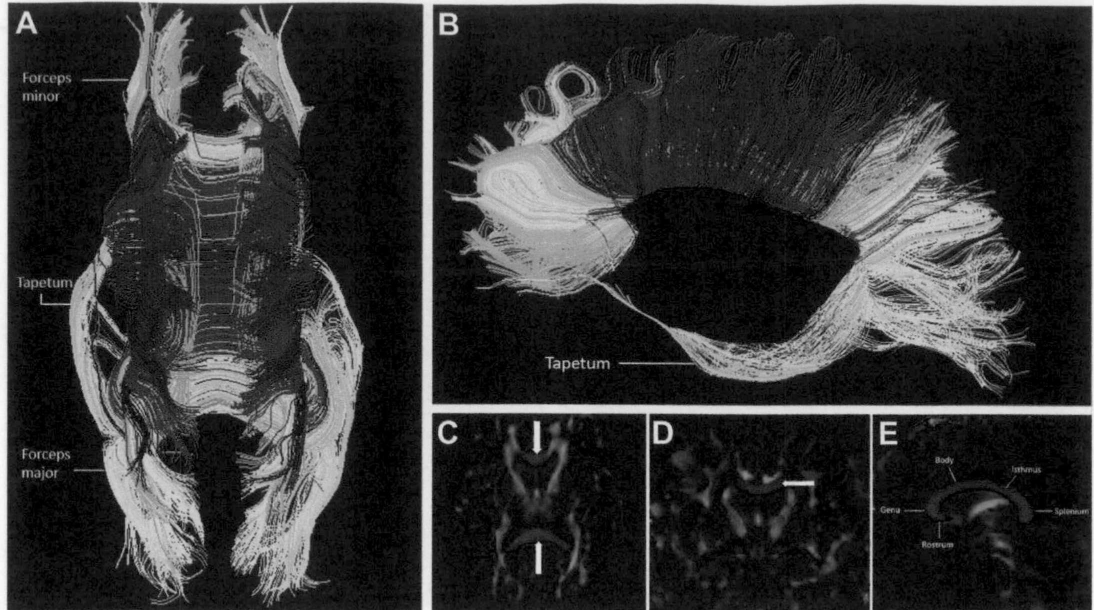

Fig. 12. 3D DTI tractography depicting the corpus callosum from above (*A*), and from the side (*B*). Note fibers of the minor forceps, tapetum, and major forceps and their relationship to the genu, temporal horns, and splenium, respectively. Trajectory of the corpus callosum in the axial (*C*), coronal (*D*), and sagittal (*E*) planes.

cortical areas traverse the rostrum, genu, and anterior body.[46] Although no clear demarcation exists between the segments of the corpus callosum, it can be divided into the following based on morphology and topography (see Fig. 12E).

Rostrum: The rostrum represents the anteroinferior part of the corpus callosum. It forms the floor of the frontal horn and is contiguous caudally with the lamina terminalis. It is usually the thinnest portion of the CC and connects the orbital surfaces of the frontal lobes.

Genu: The anterior bend of the corpus callosum is formed by the genu, the fibers of which curve forward as *forceps minor* (see Fig. 12A) connecting the medial and lateral surfaces of the frontal lobes.

Body: The bulk of the corpus callosum is formed by the body, the fibers of which pass laterally intersecting with the projection fibers of the corona radiata, and connect wide areas of the cerebral hemispheres.

Isthmus: The isthmus represents the normal constriction of the corpus callosum at the junction of the body and the splenium, and carries primary motor, somatosensory and auditory fibers.

Splenium: The splenium forms the posterior most part of the corpus callosum, and consists primarily of visual and association temporo-occipital and parietal commissural fibers. The *tapetum* (see Figs. 12A and B) is formed by fibers of the body and splenium that course around the lateral wall of the ventricular trigones and posterior horns of the lateral ventricles. The fibers interconnecting the occipital lobes curve posteriorly from the splenium forming the *forceps major* (see Fig. 12A).

Anterior Commissure

The anterior commissure contains decussating olfactory fibers that connect the olfactory bulb, anterior olfactory nucleus, and the anterior perforated substance. It also connects homologous structures of the temporal lobe, that is, the amygdala; the inferior temporal, parahippocampal, and fusiform gyri; and the inferior occipital cortex.[2]

It is represented by a compact WM tract that traverses anterior to the fornix, within the anterior wall of the third ventricle (Fig. 13). As it courses laterally, it splits into 2 bundles: an anterior bundle that connects the anterior perforated substance and olfactory tract; and a posterior bundle that fans out into the temporal lobes (see Fig. 18B).

Given its connections, the anterior commissure plays important roles in olfaction, memory, instinct, and emotion.

Posterior Commissure

The posterior commissure is a small tract that courses along the posterior wall of the third ventricle in the posterior pineal lamina to connect the midbrain, thalamus, and hypothalamus (see Fig. 13). It is postulated to play a role in the visual

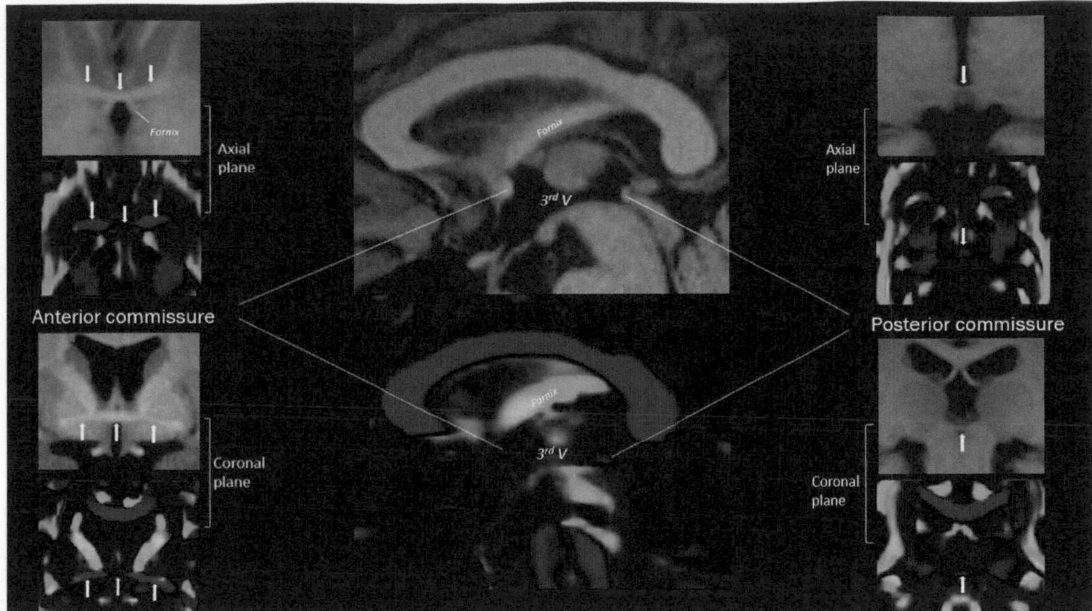

Fig. 13. Anterior and posterior commissures.

system, including the pathway for vertical gaze via reciprocal connections with the superior colliculi.[47]

Hippocampal Commissure

The hippocampal commissure contains decussating fibers of the fornix that travel to the contralateral side immediately below the posterior body and splenium of the corpus callosum and is often indistinguishable from the latter on conventional sequences. Fig. 15G shows the hippocampal commissure reconstructed via 3D tractography.

OTHER WHITE MATTER STRUCTURES

White Matter Tracts of the Limbic System

The limbic system comprises a group of cortical structures and interconnected nuclei that support a variety of functions, including emotion, memory and behavior.[8] The 3 major WM tracts of the limbic system are the cingulum, fornix, and stria terminalis. Each of these tracts forms a C-shaped loop in the sagittal plane. Depending on their connectivity, the limbic WM tracts can be classified as either association, projection, or commissural tracts.

Cingulum

The cingulum comprises of short and long association fibers that interconnect the cingulate gyrus and medial aspects of the frontal, parietal and temporal lobes with other brain areas, particularly the hippocampus.[48] From the orbital frontal cortex (at a level just below the rostrum of the corpus callosum), it courses along the dorsal surface of the corpus callosum before traversing down the temporal lobe toward the anterior temporal pole,[2,48] thereby forming a near-complete ring in the sagittal plane (Fig. 14). Many short *"U-fibers"* interlink the medial parts of the cerebral hemisphere along its sagittal course.[48] A number of classification systems for the cingulum have been described, based on its relationship with the splenium (dorsal and ventral bundles), and based on its longitudinal relationship with the corpus callosum (subgenual, anterior cingulate, midcingulate, retrosplenial, and parahippocampal subdivisions) (Figure 14E).[48] The cingulum plays vital roles in emotion and motivation as part of the limbic system, in executive function, and memory.

Fornix

The origins of the fornix can be traced to the alveus, which comprises of WM projections arising predominantly from the pyramidal cells of the hippocampus. The alveus courses posteriorly under the ependymal surface of the lateral ventricle to form the fimbria. At the level caudal to the splenium of the corpus callosum, the fimbria emerges from the hippocampus to form the crus of the fornix (Fig. 15A). Crura from either side project anterosuperiorly to course beneath the corpus callosum (see Fig. 15B). The crura connect with each other across the midline via the hippocampal commissure (see Fig. 15G). Beyond the hippocampal commissure, the crura join to form the

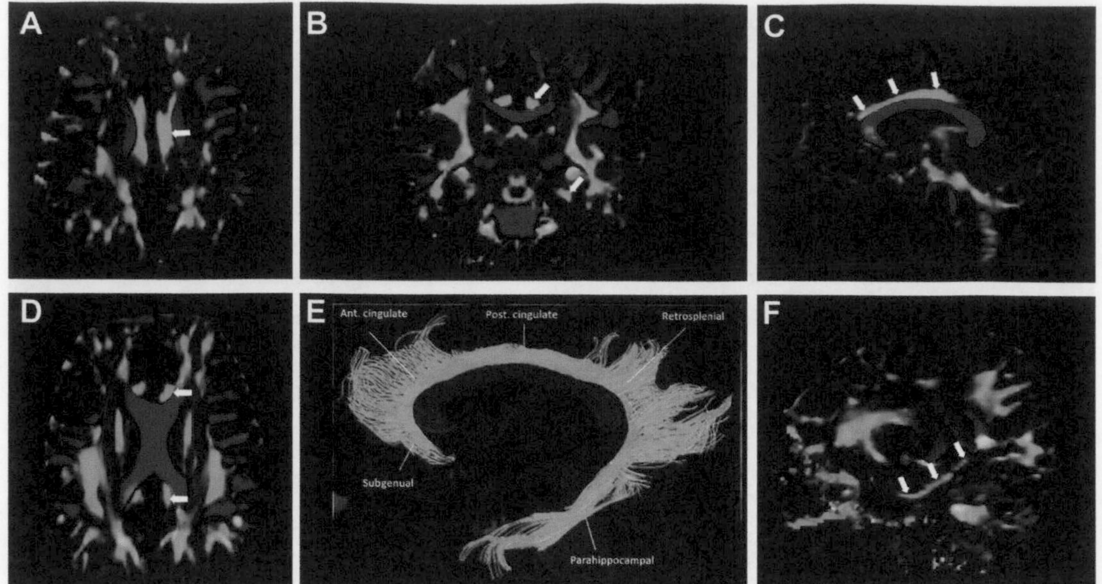

Fig. 14. Trajectory of the cingulum indicated by arrows in the axial (*A,D*), coronal (*B*), and sagittal (*C, F*) planes. Trajectory and subcomponents of the cingulum overlaid on a sagittal T1 weighted image (*E*).

body of the fornix which courses anteriorly beneath the septum pellucidum (see Fig. 15C). At the level of the foramen of Monro, the forniceal body bifurcates into the right and left forniceal columns, which descend inferiorly, and divide at the level of the anterior commissure into the precommissural and the postcommissural fibers (see Figs. 15E and F). The precommissural fibers comprise mainly fibers originating in the pyramidal cell layer of the hippocampus and terminate in the septal area and basal forebrain; whereas the postcommissural fibers arise from the subiculum of the hippocampus and terminate in the mammillary bodies and anterior nuclei of the thalamus.[49] Given

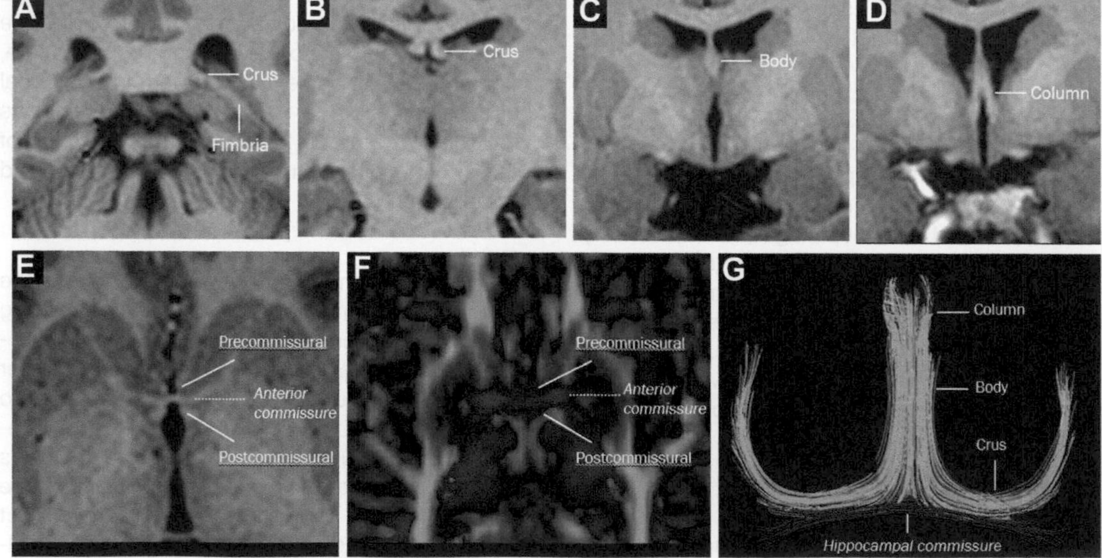

Fig. 15. Trajectory of the fornix from posterior to anterior levels in the coronal plane (*A–D*). Axial T1 weighted image (*E*) and axial color-coded FA image (*F*) show the relationship of the pre and postcommissural fibers of the fornix to the anterior commissure. 3D DTI tractography shows the course and components of the fornix along with the hippocampal commissure (*G*).

that the fornix begins as a projection tract but also forms an important commissural component at its body, it can be classified as both a projection and commissural tract.[49]

Stria terminalis

The stria terminalis (ST) provides afferent and efferent pathways between the amygdala and the hypothalamus as well as the septal nuclei.[2,50,51] Fibers of the ST arise from the amygdala and ascend superolateral to the fimbria and crus of fornix along the superior margin of the temporal horn of the lateral ventricle. After ascending to the level of the atrium, the ST turns in the frontal direction and courses medial to the caudate nucleus and rostral to the thalamus (Fig 16). The ST then courses in the caudothalamic groove reaching the level of the anterior commissure at which point it branches into multiple hypothalamic and septal nuclei.[51]

Major White Matter Conduits

The WM "*conduits*" are comprised of different WM tracts that travel in close contiguity and occupy similar positions and directions in space, thereby forming important anatomic landmarks. Involvement of these conduits or WM *"crossroads,"* therefore, often leads to multiple functional deficits related to the tracts that traverse them. We describe these further below.

Corona radiata

The corona radiata represents the caudal continuum of the centrum semiovale and comprises most of the cortico-afferent and cortico-efferent tracts and commissural fibers (Fig. 2).

Internal capsule

The internal capsules are paired WM structures that serve as the main conduit for projection fibers. It comprises of tightly packed ascending and descending fiber tracts that course between the head of the caudate nucleus, thalamus, and the lentiform nucleus, forming a V shaped structure with its apex directed medially. The internal capsule can be subdivided into the anterior limb, genu, posterior limb, retrolenticular, and sublenticular segments (Fig 17).

The anterior limb courses between the head of the caudate nucleus and the lentiform nucleus, and contains fibers of the anterior thalamic radiation and the frontopontine fibers. In addition, the anterior limb contains transversely oriented fibers that connect the caudate nucleus and the putamen (the caudolenticular gray bridges). The apex of the internal capsule at the junction of the anterior and posterior limbs is formed by the genu, which contains corticobulbar and corticoreticular tracts and some fibers of the superior thalamic radiation. The posterior limb of the internal capsule is bounded by the thalamus medially and the lentiform nucleus laterally, and contains fibers of the corticospinal, corticorubral, and corticopontine tracts, and the posterior thalamic radiation. The retrolenticular segment represents the portion of the internal capsule situated dorsal to the posterior margin of the lentiform nucleus, and contains fibers of the optic radiation, parietopontine, and occipitopontine fibers. The sublenticular segment courses inferior to the lentiform nucleus and is comprised of the auditory radiation, temporopontine fibers, and the inferior thalamic radiation.

External and extreme capsules

The thin sheet of WM that traverses between the putamen and claustrum is the external capsule; whereas the extreme capsule courses between the claustrum and the insular cortex (Fig. 17C). The external and extreme capsules serve as conduits for association fibers (external capsule-SLF, IFOF, and UF; extreme capsule-IFOF and UF).

Temporal stem

The temporal stem is a WM conduit that bridges the temporal lobe with the frontal lobe, corpus striatum, thalamus, hypothalamus, and septal

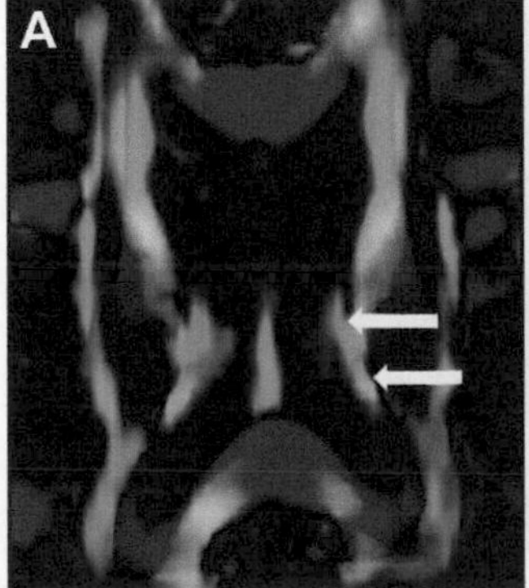

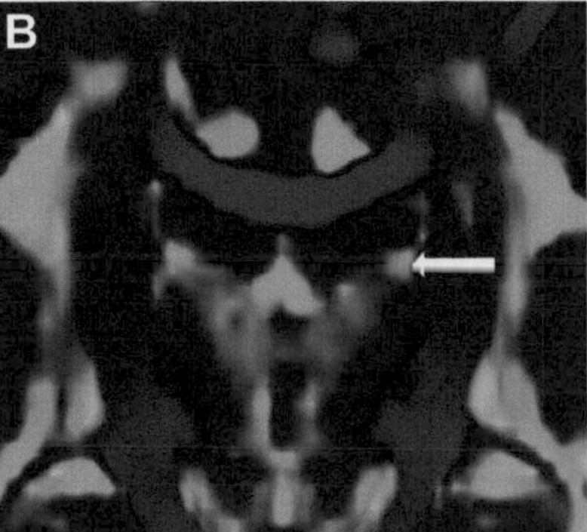

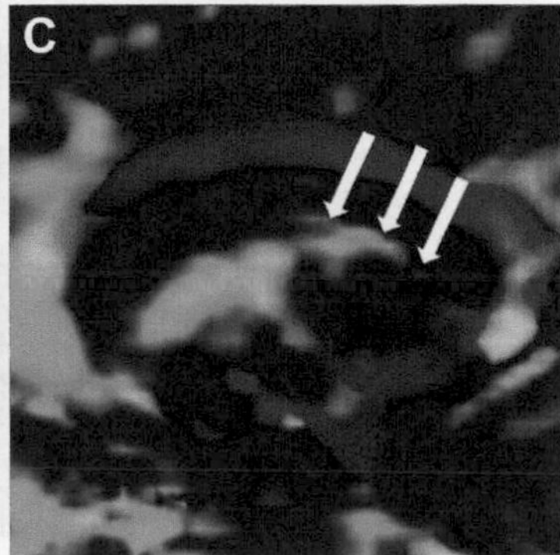

Fig. 16. Trajectory of the stria terminalis indicated by arrows in the axial (*A*), coronal (*B*), and sagittal (*C*) planes.

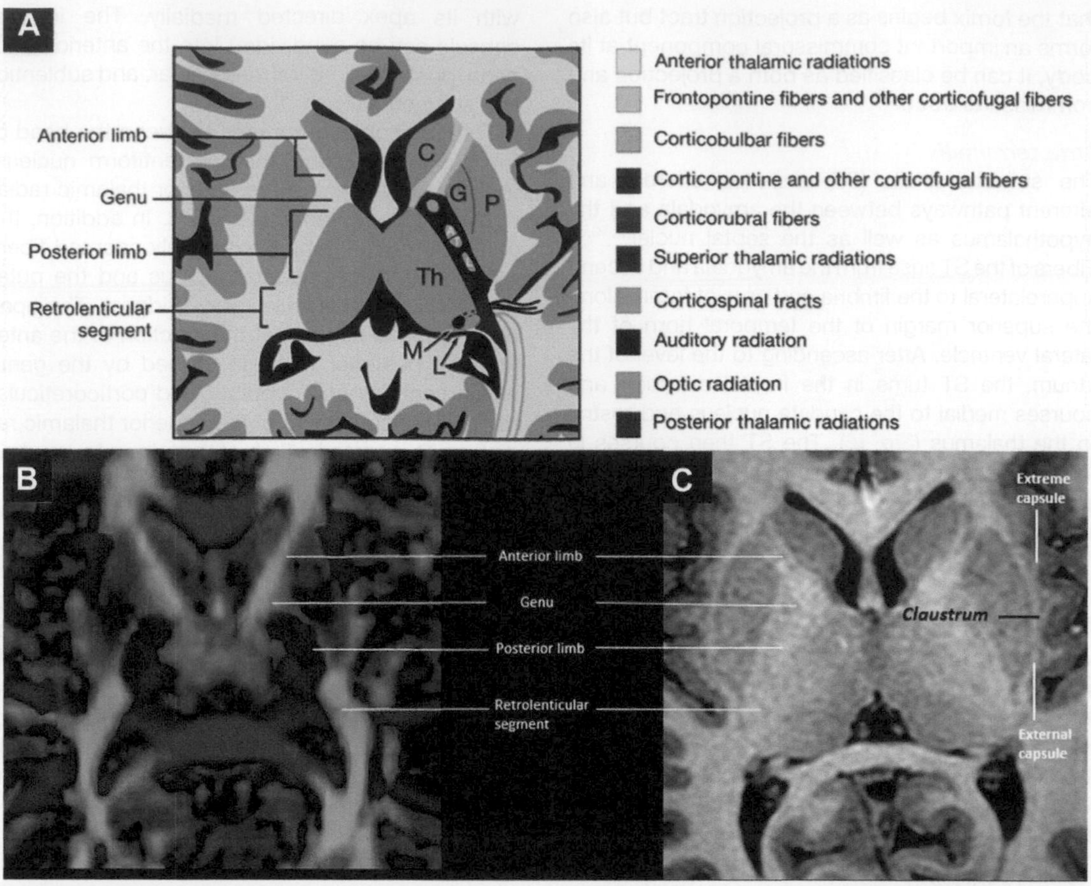

Fig. 17. Schematic diagram depicting the components of the internal capsule and various tracts that pass through it (*A*). Axial color-coded FA image (*B*) and axial T1 weighted image (*C*) shows the internal, external, and extreme capsules. Note relationship of the external and extreme capsules with the claustrum (*C*).

region. In coronal images, the temporal stem can be identified as the WM structure between the circular sulcus of the insula and the superolateral margin of the temporal horn (**Fig. 18**).[52] The major WM tracts that form the temporal stem include the IFOF, the UF, posterior bundle of the anterior commissure, and Meyer's loop of the optic radiation (see **Fig. 18**B).[52]

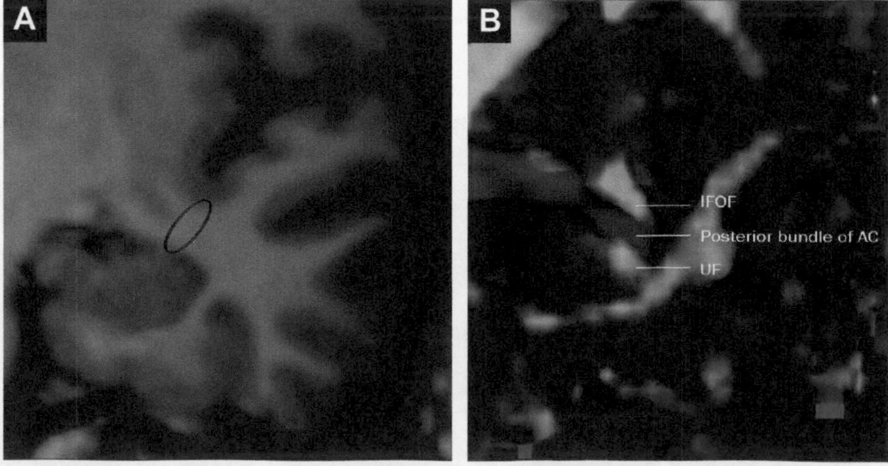

Fig. 18. Coronal T1 weighted shows the left temporal stem (*A*). Color-coded FA image at the same level shows the component tracts of the temporal stem (*B*).

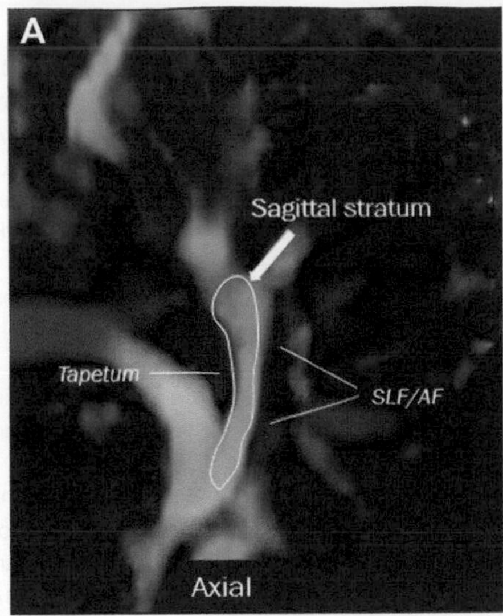

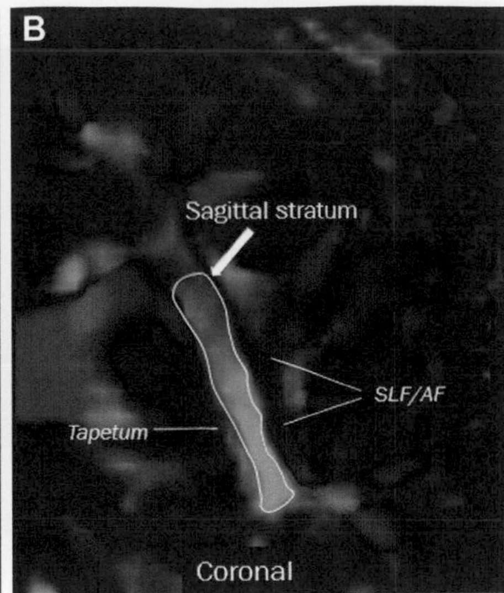

Fig. 19. Axial (*A*) and coronal (*B*) color-coded FA images show the sagittal stratum which is bound by the tapetum medially and the SLF/AF laterally.

Sagittal stratum

The sagittal stratum (SS) is a WM structure that courses lateral to the ventricular trigone (Fig. 19). The superficial layer of the SS is formed by the MdLF and ILF, the middle layer is formed by the IFOF, and the deep layer is formed predominantly by the optic radiations.[29,53] The SS can be identified on color-coded FA images as a polygonal shaped WM structure that is bounded medially by the tapetum, and laterally by the fibers of the SLF/AF (see Fig. 19).

Cerebral peduncle

The cerebral peduncles lie at the junction of the supratentorial and infratentorial compartments, thereby forming an important crossroad for long projection tracts such as the corticospinal, corticobulbar, and corticopontine fibers (see Figs. 2 and 3).

CLINICS CARE POINTS 1: LIMITATIONS OF DIFFUSION TENSOR IMAGING

- Cannot distinguish afferent from efferent tracts.
- Cannot trace the trajectory of specific axons, rather provides a macroscopic delineation of tract configurations.
- In a pixel that contains a dominant population of one tract intermixed with smaller population of another tract, the DTI results typically only provide information for the dominant tract.
- If two tracts within a pixel are of equal population but with differing orientations, the result is lower anisotropy, which can lead to a false premature termination of the tract.

CLINICS CARE POINTS 2

- In axon path finding disorders (eg, Joubert syndrome and related disorders, horizontal gaze palsy with progressive scoliosis), mutations in certain genes lead to abnormal trajectory of white matter tracts, such as failure of normal decussation of corticospinal tracts and the superior cerebellar peduncles.[54]

CLINICS CARE POINTS 3

- Disruption of thalamocortical function and connectivity contributes to loss of consciousness of patients in vegetative states.[55]
- Structural abnormalities in thalamic radiations have been described in a number of psychiatric disorders such as obsessive-compulsive disorder,[56] anorexia nervosa,[57] and schizophrenia.[17]

CLINICS CARE POINTS 4

- Damage to the Meyer loop during surgery can result in homonymous upper quadrantanopia, which occurs in 15% to 90% of cases following anterior temporal lobectomies.[58]

CLINICS CARE POINTS 5

- Agenesis of the corpus callosum may be partial or complete and may result from inherited or acquired (infection, ischemia) etiologies. Affected individuals may present with a range of deficits, depending on the severity and associated malformations, and can include sensorimotor deficits, language and developmental delay, cognitive impairment, and seizures.

CLINICS CARE POINTS 6

- The temporal stem plays an important role in seizure propagation and in the spread of infection and tumors.[2]
- Transection of the temporal stem during surgery may result in quadrantanopia or hemianopia.[52]
- Precise knowledge of the sagittal stratum is vital for surgical approaches to the ventricular atrium and in temporal lobectomies, for example, preservation of the optic radiations and posterior portion of the ILF is typically performed during surgery as these can result in severe visual deficits and reading disorders, respectively.[53]
- The cerebral peduncles serve as an important pathway for the spread of aggressive gliomas from the thalamus to the brainstem and vice versa.

DISCLOSURE

The authors have nothing to disclose.

ACKNOWLEDGMENTS

Asthik Biswas and Logi Vidarsson are partially funded by Ontasian Imaging Laboratory (OIL), Toronto.

REFERENCES

1. Mandonnet E, Sarubbo S, Petit L. The nomenclature of human white matter association pathways: proposal for a systematic taxonomic anatomical classification. Front Neuroanat 2018;12:94.
2. Wycoco V, Shroff M, Sudhakar S, et al. White matter anatomy: what the radiologist needs to know. Neuroimaging Clin N Am 2013;23(2):197–216.
3. Ramos-Fresnedo A, Segura-Duran I, Chaichana KL, et al. Chapter 2 - supratentorial white matter tracts. In: Chaichana K, Quiñones-Hinojosa A, editors. Comprehensive overview of modern surgical approaches to intrinsic brain tumors. Academic Press; 2019. p. 23–35. https://doi.org/10.1016/B978-0-12-811783-5.00002-1.
4. Dum RP, Strick PL. The origin of corticospinal projections from the premotor areas in the frontal lobe. J Neurosci 1991;11(3):667–89.
5. Jane JA, Yashon D, DeMyer W, et al. The contribution of the precentral gyrus to the pyramidal tract of man. J Neurosurg 1967;26(2):244–8.
6. Kwon HG, Hong JH, Jang SH. Anatomic location and somatotopic arrangement of the corticospinal tract at the cerebral peduncle in the human brain. AJNR Am J Neuroradiol 2011;32(11):2116–9.
7. Martin JH. The corticospinal system: from development to motor control. Neuroscientist 2005;11(2):161–73.
8. Wakana S, Jiang H, Nagae-Poetscher LM, et al. Fiber tract-based atlas of human white matter anatomy. Radiology 2004;230(1):77–87.
9. Waragai M, Watanabe H, Iwabuchi S. The somatotopic localisation of the descending cortical tract in the cerebral peduncle: a study using MRI of changes following Wallerian degeneration in the cerebral peduncle after a supratentorial vascular lesion. Neuroradiology 1994;36(5):402–4.
10. Hong JH, Son SM, Jang SH. Somatotopic location of corticospinal tract at pons in human brain: a diffusion tensor tractography study. Neuroimage 2010;51(3):952–5.
11. Kwon HG, Hong JH, Lee MY, et al. Somatotopic arrangement of the corticospinal tract at the medullary pyramid in the human brain. Eur Neurol 2011;65(1):46–9.
12. Angstmann S, Madsen KS, Skimminge A, et al. Microstructural asymmetry of the corticospinal tracts predicts right–left differences in circle drawing skill in right-handed adolescents. Brain Struct Funct 2016;221(9):4475–89.
13. Kumar A, Juhasz C, Asano E, et al. Diffusion tensor imaging study of the cortical origin and course of the corticospinal tract in healthy children. AJNR Am J Neuroradiol 2009;30(10):1963–70.
14. Bhardwaj N, Yadala S. Neuroanatomy, corticobulbar tract. In: StatPearls. StatPearls Publishing; 2021. Available at: http://www.ncbi.nlm.nih.gov/books/NBK555891/. Accessed October 4, 2021.
15. Rea P. Chapter 10 - Brainstem Tracts. In: Rea P, editor. Essential clinical anatomy of the nervous system. Academic Press; 2015. p. 177–92.
16. Kamali A, Kramer LA, Frye RE, et al. Diffusion tensor tractography of the human brain cortico-ponto-cerebellar pathways: a quantitative preliminary study. J Magn Reson Imaging 2010;32(4):809–17.

17. George K, Das MJ. Neuroanatomy, thalamocortical radiations. In: StatPearls. StatPearls Publishing; 2021. Available at: http://www.ncbi.nlm.nih.gov/books/NBK546699/. Accessed September 2, 2021.
18. Párraga RG, Ribas GC, Welling LC, et al. Microsurgical anatomy of the optic radiation and related fibers in 3-dimensional images. Oper Neurosurg 2012;71(suppl_1):ons160–72.
19. Petrides M, Pandya DN. Projections to the frontal cortex from the posterior parietal region in the rhesus monkey. J Comp Neurol 1984;228(1):105–16.
20. Wang X, Pathak S, Stefaneanu L, et al. Subcomponents and connectivity of the superior longitudinal fasciculus in the human brain. Brain Struct Funct 2016;221(4):2075–92.
21. Nakajima R, Kinoshita M, Shinohara H, et al. The superior longitudinal fascicle: reconsidering the fronto-parietal neural network based on anatomy and function. Brain Imaging Behav 2020;14(6):2817–30.
22. Dick AS, Tremblay P. Beyond the arcuate fasciculus: consensus and controversy in the connectional anatomy of language. Brain 2012;135(12):3529–50.
23. Makris N, Preti MG, Wassermann D, et al. Human middle longitudinal fascicle: segregation and behavioral-clinical implications of two distinct fiber connections linking temporal pole and superior temporal gyrus with the angular gyrus or superior parietal lobule using multi-tensor tractography. Brain Imaging Behav 2013;7(3):335–52.
24. Kalyvas A, Koutsarnakis C, Komaitis S, et al. Mapping the human middle longitudinal fasciculus through a focused anatomo-imaging study: shifting the paradigm of its segmentation and connectivity pattern. Brain Struct Funct 2020;225(1):85–119.
25. Latini F, Trevisi G, Fahlström M, et al. New insights into the anatomy, connectivity and clinical implications of the middle longitudinal fasciculus. Front Neuroanat 2021;14:106.
26. Maldonado IL, Champfleur NM de, Velut S, et al. Evidence of a middle longitudinal fasciculus in the human brain from fiber dissection. J Anat 2013;223(1):38–45.
27. Wang Y, Fernández-Miranda JC, Verstynen T, et al. Rethinking the role of the middle longitudinal fascicle in language and auditory pathways. Cereb Cortex 2013;23(10):2347–56.
28. Herbet G, Zemmoura I, Duffau H. Functional anatomy of the inferior longitudinal fasciculus: from historical reports to current hypotheses. Front Neuroanat 2018;12:77.
29. Di Carlo DT, Benedetto N, Duffau H, et al. Microsurgical anatomy of the sagittal stratum. Acta neurochirurgica 2019;161(11):2319–27.
30. Latini F, Mårtensson J, Larsson EM, et al. Segmentation of the inferior longitudinal fasciculus in the human brain: A white matter dissection and diffusion tensor tractography study. Brain Res 2017;1675:102–15.
31. Panesar SS, Yeh FC, Jacquesson T, et al. A Quantitative Tractography Study Into the Connectivity, Segmentation and Laterality of the Human Inferior Longitudinal Fasciculus. Front Neuroanat 2018;12:47.
32. Feinberg TE, Schindler RJ, Ochoa E, et al. Associative visual agnosia and alexia without prosopagnosia. Cortex 1994;30(3):395–411.
33. Thomas C, Avidan G, Humphreys K, et al. Reduced structural connectivity in ventral visual cortex in congenital prosopagnosia. Nat Neurosci 2009;12(1):29–31.
34. Türe U, Yaşargil MG, Pait TG. Is there a superior occipitofrontal fasciculus? a microsurgical anatomic study. Neurosurgery 1997;40(6):1226–32.
35. Meola A, Comert A, Yeh FC, et al. The controversial existence of the human superior fronto-occipital fasciculus: Connectome-based tractographic study with microdissection validation. Hum Brain Mapp 2015;36(12):4964–71.
36. Bao Y, Wang Y, Wang W, et al. The superior fronto-occipital fasciculus in the human brain revealed by diffusion spectrum imaging tractography: an anatomical reality or a methodological artifact? Front Neuroanat 2017;11:119.
37. Conner AK, Briggs RG, Sali G, et al. A connectomic atlas of the human cerebrum-chapter 13: tractographic description of the inferior fronto-occipital fasciculus. Oper Neurosurg (Hagerstown) 2018;15(suppl_1):S436–43.
38. Hau J, Sarubbo S, Perchey G, et al. Cortical Terminations of the Inferior Fronto-Occipital and Uncinate Fasciculi: Anatomical Stem-Based Virtual Dissection. Front Neuroanat 2016;10:58.
39. Wu Y, Sun D, Wang Y, et al. Subcomponents and connectivity of the inferior fronto-occipital fasciculus revealed by diffusion spectrum imaging fiber tracking. Front Neuroanat 2016;10:88.
40. Briggs RG, Rahimi M, Conner AK, et al. A connectomic atlas of the human cerebrum-chapter 15: tractographic description of the uncinate fasciculus. Oper Neurosurg (Hagerstown) 2018;15(suppl_1):S450–5.
41. Papagno C, Miracapillo C, Casarotti A, et al. What is the role of the uncinate fasciculus? Surgical removal and proper name retrieval. Brain 2011;134(2):405–14.
42. Oishi K, Faria AV, Hsu J, et al. Critical role of the right uncinate fasciculus in emotional empathy. Ann Neurol 2015;77(1):68–74.
43. Highley JR, Walker MA, Esiri MM, et al. Asymmetry of the uncinate fasciculus: a post-mortem study of normal subjects and patients with schizophrenia. Cereb Cortex 2002;12(11):1218–24.
44. La Corte E, Eldahaby D, Greco E, et al. The frontal aslant tract: a systematic review for neurosurgical applications. Front Neurol 2021;12:51.

45. Dick AS, Garic D, Graziano P, et al. The frontal aslant tract (FAT) and its role in speech, language and executive function. Cortex 2019;111:148–63.
46. Fabri M, Pierpaoli C, Barbaresi P, et al. Functional topography of the corpus callosum investigated by DTI and fMRI. World J Radiol 2014;6(12):895–906.
47. Bhidayasiri R, Plant GT, Leigh RJ. A hypothetical scheme for the brainstem control of vertical gaze. Neurology 2000;54(10):1985–93.
48. Bubb EJ, Metzler-Baddeley C, Aggleton JP. The cingulum bundle: Anatomy, function, and dysfunction. Neurosci Biobehav Rev 2018;92:104–27.
49. Thomas AG, Koumellis P, Dineen RA. The fornix in health and disease: an imaging review. Radiographics 2011;31(4):1107–21.
50. Mori S, Aggarwal M. In vivo magnetic resonance imaging of the human limbic white matter. Front Aging Neurosci 2014;6:321.
51. Kamali A, Yousem DM, Lin DD, et al. Mapping the trajectory of the stria terminalis of the human limbic system using high spatial resolution diffusion tensor tractography. Neurosci Lett 2015;608:45–50.
52. Kier EL, Staib LH, Davis LM, et al. MR imaging of the temporal stem: anatomic dissection tractography of the uncinate fasciculus, inferior occipitofrontal fasciculus, and Meyer's loop of the optic radiation. AJNR Am J Neuroradiol 2004;25(5):677–91.
53. Maldonado IL, Destrieux C, Ribas EC, et al. Composition and organization of the sagittal stratum in the human brain: a fiber dissection study. J Neurosurg 2021;8:1–9. https://doi.org/10.3171/2020.7.JNS192846. Published online January.
54. Welniarz Q, Dusart I, Roze E. The corticospinal tract: evolution, development, and human disorders. Dev Neurobiol 2017;77(7):810–29.
55. Zhou J, Liu X, Song W, et al. Specific and nonspecific thalamocortical functional connectivity in normal and vegetative states. Conscious Cogn 2011;20(2):257–68.
56. Wang R, Fan Q, Zhang Z, et al. Anterior thalamic radiation structural and metabolic changes in obsessive-compulsive disorder: A combined DTI-MRS study. Psychiatry Res Neuroimaging 2018;277:39–44.
57. Frieling H, Fischer J, Wilhelm J, et al. Microstructural abnormalities of the posterior thalamic radiation and the mediodorsal thalamic nuclei in females with anorexia nervosa–a voxel based diffusion tensor imaging (DTI) study. J Psychiatr Res 2012;46(9):1237–42.
58. van Lanen RHGJ, Hoeberigs MC, Bauer NJC, et al. Visual field deficits after epilepsy surgery: a new quantitative scoring method. Acta Neurochir (Wien) 2018;160(7):1325–36.

MRI-Visible Anatomy of the Basal Ganglia and Thalamus

Michael J. Hoch, MD[a], Timothy M. Shepherd, MD, PhD[b,*]

KEYWORDS

• DBS • Diencephalon • FGATIR • Functional neurosurgery • Neuroanatomy • Parkinson's disease • Subthalamic nucleus • Track-density imaging

KEY POINTS

- Functional neurosurgery relies on indirect targeting methods to optimize therapeutic profile and minimize side effects.
- The excellent contrast resolution for deep brain structures provided by the FGATIR sequence allows for better visualization of functional neurosurgery targets.
- Probabilistic tractography methods, such as track density imaging, seem to demonstrate many internal nuclei of the thalamus based on the functional organization of the tissue on a mesoscopic scale.

INTRODUCTION

Diencephalic structures (**Table 1**) are key regulators of autonomic, motor, sensory, limbic, and endocrine functions.[1,2] The basal ganglia and thalamus are critical components in complex recurrent circuits between the cortex and subcortical brain probably best understood for movement disorders,[3] but also relevant to mood, learning and other fundamental aspects of human cognition.[4–6] Pathologic changes in small structures within these complex circuits can have profound clinical impact in multiple cognitive domains. For example, loss of dopaminergic neurons in substantia nigra results in the classic triad of rigidity, tremor, and bradykinesia of Parkinson's disease (PD), but also leads to changes in sleep, mood, weight, and cognition.[7] This neuroanatomy is complex—it is hard to make progress in understanding the functional organization of human subcortical anatomy if we are unable to see basic components in living patients. The rapidly evolving field of functional neurosurgery aims to modulate selected diencephalic structures with deep brain stimulation (DBS) or ablate those targets with MR imaging-guided focused ultrasound for therapeutic benefit. The globus pallidus internus (GPi), subthalamic nucleus (STN) and ventrointermedius nucleus (Vim) are common targets to treat movement disorders.[8] DBS placement within the thalamic structures, like the anterior nucleus, also can reduce seizures in patients with epilepsy.[9]

To understand the best anatomic targets for clinical improvement observed with functional neurosurgery, ideally we need to *directly* visualize the relevant neuroanatomy. However, this is challenging owing to the poor contrast resolution of diencephalic structures with conventional MR imaging. Atlases of the basal ganglia and thalami

[a] Department of Radiology, University of Pennsylvania, 3400 Spruce Street, Suite 130, Philadelphia, PA 19104, USA; [b] Department of Radiology, New York University Langone School of Medicine, 660 First Avenue, Room 226, New York, NY 10016, USA
* Corresponding author.
E-mail address: timothy.shepherd@nyulangone.org
Twitter: @RVUhound (M.J.H.); @tim0shepherd (T.M.S.)

Neuroimag Clin N Am 32 (2022) 529–541
https://doi.org/10.1016/j.nic.2022.05.003

Table 1
List of anatomic assignments of labeled structures in Figures

A	Anterior Nucleus	NA	Nucleus Accumbens
AC	Anterior Commissure	OC	Optic Chiasm
AL	Ansa Lenticularis	OT	Optic Tract
BSC	Brachium of the Superior Colliculus	OTub	Olfactory Tubercle
C	Caudate	PC	Posterior Commissure
Ce	Centromedian Nucleus	Pf	Parafascicularis Nucleus
Cl	Claustrum	Post F	Postcommissural Fornix
CP	Cerebral Peduncle	PPN	Pedunculopontine Nucleus
DBB	Diagonal Band of Broca	Pre F	Precommissural Fornix
Do	Dorsal Oralis Nucleus	PTT	Pallidotegmental Tract
DRT	Dentatorubrothalamic Tract	Pul	Pulvinar Lateralis Nucleus
DSCP	Decussation of the Superior Cerebellar Peduncle	Pum	Pulvinar Medialis Nucleus
EC	External Capsule	Puo	Pulvinar Oralis Nucleus
Ex	Extreme Capsule	Put	Putamen
F	Fornix	RN	Red Nucleus
FF	Forel's Field (H)	SM	Stria Medullaris
GPe	Globus Pallidus Externa	SN	Substantia Nigra
GPi	Globus Pallidus Interna	STF	Subthalamic Fasciculus
Gm	Medial Geniculate Nucleus	STN	Subthalamic Nucleus
H	Habenular Nucleus	TF	Thalamic Fasciculus (H1)
IC	Internal Capsule	Thal	Thalamus
LF	Lenticular Fasciculus (H2)	Vce	Ventrocaudalis Externus Nucleus
Lpo	Lateropolaris Nucleus	Vci	Ventrocaudalis Internus Nucleus
M	Medialis Nucleus	Vim	Ventrointermedius Nucleus
MB	Mammillary Body	Voe	Ventro-oralis Externus Nucleus
ML	Medial Lemniscus	Voi	Ventro-oralis Internus Nucleus
MTT	Mammillothalamic Tract	ZI	Zona Incerta

based on myelin or other histology stains of individual brains[10–12] are difficult to juxtapose onto MR images in individual patients with any spatial accuracy. Group-based atlases based on MR images are helpful, but also do not account for known individual variability.[12,13] The ideal solution is to visualize targets and off-targets for functional neurosurgery directly in the individual patient's brain. While the complete anatomy of the basal forebrain is too detailed to cover in this review, we aim to emphasize the anatomic relationships of the 3 most common targets (GPi, STN, and Vim) in functional neurosurgery with the best available translational MR imaging sequences applicable to patients.

The primate or human brain has a unique flexion in the subthalamic region at the junction between the midbrain and thalamus that may represent an evolutionary adaptation to upright posture or bipedal motion. This makes comparative neuroanatomy and terminology confusing in these regions, especially the terms "ventral" and "dorsal." For example, both the oculomotor nucleus and parafascicularis nucleus of the thalamus are "dorsal" to the red nucleus, but occupy very different positions in 3D space. The terms "cranial" and "caudal" also can create confusion above this flexure. We have avoided these terms except when used for the specific name of a structure. We also clarify the Fields of Forel in relation to the pallidothalamic tracts (a reemerging target for functional neurosurgery in movement disorders). We try to clarify the very confusing nomenclature of the thalamic motor nuclei. Note, clinical MR imaging does not resolve internal anatomy of the hypothalamus, another diencephalic structure, and it is not discussed further due to space limitations. Ultimately, we hope this review can be an effective first reference for trainees and clinicians interested in the basal ganglia and thalamus, particularly regarding current functional neurosurgery applications.

IMAGING THE THALAMUS AND BASAL GANGLIA

Conventional MR imaging poorly depicts internal functional divisions and myelinated tracts within the basal ganglia and thalamus.[14] Functional neurosurgery, therefore, relies on indirect targeting of subcortical structures using measurements of intercommissural distances, third ventricular widths, or other mathematical calculations originally derived from pneumoencephalography (**Table 2**). Stereotactic atlases provide coordinates based on the positions and distances between the anterior and posterior commissures of individual patients even though there is known variability in subcortical nuclei positions across individuals, and sometimes right-left differences in the same individual.[10,12,13] This can result in decreased therapeutic profile and increased risk of side effects.[15] In this review, we explain MR imaging sequence and postprocessing developments over the past ~15 years that have improved our ability to visualize basal ganglia and thalamic anatomy *directly* in patients and research subjects. The basic NYU MR imaging protocol for subcortical anatomy is summarized in our companion chapter on brainstem anatomy. We emphasize sequences that are easy to translate into clinical practice using widely- available 3-T MR imaging systems.

The 3D Fast Gray Matter Acquisition T1 Inversion Recovery (FGATIR) sequence uses a different inversion pulse than MPRAGE (180 vs 90 degrees, and 410 vs 900 ms, respectively) to better suppress the signal from myelinated structures in the subcortical brain. FGATIR was created to improve direct targeting of thalamic nuclei for functional neurosurgery[16] and is now in widespread use for this purpose. We have observed that FGATIR contrast is greatly improved with multiple signal averages (ie, 25–50 minute scan times) or with 7-T acquisitions, but this creates clinical feasibility issues for many practices. We have developed a denoising approach using a convolutional neural network (CNN) trained on multiple average data from controls to improve the image contrast resolution of FGATIR in patients. Single average CNN-denoised FGATIR images appeared equivalent to 3 to 4 averages on quantitative image measurements and subjective rater assessment.[17] The thalamus and basal ganglia images shown here use this new FGATIR protocol with 1 acquired average (~13-min scan time) then CNN-denoising. **Figs. 1–5** and **Fig. 9** demonstrate multiplanar FGATIR images for the potential targets of current or investigational functional neurosurgery. The actual stereotactic coordinates for 3 DBS electrode tip targets in current clinical practice at NYU are depicted with yellow circles—Gpi (**Fig. 1**), STN (**Fig. 4**), and Vim (**Fig. 5**). Note a similar position for the Vim is also targeted for MR imaging-guided focus ultrasound ablation.

Table 2
NYU-Specific Initial Targeting Coordinates for Common Functional Neurosurgery Targets (these will vary slightly between institutions and neurosurgeons)

Structure	Disease	Axial	Coronal	Sagittal	Description of Electrode tip Location
Subthalamic nucleus (STN)	PD	4–5 mm below AC-PC plane	4 mm posterior to mid AC-PC point	10–13 mm lateral to midline	Posterolateral inferior aspect of STN
Ventrointermedius nucleus (Vim)	ET or PD tremor	0–3 mm above AC-PC plane	3/4 posterior to AC along AC-PC line	11 mm lateral to 3rd ventricle wall	Medial to PLIC
Globus pallidus interna (GPi)	PD, dystonia and Tourette's syndrome	4–5 mm below AC-PC plane	2 mm anterior to mid AC-PC point	18–21 mm lateral to midline	Posterior inferior corner of GPi above optic tract

Abbreviations: AC & PC, anterior and posterior commissure; ET, essential tremor; GPi, globus pallidus interna; PD, Parkinson's disease; PLIC, posterior limb internal capsule; STN, subthalamic nucleus.

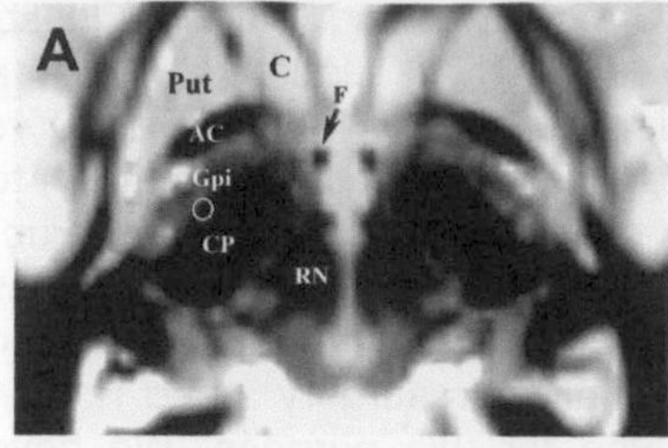

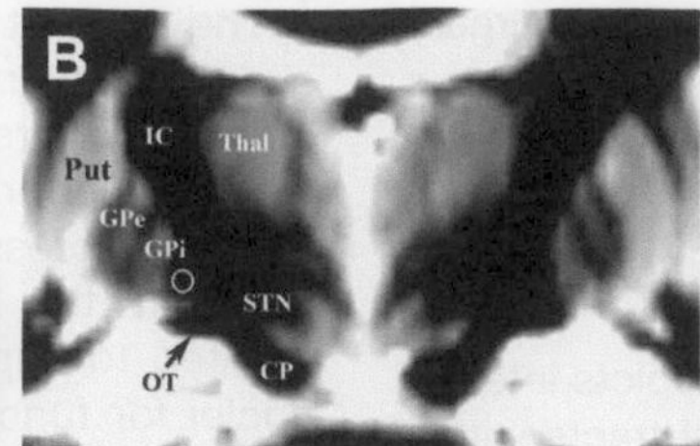

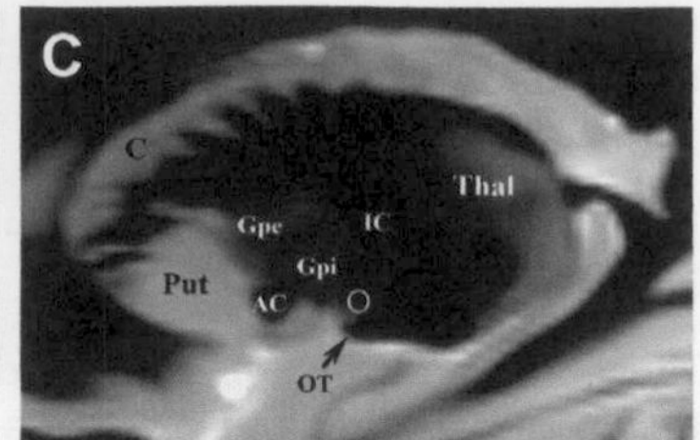

Fig. 1. (*A*) Axial, (*B*) coronal, and (*C*) sagittal FGATIR images showing the globus pallidus interna (GPi) and surrounding structures. The yellow circle represents approximate DBS electrode tip placement in the posterior inferior corner of the GPi just above the optic tract (OT) (see Table 2). If electrode is too medial or posterior in the cerebral peduncle (CP), the patient may experience muscle contractions of the contralateral body. FGATIR can reveal fine lamina separating the putamen, globus pallidus externa and interna on the coronal image.

Diffusion MR imaging also shows great promise for parcellating thalamic nuclei,[18,19] but is signal-to-noise limited such that it is challenging to acquire better than 2 mm isotropic resolution data in most patients—detailed image contrast resolution of internal thalamic features then may be limited by partial volume effects. Alternatively, super-resolution of the acquired data can be generated by postprocessing analysis of probabilistic tractography. We have explored one such method called Track Density Imaging (TDI)[20] in the human thalamus.[21] High angular resolution diffusion-weighted MR imaging sequence was acquired (3 mm isotropic resolution, 2-slice acceleration, iPAT = 2, TR/TE = 3300/99 ms, 8 averages without diffusion weighting, monopolar diffusion gradients with b-value = 2500 s/mm^2 with 256 directions) over a 15 min acquisition. To generate the track-density maps, whole-brain probabilistic fiber tracking was performed by randomly seeding 4,000,000 tracks throughout the brain using MRtrix software package (Brain Research Institute, Melbourne, Australia).[20] The constrained spherical deconvolution (CSD) technique[22] was used to model multiple fiber orientations. The relevant fiber tracking parameters were: 0.2 mm stepsize, 20° maximum angle between steps, 1 cm minimum track length, maximum harmonic order lmax = 8 and with track termination criteria if track exited the brain or when the CSD fiber orientation distribution amplitude was less than 0.1. Super-resolution TDI and direction-encoded color track density (DEC-TDI) maps were generated by calculating the total number of tracks present in each element of a 500 μm isotropic grid.

NORMAL ANATOMY

Basal Ganglia - Globus Pallidus Interna (GPi) and Pallidothalamic Tracts

The best-understood function of the basal ganglia (caudate, putamen, and globus pallidus) is to regulate motor control. The globus pallidus is separated by a thin internal medullary lamina into the

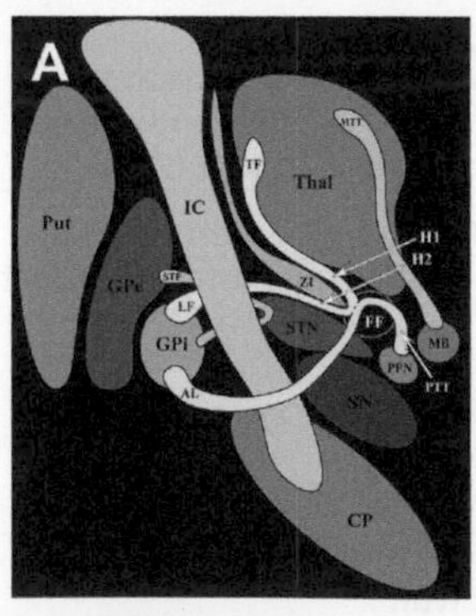

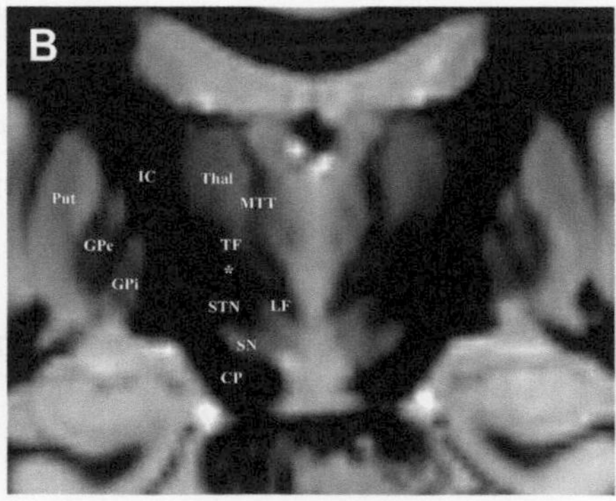

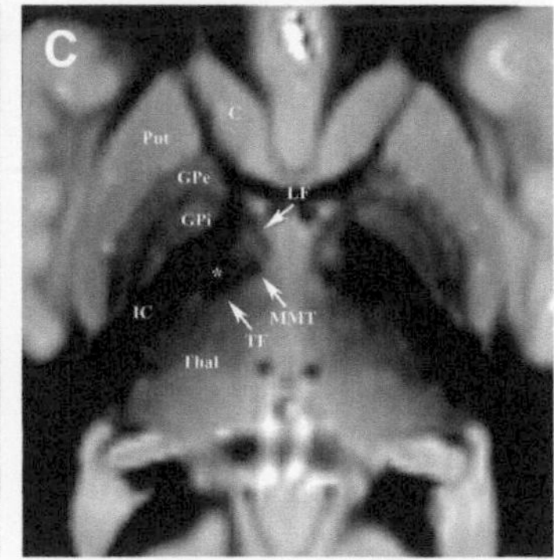

Fig. 2. (*A*) Coronal schematic showing the complex relationships of the pallidothalamic tracts and the Fields of Forel. The Lenticular fasciculus (H2) joins the Ansa lenticularis in the Forel's Field H and becomes the Thalamic fasciculus (H1) which projects to the motor thalamus. The subthalamic fasciculus (STF) and mammillothalamic tract (MTT) are also shown. Oblique coronal FGATIR (*B*) (9° anterosuperior to posteroinferior) and (*C*) oblique axial FGATIR (7° anteroinferior to posterosuperior and through the AC) show these pallidothalamic relationships in living subject. Asterisk = zona incerta. For the interested reader, T2-weighted MR imaging in ex vivo brain shows all 3: AL, LF, TF in one oblique image (see Fig. 5B in prior publication).[60]

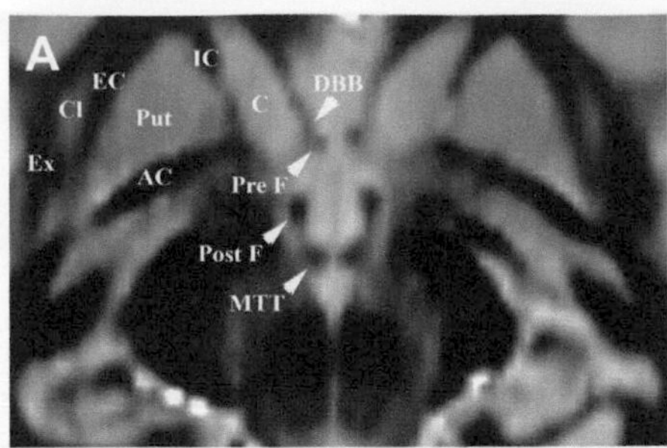

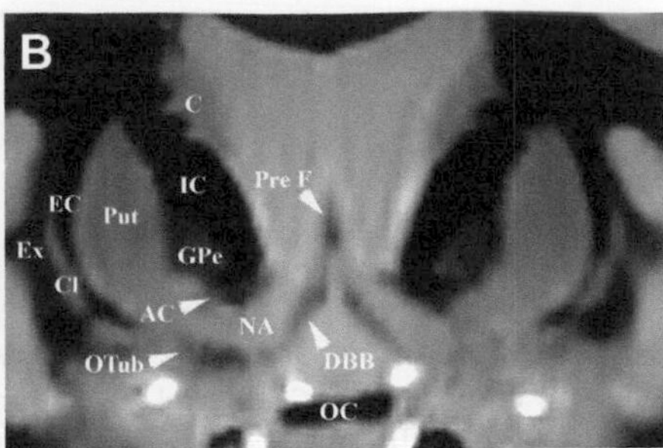

Fig. 3. (*A*) Axial and (*B*) coronal FGATIR images of the "ventral striatum," pre and postcommissural projections of the fornix. The nucleus accumbens (NA) is important to the reward circuit and an investigational DBS target for functional neurosurgery. The Nucleus accumbens is bordered by the putamen (Put) laterally and the caudate nucleus medially ("C"), and its superior surface abuts the anterior commissure (AC) and anterior limb internal capsule (IC). The dark diagnonal band of Broca (DBB) is anteroinferior to the anterior commissure (AC; not seen near midline in these images) and has an inferior–lateral–posterior to superior–medial–anterior orientation (it appears more compact and myelinated in its superior aspect). The diagonal band of Broca projects to the hippocampus, and contains vertical and horizontal cholinergic nuclei that are affected by Lewy body pathology.[58]

globus pallidus externa (GPe) and the interna (GPi). The GPi can be further subdivided into medial and lateral components by an accessory lamina. The optic tract lies along the inferior border of the GPi and the posterior limb of the internal capsule along its medial border (see Fig. 1). The GPi is targeted for the treatment of Parkinson's disease (PD), dystonia and Tourette's syndrome.[8,23] Surgeons try to stimulate the posterior inferior corner of the Gpi just above the lateral edge of the optic tract. On an axial slice parallel to the AC-PC plane, the trajectory should be about 2 mm lateral to the internal capsule. If the electrode tip is too deep, visual phenomena (ie, phosphenes) can occur from stimulating the optic tract. If too medial or posterior, the patient can suffer muscle contractions of the contralateral body.

In simplest terms the basal ganglia function in a feedback loop: cerebral cortex → basal ganglia → thalamus → cerebral cortex. It is here that we encounter the Field of Forel terminology, which is less commonly used today, but can be confusing to readers of older publications. The major inputs to the GPi are the striatum (caudate and putamen) and the subthalamic nucleus (STN). The major outflow of the basal ganglia is the pallidothalamic tracts. The first pallidothalamic tract emerges from the medial aspect of the GPi as a discrete myelinated pathway called the lenticular fasciculus (Forel's Field H2). The lenticular fasciculus passes through the internal capsule near its genu and travels between the STN and zona incerta (ZI) to the H Field of Forel. The H Field of Forel is located just anterior–superior to the red nucleus ("prerubral") and medial to the STN. A second pallidothalamic tract called the ansa lenticularis projects from the inferior GPi and loops around the inferior edge of the anterior limb internal capsule. The ansa lenticularis then merges in the H Field of Forel with the lenticular fasciculus and the contralateral dentatorubrothalamic tract to become the thalamic fasciculus (Forel's Field H1) that then projects onto motor thalamic nuclei (Lpo & Vo; Fig. 2). The thalamic nuclei then project

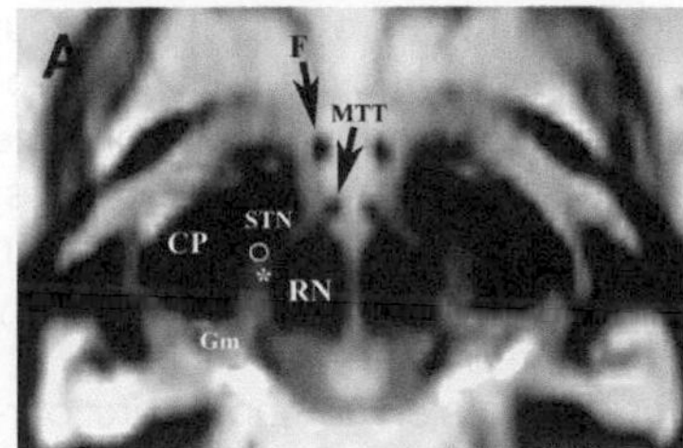

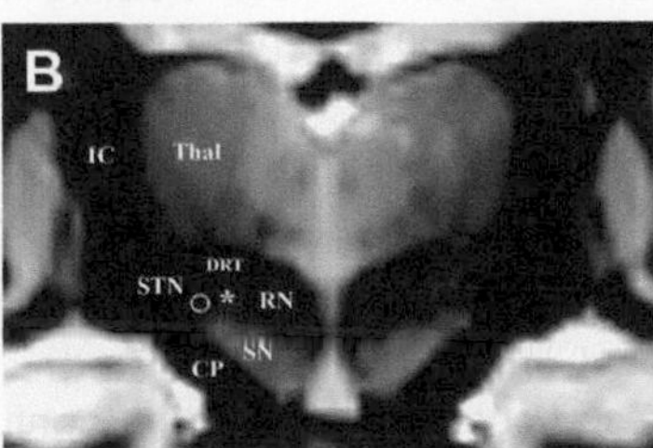

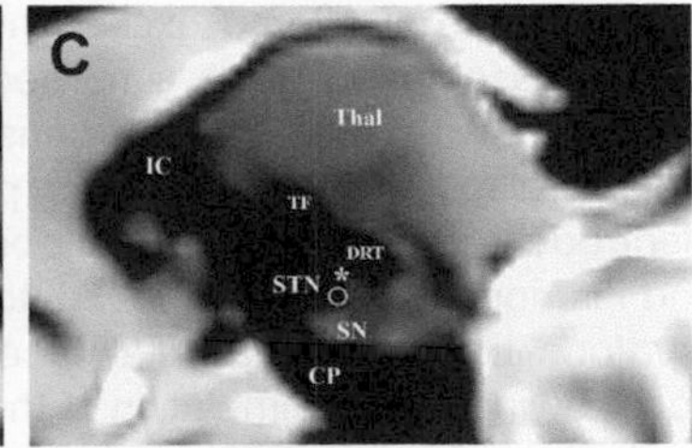

Fig. 4. (*A*) Axial, (*B*) coronal and (*C*) sagittal FGATIR images showing the Subthalamic nucleus (STN) and surrounding structures. The STN is a lenticular-shaped structure oriented obliquely in all three standard planes. The yellow circle (see Table 2) represents approximate DBS electrode tip placement in the posterior–lateral–inferior aspect of the STN. If electrode tip is too lateral, stimulation of the corticospinal tract results in contractions of the contralateral face or arm. DBS current spread into the mid and inferior portions of the adjacent zona incerta (*asterisk*) may represent a bystander therapeutic target for PD.[34]

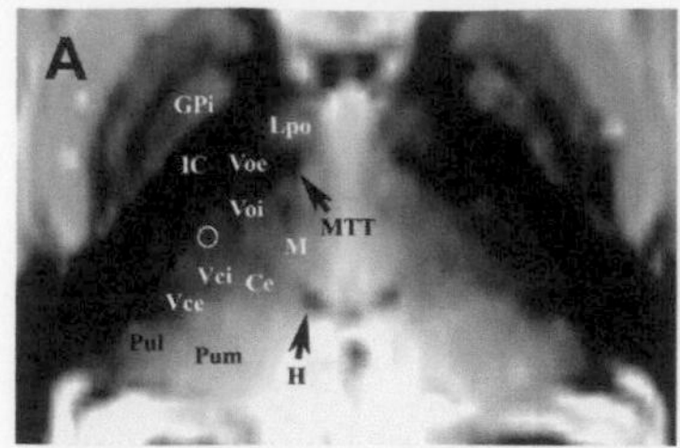

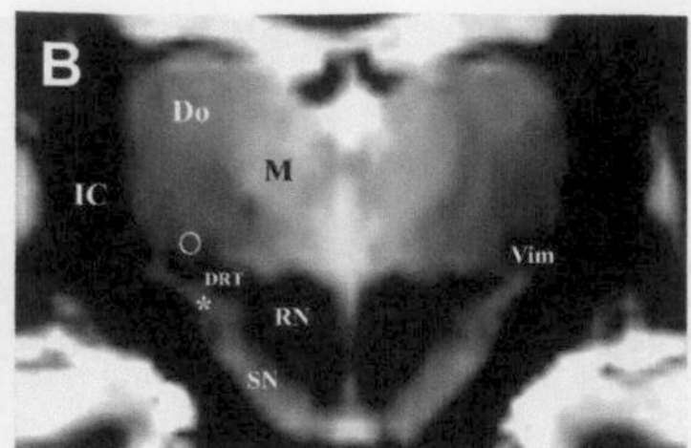

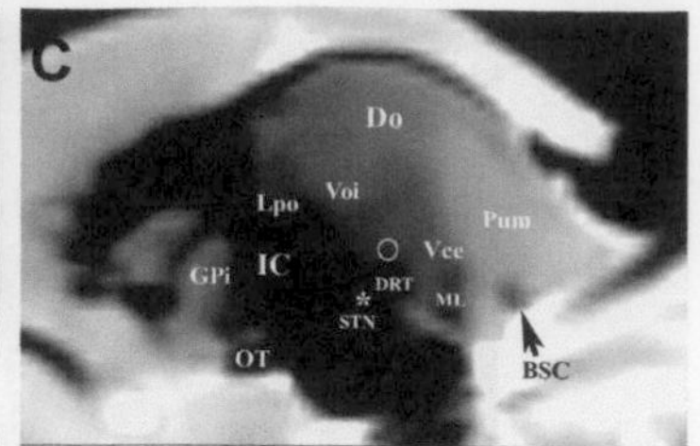

Fig. 5. (*A*) Axial, (*B*) coronal, and (*C*) sagittal FGATIR images showing the ventrointermedius nucleus (Vim) and surrounding structures. FGATIR images allow thalamic nuclei parcellation sufficient for DBS direct localization. The yellow circle represents approximate DBS electrode tip placement or MR imaging-guided focused ultrasound ablation zone for the Vim just medial to the posterior limb of the internal capsule and just above the DRT terminations (see Table 2). Asterisk = Zona incerta.

to the cortex. A third track called the pallidotegmental tract also projects from the GPi to the pedunculopontine nucleus in the midbrain to help regulate posture (we cannot see this tract on MR imaging). Altered basal ganglia function can result in movement disorders (Parkinson's, Huntington, and Wilson diseases) or neuropsychiatric conditions (Tourette syndrome and obsessive–compulsive disorder).[24,25] The ventral striatum, such as nucleus accumbens and adjacent structures (Fig. 3), form the complex reward circuit important to rational decision making and goal-directed behavior.[26] This region also is an emerging investigational target for functional neurosurgery.[27]

Subthalamus - Subthalamic Nucleus

The subthalamic region is inferior to the larger "dorsal thalamus" and includes the STN, adjacent prerubral area, and posteriorly the Zona Incerta (ZI). The STN is a biconvex structure, oriented oblique to all three standard planes, with the lenticular fasciculus (H2) along its superior border and the substantia nigra along its inferomedial margin (see Fig. 4). The STN modulates basal ganglia output and is the most common DBS target for the treatment of PD.[28] In PD, loss of dopaminergic neurons in the substantia nigra results in a complex cascade of altered excitation and inhibition in the basal ganglia. In simplified terms, DBS placement within the STN dampens excess excitatory projections to the globus pallidus.[29] The electrode tip should be in the posterior, lateral, and inferior aspects of the STN. If too lateral, contractions of the contralateral face or arm may occur owing to the stimulation of the corticospinal tract. The cells of the STN receive input from motor cortex, project to the substantia nigra, and have a bidirectional tract connecting to the globus pallidus called the subthalamic fasciculus which traverses the internal capsule (we cannot see this tract on MR imaging). Ischemic injuries of the STN involving the perforating branches of the posterior cerebral artery or posterior communicating artery can result in hemiballismus, but this is now considered a rare clinical presentation.[30,31]

The zona incerta (ZI) is a thin component of gray matter situated superior to the STN and between the lenticular and thalamic fasciculi.[32] The functions of the ZI are poorly understood, but it seems to be a superior extension of the reticular formation involved in motor and sensory processing.[33] The ZI projects to the cerebral cortex, superior colliculus, pretectal region, and basilar pons. Inputs arise from the basal ganglia, motor cortex, and sensory medial lemniscus.[31,32] Previous studies have suggested current from DBS contact points in the mid and inferior portions of the ZI may contribute to effective treatment of PD.[34]

Thalamus - Ventrointermedius Nucleus

The thalamus serves as a key anatomic gateway and regulator between the cerebrum and other subcortical structures.[35,36] Describing the many nuclei and their complex functional connections is beyond the scope of this review (or current understanding!), but key specific nuclei are summarized in Table 3.[4] The "ventrolateral" thalamus or motor group is an important stereotactic target for treating movement disorders in functional neurosurgery and is the focus of this report. Our knowledge of the afferent and efferent connections of the thalamus comes from primate studies.[37–41] Unfortunately, the terminology most frequently applied to the motor nuclei of the human thalamus[42] differs substantially from terminology used for the thalamus of other primates,[11,43,44] creating confusion.[45] Hassler nomenclature parcellates thalamic nuclei well beyond the resolution of current state-of-the-art MR imaging based on cyto- and myeloarchictecture differences. We prefer the nomenclature of Van Buren and Borke,[12] later refined by Ohye,[46] as it is commonly known and not overly complicated relative to the

Table 3
Thalamic nuclei functional connections

Nucleus[a]	Afferent Input	Efferent Connection		Function
Lpo (VA)	Basal ganglia	Premotor cortex	Motor	Initiation & planning
Vo (VL)	Basal ganglia & Cerebellum	Primary motor cortex		Modulation & coordination
Vim (VIM)	Cerebellum (DRT)	Primary motor cortex		Coordination
Vce (VPL)	Spinothalamic tract & Medial Lemniscus	Primary sensory cortex	Sensory	Contralateral body somatic sensation
Vci (VPM)	Trigeminothalamic tract, Rostral part of the Solitary nucleus	Primary sensory cortex		Contralateral face somatic sensation, taste
Gm (MG)	Brachium of Inferior colliculus	Primary auditory cortex (STG)		Hearing
Gl (LG)	Optic Tract	Primary visual cortex (calcarine)		Vision
Pulvinar	Gm, Gl, Superior & Inferior colliculi	Visual association cortex (occipital)		Visual processing
Anterior	Mammillothalamic tract, Fornix	Cingulate cortex	Limbic	Memory, emotion

Abbreviations: DRT, dentatorubrothalamic tract; Gl, lateral geniculate; Gm, medial geniculate; STG, superior temporal gyrus.
[a] Van Buren & Borke (Walker) classifications.

structures that can be seen directly using MR imaging (**Table 4**).

The Vim nucleus is located in the midportion of the inferolateral thalamus and serves as a common target for the DBS treatment of essential tremor (ET) and tremor-dominant PD.[8] It is posterior to the inferior half of the Vo (VL) nucleus and anterior to the Vce (VPL) nucleus (see **Fig. 5**). The dentatorubrothalamic tract (DRT) projects to the Vim via a complicated trajectory, beginning as a projection from the contralateral dentate nucleus of the cerebellum through the superior cerebellar peduncles and their decussation. This projection envelopes the contralateral red nucleus and then seems to terminate along the inferomedial surface of the Vim. The Vim is not visualized well with conventional MR imaging sequences and instead is targeted indirectly based on the AC-PC coordinate system. Lateral target position can be challenging in elderly patients with atrophy and ventricular enlargement such that lateral measurements are made from the 3rd ventricle medial wall instead of the midsagittal plane defined by the commissures. It is important that current spread from the DBS electrode tip should remain medial to the posterior limb internal capsule, otherwise contractions of the contralateral face or arm may occur. If the DBS electrode is too posterior, it will stimulate the Vce (VPL) nucleus and cause perioral or hand paresthesia. Another Vim targeting approach uses diffusion tractography where the lateral and posterior surfaces of the Vim are defined by the ipsilateral corticospinal tract and medial lemniscus margins, respectively.[47] A tractography seed point can also be placed within these margins to verify the putative target involves the terminations of the DRT (**Fig. 6**).

Several groups have focused on diffusion anisotropy and/or tractography to improve the MR imaging detection of internal thalamic anatomy.[18,19,48–50] Unlike previous parcellations based on histologic stains, diffusion anisotropy reflects coherent orientations of axons and dendrites within the thalamic nuclei and may better correlate to selective aspects of their functional organization. We previously described the use of Track Density Imaging (TDI)[20] to directly visualize thalamic nuclei.[21] While most targeting is conducted in the axial plane, **Fig. 7** shows that TDI and DEC-TDI data can also be displayed in coronal and sagittal planes to confirm target location orthogonally (in this case Vim). The DEC TDI maps show consistent internal divisions of the thalamus across individuals not previously visualized in vivo using 3-T MR imaging. These anatomic boundaries appear largely consistent with the location and areas/volumes of the thalamic nuclei in historical atlases based on histology in individual subjects,[12,46] but there are some minor

Table 4
Streamlined terminology comparison of the ventrolateral thalamic nuclei

		Humans		
Primates		German Terminology	Anglosaxon Terminology	
Walker	**Jones**	**Hassler**	**Van Buren & Borke**	**Ohye**
VA	VA	Do, Lpo	Lpo	Lpo
VAmc	VAmc	Lpo (mc)	Lpo (mc)	
VM	VMp	Vo medialis		
VL	VLa	Vo anterior	Vo externus (a)	Vo externus (a)
		Vo posterior	Vo externus (p)	Vo externus (p)
	VLp	Vo internus	Vo internus	Vo internus
		Dim externus	Do	
		Dim internus		
		Dim superior		
LPpa		Dim externus (mc)		
VIM		Vim externus	Vim externus	Vim
		Vim internus	Vim internus	
VPL	VPLa	Vca externus	Vc externus	Vc externus
		Vca internus		
VPM	VPLp	Vcp externus	Vc internus	Vc internus
		Vcp internus		

Nuclei Key: Dim-dorsointermedius, Do-Dorsalis oralis, LP-lateralis posterior, Lpo-lateropolaris, mc-magnocellularis, VA-ventralis anteior, Vc-Ventrocaudalis, Vca-ventrocaudalis anterior, Vcp-ventrocaudalis posterior, VIM-ventralis intermedius, Vim-ventrointermedius, VL-ventralis lateralis, VM-ventralis medialis, Vo-ventro-oralis, VPL-ventralis posterolateralis, VPM-ventralis posteromedialis, a-anterior, p-posterior.

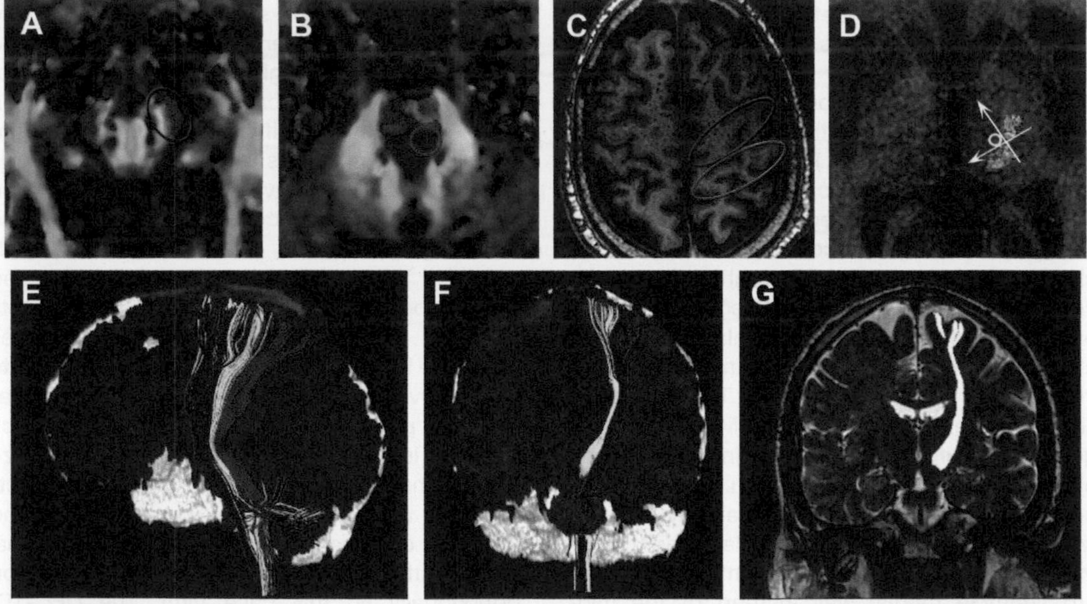

Fig. 6. Step-by-step diffusion tractography for targeting the Vim to treat essential tremor.[47] Axial DEC-FA images of the brain at the level of the (*A*) inferior midbrain and (*B*) mid-pons showing initial seed placements for the left corticospinal tract (CST) (*blue oval*) and medial lemniscus (ML) (*red circle*). Axial MPRAGE (*C*) showing second seed points for both tracts in the primary motor (*blue oval*) and sensory (*red oval*) gyri. Axial MPRAGE image at the level of the AC-PC plane (*D*) showing the placement of the seed point for the dentatorubrothalamic tract (DRT; *yellow circle*) in the angle formed from the margins of the CST and ML tracts. Sagittal (*E*) and coronal (*F*) 3D tractography streamlines of the DRT (yellow), CST (*blue*) and ML (*red*). (*G*) Coronal 3D surgical navigation fibers of the left DRT.

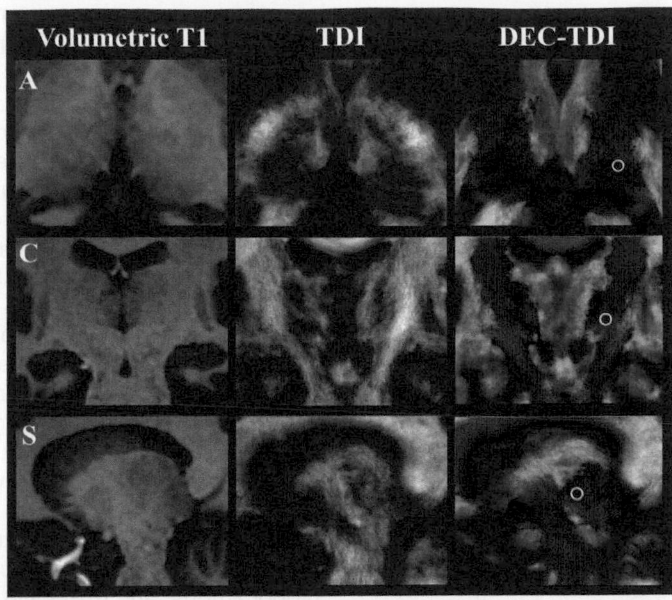

Fig. 7. Side-by-side comparison of internal thalamic detail for cropped, magnified images of volumetric 3D T1, track density (TDI) and direction-encoded track density (DEC-TDI) maps in the axial (*A*), coronal (*C*) and sagittal (S) planes for a healthy control subject [for TDI & DEC-TDI: pixel intensity = number of probabilistic streamlines; red = left–right, green = anterior–posterior & blue = superior–inferior orientations]. Image planes intersect with approximate indirect targeting coordinates (see Table 2) for DBS electrode tip placement or ablation of the Vim (*yellow circle*). TDI is a super-resolution technique that demonstrates consistent internal features of thalamic anatomy across subjects similar to other whole-brain probabilistic tractography methods.

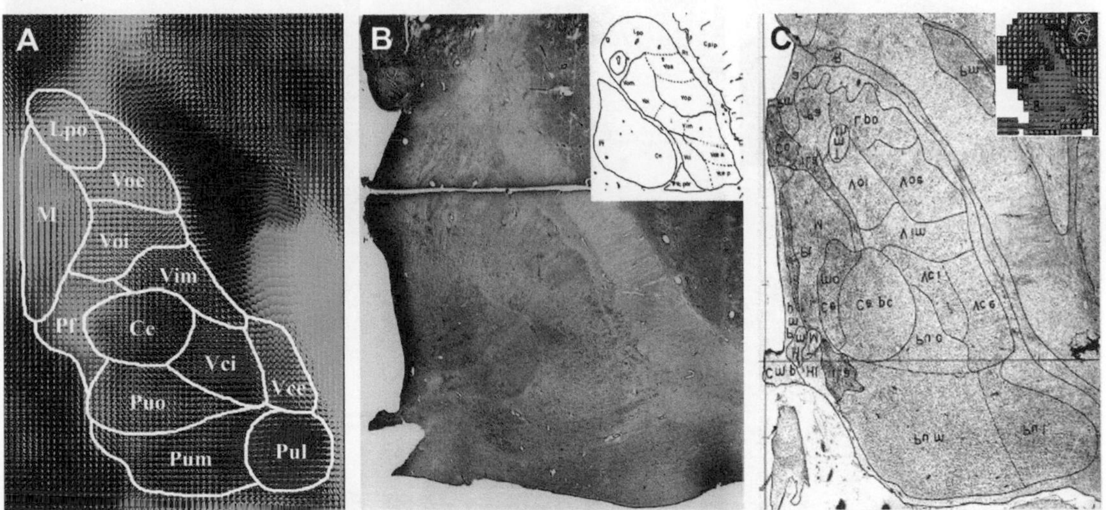

Fig. 8. Direct comparison of TDI-derived orientation distribution function (ODF) map of the thalamus to atlases based on cytoarchitecture and myeloarchictecture. (*A*) The axial ODF map from Fig. 7 is cropped to show the left thalamus and then compared with similar atlas images parallel to the intercommissural plane (*B*) from Ohye C. Thalamus, in Paxinos G (ed): The Human Nervous System. San Diego: Academic Press, 1990, pp 439–468[12] and (*C*)adapted from Wiegell MR, Tuch DS, Larsson HB, Wedeen VJ. Automatic segmentation of thalamic nuclei from diffusion tensor magnetic resonance imaging. Neuroimage. 2003 Jun;19(2 Pt 1):391–401.[19] There seems to be some concordance between putative TDI thalamic nuclei assignments and histology. TDI contrast is more visually obvious than conventional histology and reflects local tissue anisotropy from the functional organization of axons and dendrites on a mesoscopic scale.

differences. Fig. 8 compares an in vivo axial Fiber Orientation Distribution (FOD) map derived from TDI to human thalamus histology atlas images in the same axial plane. A consistent feature of both diffusion-based segmentation and histology is that not all borders between nuclei are sharp. Also note similar cytoarchitectural areas in border regions have been sometimes assigned to different nuclei by different historical references[12,46,51,52]. The boundaries between the globus pallidus, PLIC, and thalamus are clearly demarcated on DEC-TDI maps. An important potential limitation of TDI and most diffusion-based approaches to the parcellation of the thalamus or basal ganglia is that contrast based on whole-brain probabilistic tractography may be affected by pathology in *any* brain region,[53] especially since the thalamus has such extensive reciprocal connections.

Thalamus – Fornix, Mammillary Bodies and Anterior Nucleus

Clinicians may underestimate the functional importance of limbic structures within the thalamus that are increasingly targets of interest to functional neurosurgery. For instance, hippocampal disconnection fails to produce deficits as severe as direct injury to the mammillary bodies or mammillothalamic tract (MTT). Mammillary body injury alone results in debilitating Korsakoff's syndrome.[54] The development of neurofibrillary tangle and amyloid pathology in the anterior nucleus also may herald initial clinical symptoms of Alzheimer's disease.[55] Hence, these anterior thalamic structures also are being investigated as a DBS target for neurodegenerative disease.[9] DBS contacts in the mammillary body, MTT or anterior nucleus of the thalamus also seem effective for treating medically refractory epilepsy.[56]

The fornix is the major output pathway from the hippocampus and serves episodic memory.[57] The fornix divides around the anterior commissure. The precommissural fornix projects to the anterior septal nuclei and adjacent structures. The FGATIR sequence also seems to resolve the diagonal band of Broca just anterolateral to precommissural fornix (see Fig. 3). This structure contains vertical and horizontal cholinergic nuclei, projects to the hippocampus, and may have an important role in Lewy body pathology.[58] The postcommissural fornix projects to the superolateral surface of the mammillary body. The major projection of the mammillary body, the MTT, emerges from the superomedial surface of the mammillary body and projects first posteriorly ~3 mm, then turns 90° superiorly toward the anterior nucleus of the

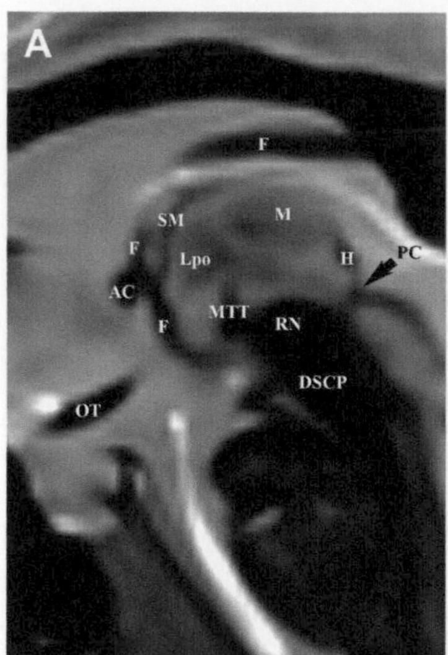

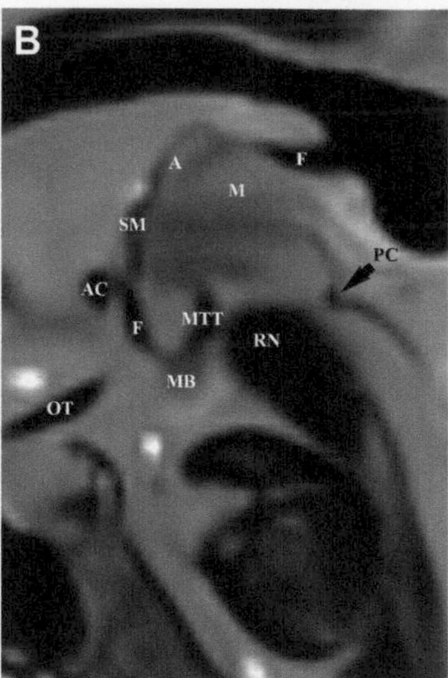

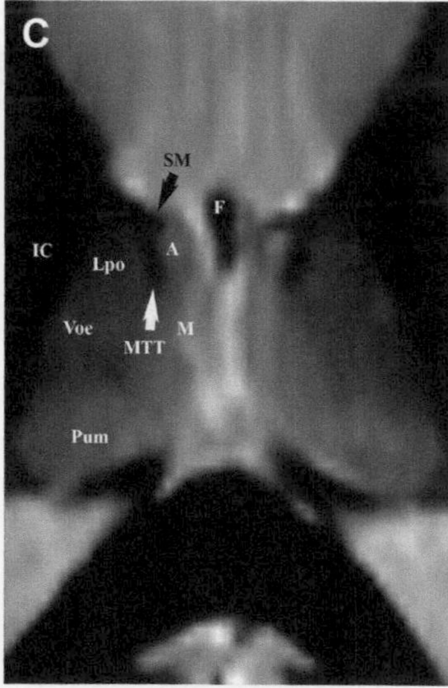

Fig. 9. FGATIR (*A*) sagittal 3 mm lateral to midline and (*B*) double-oblique sagittal (4° anterolateral to posteromedial, and 5° inferomedial to superolateral) demonstrate positions of fornix (F), mammillary body (MB) and mammillothalamic tract (MTT) that form complex circuit and projection to the anterior nucleus (*A*) of the thalamus. (*C*) Axial image ~13 mm superior to the AC-PC plane shows stria medullaris (SM) along the anterolateral border and the distal MTT along the posterolateral border of the anterior nucleus (*A*). A direct posterolateral projection of the fornix above the anterior commissure (not shown) spreads superiorly across the anterior surface of the anterior nucleus (see dark anteromedial surface). (*C*) This represents the hippocampal-thalamic pathway important for recollective, recognition memory.[57] DBS electrode placement in the anterior nucleus has recently been reported effective for refractory epilepsy.

thalamus (Fig. 9). It is intriguing that this sharp proximal MTT turn also abuts the medial border of the Forel's Field H. A recent study also reported interesting 12% to 14% right–left and male–female asymmetries in the more distal MTT 5 mm above the commissural plane.[59] The less well-known third fornix projection visible with FGATIR and postmortem MR imaging[60] arises just superior to its division around the anterior commissure and projects posterolaterally onto the anterior nucleus of the thalamus. This represents a direct hippocampal-thalamic pathway that bypasses the mammillary bodies and seems important for recollective, recognition memory.[57] Together, the precommissural fornix and this direct projection to the anterior nucleus may represent ~40% of the total fornix projection from the hippocampus.[60]

SUMMARY

The FGATIR sequence, especially after denoising with a convolutional neural network, improves the visualization of internal anatomy of the basal ganglia and thalamus important for current functional neurosurgery applications. Track density imaging, a super-resolution technique based on whole-brain probabilistic tractography, also demonstrates detailed internal features of the thalamus based on diffusion anisotropy that reflects the local functional organization of axons and dendrites. Both imaging techniques and other diffusion MR imaging approaches based on tractography, improve our ability to directly visualize anatomy in living subjects using widely available 3-T MR imaging. This review of basal ganglia and thalamic anatomy should serve as an introductory guide for radiology trainees and neuroradiologists interested in basal ganglia and thalamus function, and emerging functional neurosurgery applications in these regions.

CLINICS CARE POINTS

- Conventional MR imaging does not discriminate internal anatomic features of the basal ganglia and thalamic well. Functional neuro surgery instead uses indirect targeting as the clinical standard based on intercommissural distances or atlas-based coordinates.
- Atlas-based approaches do not fully account for variability in subcortical anatomy across individuals or asymmetries in the same individual. This can result in decreased therapeutic benefit and increased risk of side effects.
- Recent 3-T MR imaging sequence innovations such as FGATIR and whole-brain probabilistic tractography may directly reveal clinically relevant targets and off-targets for functional neurosurgery previously only detected with high-field scanners or autopsy samples.
- Thalamic nuclei nomenclature is complex and varies among primate and human subjects. Familiarity with these classifications will promote clear communication between different clinical specialists.

ACKNOWLEDGMENTS

The authors wish to thank Sohae Chung for her help with TDI figures.

DISCLOSURE

T.M. Shepherd is cofounder and equity holder for MICroStructure Imaging (MICSI). M.J. Hoch has nothing to disclose.

REFERENCES

1. Carpenter MB, Strong OS, Truex RC. Human neuroanatomy: (formerly Strong and Elwyn's human neuroanatomy). 7th edition. Baltimore (MD): Lippincott Williams and Wilkins; 1976.
2. Haines DE. Neuroanatomy: an atlas of structures, sections and systems. 6th edition. Philadelphia (PA): Lippincott Williams and Wilkins; 2004.
3. DeLong MR, Wichmann T. Circuits and circuit disorders of the basal ganglia. Arch Neurol 2007;64(1): 20–4.
4. Nieuwenhuys R, Voogd J, van Huijzen C. The human central nervous system. 4th edition. Berlin (Germany): Springer-Verlag; 2008.
5. Ring HA. Serra-Mestres J Neuropsychiatry of the basal ganglia. J Neurol Neurosurg Psychiatry 2002;72:12–21.
6. Nagano-Saito A, Martinu K, Monchi O. Function of basal ganglia in bridging cognitive and motor modules to perform an action. Front Neurosci 2014;8: 187.
7. Tolosa E, Compta Y, Gaig C. The premotor phase of Parkinson's disease. Parkinsonism Relat Disord 2007;(13 Suppl):S2–7.
8. Miocinovic S, Somayajula S, Chitnis S, et al. History, applications, and mechanisms of deep brain stimulation. JAMA Neurol 2013;70:163–71.
9. Fisher R, Salanova V, Witt T, et al, SANTE Study Group. Electrical stimulation of the anterior nucleus of thalamus for treatment of refractory epilepsy. Epilepsia 2010;51:899–908.

10. Schaltenbrand G, Wahren W. Atlas of stereotaxy of the human brain. 2nd ed. Stuttgart, Germany: Thieme; 1977.
11. Hirai T, Jones EG. A new parcellation of the human thalamus on the basis of histochemical staining. Brain Res Brain Res Rev 1989;14:1–34.
12. Van Buren JM, Borke RC. Variations and connections of the human thalamus, 2 Vols. Heidelberg: Springer; 1972.
13. Brierley JB, Beck E. The significance in human stereotactic brain surgery of individual variation in the diencephalon and globus pallidus. J Neurol Neurosurg Psychiatr 1959;22:287–98.
14. Guridi J, Rodriguez-Oroz MC, Lozano AM, et al. Targeting the basal ganglia for deep brain stimulation in Parkinson's disease. Neurology 2000;55(12 Suppl 6):S21–8.
15. Ohye C. Selective Thalamotomy and Gamma Thalamotomy for Parkinson Disease. In: Lozano AM, Gildenberg PL, Tasker RR, editors. Textbook of stereotactic and functional neurosurgery. 2nd edition. Berlin (Germany): Springer; 2009. p. 1549–657.
16. Sudhyadhom A, Haq IU, Foote KD, et al. A high resolution and high contrast MRI for differentiation of subcortical structures for DBS targeting: the fast gray matter acquisition t1 inversion recovery (FGATIR). Neuroimage 2009;47(Suppl 2):T44–52.
17. Ades-aron B, Elsayed M, Hoch M, et al. CNN denoising of FGATIR MRI improves visualization of subcortical anatomy. ISMRM 2022.
18. Behrens TE, Johansen-Berg H, Woolrich MW, et al. Non-invasive mapping of connections between human thalamus and cortex using diffusion imaging. Nat Neurosci 2003;6(7):750–7.
19. Wiegell MR, Tuch DS, Larsson HB, et al. Automatic segmentation of thalamic nuclei from diffusion tensor magnetic resonance imaging. Neuroimage 2003;19(2 Pt 1):391–401.
20. Calamante F, Tourneir JD, Jackson GD, et al. Track density imaging (TDI): super-resolution white matter imaging using whole-brain track density mapping. NeuroImage 2010;53:1233–43.
21. Shepherd TM, Chung S, Glielmi C, et al. 3-T MRI tract density imaging to identify thalamic nuclei for functional neurosurgery. Neurosurgery 2014;61: S1–221.
22. Tournier JD, Calamante F, Connelly A. Robust determination of the fibre orientation distribution in diffusion MRI: non-negativity constrained super resolved spherical deconvolution. Neuroimage 2007;35(4):1459–72.
23. Middlebrooks EH, Domingo RA, Vivas-Buitrago T, et al. Neuroimaging advances in deep brain stimulation: review of indications, anatomy, and brain connectomics. AJNR Am J Neuroradiol 2020;41(9): 1558–68.
24. Anderson JC, Costantino MM, Stratford T. Basal ganglia: anatomy, pathology, and imaging characteristics. Curr Probl Diagn Radiol 2004;33:28–41.
25. Walkup JT, Mink JW, Hollenbeck PJ, editors. Advances in neurology: tourette disorder, 99. Philadelphia (PA): Lippincott Williams and Wilkins; 2006.
26. Haber SN. Neuroanatomy of reward: a view from the ventral striatum. In: Gottfried JA, editor. Neurobiology of sensation and reward. Boca Raton (FL): CRC Press/Taylor & Francis; 2011. Chapter 11. Available from https:www.ncbi.nlm.nih.gov/books/NBK92777/.
27. Wu H, Miller KJ, Blumenfeld Z, et al. Closing the loop on impulsivity via nucleus accumbens delta-band activity in mice and man. Proc Natl Acad Sci U S A 2018;115(1):192–7.
28. Hamani C, Saint-Cyr JA, Fraser J, et al. The subthalamic nucleus in the context of movement disorders. Brain 2004;127:4–20.
29. Okun MS. Deep-brain stimulation–entering the era of human neural-network modulation. N Engl J Med 2014;371(15):1369–73.
30. Etemadifar M, Abtahi SH, Abtahi SM, et al. Hemiballismus, hyperphagia, and behavioral changes following subthalamic infarct. Case Rep Med 2012; 2012:768580.
31. Mihailoff GA, Haines DE. The Diencephalon, in Fundamental Neuroscience for Basic and Clinical Applications (Fifth Edition), 2018.
32. Zrinzo L, Hyam JA. Deep Brain Stimulation for Movement Disorders, in Principles of Neurological Surgery (Fourth Edition), 2018.
33. Mitrofanis J. Some certainty for the "zone of uncertainty"? Exploring the function of the zona incerta. Neuroscience 2005;130:1–15.
34. Plaha P, Ben-Shlomo Y, Patel NK, et al. Stimulation of the caudal zona incerta is superior to stimulation of the subthalamic nucleus in improving contralateral parkinsonism. Brain 2006;129:1732–47.
35. Sherman SM. Thalamic relays and cortical functioning. Prog Brain Res 2005;149:107–26.
36. McFarland NR, Haber SN. Thalamic relay nuclei of the basal ganglia from both reciprocal and nonreciprocal cortical connections, linking multiple frontal cortical areas. J Neurosci 2002;22(18):8117–32.
37. Walker AE. The primate thalamus. Chicago (IL): University of Chicago Press; 1938.
38. Percheron G, François C, Talbi B, et al. The primate motor thalamus analyzed with reference to subcortical afferent territories. Stereotact Funct Neurosurg 1993;60:32–41.
39. Olszewski J. The thalamus of the Macaca mulatta. An atlas for use with the stereotaxic instrument. Basel (Switzerland): Karger; 1952.
40. Ilinsky IA, Kultas-Ilinsky K. Sagittal cytoarchitectonic maps of the Macaca mulatta thalamus with a revised nomenclature of the motor-related nuclei validated

by observations on their connectivity. J Comp Neurol 1987;262:331–64.

41. Jones EG. Correlation and revised nomenclature of ventral nuclei in the thalamus of human and monkey. Stereotact Funct Neurosurg 1990;54/55:1–20.
42. Hassler R. Anatomy of the thalamus. In: Schaltenbrand G, Bailey P, editors. Introduction to stereotaxis with an atlas of the human brain. Stuttgart (Germany): Thieme; 1959. p. 230–90.
43. Walker AE. Normal and pathological physiology of the human thalamus. In: Schaltenbrand G, Walker AE, editors. Stereotaxy of the human brain. Anatomical, physiological and clinical applications. 2nd edition. Stuttgart (Germany): Thieme; 1982. p. 181–217.
44. Dewulf A. Anatomy of the normal human thalamus, topometry and standardized nomenclature. Amsterdam (the Netherlands): Elsevier; 1971.
45. Macchi G, Jones EG. Toward an agreement on terminology of nuclear and subnuclear divisions of the motor thalamus. J Neurosurg 1997;86:670–85.
46. Ohye C. Thalamus. In: Paxinos G, editor. The human nervous system. San Diego: Academic Press; 1990. p. 439–68.
47. Sammartino F, Krishna V, King NK, et al. Tractography-based ventral intermediate nucleus targeting: novel methodology and intraoperative validation. Mov Disord 2016;31(8):1217–25.
48. Tian Q, Wintermark M, Jeffrey Elias W, et al. Diffusion MRI tractography for improved transcranial MRI-guided focused ultrasound thalamotomy targeting for essential tremor. Neuroimage Clin 2018;19: 572–80.
49. Middlebrooks EH, Holanda VM, Tuna IS, et al. A method for pre-operative single-subject thalamic segmentation based on probabilistic tractography for essential tremor deep brain stimulation. Neuroradiology 2018;60(3):303–9.
50. Calabrese E. Diffusion tractography in deep brain stimulation surgery: a review. Front Neuroanat 2016;10:45.
51. Duvernoy H. The human brain. Surface, three-dimensional sectional anatomy and MRI. New York: Springer-Verlag; 1991.
52. Morel A, Magnin M, Jeanmonod D. Multiarchitectonic and stereotactic atlas of the human thalamus. J Comp Neurol 1997;387:588–630.
53. Calamante F, Smith RE, Tournier JD, et al. Quantification of voxel wise total fibre density: investigating the problems associated with track-count mapping. Neuroimage 2015;117:284–93.
54. Dillingham CM, Milczarek MM, Perry JC, et al. Time to put the mammillothalamic pathway into context. Neurosci Biobehav Rev 2021;121:60–74.
55. Aggleton JP, Pralus A, Nelson AJ, et al. Thalamic pathology and memory loss in early Alzheimer's disease: moving the focus from the medial temporal lobe to Papez circuit. Brain 2016;139(Pt 7):1877–90.
56. Balak N, Balkuv E, Karadag A, et al. Mammillothalamic and mammillotegmental tracts as new targets for dementia and epilepsy treatment. World Neurosurg 2018;110:133–44.
57. Aggleton JP, O'Mara SM, Vann SD, et al. Hippocampal-anterior thalamic pathways for memory: uncovering a network of direct and indirect actions. Eur J Neurosci 2010;31:2292–307.
58. Liu AKL, Lim EJ, Ahmed I, et al. Review: Revisiting the human cholinergic nucleus of the diagonal band of Broca. Neuropathol Appl Neurobiol 2018; 44(7):647–62.
59. Ghaderi Niri S, Khalaf AM, Massoud TF. The mammillothalamic tracts: Age-related conspicuity and normative morphometry on brain magnetic resonance imaging. Clin Anat 2020;33(6):911–9.
60. Hoch MJ, Bruno MT, Faustin A, et al. 3T MRI whole-brain microscopy discrimination of subcortical anatomy, part 2: basal forebrain. AJNR Am J Neuroradiol 2019;40(7):1095–105.

Brain Connectomics

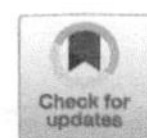

Erik H. Middlebrooks, MD[a,b,*], Sanjeet S. Grewal, MD[b]

KEYWORDS

• Connectomics • Functional MRI • Deep brain stimulation • Epilepsy • Essential tremor
• Parkinson's disease

KEY POINTS

- Traditional "localizationist" models of the brain are increasingly obsolete in favor of the conception of the brain as a "circuit."
- "Connectomics" is the study of the connectome, which represents the sum total of connectivity within the brain consisting of cortical or subcortical hubs linked by white matter tracts.
- Many neurologic disorders can be defined by abnormalities within specific brain circuits or "circuitopathies," which may be amenable to neuromodulation.

INTRODUCTION

For millennia, the complexity and elegance of the brain have fascinated humankind. Rudimentary attempts at brain surgery have been found as far back as the Neolithic period, but the greatest advances in understanding began in the nineteenth and twentieth centuries. During this span, revolutionary observations made by pioneers of neuroscience, such as Pierre Paul Broca, John Martyn Harlow, and Brenda Milner, were a driving force in the attempt to assign specific "locations" to brain functions. According to this localizationist theory, particular cognitive functions, such as language, were discretely represented in isolated brain regions. Damage to these critical cortical regions would result in cessation of function.

With further studies throughout the twentieth century and the advent of neuroimaging, it became apparent that many deficits were unable to be explained by these localizationist models.[1] These "extended" areas became less anatomically defined while shifting more toward a functional concept with a loose anatomic definition.[2] Toward the end of the twentieth century, advances in neuroimaging, EEG, MEG, and so forth greatly expanded our ability to understand brain function. The science of "connectomics," or the study of the connectome (the sum total of connectivity within the brain), has helped reshape our understanding of how the brain functions. Within connectomics, we must consider both structural and functional connectivity. Functional connectivity is a measure of temporal synchronicity between the local or distant brain regions without consideration of direct anatomic connectivity. As such, functional connectivity can be theoretically mediated by direct monosynaptic connection but also by second- or third-order synapses and so forth. On the macroscale, structural connectivity considers both short- and long-fiber connections within the brain. Both functional and structural connectivity form the basis of these widespread brain networks.

Leveraging Connectomics to Understand Human Disease

Two of the most common imaging measurements of functional connectivity are task-based functional MRI (fMRI) and resting-state fMRI (rs-fMRI). Task-based fMRI relies on subjects performing specific tasks that reliably activate the network of interest (eg, motor, vision, language, and so forth) while controlling for effects of no interest. In contrast to the task-based fMRI, rs-fMRI signals arise from intrinsic brain activity in the absence of an external task. Many of the brain networks described in the prior articles,

[a] Department of Radiology, Mayo Clinic, 4500 San Pablo Road, Jacksonville, FL 32224, USA; [b] Department of Neurosurgery, Mayo Clinic, 4500 San Pablo Road, Jacksonville, FL 32224, USA
* Corresponding author. Department of Radiology, Mayo Clinic, 4500 San Pablo Road, Jacksonville, FL 32224.
E-mail address: middlebrooks.erik@mayo.edu
Twitter: @EMiddlebrooksMD (E.H.M.)

Neuroimag Clin N Am 32 (2022) 543–552
https://doi.org/10.1016/j.nic.2022.04.002

Abbreviations	
ALIC	anterior limb of the internal capsule
ANT	anterior nucleus of thalamus
CM	centromedian nucleus
DBS	deep brain stimulation
DMN	default mode network
DRTT	dentato-rubro-thalamic tract
ET	essential tremor
GPe	globus pallidus externus
GPi	globus pallidus internus
OCD	obsessive-compulsive disorder
MMT	mammillothalamic tract
PD	Parkinson's disease
PSA	posterior subthalamic areas
IMFB	superolateral branch of the medial forebrain bundle
SMA	supplementary motor area
STN	subthalamic nucleus
UPDRS	Unified Parkinson's Disease Rating Scale
VIM	ventral intermediate nucleus
VOp	ventralis oralis posterior nucleusZI = zona incerta

such as those involved with language and vision, can be elicited in rs-fMRI. In addition, a widely distributed network, known as the default mode network (DMN),[3] is heavily engaged at rest and frequently referred to as a "task-negative network," although evidence suggests it also plays an active role during goal-directed cognition. In addition, rs-fMRI signals can be used to identify brain networks that represent sensory and higher order cognitive function or higher order social function. For example, the visual network typically corresponds to the medial occipital pole and lateral visual areas, although the sensory motor network includes the supplementary motor cortex, sensorimotor cortex, and the secondary somatosensory cortex. Similarly, there is an auditory network that includes the superior temporal gyrus, Heschl's gyrus, and the posterior insula. Many neurologic disorders have been shown to affect these resting-state networks and may provide insight into the pathophysiology of disease.

One of the most widely studied resting networks is the DMN. This network was first identified using PET studies, in which it was noted to be connected areas that would be suppressed when subjects were asked to perform external tasks, such as word judgments or object classification. The DMN is a widespread, cortical and subcortical network with primary components including the posterior and anterior cingulate cortex, inferior parietal lobule, precuneus, medial prefrontal cortex, hippocampus, parahippocampal cortex, anterior, medial, and posterior thalamic nuclei, putamen, pallidum, caudate, ventral tegmental area, and cerebellum, among others.[4,5] This network has been noted to be involved in multiple disease states such as epilepsy, which will be discussed in further detail later.

Although the traditional neuroscience focused on the amalgamation of lesion data to identify a discrete brain area responsible for function, this approach has seen a dramatic revolution in recent years. With the advent of functional neuroimaging, these tools have been used to assign brain lesions to *networks* rather than discrete regions. One commonly applied approach is *lesion network mapping.* In this approach, brain lesions producing specific neurologic or neuropsychiatric symptoms are mapped in a common template space and used as seed regions for connectivity measures in the large sets of normative connectomic imaging data, including fMRI and MR tractography. This approach has led to improve an understanding of numerous neurologic conditions, including various movement disorders, disorders of consciousness, pain, aphasia, depression, hallucinations, and many other neurologic conditions.[6–12]

In addition to providing a mechanistic framework to better understand neurologic disorders, connectomics also serves to inform new advances in treatment, such as neuromodulation. A so-called "connectomic surgery" is a growing concept that aims to integrate an understanding of pathologic brain circuits, or "circuitopathies," with technology that allows the intentional alteration of these anomalous brain circuits.[13] The concluding section provides clinical examples of how these circuits may go awry and how recent advances in the integration of connectomics and deep brain stimulation (DBS) may provide a revolutionary tool for "correcting" these alterations.

Clinical applications

Essential Tremor

Essential tremor (ET) is one of the most common indications for DBS, initially approved by the Food and Drug Administration (FDA) in 1997. Historically, the target was considered the ventral intermediate nucleus (VIM) of the thalamus.[14] However, subsequent studies have suggested multiple other targets from the posterior subthalamic area (PSA), namely the caudal zona incerta) and the ventralis oralis posterior (VOp) nucleus of the thalamus.[15–20] Importantly, these debates centered on the localizationist concept of brain function. More recently, the connectomic concept has been applied to tremor treatment and has shown network-specific changes within the brain in ET patients. In particular, abnormalities in the cerebello-thalamo-cortical pathway have been shown, with increased functional connectivity between the VIM and motor cortex and decreased connectivity with the cerebellum.[21] These findings would support a circuitopathy mediated by the dentato-rubro-thalamic tract (DRTT), a tract connecting the dentate nucleus of the cerebellum with the contralateral thalamus and motor cortex (Fig. 1), which may be a primary mediator of tremor improvement.[18]

Recently, many studies have retrospectively shown a correlation between tremor improvement and stimulation of this cerebello-thalamic motor network.[18,22–25] The role of the DRTT was also highlighted in a prospective blinded, crossover trial showing superiority of direct stimulation targeting of DRTT versus sham and standard-of-care programming.[26] Middlebrooks and colleagues,[18] in the largest study to date, showed that the DRTT was predictive of tremor improvement in a large, single-center cohort and the resulting network "*fingerprint*" was able to predict outcomes in a separate cohort from another center. Importantly, they also showed that the previously reported stimulation "sweet spots" spanning the ventral thalamus and PSA all lie on the course of the DRTT, providing a unification of these targets and reinforcing the concept of a connectomic theory of treatment rather than a localizationist theory.[18]

The connectomic basis of treatment is an important milestone in DBS. First, it reconciles decades of debate on the "ideal" target by showing that tremor improvement is strongly driven by a tract that traverses all of the regions, not necessarily just the local nucleus stimulation. Second, it provides a patient-specific biomarker that can reduce the reliance on less accurate coordinate-based targeting approaches that do not account for the variability between the patients.[19] Third, alternative noninvasive treatments, such as MR-guided focused ultrasound and stereotactic radiosurgery, lack the robust electrophysiological data and ability to fine-tune settings in the long-term as present in DBS, which makes targeting accuracy even more critical. Although more prospective studies and long-term outcomes are needed to fully understand the role of DRTT in tremor reduction, it is clear that connectomics will have a lasting role in treatment of ET.

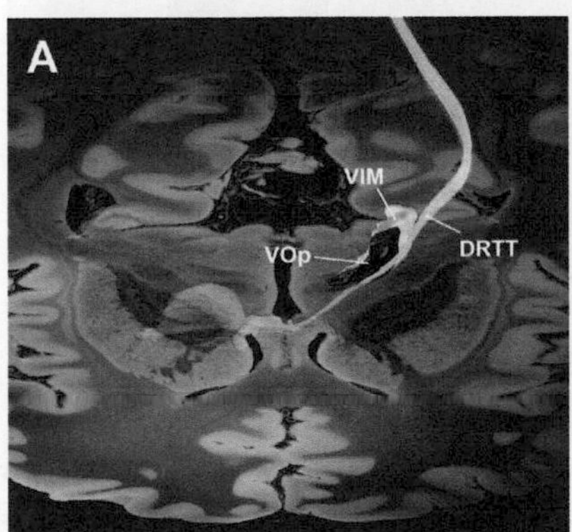

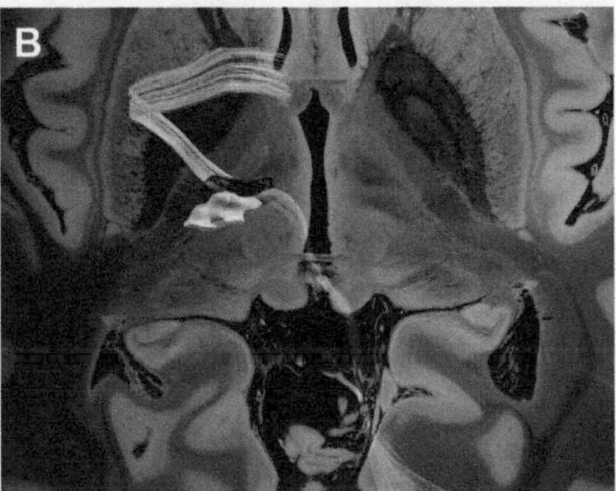

Fig. 1. (*A*) Coronal and (*B*) axial images showing the relationship of the DRTT (green) with the VIM (yellow), and VOp (purple) nucleus of the thalamus. ROIs from the DBS Intrinsic Template Atlas[50]; DRTT from Middlebrooks and colleagues[51]. *Brain backdrop from* Edlow BL, Mareyam A, Horn A, et al. 7 T MRI of the ex vivo human brain at 100 micron resolution. Sci Data. Oct 30 2019;6(1):244.])

Parkinson's Disease

The most common targets for treatment of Parkinsonism have been the globus pallidus internus and subthalamic nucleus (STN) (**Fig. 2**). Within these nuclei, there has been establishment of a functional gradient of network connectivity with a posterior motor division, middle associative division, and anterior limbic division.[27,28] Similar to ET, the shift from a localizationist model to a connectomic model has shown the importance of this functional gradient, as well as adjacent white matter tracts, in understanding the network effect of DBS.

Similar to ET, DBS in Parkinson's disease (PD) has also shown network-specific *"fingerprints"* that correlate with outcome. Horn and colleagues[29] used connectomics to predict improvement in Unified Parkinson's Disease Rating Scale Part III (UPDRS-III) motor scores and found predictions within 15% of ground truth. With STN DBS, connectivity to the supplementary motor area (SMA), prefrontal cortex, and cerebellum, as well as anticorrelation with the primary motor cortex, was predictive of overall UPDRS motor score improvement.[29] However, symptomatology of PD is more complex than ET, with PD patients exhibiting variable phenotypes. Connectomics sheds light on the variation in treatment effect on different parkinsonian symptoms. Rigidity has been shown to correlate with greater prefrontal and SMA connectivity, bradykinesia with connectivity to SMA, and tremor with connectivity to the primary motor cortex.[30]

Two important pathways that may explain response of specific symptoms to DBS are the pallidofugal pathway (connecting the pallidum with the STN, thalamus, substantia nigra, and pedunculopontine nucleus) and the striatofugal pathways (connecting the substantia nigra [SN] with the pallidum and striatum).[31] Stimulation dorsal to the STN and to the ventral globus pallidus internus (GPi) has both been shown to improve rigidity, suppress dyskinesia, and reduce tremor.[31–33] Both areas correspond to the course of the pallidofugal pathways (**Fig.** 3A, B), including the thalamic fasciculus, lenticular fasciculus, pallidosubthalamic tracts, and ansa lenticularis, which suggests a common network for both targets. Meanwhile, the ventral STN and the dorsal GPi/globus pallidus externus (GPe) have both been shown to improve bradykinesia but also worsen dyskinesia.[31–33] Likewise, both targets have a tract in common—the nigrofugal pathway (**Fig. 3**C, D), which courses from the SN along the ventrolateral STN and the dorsal GPi/GPe to the putamen.[34] Lastly, the hyperdirect pathway, connecting the STN directly to the cortex, has been implicated in symptomatology of PD and associated with motor improvement seen with STN DBS in PD, as well as various nonmotor effects of STN DBS.[34]

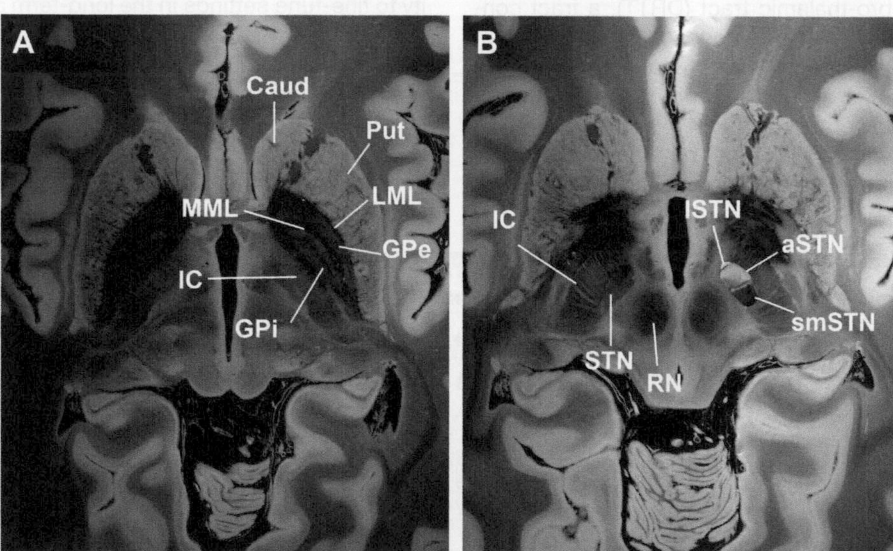

Fig. 2. Axial images at the level of the (*A*) pallidum and (*B*) subthalamic region showing the anatomy of the basal ganglia structures. aSTN = associate portion of subthalamic nucleus; Caud = caudate nucleus; GPe = globus pallidus externus; GPi = globus pallidus internus; IC = internal capsule; LML = lateral medullary lamina; lSTN = limbic portion of the subthalamic nucleus; MML = medial medullary lamina; Put = putamen; RN = red nucleus; smSTN = sensorimotor portion of the subthalamic nucleus. ROIs from the DBS Intrinsic Template Atlas.[50] (*Brain backdrop from* [Edlow BL, Mareyam A, Horn A, et al. 7 T MRI of the ex vivo human brain at 100 micron resolution. Sci Data. Oct 30 2019;6(1):244.])

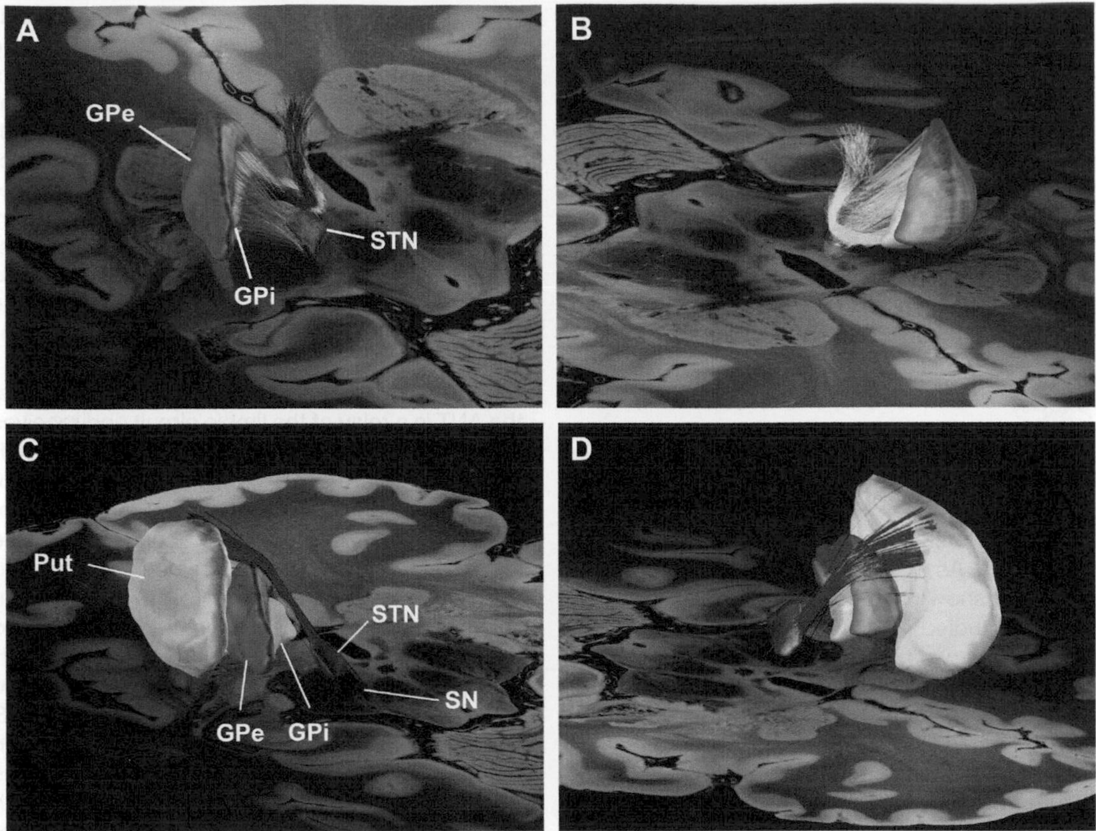

Fig. 3. (*A*) Posterior oblique and (*B*) anterior oblique images showing the pallidofugal fibers including the fasciculus subthalamicus (blue fibers) and ansa subthalamica (purple fibers), connecting the pallidum to the STN, and the ansa lenticularis (yellow fibers) and fasciculus lenticularis (orange fibers), which join to form the thalamic fasciculus inserting into the ventral thalamus. (*C*) Posterior oblique and (*D*) anterior oblique images of the course of the striatofugal fibers (red tracts) connecting the SN to the putamen (Put). The fibers course ventral and lateral to the STN before passing superior to the globus pallidus internus (GPi) and externus (GPe). ROIs from the DBS Intrinsic Template Atlas[50]; pallidofugal fibers from Petersen and colleagues[52]. (*Brain backdrop from* [Edlow BL, Mareyam A, Horn A, et al. 7 T MRI of the ex vivo human brain at 100 micron resolution. Sci Data. Oct 30 2019;6(1):244.])

Obsessive-Compulsive Disorder

In 2009, the FDA issued a humanitarian device exemption for DBS in the treatment of obsessive-compulsive disorder (OCD) by targeting the anterior limb of the internal capsule (ALIC). However, the treatment outcomes were initially quite variable resulting in the exploration of other targets, such as the anteriomedial STN, nucleus accumbens, and ventral striatum. Nevertheless, the variation in outcome with differing targets led to confusion regarding the optimal stimulation target.

As with many neuropsychiatric disorders, localizationist theories have historically provided little insight into the pathogenesis. However, connectomics provides new insights into the mechanistic basis of OCD. Both patients with OCD and their first-degree relatives have been shown to have alterations in functional connectivity compared with controls. Widespread network disturbances are observed in OCD, particularly within the limbic network and mediated by cortical-striatal-thalamic-cortical connections.[35] These limbic network alterations may serve as a substrate for the effects of neuromodulation.

Initial interest in connectomics suggested several potential pathways that may mediate response to DBS. One target includes what was originally named the "superolateral branch of the medial forebrain bundle."[36] Importantly, this tract was only identified by MR diffusion tractography and had an anatomic description that did not follow the traditional, established anatomy of the medial forebrain bundle. Subsequently, a common tract was identified along the course of many described OCD DBS targets corresponding to the hyperdirect pathways from the anteromedial

STN to the frontal cortex, particularly dorsal anterior cingulate cortex and ventrolateral prefrontal cortex, which traverse within the ventral ALIC (Fig. 4).[37] As discussed earlier, the anterior portion of the STN corresponds to the limbic subdivision, which reconciles the network stimulation effect with prior observations regarding limbic network disturbances in OCD.[35] Indeed, the connectomic model is able to provide a unifying hypothesis for decades of debate on the optimal "localizationist" targets by showing they are all ultimately nodes along the same network.

Epilepsy

One of the most highly studied "circuitopathies" in the history of medicine is epilepsy. Epilepsy is one of the most complex "circuitopathies" because of the heterogeneity of pathogenesis, onset zone, and so forth. As expected, numerous brain circuits have been shown to go awry in epilepsy.[38] One of the most studied networks is the DMN. The DMN is the primary "task-negative" network, which means that it is engaged in the absence of any other active task (rest). In epilepsy, the DMN has been shown to deactivate during interictal epileptiform discharges and seizures. Cessation of seizure activity has also been shown to correlate with the onset of recovery of DMN connectivity.[39,40]

DBS for treatment of drug-resistant epilepsy is the most recent US FDA approved DBS indication (2018). Unlike many movement disorders, such as ET and PD, there is no immediate response feedback to use as a biomarker to guide optimal device programming. Therefore, alternative biomarkers are vital to successful outcomes. The most common target has been the anterior nucleus of thalamus (ANT) after the Stimulation of the Anterior Nucleus of the Thalamus in Epilepsy trial, which reported a five-year responder rate of 68%.[41] Importantly, patients with temporal or frontal lobe onset of seizures had a higher response rate, which is not surprising given that the ANT is part of the limbic network and may potentially be the substrate for connectomic effects.

Situated in the anterior dorsomedial thalamus, the ANT is a relay of the limbic circuit and receives input from the mammillary bodies via the mammillothalamic tract (MMT) (Fig. 5A, B), with output from the anterior pole of the nucleus to the anterior cingulate cortex.[42,43] These connections are important as patients with greatest response to ANT DBS have been shown to have stimulation volumes located at the termination of MMT and the anterior ANT, suggesting that the modulation of these pathways may serve as the physiologic basis of seizure control.[44,45] fMRI studies of DBS effect have supported this mechanism of action by showing ANT stimulation primarily modulates the limbic and DMNs, and a greater overlap with these networks correlates with a higher rate of treatment response.[45–48]

As many nonresponders to ANT DBS had extratemporal onset, this suggests that, based on connectomic theory, modulating the limbic circuit may

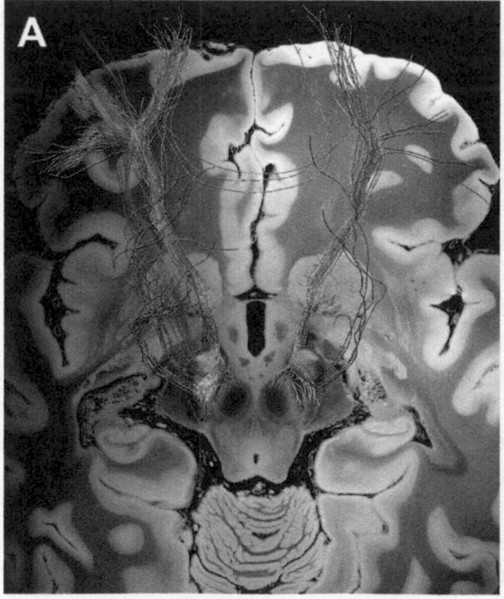

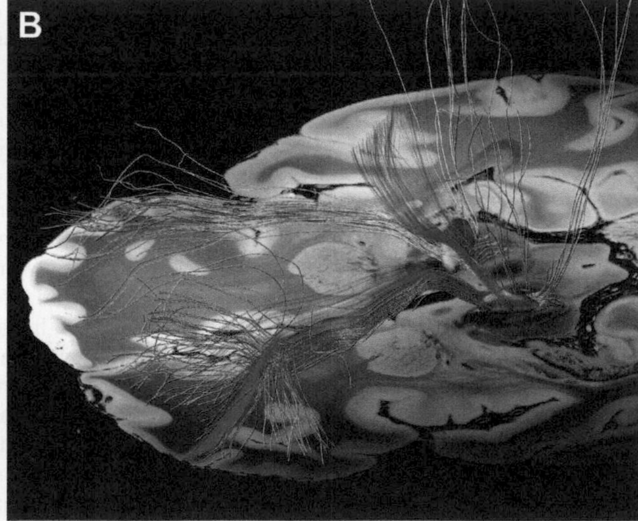

Fig. 4. (*A*) Axial and (*B*) oblique sagittal images showing the tracts (red) predictive of response to deep brain stimulation in OCD.[37] The limbic hyperdirect fibers[51] (blue tracts) from the subthalamic nucleus (orange) are shown for reference and correspond to a similar fiber distribution. ROIs from the DBS Intrinsic Template Atlas[50]; tracts from Li and colleagues[37] and Middlebrooks and colleagues.[51] (*Brain backdrop from* [Edlow BL, Mareyam A, Horn A, et al. 7 T MRI of the ex vivo human brain at 100 micron resolution. Sci Data. Oct 30 2019;6(1):244.])

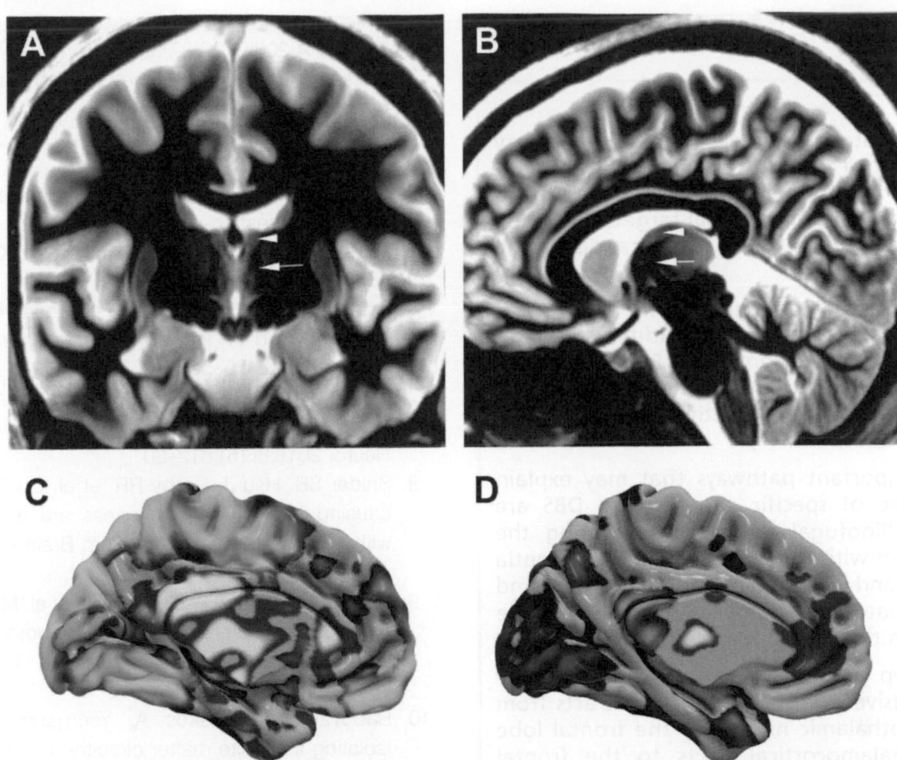

Fig. 5. (*A*) Coronal and (*B*) sagittal fast gray matter acquisition T1 inversion recover (FGATIR) MRI shows the course of the MMT (*arrow*) as it traverses through the thalamus to terminate at the anterior nucleus of the thalamus (ANT; *arrowhead*). (*C*) fMRI activation (red-orange) and deactivation (blue-green) pattern from ANT DBS stimulation in a responder shows activation in nodes of the DMN and limbic network, including anterior and posterior cingulate, anterior nucleus, hippocampus, and amygdala. (*D*) fMRI activation and deactivation in an ANT DBS nonresponder shows a largely opposite pattern with deactivation in the posterior cingulate, hippocampus, and amygdala.

not provide an ideal network effect in patients with seizures originating in other networks. As such, there has been an increasing interest in other thalamic targets, such as the centromedian nucleus in Rolandic epilepsy and Lennox-Gestaut syndrome and pulvinar in posterior quadrant epilepsy. Although data are currently limited, the reported response to such therapy supports the notion that seizure response to thalamic DBS may indeed be network-specific and provides a connectomic basis for selection of the ideal target for each individual patient. Importantly, Middlebrooks and colleagues[47] have shown variable activation patterns in ANT DBS despite similar target locations (Fig. 5C, D) suggesting that disease-related network changes may prevent adequate stimulation effect and therapeutic outcome.[49] In the future, presurgical functional imaging could perhaps provide a noninvasive measure of these network changes and serves as a biomarker to predict those patients who may not respond to neuromodulation.

SUMMARY

In conclusion, neuroradiologists must be willing to abandon the traditional concepts of human brain function in the face of mounting evidence for the science of connectomics. Although connectomics is in its infancy, solid examples of the impact on clinical medicine already exist. Historically, these updated models have improved our risk assessment for surgical planning. However, the next evolutionary leap in neuroscience may be in the arena of neuromodulation. The impact of connectomics on neuromodulation has already been shown, including the reconciliation of historical targeting differences, increased understanding of the mechanism of action, improved patient outcomes, and even the determination of new network targets. Our increasing understanding of connectomics will pave the way for patient-specific network modulation for treatment of many neurologic and neuropsychiatric disorders.

CLINICS CARE POINTS

- The dentato-rubro-thalamic tract is a primary mediator of tremor control in the treatment of essential tremor and provides a unifying explanation for traditional targets of ventral intermediate nucleus and caudal zona incerta.
- In deep brain stimulation for Parkinson's disease, improvement in rigidity correlates with greater prefrontal and SMA connectivity, bradykinesia with connectivity to SMA, and tremor with connectivity to the primary motor cortex.
- Two important pathways that may explain response of specific symptoms to DBS are the pallidofugal pathway (connecting the pallidum with the STN, thalamus, substantia nigra, and pedunculopontine nucleus) and the striatofugal pathways (connecting the SN with the pallidum and striatum).
- In deep brain stimulation for obsessive-compulsive disorder, hyperdirect tracts from the subthalamic nucleus to the frontal lobe and thalamocortical tracts to the frontal lobe may explain the effect of multiple targets from subthalamic nucleus, thalamus, anterior limb of the internal capsule, and nucleus accumbens.
- Deep brain stimulation is an effective palliative therapy for medication-refractory epilepsy, and the anterior nucleus of the thalamus is the most used target to date. Stimulation of the mammillothalamic tract and anterior pole of the anterior nucleus is likely the primary mechanism of action.

DISCLOSURE

E.H. Middlebrooks receives research support and consultant fees from Boston Scientific Corp. and Varian Medical Systems. S.S. Grewal. receives research support and consultant fees from Boston Scientific Corp. and Medtronic, Inc.

REFERENCES

1. Binder JR. The wernicke area: modern evidence and a reinterpretation. Neurology 2015;85(24): 2170–5.
2. Tremblay P, Dick AS. Broca and Wernicke are dead, or moving past the classic model of language neurobiology. Brain Lang 2016;162:60–71.
3. Fox MD, Snyder AZ, Vincent JL, et al. The human brain is intrinsically organized into dynamic, anticorrelated functional networks. Proc Natl Acad Sci U S A 2005;102(27):9673–8.
4. Buckner RL, Andrews-Hanna JR, Schacter DL. The brain's default network: anatomy, function, and relevance to disease. Ann N Y Acad Sci 2008;1124: 1–38.
5. Damoiseaux JS, Rombouts SA, Barkhof F, et al. Consistent resting-state networks across healthy subjects. Proc Natl Acad Sci U S A 2006;103(37): 13848–53.
6. Joutsa J, Horn A, Hsu J, et al. Localizing parkinsonism based on focal brain lesions. article. Brain 2018;141(8):2445–56.
7. Joutsa J, Shih LC, Fox MD. Mapping holmes tremor circuit using the human brain connectome. Ann Neurol 2019;86(6):812–20.
8. Snider SB, Hsu J, Darby RR, et al. Cortical lesions causing loss of consciousness are anticorrelated with the dorsal brainstem. Hum Brain Mapp 2020; 41(6):1520–31.
9. Elias GJB, De Vloo P, Germann J, et al. Mapping the network underpinnings of central poststroke pain and analgesic neuromodulation. Pain 2020; 161(12):2805–19.
10. Baboyan V, Basilakos A, Yourganov G, et al. Isolating the white matter circuitry of the dorsal language stream: connectome-symptom mapping in stroke induced aphasia. Hum Brain Mapp 2021; 42(17):5689–702.
11. Kim NY, Hsu J, Talmasov D, et al. Lesions causing hallucinations localize to one common brain network. Mol Psychiatry 2021;26(4):1299–309.
12. Padmanabhan JL, Cooke D, Joutsa J, et al. A human depression circuit derived from focal brain lesions. Biol Psychiatry 2019;86(10):749–58.
13. Lozano AM, Lipsman N, Bergman H, et al. Deep brain stimulation: current challenges and future directions. Nat Rev Neurol 2019;15(3):148–60.
14. Flora ED, Perera CL, Cameron AL, et al. Deep brain stimulation for essential tremor: a systematic review. Mov Disord 2010;25(11):1550–9.
15. Blomstedt P, Stenmark Persson R, Hariz GM, et al. Deep brain stimulation in the caudal zona incerta versus best medical treatment in patients with Parkinson's disease: a randomised blinded evaluation. J Neurol Neurosurg Psychiatry 2018;89(7):710–6.
16. Elias GJB, Boutet A, Joel SE, et al. Probabilistic mapping of deep brain stimulation: insights from 15 years of therapy. Ann Neurol 2021;89(3):426–43.
17. Middlebrooks EH, Grewal SS, Holanda VM. Complexities of connectivity-based DBS targeting: Rebirth of the debate on thalamic and subthalamic treatment of tremor. NeuroImage Clin 2019;22: 101761.
18. Middlebrooks EH, Okromelidze L, Wong JK, et al. Connectivity correlates to predict essential tremor deep brain stimulation outcome: Evidence for a

common treatment pathway. NeuroImage Clin 2021; 32:102846.
19. Middlebrooks EH, Holanda VM, Tuna IS, et al. A method for pre-operative single-subject thalamic segmentation based on probabilistic tractography for essential tremor deep brain stimulation. Neuroradiology 2018;60(3):303–9.
20. Middlebrooks EH, Tuna IS, Almeida L, et al. Structural connectivity-based segmentation of the thalamus and prediction of tremor improvement following thalamic deep brain stimulation of the ventral intermediate nucleus. article. NeuroImage Clin 2018;20:1266–73.
21. Fang W, Chen H, Wang H, et al. Essential tremor is associated with disruption of functional connectivity in the ventral intermediate Nucleus–Motor Cortex–Cerebellum circuit. Hum Brain Mapp 2016;37(1): 165–78.
22. Al-Fatly B, Ewert S, Kubler D, et al. Connectivity profile of thalamic deep brain stimulation to effectively treat essential tremor. Brain 2019;142(10): 3086–98.
23. Coenen VA, Sajonz B, Prokop T, et al. The dentato-rubro-thalamic tract as the potential common deep brain stimulation target for tremor of various origin: an observational case series. Acta Neurochir (Wien) 2020;162(5):1053–66.
24. Coenen VA, Madler B, Schiffbauer H, et al. Individual fiber anatomy of the subthalamic region revealed with diffusion tensor imaging: a concept to identify the deep brain stimulation target for tremor suppression. Neurosurgery 2011;68(4):1069–75. Discussion 1075-6.
25. Coenen VA, Allert N, Paus S, et al. Modulation of the cerebello-thalamo-cortical network in thalamic deep brain stimulation for tremor: a diffusion tensor imaging study. Neurosurgery 2014;75(6):657–69. Discussion 669-70.
26. Middlebrooks EH, Okromelidze L, Carter RE, et al. Directed stimulation of the dentato-rubro-thalamic tract for deep brain stimulation in essential tremor: a blinded clinical trial. Neuroradiology J 2021; 35(2):203–12.
27. Parent A, Hazrati L-N. Functional anatomy of the basal ganglia. II. the place of subthalamic nucleus and external pallidium in basal ganglia circuitry. Brain Res Rev 1995;20(1):128–54.
28. Grewal SS, Holanda VM, Middlebrooks EH. Corticopallidal connectome of the globus pallidus externus in humans: an exploratory study of structural connectivity using probabilistic diffusion tractography. AJNR Am J Neuroradiol 2018;39(11):2120–5.
29. Horn A, Reich M, Vorwerk J, et al. Connectivity predicts deep brain stimulation outcome in Parkinson disease. Article. Ann Neurol 2017;82(1):67–78.
30. Akram H, Sotiropoulos SN, Jbabdi S, et al. Subthalamic deep brain stimulation sweet spots and hyperdirect cortical connectivity in Parkinson's disease. Neuroimage 2017;158:332–45.
31. Avecillas-Chasin JM, Honey CR. Modulation of nigrofugal and pallidofugal pathways in deep brain stimulation for Parkinson disease. Neurosurgery 2020;86(4):E387–97.
32. Dembek TA, Roediger J, Horn A, et al. Probabilistic sweet spots predict motor outcome for deep brain stimulation in Parkinson disease. Ann Neurol 2019; 86(4):527–38.
33. Tsuboi T, Charbel M, Peterside DT, et al. Pallidal connectivity profiling of stimulation-induced dyskinesia in Parkinson's disease. Mov Disord 2021;36(2): 380–8.
34. Holanda VM, Okun MS, Middlebrooks EH, et al. Postmortem dissections of common targets for lesion and deep brain stimulation surgeries. Neurosurgery 2020;86(6):860–72. https://doi.org/10.1093/neuros/nyz318.
35. Hou JM, Zhao M, Zhang W, et al. Resting-state functional connectivity abnormalities in patients with obsessive-compulsive disorder and their healthy first-degree relatives. J Psychiatry Neurosci 2014; 39(5):304–11.
36. Coenen VA, Schlaepfer TE, Goll P, et al. The medial forebrain bundle as a target for deep brain stimulation for obsessive-compulsive disorder. CNS Spectr 2017;22(3):282–9.
37. Li N, Baldermann JC, Kibleur A, et al. A unified connectomic target for deep brain stimulation in obsessive-compulsive disorder. Nat Commun 2020;11(1):3364.
38. Cataldi M, Avoli M, de Villers-Sidani E. Resting state networks in temporal lobe epilepsy. Epilepsia 2013; 54(12):2048–59.
39. Danielson NB, Guo JN, Blumenfeld H. The default mode network and altered consciousness in epilepsy. Behav Neurol 2011;24(1):55–65.
40. Fahoum F, Zelmann R, Tyvaert L, et al. Epileptic discharges affect the default mode network–FMRI and intracerebral EEG evidence. PLoS One 2013;8(6): e68038.
41. Salanova V, Witt T, Worth R, et al. Long-term efficacy and safety of thalamic stimulation for drug-resistant partial epilepsy. Neurology 2015;84(10):1017–25.
42. Grewal SS, Middlebrooks EH, Kaufmann TJ, et al. Fast gray matter acquisition T1 inversion recovery MRI to delineate the mammillothalamic tract for preoperative direct targeting of the anterior nucleus of the thalamus for deep brain stimulation in epilepsy. article. Neurosurg Focus 2018;45(2):E6.
43. Ferreira TA Jr, Middlebrooks EH, Tzu WH, et al. Postmortem dissections of the papez circuit and nonmotor targets for functional neurosurgery. World Neurosurg 2020;144:e866–75.
44. Schaper F, Plantinga BR, Colon AJ, et al. Deep brain stimulation in epilepsy: a role for modulation of the

mammillothalamic tract in seizure control? Neurosurgery 2020;87(3):602–10.
45. Middlebrooks EH, Grewal SS, Stead M, et al. Differences in functional connectivity profiles as a predictor of response to anterior thalamic nucleus deep brain stimulation for epilepsy: a hypothesis for the mechanism of action and a potential biomarker for outcomes. article. Neurosurg Focus 2018;45(2):E7.
46. Middlebrooks EH, Lin C, Okromelidze L, et al. Functional activation patterns of deep brain stimulation of the anterior nucleus of the thalamus. World Neurosurg 2020;136:357–363 e2.
47. Middlebrooks EH, Jain A, Okromelidze L, et al. Acute brain activation patterns of high- versus low-frequency stimulation of the anterior nucleus of the thalamus during deep brain stimulation for epilepsy. Neurosurgery 2021;89(5):901–8.
48. Sarica C, Yamamoto K, Loh A, et al. Blood oxygen level-dependent (BOLD) response patterns with thalamic deep brain stimulation in patients with medically refractory epilepsy. Epilepsy Behav 2021;122:108153.
49. Wang YC, Kremen V, Brinkmann BH, et al. Probing circuit of Papez with stimulation of anterior nucleus of the thalamus and hippocampal evoked potentials. Epilepsy Res 2020;159:106248.
50. Ewert S, Plettig P, Li N, et al. Toward defining deep brain stimulation targets in MNI space: a subcortical atlas based on multimodal MRI, histology and structural connectivity. review. Neuroimage 2018;170:271–82.
51. Middlebrooks EH, Domingo RA, Vivas-Buitrago T, et al. Neuroimaging advances in deep brain stimulation: review of indications, anatomy, and brain connectomics. AJNR Am J Neuroradiol 2020;41(9):1558–68.
52. Petersen MV, Mlakar J, Haber SN, et al. Holographic reconstruction of axonal pathways in the human brain. Neuron 2019;104(6):1056–64. e3.

MRI-Visible Anatomy of the Brainstem

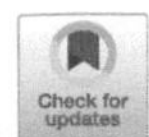

Timothy M. Shepherd, MD, PhD[a,*], Michael J. Hoch, MD[b]

KEYWORDS

• Parkinsonism • Nigrosome • Locus coeruleus • Tractography • FGATIR • Neuromelanin

KEY POINTS

- Despite appearing homogeneous on conventional sequences, every MRI voxel within the brainstem contains eloquent structures associated with different clinical signs and symptoms.
- The fast gray matter acquisition T1 inversion recovery (FGATIR) MRI sequence provides excellent contrast resolution for many brainstem structures based on myelination and can serve as clinical index standard for evaluating other MRI sequences.
- Diffusion MRI provides incomplete contrast resolution of brainstem structures owing to their small size relative to feasible image voxel size and often similar diffusion anisotropy (magnitude and orientation) to adjacent structures.
- Neuromelanin and susceptibility-weighted imaging sequences provide novel contrasts in selected upper brainstem structures that may improve detection of early neurodegenerative disease.

INTRODUCTION

The brainstem and upper cervical spinal cord are the only nervous system structures absolutely necessary for life. The brainstem contains nuclei that control essential functions such as respiration, eye movements, hearing, interoception, taste, and swallowing. Further, the brainstem is a critical nexus for axonal projections between the cerebral cortex, basal ganglia, thalamus, cerebellum, and spinal cord—brainstem nuclei further modulate or regulate these traversing pathways.[1] Isodendritic cores within the brainstem, such as the locus coeruleus or raphe nuclei, project extensively to other subcortical brain structures to modulate their function by altering local neurotransmitter availability and homeostasis.[2] These same brainstem structures are the first to show histopathologic changes in Alzheimer or Parkinson disease.[3,4] The brainstem can be affected by other common neurologic diseases such as demyelination, ischemia and tumor.[5–7] Even focal 1-mm pathologic condition or lesions can have profound clinical consequences because of the inherently dense and compact nature of brainstem neuroanatomy. Better direct visualization of this anatomy has the potential to improve focal lesion location, neurosurgical treatments, and accuracy of quantitative MRI analysis for local histopathology.

The intricate neuroanatomy of the brainstem is obvious on postmortem histology but the current state-of-the-art clinical MRI depicts the internal contrast of the brainstem anatomy poorly. Trainees, instead, learn brainstem anatomy from histology atlases usually based on a single postmortem sample with limited clinical validity except to future neuropathologists. Clinicians infer the location of specific structures based on their knowledge of histology-defined anatomy relative to the patient's brainstem surface anatomy and a few internal landmarks visible on conventional MRI. We suggest many radiologists eventually forget most brainstem anatomy because it is rarely visible on imaging studies! Postmortem MRI using clinically impossible scan times (eg, 8–100 hours),

[a] Department of Radiology, New York University Langone School of Medicine, 660 First Avenue, Room 230D, New York, NY 10016, USA; [b] Department of Radiology, University of Pennsylvania, 3400 Spruce Street, Suite 130, Philadelphia, PA 19104, USA
* Corresponding author.
E-mail address: timothy.shepherd@nyulangone.org
Twitter: @tim0shepherd (T.M.S.); @RVUhound (M.J.H.)

Neuroimag Clin N Am 32 (2022) 553–564
https://doi.org/10.1016/j.nic.2022.04.003

Abbreviations	
MRI	Magnetic Resonance Imaging
CSF	CerebroSpinal Fluid
NYU	New York University
MPRAGE	Magnetization Prepared RApid Gradient Echo
DESIGNER	Diffusion parameter EStImation with Gibbs and NoisE Removal
FSL	FMRIB Software Library
FLIRT	FMRIB's Linear Image Registration Tool
FDA	Food & Drug Administration
PD	Parkinson's Disease

high static magnetic fields (7-T or greater), and radiofrequency coils smaller than the human head can generate truly exquisite contrast resolution of internal brainstem anatomy.[8–11] These results can be coregistered to in vivo MRI[12] and have potential advantages over histology for quantitative research investigations. These studies also prove that MRI contrasts have the intrinsic potential to depict internal brainstem anatomy well. To achieve this in vivo, however, MRI of the brainstem must overcome the scan-time tolerances of living patients, CSF flow, brainstem motion, adjacent skull base artifacts, and signal-to-noise limitations that affect both spatial and contrast image resolution. There are several potential approaches to improving in vivo visualization of internal brainstem anatomy including increased image resolution, atlas-based segmentation, or even coregistration to higher resolution ex vivo MRI microscopy data. During the past 7 years, we have borrowed, modified, or developed clinically feasible sequences for improved imaging of in vivo brainstem neuroanatomy using widely available 3-T MRI.[13,14] These sequences converge around 1-mm isotropic resolution that is probably the limit for clinical feasibility at this time. Such "limited" spatial and contrast resolution also has the advantage of not revealing too much; hence, we are able to focus this report on the most clinically relevant MRI-visible brainstem neuroanatomy.

IMAGING THE BRAINSTEM

Visualizing brainstem anatomy in vivo using MRI is not easy. Unlike the cerebral hemispheres, the brainstem is a highly compact 3D arrangement of many nuclei and small-diameter myelinated axonal pathways. Even a 1-mm increment in any direction within the brain stem produces a high probability of moving to an adjacent, functionally distinct structure. It is unlikely that in vivo MRI spatial resolution will ever be adequate to reveal the "complete" functional organization of the brainstem. The reticular formation is composed of numerous important nuclei that often have obscure names, some of which are just subtle clusters of neurons only distinct from their surroundings using specific immunohistological stains. Most of these small nuclei have very similar signal characteristics using conventional MRI contrasts such as T1, T2, and FLAIR sequences. Unlike the corpus callosum or internal capsule, traversing and internally connecting axonal projections can be much smaller but also vary more in myelination and the compactness of their fascicles along the superior-inferior axis of the brainstem. The in vivo brainstem moves more than the cerebrum because of a complex interaction of CSF flow with overlapping periodic motions from respiration and cardiac pulsation. Finally, the brainstem is situated in the posterior fossa where adjacent bone, air spaces, and ligamentous structures create magnetic field inhomogeneities that degrade multiple MRI sequences, especially at higher static magnetic fields (eg, 7T).

Table 1 provides key details of the current NYU clinical MRI protocol we have developed for imaging subcortical anatomy (brainstem, basal ganglia, and thalamus) using an outpatient 3-T MRI Prisma system with 20-channel head and neck coil (Siemens Healthcare, Erlangen, Germany). This clinical protocol is currently used for localizing brainstem lesions in selected cases (stroke, multiple sclerosis, or other), surgical planning for resection or biopsy of brainstem masses (eg, cavernomas), and for research protocols in neurodegeneration. The 3D MPRAGE and 2D axial T2 sequences are widely used standards. The susceptibility-weighted imaging (SWI) and neuromelanin sequences are based on prior publications—the latter sequence is not obtained for all clinical applications (eg, not for surgical planning).

Table 1
NYU Subcortical Anatomy Clinical MRI protocol (Brainstem, basal ganglia, and thalamus)[a]

Sequence	Time	Resolution	TR/TE/TI (ms)	FA	NEX	iPAT	Additional Details
MPRAGE	5:06	3D: 1-mm isotropic	2200/3.17/900	9°	1	2	90 degree inversion pulse
T2	4:29	2D: 0.6 × 0.6 × 2 mm	6520/110/–	150°	2	–	ETL = 20, TF = 14
FGATIR	12:50	3D: 0.8-mm isotropic	3000/1.95/410	6°	1	2	180 degree inversion pulse
DTI	8:58	3D: 2-mm isotropic	5200/84/–	–	1	2	2-shell, b = 1000 × 21 and 2000 × 65 + b = 0 PA reversal
SWI	11:44	3D: 0.7-mm isotropic	64/35/-	10°	2	–	–
NM	6:57	2D: 0.5 × 0.5 × 3 mm	270/2.76/–	40°	7	2	MT offset = 1200 Hz, pulse duration = 10.24 ms

Abbreviations: b, diffusion weighting (s/mm^2); ETL, echo train length; FA, flip angle; iPAT, parallel imaging factor; MT, magnetization transfer; NEX, averages; TE, echo time; TF, turbo factor; TI, inversion time; TR, repetition time.
[a] 3T Prisma MRI, 20-channel head and neck coil; total time = 50 min 4 s; full protocol available on reasonable request

Although it can be helpful for localization and clinical decision-making, it is beyond the scope of the current presentation to show penetrating, surface, and overlying vessels of the brainstem or the cranial nerve anatomy in the basal cisterns. A 3D FLAIR sequence accelerated by compressed sensing reconstructions (~3–4 minutes) also can be helpful for detecting white matter changes and supratentorial pathologic condition. This protocol also was used for our companion report on basal ganglia and thalamus—full details will be provided on reasonable request.

Multishell diffusion MRI data were acquired with parallel imaging and simultaneous multislice technique to accelerate acquisition times.[15,16] Our up-to-date analysis pipeline for 1-mm isotropic resolution diffusion MRI data has been recently described.[17] Raw complex diffusion data were denoised using Marchenko-Pasteur Principle Component Analysis.[18] These diffusion data were further preprocessed using DESIGNER, which includes correction for partial Fourier (6/8) induced Gibb ringing, eddy current, and echoplanar imaging distortion corrections.[19] Diffusion data then were coregistered to MPRAGE using a 6-degrees of freedom rigid transform using FSL-FLIRT.[20] The multishell diffusion data can be used for diffusion tensor or kurtosis fitting, advanced models of nervous tissue, and tractography. For this report, we chose direction-encoded color tractography to illustrate diffusion-based contrast of normal brainstem anatomy. Whole brain fiber tracking was performed for the diffusion dataset using the probabilistic tensor-tracking algorithm with matrix3, 100,000 selected streamlines, and flip angle (FA) cutoff of 0.30. Direction-encoded color probabilistic streamlines were superimposed on background fast gray matter acquisition T1 inversion recovery (FGATIR) images for the figures in this report. Streamlines were color-coded where red = left–right, green = anterior–posterior, and blue—superior–inferior tract orientation.

The 3D FGATIR sequence uses a shorter inversion time than MPRAGE (410 vs 900 ms, respectively) to better suppress signal from myelinated structures in the subcortical brain. FGATIR was created to improve direct targeting of thalamic nuclei for functional neurosurgery.[21] We recently reported that FGATIR also generates excellent contrast resolution of internal brainstem anatomy in living subjects.[14] However, in that initial report multiple signal averages were coregistered and averaged outside k-space to generate sufficient contrast for seeing smaller structures and resolving internal features of the tegmentum. This was a long acquisition (eg, 3–4 individual averages taking 12–15 minutes each) limiting its widespread application in patients. We have recently developed a denoising approach using a convolutional neural network (CNN) trained on multiaverage data from controls to improve the image contrast resolution of FGATIR using a single average. Single average CNN-denoised FGATIR images seem equivalent to 3 to 4 averages on quantitative image measurements and subjective rater assessment.[22] The brainstem images shown here use this newer CNN-denoised single-average FGATIR acquisition.

NORMAL ANATOMY

It is beyond the scope of this review to show "all" MRI contrasts at multiple levels of the brainstem, so we have focused on the contrasts that we think are the most promising overall clinically—FGATIR and direction-encoded color diffusion tractography (DEC-DT). **Fig. 1** shows imaging planes for **Figs. 2–6** and **Box 1** provides the legend for labels in all figures. We demonstrate canonical axial

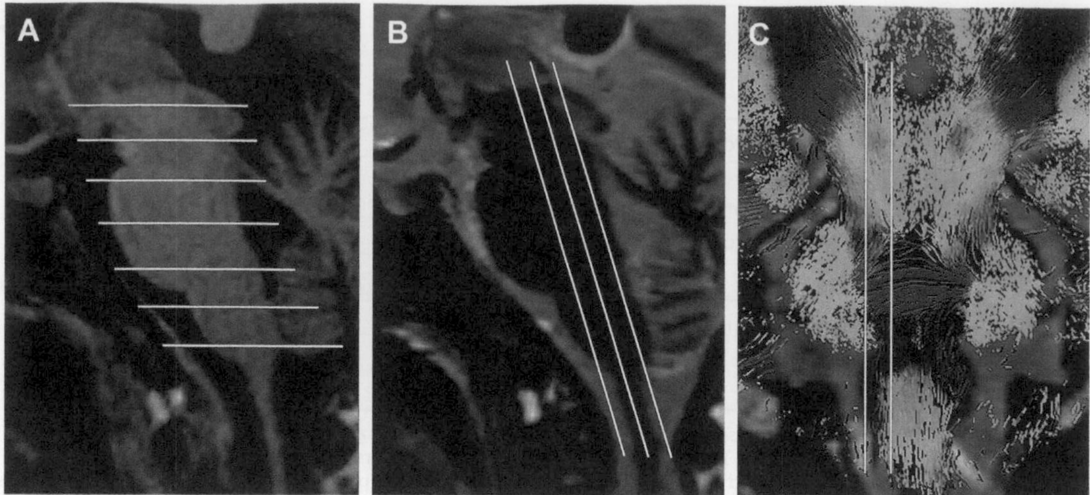

Fig. 1. Roadmap for subsequent figures/images of human brainstem anatomy using 3-T MRI. Axial lines overlaid on the parasagittal MPRAGE image (*A*) depict canonical axial planes parallel to the commissural plane used for midbrain, pons, and medulla (see Figs. 2–4 respectively). Oblique coronal lines overlaid on the parasagittal FGATIR image (*B*) depict coronal planes parallel and 2, 4, or 6-mm deep to the rhomboid fossa in Fig. 5. Parasagittal lines overlaid on a coronal DEC-DT image registered to an FGAITR background image (*C*) depict parasagittal planes in Fig. 6.

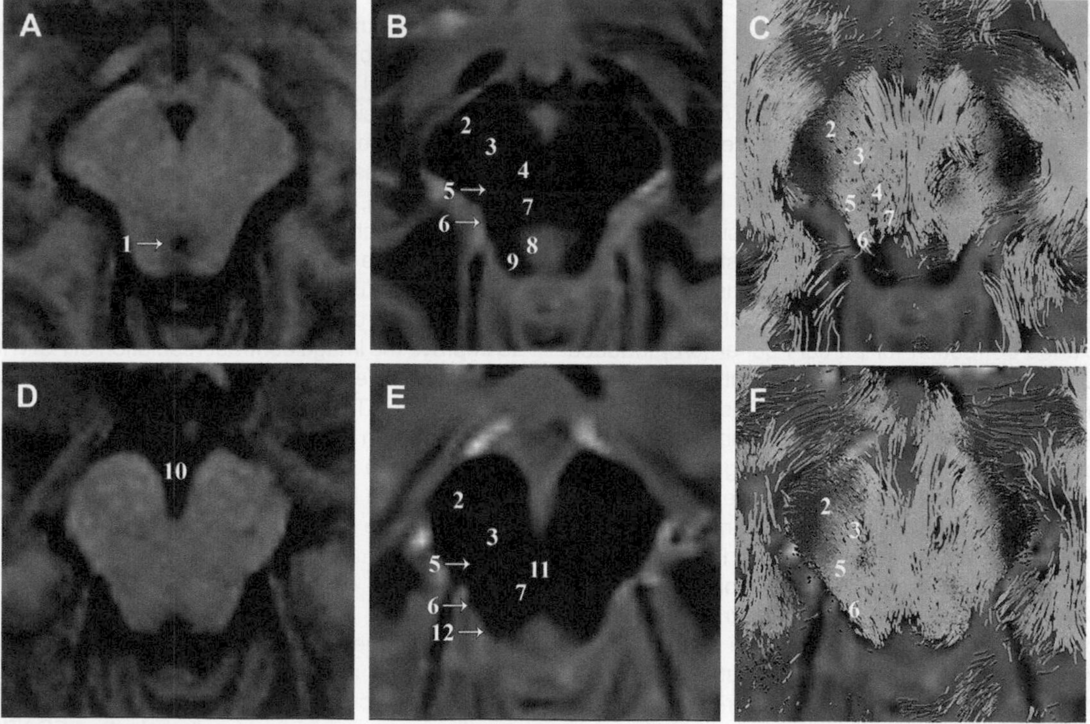

Fig. 2. Axial MPRAGE, FGATIR, and DEC-DT images of the superior (*A–C*) and inferior midbrain (*D–F*), respectively (see Box 1 for legend). Fibers of the dentatorubrothalamic tract pass through and around the red nucleus (4; panel *C*) resulting in superior–inferior anisotropy. Despite their myelination and high anisotropy on histology and postmortem MRI, the medial lemniscus (5) and spinothalamic tract (6) visualized on FGATIR (*B, E*) are not resolved well with in vivo 2-mm isotropic DEC-DT (*C, F*).

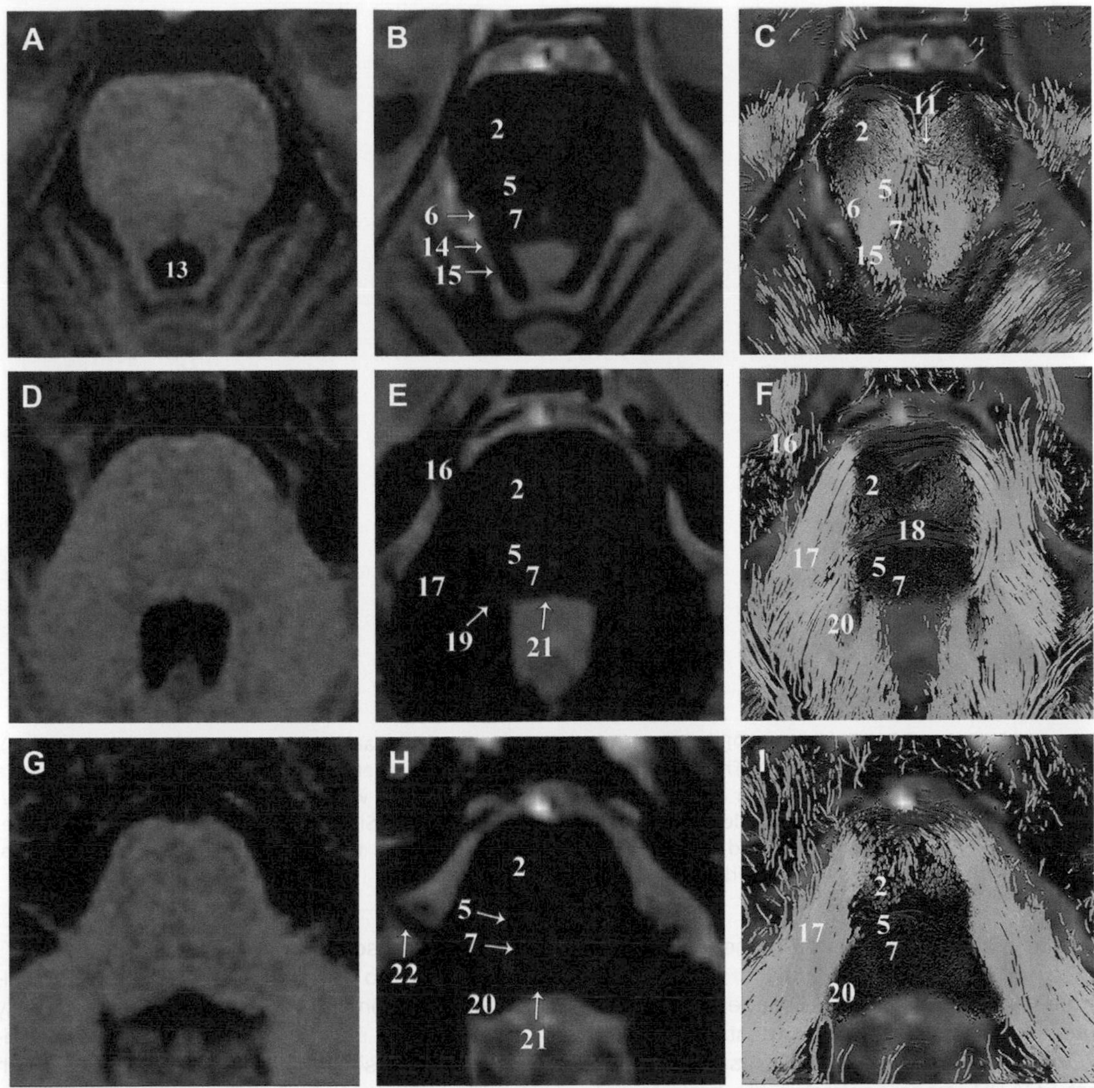

Fig. 3. Axial MPRAGE, FGATIR, and DEC-DT images of the superior (*A–C*), mid (*D–F*), and inferior pons (*G–I*), respectively (see Box 1 for legend). The FGATIR and DEC-DT images both resolve the corticospinal tracts (2). The medial lemniscus (%) seems as a horizontal dark band on FGATIR images (*B,E,H*) that helps define the anterior border of the pontine tegmentum. DEC-DT of the normal tegmentum lacks contrast resolution of individual structures compared with FGATIR (that emphasizes myelination) because most structures in this region have similar magnitude of superior-inferior anisotropy (*blue*; *C,F,I*).

anatomy using coregistered MPRAGE, FGATIR, and DEC-DT (superimposed on background FGATIR image) in the superior and inferior midbrain (see Fig. 2); superior, middle, and inferior pons (see Fig. 3); and superior and inferior medulla (see Fig. 4). Many of the MRI sequences in the NYU subcortical anatomy protocol generate isotropic resolution that improves localization and understanding of spatial relationships of structures or potential lesions in multiple imaging planes. Simultaneous multiplane visualization was essential to us when initially identifying some of the smaller individual structures labeled here and in our recent publications. Fig. 5 demonstrates coronal brainstem anatomy visible with FGATIR using an imaging plane that parallels the rhomboid fossa (ie, floor of the fourth ventricle). Fig. 6 demonstrates sagittal brainstem anatomy in 2 parasagittal images with direction-encoded color diffusion tractography (superimposed on background FGATIR image). We also have included 2 additional MRI sequences for readers interested in movement disorders using a healthy control subject. Fig. 7 demonstrates a slightly

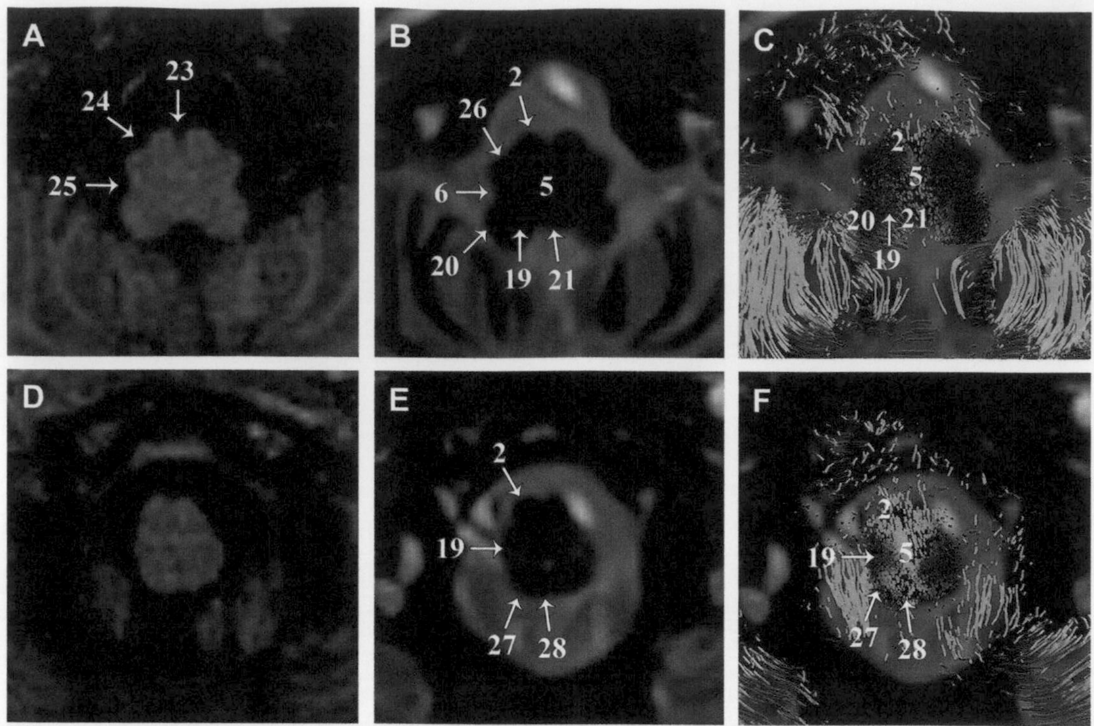

Fig. 4. Axial MPRAGE, FGATIR, and DEC-DT images of the superior (*A–C*) and inferior medulla oblongata (*D–F*), respectively (see Box 1 for legend). The X-shaped dark signal in the center of the inferior or "closed" medulla is the sensory decussation. The motor decussation also can be clearly seen with FGATIR (not shown). The left pyramidal tract (2) is deformed by the left intradural vertebral artery (*E,F*). Similar to sulcation patterns in the cerebrum, we have previously reported substantial individual variability in the size and shape of the pyramidal tracts and other structures in the medulla.

oblique axial plane relative to the commissural plane using neuromelanin MRI. Fig. 8 demonstrates axial and coronal SWI images that both traverse nigrosome-1 within the substantia nigra.

Comparison to histology atlases demonstrates that FGATIR image contrast in the brainstem depends on the amount of myelin present. Densely myelinated structures (eg, corticospinal tract or medial lemniscus) seem dark, whereas brainstem nuclei (substantia nigra or inferior olivary nucleus) seem bright. Structures with less densely packed myelin, such as the central tegmental tract (see Fig. 2B or 5C), demonstrate intermediate signal intensity that is distinguishable from the background pontine tegmentum. It is remarkable to see all the internal features FGATIR shows in the brainstem compared with the coregistered T1-weighted MPRAGE. We previously reported highly detailed analysis of the brainstem anatomy based on ~1 to 2 hours of FGATIR acquisitions at 800-μm isotropic resolution.[14] The present CNN-denoised single average FGATIR shows less detail, and there is the appearance of image smoothing but it is much more feasible to acquire in patients (and requires less recall of neuroanatomy knowledge from medical school!). Recently FDA-approved 7-T MRI[23,24] also can be used for FGATIR acquisitions but T1 contrast is diminished, 7T is not widely available, and skull base artifacts make complementary MRI sequences such as diffusion much harder in the posterior fossa.

We encourage readers to review and identify long white matter tracts that traverse large portions of the brainstem first, including the corticospinal tract, medial lemniscus, central tegmental tract, and proximal portions of the dentatorubrothalamic tract. We have previously observed asymmetries in signal intensity for the corticospinal tracts with left appearing darker on in vivo FGATIR and ex vivo T2-weighted MRI sequences (eg, compare right and left on Fig. 3H). This may reflect asymmetries in myelination or the relative compactness of the corticospinal tract. Further research is needed to determine if this also correlates with some component of handedness. The FGATIR sequence also demonstrates smaller or less distinct myelinated tracts such as the medial longitudinal fasciculus, spinothalamic tract, and lateral lemniscus. Larger brainstem nuclei, such as the substantia nigra and inferior olivary nucleus,

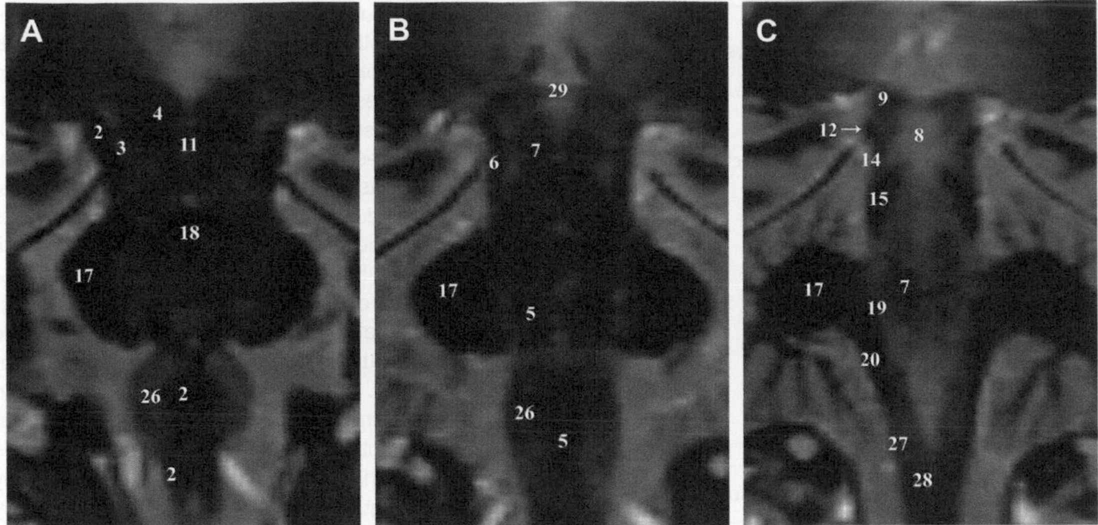

Fig. 5. Oblique coronal FGATIR images of the brainstem ordered anterior to posterior approximately 6, 4, and 2-mm deep and parallel to the rhomboid fossa (*A*, *B*, and *C*, respectively). Similar to supratentorial white matter pathways, the corticospinal tract (2; *A*) and medial lemniscus (5; *B*) bend, twist, rotate, and translate their positions relative to the center and surface of the brainstem along its superior–inferior axis making it difficult to demonstrate entire tracts in a single planar image. Gray matter in the vagal and hypoglossal trigone (V-shaped bright region in lower panel *C*) have subtle contrast differences to CSF in the fourth ventricle better appreciated in axial images (see Fig. 4B).

appear more hyperintense and then are defined by location and adjacent myelinated regions. Finally, the visual brainstem structures can be used to better infer the locations of additional structures not clearly seen such as the locus coeruleus lateral to the central tegmental tract in Fig. 3B, or the trapezoid body (auditory pathway) along the anterolateral margin of the medial lemniscus in Fig. 3H.

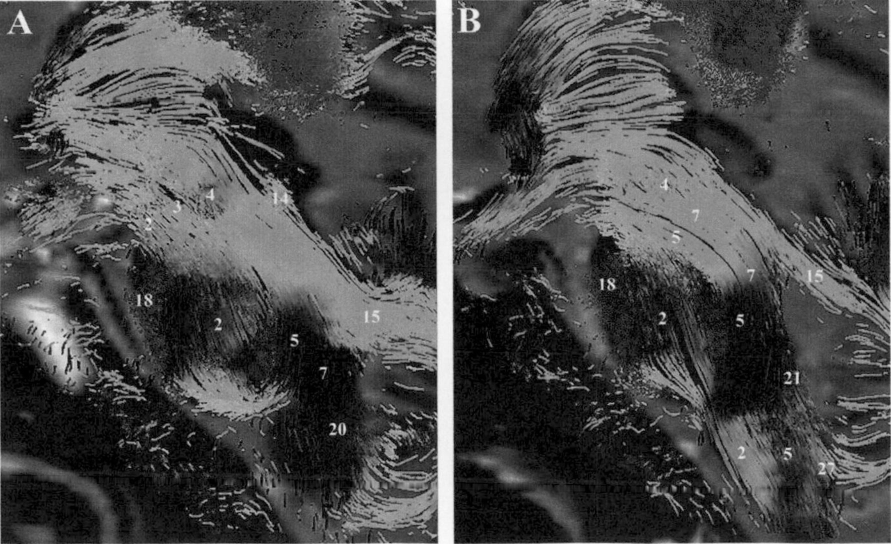

Fig. 6. Sagittal DEC-DT images through the lateral (*A*) and medial (*B*) aspects of the red nucleus (4; blue structure). The midbrain/thalamus and pons/medulla are dominated by anterior–posterior and superior–inferior anisotropy, respectively. In the lower brainstem, the corticospinal tract (2), medial lemniscus (5), central tegmental tract (7), inferior cerebellar peduncle (20), and medial longitudinal fasciculus (21) have similar anisotropy (magnitude and orientation; blue) and can only be distinguished by position within the brainstem relative to the surface and traversing ponto-cerebellar fibers (18; red structure).

Box 1
Anatomic assignments of brainstem structures labeled in the figures

1. Cerebral Aqueduct
2. Corticospinal—Pyramidal Tract
3. Substania Nigra
4. Red Nucleus
5. Medial Lemniscus
6. Spinothalamic Tract
7. Central Tegmental Tract
8. Periaqueductal Gray Matter
9. Superior Colliculus
10. Interpeduncular Cistern
11. Decussation of the Superior Cerebellar Peduncles
12. Brachium of the Inferior Colliculus
13. Fourth Ventricle
14. Lateral Lemniscus
15. Superior Cerebellar Peduncle
16. Trigeminal Nerve
17. Middle Cerebellar Peduncle
18. Ponto-cerebellar Fibers
19. Trigeminal Nucleus and Tract
20. Inferior Cerebellar Peduncle
21. Medial Longitudinal Fasciculus
22. Facial and Vestibulocochlear Nerves
23. Median Sulcus
24. Preolivary Sulcus
25. Postolivary Sulcus
26. Inferior Olivary Nucleus
27. Cuneate Fasciculus
28. Gracile Fasciculus
29. Posterior Commissure
30. Cerebral Peduncle
31. Substantia Nigra Pars Reticulata
32. Substantia Nigra Pars Compacta (anterior)
33. Substantia Nigra Pars Compacta (posterior)
34. Intermediate Area/Parabrachial Pigmented Nucleus
35. Subthalamic Nucleus
36. Ventral Tegmental Area
37. Locus Coeruleus

We hypothesize that the accuracy of indirect localization is improved by the visibility of adjacent internal structures.

Multiple groups have used high angular resolution diffusion MRI to depict normal brainstem anatomy.[25–27] We previously used track density imaging (TDI), a superresolution technique based on whole-brain probabilistic tractography,[28] to generate 500-μm isotropic resolution images of the in vivo brainstem.[13] TDI has limitations and brainstem contrast may be altered by pathologic condition or artifacts anywhere in the brain.[29] This could ultimately limit the use of TDI in patients. Here, we chose to illustrate direction-encoded color probabilistic tractography images of the brainstem derived from simple DTI representations of source 2mm isotropic diffusion MRI data. Similar to FGATIR, these diffusion tractography images consistently provide better contrast resolution of internal brainstem structures compared with the MPRAGE images (and many other MRI sequences not shown). We admittedly have kept the tractography relatively simple—more advanced models of diffusion, different tractography algorithms, or conditions may show additional structures but this is beyond the scope of this report and may require too much scan time in real patients.

The corticospinal tract and cerebellar peduncles are well visualized throughout the brainstem. The red nucleus is in fact "blue" (see **Figs.** 1C and 2C) owing to the superior orientation of the dentatorubrothalamic tract that surrounds and passes through the red nucleus. Interestingly, we see only a small volume of left–right orientation within the inferior aspect of the decussation of the superior cerebellar peduncle (see **Fig.** 3C). The more anterior orientation in the midbrain tegmentum is attributed to the anterior–superior curvature of the superior medial longitudinal fasciculus and central tegmental tract, and the anterior direction for the roots of the oculomotor nerves. The medullary and pontine tegmentum is dominated by superior–inferior diffusion anisotropy or "tracts." The medial lemniscus and central tegmental tract cannot be individually discriminated with diffusion tractography. This problem may be partially resolved with other DTI parameter maps but it is much easier to recognize the tracts with FGATIR. This suggests relative differences in myelination within the tegmentum provide better contrast than differences in anisotropy magnitude and orientation. We suggest FGATIR can be used as an in vivo index standard for validating tractography in the brainstem and other subcortical regions for some myelinated axonal projections such as the medial lemniscus. Conversely, neither diffusion tractography or FGATIR can visually discriminate the adjacent medial lemniscus, tectospinal tract, and medial longitudinal fasciculus that form paired inverted triangles in the midline of the

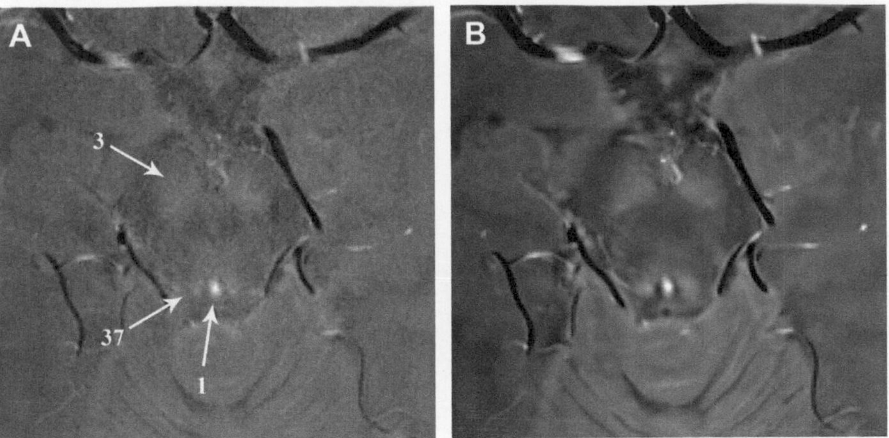

Fig. 7. Oblique axial neuromelanin-sensitive MRI image of the midbrain before and after image denoising with a convolutional neural network (*A* and *B*, respectively) in a healthy adult subject. Quantitative reductions in Neuromelanin signal intensity within the substantia nigra (3) are associated with Parkinson disease and Parkinson-plus syndromes but not essential tremor. Reductions in signal intensity within the locus coeruleus may be associated with depression, Parkinson disease, or neurofibrillary tangle pathologic condition in Alzheimer disease.

medulla (nor resolve the different components of the cerebral peduncles).

The tegmentum also contains the reticular formation made of multiple small nuclei that are difficult to discriminate even in postmortem samples with immunohistochemistry or MRI microscopy. We consider these regions the "dark matter" of the brainstem that contain structures of great importance to functional neurosurgery, such as the pedunculopontine nucleus[30] or great importance to neurodegenerative disease, such as the locus coeruleus.[2] We previously described how some of these regions can be indirectly localized based on proximity to visible boundaries on MRI sequences such as FGATIR.[14] The neuromelanin MRI sequence in fact can define the location of the locus coeruleus, the earliest brain site for neurofibrillary tangles in Alzheimer disease, within the dorsolateral brainstem at the junction of the pons and midbrain (see Fig. 7A). Neuromelanin is a protein byproduct of catecholamine synthesis that also can be detected in the ventral tegmental

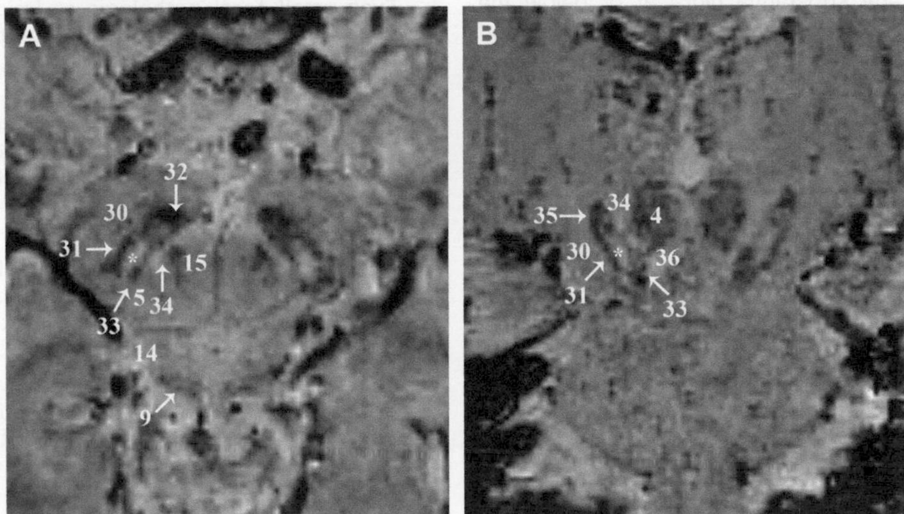

Fig. 8. Axial (*A*) 1-mm isotropic SWI of the midbrain just below the red nucleus demonstrates a "swallow-tail" formed by the bright nigrosome-1 (*) surrounded by more iron-containing and hence darker parts of the substantia nigra pars compacta. We observed a relative "swallow-tail" is also visible in the coronal plane generated from 3D SWI data (*B*). Nigrosome-1 is selectively vulnerable to Lewy body pathologic —loss of the bright signal and swallow tail can be observed in Parkinson disease, Lewy Body dementia, and other Parkinson-plus syndromes but not essential tremor.

area (VTA) and substantia nigra pas compacta.[31] This protein causes T1 relaxation that can be detected by T1-weighted MRI sequences further sensitized by magnetization transfer pulses.[32] Decreased absolute signal or relative area of neuromelanin signal in the substantia nigra (see **Fig. 7**) is observed in Parkinson disease and Parkinson-plus syndromes but not essential tremor.[33] Neuromelanin MRI seems to be valuable as a targeted MRI contrast for assessing these 3 brainstem regions (VTA not discussed) but does not provide useful contrast in other brainstem regions.

SWI is another sequence that provides selective but interesting contrast in the upper brainstem.[34] Susceptibility changes can be seen with deoxygenated blood, iron, hemosiderin, and calcium. In particular, SWI demonstrates internal features of the substantia nigra much better than MPRAGE, FGATIR, diffusion, or neuromelanin MRI (Compare **Figs. 2**D–F, **7A**, and **8A**). Low signal on SWI also defines the margins of the red nucleus (**Fig. 8**B), crus cerebri, and subthalamic nucleus.[35] SWI contrast of internal brainstem anatomy below the midbrain is limited (see lower half of **Fig. 8**B) but high-resolution 3D SWI does demonstrate large penetrating arteries and veins within the brainstem parenchyma (eg, see midline vessel **Fig. 8**A) that may be helpful for surgical planning. The substantia nigra is a primary site of a dopamine synthesis pathway that involves iron.[36] This results in mild hypointense signal in healthy controls but excess iron accumulates in Parkinson disease.[37] Nigrosome-1 is a calbindin-poor zone within the posterolateral substantia nigra at or below the margin of the red nucleus that is iron-free and seems bright on SWI sequences.[38] This is visible as a bright region bordered anteriorly and posteriorly by dark iron-richer portions of the inferior substantia nigra—the imaging appearance is called the "swallow tail." Nigrosome-1 seems disproportionately affected by dopaminergic neuron loss in early PD and results in the loss of the swallow tail.[39] This abnormality is also seen in Parkinson-plus syndromes but not essential tremor or vascular parkinsonism. SWI at 7T can also detect Nigrosomes 2, 4, and 5, which are located in the substantia nigra at the level of the red nucleus but these are smaller and so far considered less useful clinically.[33]

SUMMARY

We need to directly visualize functionally important individual nuclei and tracts to improve our understanding of in vivo brainstem function in health and disease. This report demonstrates that FGATIR, diffusion-based contrast, neuromelanin and SWI sequences all provide clinically feasible and complementary ways to improve visualization of internal brainstem anatomy in individual patients using widely available 3-T MRI. Even localization of some key brainstem structures can improve the accuracy of indirect localization for other clinically important structures, including isodendritic cores. Diffusion-based methods based on tractography, anisotropy, or other parameter maps generate beautiful maps of some normal brainstem anatomy but have spatial resolution limitations due to poor signal-to-noise and require incompletely validated modeling assumptions. Ideally, brainstem anatomy can be visualized with a contrast that is not altered by early pathologic condition or treatment—this also seems to be a limitation to relying solely on diffusion-based anatomic parcellations. We are most excited about using 1-mm isotropic FGATIR[14] with CNN denoising[22] to generate a clinically feasible index standard for imaging brainstem anatomic contrast that is intuitive to clinicians previously taught using histology. This 3D sequence is less sensitive to skull base artifacts, may be robust to early tissue pathology and serves as excellent registration target for complementary MRI sequences and surgical navigation software.

CLINICS CARE POINTS

- Even small focal pathologic or lesions can have profound clinical consequences because of the inherently dense and compact nature of brainstem neuroanatomy.
- Single average fast gray matter acquisition T1 inversion recovery denoised by a convolutional neural network is a clinically feasible 3-T MRI approach for demonstrating long brainstem tracts and some brainstem nuclei.
- Diffusion anisotropy and tractography provide useful contrast in the brainstem but have some important limitations that should be recognized.
- In patients, diffusion MRI approaches may be better suited for assessing connectivity or pathologic changes than as an index standard for localizing internal brainstem anatomy.

DISCLOSURE

T.M. Shepherd is cofounder and equity holder for MICroStructure Imaging (MICSI). M.J. Hoch has nothing to disclose.

REFERENCES

1. Carpenter MB, Strong OS, Truex RC. Human neuroanatomy (formerly Strong and Elwyn's human neuroanatomy). 7th edition. Philadelphia: Lippincott Williams & Wilkins; 1976.
2. Ramón-Moliner E, Nauta WJ. The isodendritic core of the brain stem. J Comp Neurol 1966;126(3):311–35.
3. Betts MJ, Kirilina E, Otaduy MCG, et al. Locus coeruleus imaging as a biomarker for noradrenergic dysfunction in neurodegenerative diseases. Brain 2019;142(9):2558–71.
4. Matchett BJ, Grinberg LT, Theofilas P, et al. The mechanistic link between selective vulnerability of the locus coeruleus and neurodegeneration in Alzheimer's disease. Acta Neuropathol 2021;141(5):631–50.
5. Tintore M, Rovira A, Arrambide G, et al. Brainstem lesions in clinically isolated syndromes. Neurology 2010;75:1933–8.
6. Ortiz de Mendivil A, Alcalá-Galiano A, Ochoa M, et al. Brainstem stroke: anatomy, clinical and radiological findings. Semin Ultrasound CT MR 2013;34:131–41.
7. Donaldson SS, Laningham F, Fisher PG. Advances toward an understanding of brainstem gliomas. J Clin Oncol 2006;24:1266–72.
8. Aggarwal M, Zhang J, Pletnikova O, et al. Feasibility of creating a high-resolution 3D diffusion tensor imaging based atlas of the human brainstem: a case study at 11.7 T. Neuroimage 2013;74:117–27.
9. Hoch MJ, Bruno MT, Faustin A, et al. 3T MRI whole-brain microscopy discrimination of subcortical anatomy, part 1: brain stem. AJNR Am J Neuroradiol 2019;40(3):401–7.
10. Edlow BL, Mareyam A, Horn A, et al. 7 Tesla MRI of the ex vivo human brain at 100 micron resolution. Sci Data 2019;6(1):244.
11. Ford AA, Colon-Perez L, Triplett WT, et al. Imaging white matter in human brainstem. Front Hum Neurosci 2013;7:400.
12. Shepherd TM, Hoch MJ, Bruno M, et al. Inner SPACE: 400-Micron Isotropic Resolution MRI of the Human Brain. Front Neuroanat 2020;14:9.
13. Hoch MJ, Chung S, Ben-Eliezer N, et al. New clinically feasible 3T MRI protocol to discriminate internal brain stem anatomy. AJNR Am J Neuroradiol 2016;37(6):1058–65.
14. Shepherd TM, Ades-Aron B, Bruno M, et al. Direct in vivo MRI discrimination of brain stem nuclei and pathways. AJNR Am J Neuroradiol 2020;41(5):777–84.
15. Setsompop K, Gagoski BA, Polimeni JR, et al. Blipped-controlled aliasing in parallel imaging for simultaneous multislice echo planar imaging with reduced g-factor penalty. Magn Reson Med 2012;67:1210–24.
16. Hoch MJ, Bruno M, Pacione D, et al. Simultaneous multislice for accelerating diffusion MRI in clinical neuroradiology protocols. AJNR Am J Neuroradiol 2021;42(8):1437–43.
17. Ades-aron B, Coelho S, Lemberskiy G, et al. MP-PCA denoising of complex imaging data for direct visualization of the dentatorubrothalamic tract using diffusion MRI at 3T. Proc ISMRM 2022;2105.
18. Veraart J, Novikov DS, Christiaens D, et al. Denoising of diffusion MRI using random matrix theory. Neuroimage 2016;142:394–406.
19. Ades-Aron B, Veraart J, Kochunov P, et al. Evaluation of the accuracy and precision of the diffusion parameter estimation with Gibbs and noise removal pipeline. Neuroimage 2018;183:532–43.
20. Jenkinson M, Bannister P, Brady M, et al. Improved optimization for the robust and accurate linear registration and motion correction of brain images. Neuroimage 2002;17(2):825–41.
21. Sudhyadhom A, Haq IU, Foote KD, et al. A high resolution and high contrast MRI for differentiation of subcortical structures for DBS targeting: the fast gray matter acquisition t1 inversion recovery (FGATIR). Neuroimage 2009;47(Suppl 2):T44–52.
22. Ades-aron B, Elsayed M, Hoch M, et al. CNN denoising of FGATIR MRI improves visualization of subcortical anatomy. Proc ISMRM 2022;1913.
23. Gizewski ER, Maderwald S, Linn J, et al. High-resolution anatomy of the human brain stem using 7-T MRI: improved detection of inner structures and nerves? Neuroradiology 2014;56:177–86.
24. Deistung A, Schäfer A, Schweser F, et al. High resolution MR imaging of the human brainstem in vivo at 7 Tesla. Front Hum Neurosci 2013;7:710.
25. Soria G, De Notaris M, Tudela R, et al. Improved assessment of ex vivo brainstem neuroanatomy with high-resolution MRI and DTI at 7 Tesla. Anat Rec (Hoboken) 2011;294:1035–44.
26. Nagae-Poetscher LM, Jiang H, Wakana S, et al. High-resolution diffusion tensor imaging of the brain stem at 3 T. AJNR Am J Neuroradiol 2004;25:1325–30.
27. Naganawa S, Yamazaki M, Kawai H, et al. Anatomical details of the brainstem and cranial nerves visualized by high resolution read- out-segmented multi-shot echo-planar diffusion-weighted images using unidirectional MPG at 3 T. Magn Reson Med Sci 2011;10:269–75.
28. Calamante F, Tourneir JD, Jackson GD, et al. Track-densityimaging (TDI): super-resolution white matter imaging using whole-brain track density mapping. Neuroimage 2010;53:1233–43.
29. Calamante F, Smith RE, Tournier JD, et al. Quantification of voxel- wise total fibre density: investigating

the problems associated with track-count mapping. Neuroimage 2015;117:284–93.
30. Thevathasan W, Debu B, Aziz T, et al. Movement Disorders Society PPN DBS Working Group in collaboration with the World Society for Stereotactic and Functional Neurosurgery. Pedunculopontine nucleus deep brain stimulation in Parkinson's disease: A clinical review. Mov Disord 2018;33(1):10–20.
31. Schwarz ST, Xing Y, Tomar P, et al. In vivo assessment of brainstem depigmentation in Parkinson disease: potential as a severity marker for multicenter studies. Radiology 2017;283(3):789–98.
32. Martin-Bastida A, Pietracupa S, Piccini P. Neuromelanin in parkinsonian disorders: an update. Int J Neurosci 2017;127(12):1116–23.
33. Bae YJ, Kim JM, Sohn CH, et al. Imaging the substantia nigra in parkinson disease and other parkinsonian syndromes. Radiol 2021;300:260–78.
34. Manova ES, Habib CA, Boikov AS, et al. Characterizing the mesencephalon using susceptibility-weighted imaging. AJNR Am J Neuroradiol 2009; 30(3):569–74.
35. Miocinovic S, Somayajula S, Chitnis S, et al. History, applications, and mechanisms of deep brain stimulation. JAMA Neurol 2013;70:163–71.
36. Sofic E, Paulus W, Jellinger K, et al. Selective increase of iron in substantia nigra zona compacta of parkinsonian brains. J Neurochem 1991;56(3): 978–82.
37. Sohmiya M, Tanaka M, Aihara Y, et al. Structural changes in the midbrain with aging and Parkinson's disease: an MRI study. Neurobiol Aging 2004;25(4): 449–53.
38. Damier P, Hirsch EC, Agid Y, et al. The substantia nigra of the human brain. I. Nigrosomes and the nigral matrix, a compartmental organization based on calbindin D(28K) immunohistochemistry. Brain 1999; 122(Pt 8):1421–36.
39. Schwarz ST, Afzal M, Morgan PS, et al. The 'swallow tail' appearance of the healthy nigrosome - a new accurate test of Parkinson's disease: a case-control and retrospective cross-sectional MRI study at 3T. PLoS One 2014;9(4):e93814.

Cranial Nerve Anatomy

Katie Suzanne Traylor, DO*, Barton F. Branstetter IV, MD

KEYWORDS

• Cranial nerves • Anatomy • Neuroradiology • MRI

KEY POINTS

- Discuss the entire course of the CNs and their relation to other important anatomy.
- Discuss the functions of each of the CNs.
- Discuss some important pathologies that can directly affect a CN given its location.

INTRODUCTION

Twelve pairs of cranial nerves (CNs) supply sensory, parasympathetic, and motor functions to the head and neck. All the CNs except CN11 arise within the cranium. CN anatomy is complex but necessary to understand when evaluating CN neuropathy patients. Each CN has a nucleus (brainstem), parenchymal fascicular segment (brainstem), cisternal segment (passing through the cerebrospinal fluid [CSF]), dural cave segment (transiting through several complex anatomic spaces), intradural segment (closely adherent to the periosteum before exiting the cranium), and an extracranial segment.[1,2] By evaluating each of these segments, the radiologist can ensure a complete imaging evaluation of abnormalities in the structure or function of a CN.

OLFACTORY NERVE (CN1)

CN1 is a sensory nerve used in olfaction and is located immediately superior to the cribriform plate at the anterior skull base.[3] CN1 does not have Schwann cells like most CNs. Instead, it is myelinated by olfactory ensheathing cells, a direct extension of brain white matter tracts.[2,3] Olfaction is one of the two sensory pathways in the body where the neurons do not decussate in the brain resulting in an ipsilateral deficit if injured. Without Schwann cells, schwannomas cannot develop, however, schwannomas rarely develop along the anterior skull base/olfactory groove likely from other neural structures in the vicinity.[4,5]

The olfactory bulbs are inferior to the frontal lobes and immediately below the olfactory sulcus, between the medial orbital gyrus and rectus gyrus (Fig. 1).[4] The transethmoidal segment from the distal nerve connects the olfactory neuroepithelium (upper-fifth of the nasal cavity, in the olfactory recesses) through the cribriform plate to the olfactory bulbs.[4] As the neurons track posteriorly from the olfactory bulb, sensory olfactory tracts are formed and divide, eventually tracking into the brain where processing occurs.[1,4]

OPTIC NERVE (CN2)

Similar to CN1, the optic nerve (ON) is not technically a CN as it does not contain Schwann cells but rather a direct extension of brain white matter tracts myelinated by oligodendrocytes.[3,4] The ON has four segments: retinal (or intraocular), intraorbital, intracanalicular, and cisternal (or intracranial) (Fig. 2). Axons arising from the inner retinal ganglion cells form the intraocular portion of the ON (only 1 mm thick), which exits from the optic disc via the lamina cribrosa to form the intraorbital segment extending to the orbital apex.[4,6,7] CSF within the ON sheath is directly connected to the suprasellar cistern.[4] The intraorbital segment has a slight S-shape course allowing globe mobility.[7] The intraorbital segment continues into the intracanalicular segment, best evaluated using MRI; however, CT is the best for the osseus

Neuroradiology Division, University of Pittsburgh School of Medicine, 200 Lothrop Street, South Tower, 2nd Floor, Suite 200, Pittsburgh, PA 15213, USA
* Corresponding author.
E-mail address: traylorks@upmc.edu
Twitter: @CharBranstetter (K.S.T.)

Neuroimag Clin N Am 32 (2022) 565–576
https://doi.org/10.1016/j.nic.2022.04.004

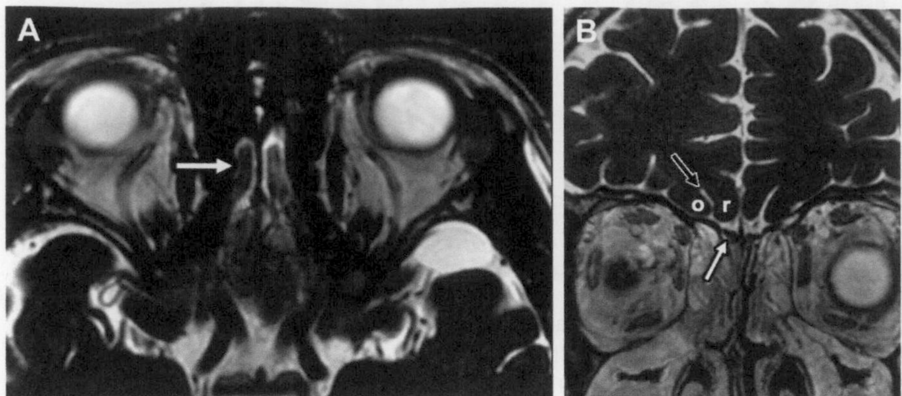

Fig. 1. CN1. Axial (*A*) and coronal (*B*) SSFP postcontrast MRI showing olfactory bulbs (*white arrow*) below the olfactory sulcus (*black arrow*), gyrus rectus (r), and medial orbital gyrus (o).

boundaries.[4] The intracanalicular segment (0.9 cm) is completely enclosed by the ON canal and, prior to its entrance, the dura is fixed on this bony canal. The canal is bounded laterally by the sphenoid wing and optic strut with the ethmoids located medially. Sometimes, the thin, medial osseus wall is dehiscent providing a potential infection route or a surgical hazard. The intracanalicular segment extends posteriorly at a 45° to form the cisternal segment (1 cm),[6,7] which is covered by the pia mater after the two ONs combine to form the optic chiasm. The chiasm is lateral to the internal carotid artery (ICA) and above the sella.[7] At the optic chiasm, the axons from the temporal hemiretinas do not decussate and continue posteriorly to the ipsilateral optic tract. The nasal hemiretinas axons decussate, coursing to the contralateral optic tract.[4] These tracts extend further posteriorly around the cerebral peduncles where most of the axons synapse with the lateral geniculate body of the thalamus, proceed through the Meyer loop, and enter the visual cortex in the occipital lobes.[3,6]

OCULOMOTOR NERVE (CN3)

CN3 has both motor and parasympathetic functions. The motor function controls the inferior rectus, superior rectus, middle rectus, inferior oblique, and levator palpebrae superioris muscles. The parasympathetic portion controls the ciliaris and sphincter pupillae muscles that mediate pupillary constriction.[6,8]

The motor fibers start at the CN3 complex (Fig. 3) at the level of the superior colliculi in the midbrain, inferior to the pineal gland, ventral to the cerebral aqueduct and periaqueductal gray matter, and dorsal to the medial longitudinal fasciculus (MLF) and red nucleus.[1,3,6] Posteriorly, the parasympathetic fibers arise from the Edinger–Westphal nucleus.[1] There are four paired subnuclei where the most medial nucleus

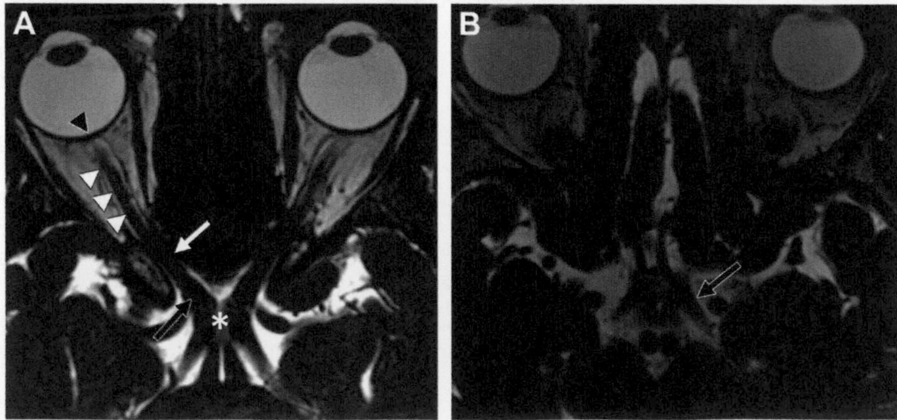

Fig. 2. CN2. (*A*) Axial SSFP MRI demonstrating CN2 segments: retinal (black *arrowhead*), intraorbital (*white arrowheads*), intracanalicular (*white arrow*), cisternal (*black arrow*) extending to the optic chiasm (*). (*B*) Axial SSFP MRI image illustrating the optic tracts (*black arrow*) coursing posteriorly from the optic chiasm.

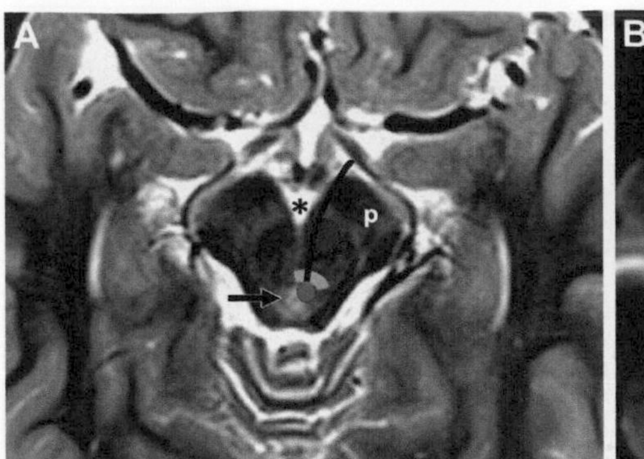

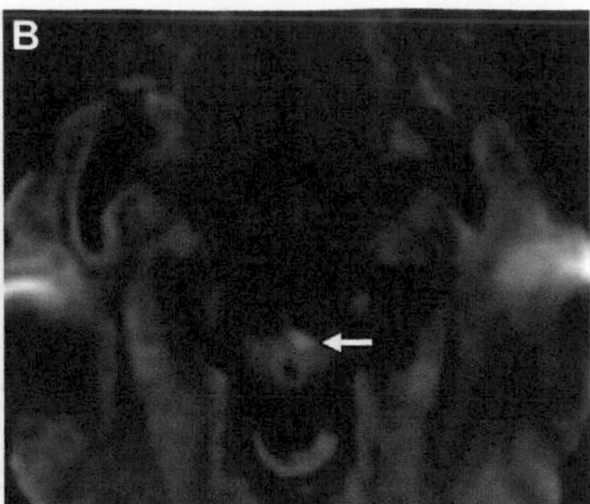

Fig. 3. CN3. (*A*) Axial T2-weighted MRI at the CN3 complex (blue circle), near the midline and ventral to the cerebral aqueduct/periaqueductal gray (*black arrow*). CN3 (black *line*) courses ventrally through the MLF (green), red nucleus (red), and medial aspect of the cerebral peduncle (P), exiting into the interpeduncular cistern (*). (*B*) Axial diffusion-weighted image with an acute infarct along the fascicular segment (*white arrow*) causing acute onset vision change and dizziness.

innervates the superior rectus muscle. This nucleus is the only nucleus that controls both orbits; therefore, a lesion occurring in one superior rectus subnucleus causes partial denervation of both superior rectus muscles.[8]

CN3 enters the interpeduncular cistern before entering the cavernous sinus (CS).[6] The anatomic location of CN3 is important as the posterior cerebral artery/posterior communicating artery is superior and the superior cerebellar artery is inferior (Fig. 4).[1,6,8] Therefore, an aneurysm here can cause CN3 palsy. CN3 will exit the prepontine cistern piercing the dura lateral to the posterior clinoid process, entering the lateral CS where CN3 is the most superior nerve (Fig. 5).[3,8] Additionally, CN3 is positioned superolateral to the ICA.[1] CN3 reaches the orbit via the superior orbital fissure (SOF).[6] CN3 enters the annulus of Zinn once beyond the SOF, splitting into superior and inferior divisions lateral to the ON.[1,3] The superior division innervates the superior rectus and levator palpebrae muscle while the inferior division innervates the inferior rectus, inferior oblique, and medial rectus muscles. The parasympathetic branches follow the inferior oblique branch terminating in the ciliary ganglion in the orbital apex at the annulus of Zinn.[1] Some authors recognize the superior tarsal muscle as a component of the levator palpebrae superioris attached to its underside near its insertion point. The superior tarsal muscle receives sympathetic innervation from the carotid plexus whose fibers join CN3 while it passes through the CS.[9]

TROCHLEAR NERVE (CN4)

CN4 is a purely motor nerve depressing, intorting, and abducting the globe.[10] The nucleus is one of the smallest motor nuclei in the brainstem, inferior to the CN3 complex at the inferior colliculus, anterior to the cerebral aqueduct, and posterior to the MLF.[1,4,10] Given the close proximity of the nucleus to the MLF, a lesion here can result in both a CN4 palsy and internuclear ophthalmoplegia.[4] The axons course posteriorly from the nucleus, around the cerebral aqueduct, decussating within the superior medullary velum before exiting the midbrain dorsally (Fig. 6) and coursing within the cerebellomesencephalic fissure to eventually traverse the quadrigeminal, ambient, crural and pontomesencephalic cisterns. CN4 courses anterolaterally along the upper pons and brachium conjunctivum inferiorly to the tentorial leaflet.[1,8,10] CN4 punctures the dura entering the cisterna basalis between the free and attached portions of the tentorium[3] and courses immediately inferior to the CN3 before entering the lateral CS, inferior to CN3.[3,10] CN4 courses with CN3 and CN6 to enter the SOF, however, CN4 courses above the annulus of Zinn before innervating the superior oblique muscle.[1]

CN4 has the longest intracranial course (6 cm), is the smallest, and is the only dorsally exiting CN. Moreover, it is the only CN to completely decussate, innervating the contralateral superior oblique muscle.[4,10] CN4 is susceptible to injury because some of its intracranial course lies between dural layers, resulting in difficulty visualizing the nerve radiologically.[3,10] Once the nerve passes beyond the free edge of the tentorial leaflet, surgeons have difficulty directly visualizing CN4; therefore, they need to presurgically plan any tentorial incision.[10]

TRIGEMINAL NERVE (CN5)

CN5 is the largest of all the CNs[4,6] and has motor and sensory functions to the muscles of

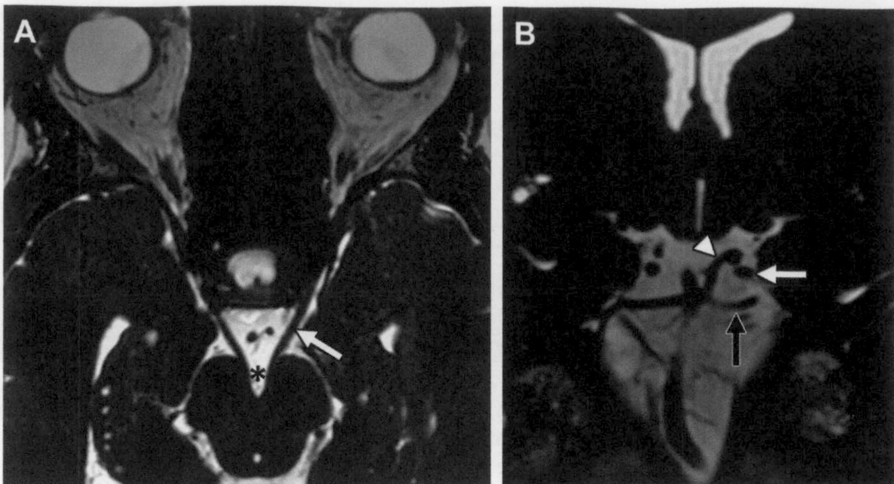

Fig. 4. CN3. Axial (*A*) and Coronal (*B*) SSFP MRI demonstrating CN3 (*white arrow*) in the interpeduncular cistern (*) between the posterior cerebral artery (white *arrowhead*) and superior cerebellar artery (*black arrow*).

mastication and a large sensory component to the face. CN5 has a complex and widespread set of nuclei; within the pons, there is one motor nucleus and three sensory nuclei (Fig. 7). The motor nucleus is in the lateral pontine tegmentum and supplies all the muscles of mastication, tensor veli palatini, and tensor tympani muscles.[4] Lateral to the motor nucleus and anterolateral to the fourth ventricle is the principal sensory nucleus providing facial touch sensation.[1] The mesencephalic nucleus is located superiorly in the midbrain up to the level of the inferior colliculus receiving afferent fibers for facial proprioception of the muscles of mastication, teeth, hard palate, and temporomandibular joints.[1,4] The peripheral processes also supply stretch receptors for the muscles of mastication and periodontal ligaments. Inferior to the principal sensory nucleus is the spinal nucleus that descends from the pons to the C3 spinous level.[4] The spinal nucleus contributes to facial pain, temperature sensation, and facial touch sensation.[1,4]

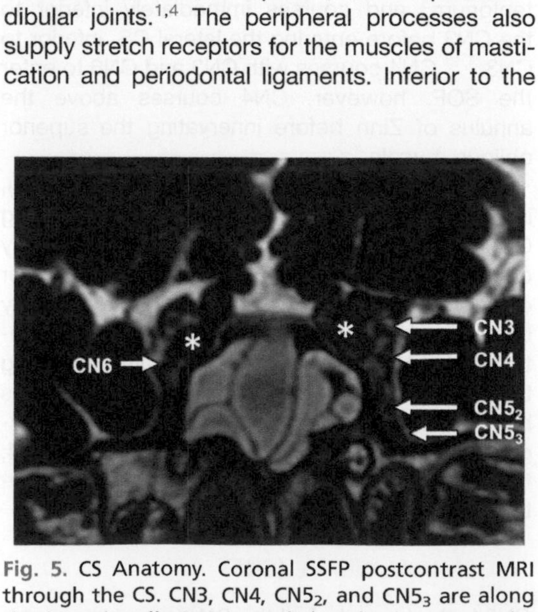

Fig. 5. CS Anatomy. Coronal SSFP postcontrast MRI through the CS. CN3, CN4, $CN5_2$, and $CN5_3$ are along the lateral wall. CN6 is medial and adjacent to the ICA (*).

CN5 exits from the lateral aspect of the midpons coursing through the prepontine cistern through the porus trigeminus into Meckel's cave. CN5 is centrally myelinated from the nerve root entry point until approximately halfway along the cisternal segment (see Fig. 7). In the setting of classical trigeminal neuralgia, neurovascular contact along this centrally myelinated segment mostly results in patient symptomatology.[11] The preganglionic segment terminates at the Gasserian ganglion along the Meckel's cave floor and contrast enhances as the blood–nerve barrier is absent. The motor portion extends underneath the ganglion exiting through the foramen ovale. The sensory root divides anteriorly at the level of the ganglion into the three divisions—ophthalmic ($CN5_1$ [V1]—exits through SOF), maxillary ($CN5_2$ [V2]—exits through foramen rotundum), and mandibular ($CN5_3$ [V3]—exits through foramen ovale). The $CN5_1$ and $CN5_2$ divisions extend along the lateral margin of the CS where $CN5_1$ is inferior to CN4 and lateral to CN6.[4] Once $CN5_1$ enters the SOF (with CN3, CN4, CN6, and superior ophthalmic vein), it divides into the frontal, lacrimal, and nasociliary nerves providing sensory innervation to the globe, nose, forehead, and scalp.[1,4,6] $CN5_2$ lies along the CS floor underneath $CN5_1$ exiting the foramen rotundum into the pterygopalatine fossa branching into the posterior superior alveolar nerve, zygomatic nerve, and two pterygopalatine nerves reaching the ganglion.

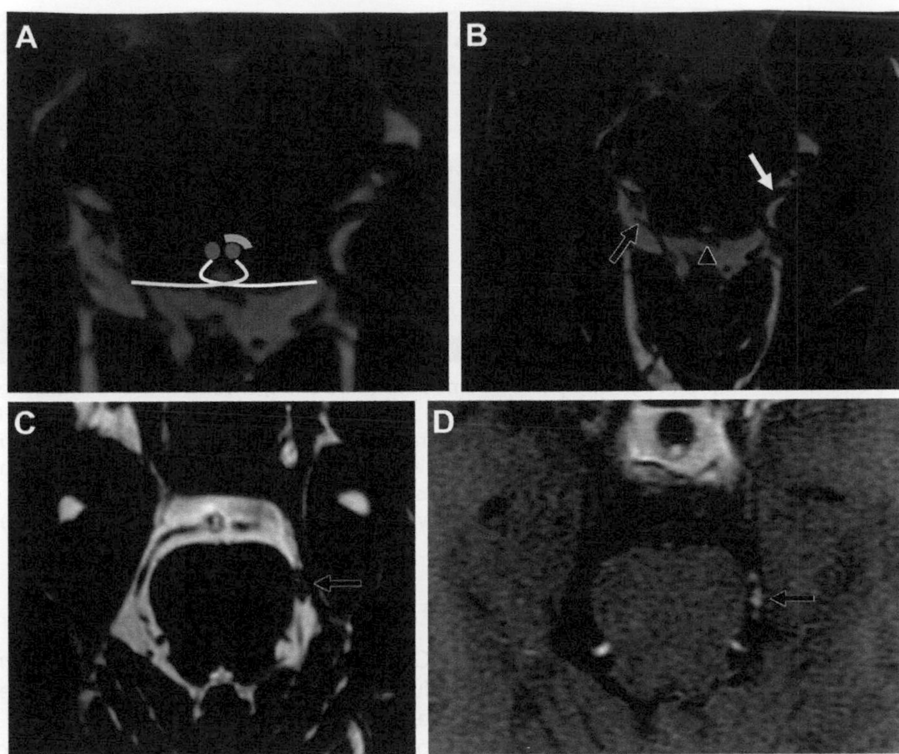

Fig. 6. CN4. (*A, B*) Axial SSFP MRI at the CN4 nuclei (blue) posterior to the MLF (green) and ventral to the periaqueductal gray in the midbrain. The left nucleus initiates the right nerve (yellow) where the right nucleus initiates the left nerve (white). CN4 exits posteriorly (*black arrow*) at the medullary velum (black *arrowhead*). The CN4 course differs from the superior cerebellar artery (*white arrow*). (*C*) Axial SSFP MRI demonstrates thickening along the cisternal segment on the left (*black arrow*). (*D*) Axial T1 postcontrast MRI demonstrating enhancement suggesting schwannoma.

$CN5_2$ extends into the orbit through the inferior orbital fissure forming the intraorbital segment and coursing along the orbital floor, exiting into the face via the infraorbital foramen. $CN5_2$ receives sensory information from the midface, cheek, and upper teeth. Unlike $CN5_1$ and $CN5_2$, $CN5_3$ does not enter the CS. $CN5_3$ joins the motor root and branches into two major nerves just below the skull base—the masticator nerve (muscles of mastication) and myohyoid nerve (mylohyoid and

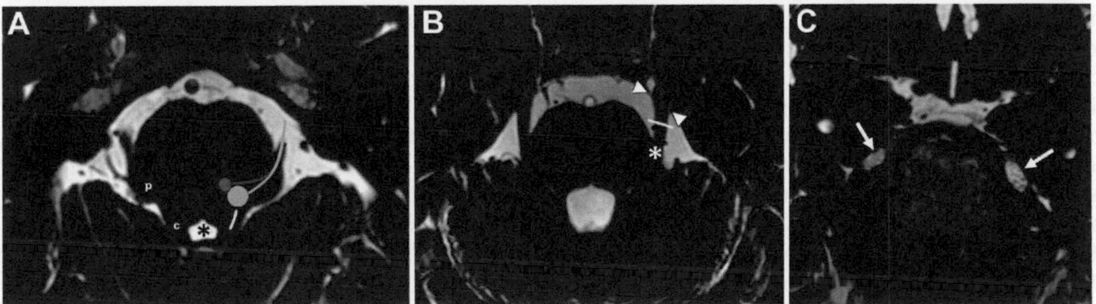

Fig. 7. CN5. (*A*) Axial SSFP MRI demonstrating the trigeminal nuclei. The motor nucleus (blue) and principal sensory nucleus (green) are medial to the branchium pontis (P). The mesencephalic nucleus (yellow) is posteriorly in the brachium conjunctivum (*C*), medial to the fourth ventricle (*). (*B*) Axial SSFP MRI showing the CN5 nerve root entry point (*). The transition (yellow) between the proximal centrally myelinated portion (dorsal) and distal peripherally myelinated portion (ventral). CN5 enters the Meckel's cave through the porus trigeminus (*white arrowheads*). (*C*) Coronal SSFP MRI showing the multiple CN5 fascicles traversing the CSF space in Meckel's caves (*white arrows*).

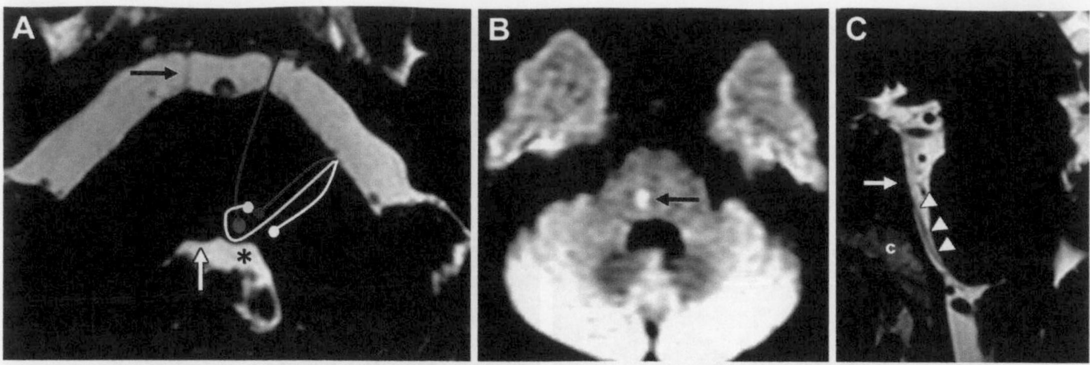

Fig. 8. CN6. (*A*) Axial SSFP MRI through mid-pons. CN6 nucleus (blue circle) is ventral to the fourth ventricle (*). CN7 motor nucleus (yellow circle) nerve fibers (yellow *line*) courses around CN6 nucleus forming the facial colliculus (*white arrow*). The cisternal segment (*black arrow*) traverses the prepontine cistern. The superior salivary nucleus (red circle) and solitary tract nucleus (white circle) are more lateral. (*B*) Axial diffusion-weighted image showing an acute infarct (*black arrow*) along the CN6 fascicular segment causing acute diplopia. C. Sagittal SSFP MRI demonstrating CN6's inferior-to-superior course (white *arrowheads*) posterior to the clivus (*C*). CN6 pierces the dura to enter Dorello's canal (*white arrow*).

anterior belly of the digastric muscles).[4] The sensory branch divides into the meningeal, medial and lateral pterygoid, masseteric, deep temporal, inferior alveolar, lingual, small buccal branch, and auriculotemporal nerves.[4,6] The auriculotemporal nerve extends into the parotid, where CN5 and CN7 communicate, providing an important pathway in perineural tumor spread. The inferior alveolar nerve courses inferiorly entering the mandibular foramen and then exits the mental foramen where it provides sensory information from the ipsilateral chin and mandibular teeth. $CN5_3$ overall provides sensory information from the floor of mouth, lower one-third of the face, tongue, and jaw.[4]

ABDUCENS NERVE (CN6)

CN6 is a purely motor nerve innervating the lateral rectus muscle resulting in globe abduction. The nucleus is in the pons near midline, below the fourth ventricle floor, and at the level of the facial colliculus (Fig. 8).[4,6] CN6 courses anteroinferiorly through the pontine tegmentum, exiting the ventral pons at the bulbopontine sulcus. CN6 courses through the prepontine cistern (1.9 cm) following an anterolateral-superior course, the only CN to have an upward course.[4,12] CN6 courses almost the entire length of the clivus before piercing dura (Dorello's canal) posterior to the sphenoid sinus between the petrous bone and petrosphenoidal ligament. This canal passes through the basilar venous plexus, traveling between two dural layers, before coursing over the petrous bone entering the medial CS.[1,3,4,13] CN6 then courses through the SOF and annulus of Zinn to reach the lateral rectus muscle.[4]

FACIAL NERVE (CN7)

CN7 has motor, sensory, and parasympathetic functions.[4,14] CN7 innervates the muscles of facial expression, stapedius, stylohyoid, and posterior belly of the digastric muscles.[4] The motor nucleus is in the ventrolateral aspect of the tegmenum of the lower pons, and the sensory nucleus is located posterolateral.[1] The motor nucleus is also medial to the nucleus of the CN5 spinal root, as discussed earlier.[4] The third sensory nucleus is lateral to the motor nucleus and provides the parasympathetic functions of the submandibular, sublingual, and lacrimal glands.[1] CN7 exits posteriorly from the motor nucleus, circles back toward the fourth ventricle floor, around (internal genu) the posterior aspect of CN6 nucleus resulting in the facial colliculus (see Fig. 8A).[1,4] CN7 exits near the pontomedullary sulcus, the most concave portion of the pons, termed the nerve root exit point. The attached segment is adherent to the undersurface of the pons extending from the root exit point to root detachment point (RDP) of the lateral pons (Fig. 9). The centrally myelinated portion of CN7 stretches from the nerve root exit point to approximately 3 mm beyond the RDP and is the only portion affected by neurovascular compression in hemifacial spasm.[15] In the cerebellopontine angle (CPA), the motor and sensory portions of the nerve separate, with the nervus intermedius being sensory.[16] The nerve travels obliquely through the CPA to enter the IAC via the porus acusticus. CN7 exits the IAC fundus to traverse the petrous portion of the temporal bone through a bony canal termed the fallopian canal or facial nerve canal. CN7 first enters the facial nerve canal via the fallopian aqueduct to form the labyrinthine

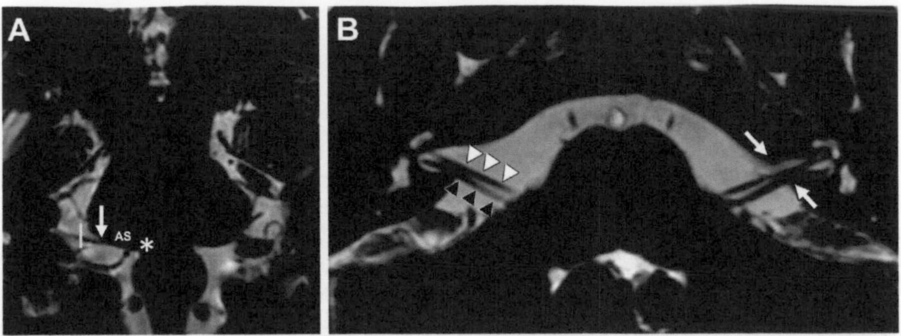

Fig. 9. CN7. (*A*) Coronal SSFP MRI demonstrates nerve root exit point (*), attached segment (AS), RDP (*white arrow*), and the transition point (yellow *line*). (*B*) Axial SSFP MRI demonstrating CN7 (white *arrowheads*) and SV nerve (black *arrowheads*) in the CPA before entering the porus acusticus (*white arrows*).

segment,[3,14] which continues to the geniculate ganglion. The greater superficial petrosal nerve travels ventromedially from the ganglion to supply the lacrimal gland, mucus membranes of the nasal cavity, and palate. CN7 takes its first external genu at the geniculate ganglion into the tympanic segment where a second genu forms marking the mastoid portion (Fig. 10).[14,16] Three separate sensory nerves branch from the mastoid segment, including the stapedius muscle nerve (stabilizes stapes), chorda tympani nerve (secretomotor innervation to both the submandibular and sublingual glands and sensory innervation to the anterior two-thirds of the tongue), and the auricular branch of CN10 (aids in sensation from the posterior auditory canal). The motor branch exits the skull base at the level of the stylomastoid foraman supplying the posterior auricular nerve (postauricular muscles) and two small motor branches (the posterior belly of the digastric and the stylohoid muscles). CN7 then courses through the parotid, immediately lateral to the retromandibular vein, supplying the muscles of facial expression.[14] The geniculate ganglion, through to the mastoid segment, can normally enhance owing to a venous plexus (Fig. 11). The five major terminal branches of the facial nerve that arise within the parotid are (from superior to inferior) the temporal, zygomatic, buccal, marginal mandibular, and cervical branches; these form a 'parotid plexus' of nerves or pes anserinus.[1]

VESTIBULOCOCHLEAR NERVE (CN8)

CN8 is a sensory nerve that detects head and body motion and sound.[1,17] The dorsal and ventral cochlear nuclei are located along the upper medulla adjacent to the restiform body.[1,18] The vestibular nuclear complex (lateral, medial, superior, inferior) is medial to the cochlear nuclei in the dorsolateral lower pons near the fourth ventricular floor (Fig. 12). The ascending and descending vestibular nerve fascicles arise from these vestibular nuclei joining with the cochlear nerve fascicles

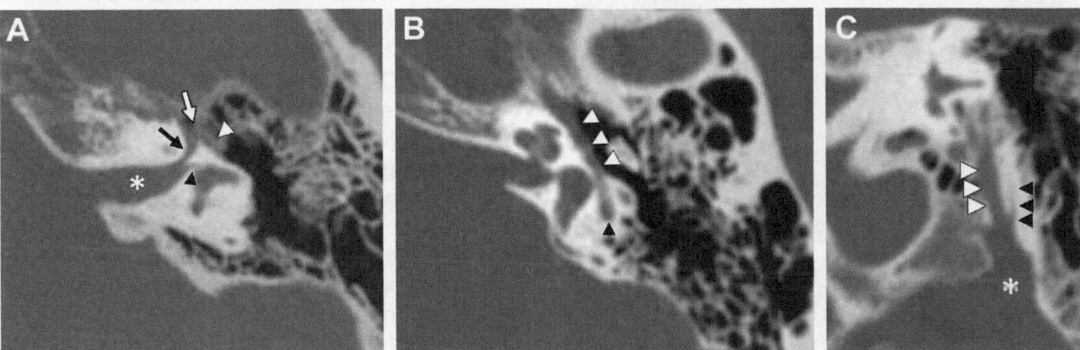

Fig. 10. CN7. (*A*) Axial CT of upper IAC (*). CN7 segments on CT—labyrinthine (*black arrow*), geniculate ganglion (*white arrow*), and tympanic (white *arrowhead*). The IV nerve branch (black *arrowhead*) is shown entering the vestibule. (*B*) Axial CT showing the tympanic segment (white *arrowheads*) to the mastoid segment (black *arrowhead*). (*C*) Coronal CT image showing the mastoid canal (white *arrowheads*) before exiting into the stylomastoid foramen (*). The chorda tympani branch (black *arrowheads*) is shown.

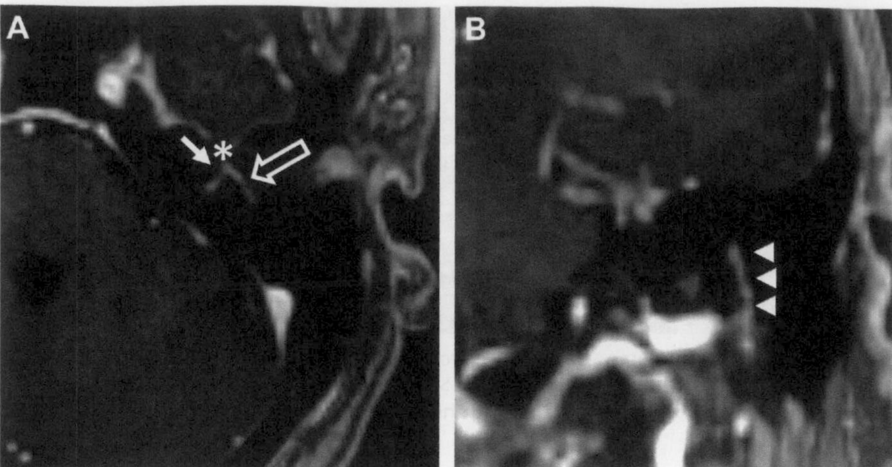

Fig. 11. CN7. Axial (*A*) and coronal (*B*) FSPGR 3D postcontrast image demonstrating a patient with abnormal enhancement of the labyrinthine segment (*white arrow*). The geniculate ganglion (*), tympanic segment (double *white arrow*), and mastoid segment of CN7 (white *arrowheads*) are also demonstrating enhancement.

before exiting at the pontomedullary junction.[1,6,19] CN8 courses posterior to CN7 in the CPA before reaching the porus acusticus where CN8 splits into three separate nerve branches—cochlear, superior vestibular (SV), and inferior vestibular (IV) nerves (**Fig. 13**).[3] The cochlear nerve is in the anteroinferior aspect of the IAC directly below CN7, although the IV nerve is located along the posteroinferior aspect of the IAC directly below the SV nerve, separated by the bony falciform crest.[3,4] At the IAC fundus, CN7 and the SV nerves are separated by Bill's bar.[4] The cochlear nerve enters the cochlea via the cochlear aperture extending to the cochlear membrane where the nerve transmits auditory sensation. The vestibular nerve enters the vestibule where the ciliary sensory cells are located in the membranous labyrinth, controlling balance.[6]

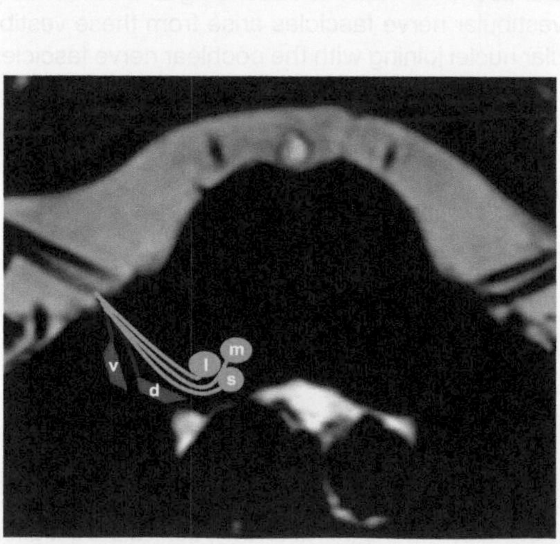

Fig. 12. CN8. Axial SSFP MRI of the cochlear nuclei (blue)—ventral (V) and dorsal (D)—and vestibular nuclei (green)—lateral (L), medial (M), and superior (S). The IV nuclei are more inferior and not shown.

GLOSSOPHARYNGEAL NERVE (CN9)

CN9 has motor, somatosensory, visceral sensory, and parasympathetic functions, with its nuclei located in the upper and middle medulla.[4,14] The preganglionic fibers arise from the nucleus ambiguous, inferior salivatory nucleus, nucleus of tractus solitarius, and spinal trigeminal nucleus (**Fig. 14**). CN9 innervates the stylopharyngeus muscle where the motor components arise from the nucleus ambiguous and are shared by CN9, CN10, and CN11. Parasympathetic fibers arise from the inferior salivatory nucleus and enter the parotid. CN9 also has a viscerosensory function to the carotid body and sinus. CN9 exits at the postolivary sulcus, posterior to the medullary olive, traversing the cistern in an anterolateral orientation with both CN10 and CN11 traveling in parallel but inferiorly. As CN9 exits the skull base, it enters the pars nervosa of the jugular foramen with the superior and inferior ganglia.[4]

CN9 enters the lateral aspect of the carotid space and stylopharyngeal muscle descending lateral to the palatine tonsil, terminating in the posterior sublingual space. The lingual branch innervates the posterior third of the tongue. Other branches of this extracranial segment include the pharyngeal branches, sinus nerve, stylopharyngeus, and tympanic branch of Jacobson's nerve. Jacobson's nerve arises from the inferior sensory ganglion ascending into the middle ear cavity, coursing over the cochlear promontory (**Fig. 15**).

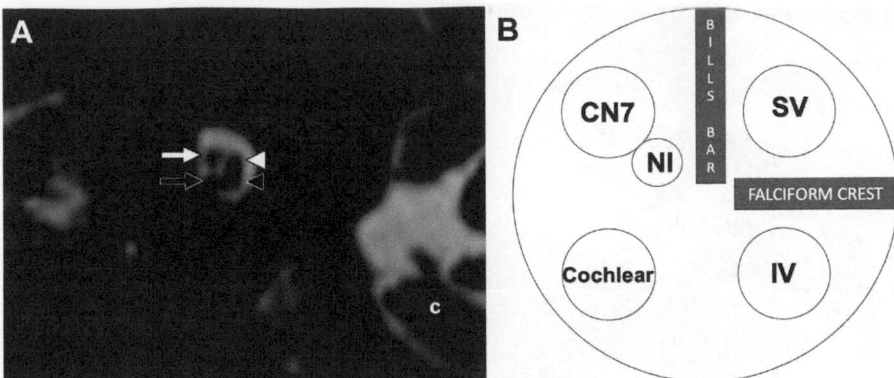

Fig. 13. IAC. (*A*) Oblique plane SSFP MRI through the IAC with CN7 (*white arrow*), cochlear nerve (*black arrow*), SV nerve (white *arrowhead*), and IV nerve (black *arrowhead*) with cerebellum (C) posterior. (*B*) Schematic of IAC contents. The nervus intermedius (NI) is a CN7 sensory branch. Bill's bar separates CN7 and SV nerves. The falciform crest separates the SV nerve from the IV nerve. Left of the diagram is anterior, and right of the diagram is posterior.

Jacobson's nerve is sensory to the middle ear and has a parasympathetic component to the parotid gland.[4]

VAGUS NERVE (CN10)

CN10 has motor, parasympathetic and sensory functions, and has the longest overall CN course.[14] The parasympathetic fibers terminate in the dorsal vagal nucleus with information from the head and neck, thoracic, and abdominal viscera. The motor portion arises from the nucleus ambiguous (Fig. 16) supplying the soft palate, pharyngeal constrictor muscle, larynx, and palatoglossus muscle of the tongue. The solitary tract nucleus also receives taste from the epiglottis. There is also sensory information terminating in the CN5 spinal nucleus from the tympanic membrane, external auditory canal, external ear, and meninges of the posterior fossa.[4,20] The nerve exits the lateral medulla/posterolateral sulcus between the olive and restiform nucleus posterior to CN9, traversing the lateral cerebellomedullary cistern parallel and inferior to CN9. CN10 enters the pars vascularis of the jugular foramen where the superior vagal ganglion is located. The inferior vagal ganglion is located just below the skull base. CN10 exits the skull base between CN9 and CN12 entering the carotid space along the posterolateral aspect of the ICA, inferiorly to the anterior wall of the aortic arch on the left and along the anterior wall of the subclavian artery on the right.[3,4,6] CN10 then exits the thorax through the esophageal hiatus entering the abdomen.[6]

The first branch of CN10, Arnold's nerve, arises from the superior vagal ganglion and courses through the mastoid canaliculus, reaching the mastoid segment of CN7.[4] Arnold's nerve provides sensory information from the external surface of the tympanic membrane, external auditory canal, and skin of the concha of the external ear.[14,19] The recurrent laryngeal nerve is the third branch from CN10 looping behind the subclavian artery (on the right) or extending between the aortopulmonary artery and ligamentum arteriosum (on the left). The recurrent laryngeal nerve then ascends into the tracheoesophageal groove providing motor innervation to all the laryngeal muscles except the cricothyroid muscle.[4,14]

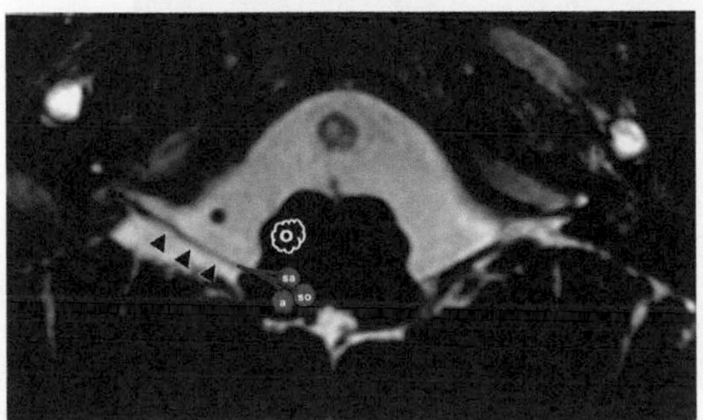

Fig. 14. CN9. Axial SSFP MRI demonstrating CN9 nuclei—nucleus ambiguous (A), solitary nucleus (so), and salivatory nucleus (sa), posterior to the olive (O) in the medulla. CN9 courses through the cistern (black arrowheads).

ACCESSORY NERVE (CN11)

CN11 is a purely motor nerve with both cranial and spinal components—bulbar motor fibers (originating in the nucleus ambiguous) and spinal motor fibers (originating in the CN11 spinal nucleus).[4,6] The spinal nucleus is lateral to the anterior horns

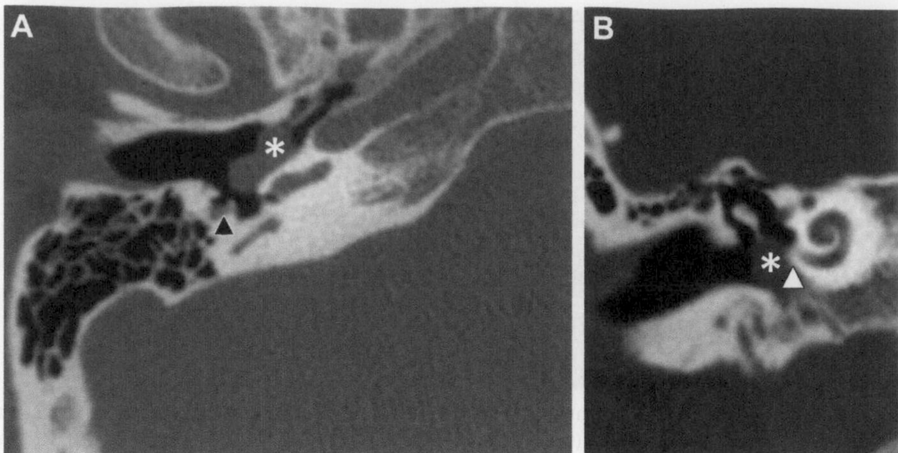

Fig. 15. Tympanicum paraganglioma. Axial (*A*) and coronal (*B*) CT with a middle ear cavity mass (*) at the cochlear promontory (white *arrowhead*), where Jacobson's nerve traverses. CN7's stapedial branch (black *arrowhead*) is shown.

of the C1–C5 levels, and CN11 rootlets exit along the lateral surface of the cervical spinal cord between the anterior and posterior roots (Fig. 17). These rootlets join and ascend through the foramen magnum into the cisterna magna, posterior to the vertebral arteries, joining the cranial rootlets in the lateral cerebellomedullary cistern. The completely formed nerve enters the pars vascularis of the jugular foramen.[3,4] The bulbar segment is inferior to CN10, exiting in the cerebellomedullary cistern, where these nerve fibers join the spinal nerve fibers in the lateral part of the basal cistern, entering the pars vascularis of the jugular foramen where the cranial roots mix with CN10 at the level of the superior vagal ganglion. The spinal roots, on the other hand, will descend laterally, exiting the skull base, entering the carotid space, traveling adjacent to CN10, and eventually innervating the soft palate and muscles of the larynx and pharynx.[14] The nerves from the spinal portion, however, continue posterolaterally to innervate the sternocleidomastoid and trapezius muscles.[4,6]

HYPOGLOSSAL NERVE (CN12)

CN12 is a motor nerve consisting of a series of rootlets innervating the intrinsic and extrinsic tongue muscles.[4,6] CN12 nucleus is in the lower medulla, medial to the dorsal nucleus of CN10, and near the midline of the anterior fourth ventricle floor (hypoglossal trigone). This results in a slight bulge into the fourth ventricle, the hypoglossal eminence, extending the entire course of the medulla (Fig. 18). The nerve fibers course

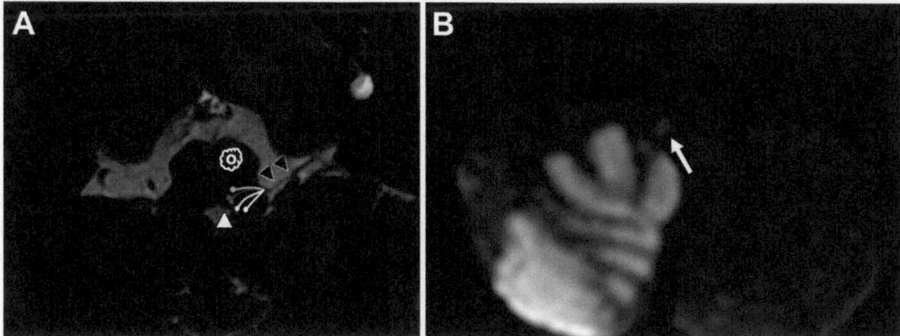

Fig. 16. CN10. (*A*) Axial SSFP MRI of the CN10 nuclei in medulla—nucleus ambiguous (green circle), inferior salivatory nucleus (blue circles), solitary tract nucleus (yellow circle), and CN5 spinal nucleus (white circle). The hypoglossal eminence (white *arrowhead*) is posteromedial, and olive (O) is ventral. The fascicular segments (colored *lines*) join, exiting the lateral medulla forming the cisternal segment (black *arrowheads*). (*B*) Axial diffusion-weighted MRI showing a lateral medullary (*white arrow*) and right posterior inferior cerebellar infarct causing right vocal fold paralysis.

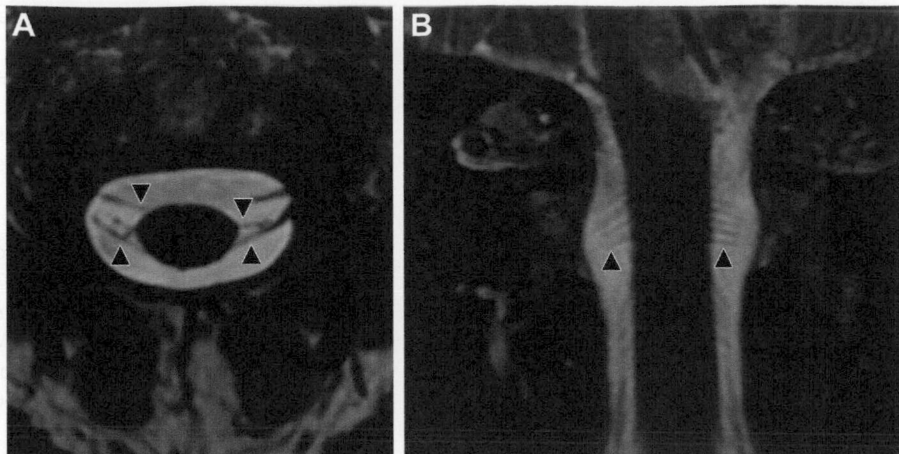

Fig. 17. CN11. (*A*) Axial SSFP MRI at the cervicomedullary junction showing CN11 rootlets (black *arrowheads*). (*B*) Coronal T2 3 mm fat-saturation showing CN11 spinal rootlets (black *arrowheads*) arising from the upper spinal cord crossing the foramen magnum joining the cranial rootlets.

anterolaterally through the medullary tegmentum traversing between the olivary nucleus and pyramid exiting at the preolivary sulcus, whereas CN9, CN10, and CN11 exit in the postolivary sulcus.[4] The nerve courses into the lateral cerebellomedullary cistern where it is anterior to the posterior inferior cerebellar artery and posterior to the vertebral artery, before entering the bony hypoglossal canal along the lateral clivus.[3,4,6] Beyond the skull base, CN12 courses lateral to CN9, CN10, and CN11 in the carotid space to the mastoid tip, exiting this space deep to the

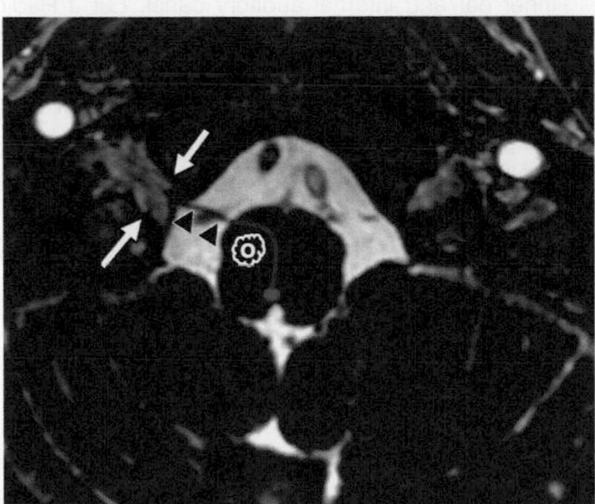

Fig. 18. CN12. Axial SSFP MRI demonstrating CN12 nuclei (blue circle) in a paramedian location. CN12 (blue *line*) travels ventrally through the medullary tegmentum before coursing laterally between the inferior olivary nucleus (O) and pyramid. CN12 exits at the preolivary sulcus and traversing through the cistern (black *arrowhead*) before entering the hypoglossal canal (*white arrow*).

margin of the posterior belly of the digastric muscle. CN12 continues inferolaterally, looping over the hyoid bone, lateral to the carotid bifurcation, and innervating the extrinsic and intrinsic tongue muscles (except the palatoglossus).[1,4,14] CN12 is susceptible to surgical injury because of its tortuous cervical course.

SUMMARY

Knowledge of CN course and function is extremely important for clinical neuroradiologists. With this knowledge, the neuroradiologist can tailor the imaging protocol to help evaluate certain parts of the brain/brainstem/nerves based on patient signs and symptoms, thus ensuring that every portion of the nerve is evaluated during image interpretation.

CLINICS CARE POINTS

- Steady-state free precession (SSFP) MRI sequence is best for CN evaluation.
- Evaluation of each CN from its nucleus through the extracranial segment is mandatory when assessing CN neuropathies.
- Only two CNs do not contain Schwann cells—the olfactory and ONs—these nerves are a direct extension of the brain.
- The trochlear nerve is the smallest CN, has the longest course, and is the only CN to exit dorsally from the brainstem. This nerve can be easily injured owing to its long course, its

location in several dural layers, and the inability to visualize it radiographically and surgically.

- The abducens nerve is the only CN to have an upward course.
- The auriculotemporal nerve is important as it connects the trigeminal and facial nerves extracranially and is an important pathway for perineural tumor spread. Intracranially, the greater superficial petrosal nerve connects the trigeminal and facial nerves and is another important pathway for perineural tumor spread.
- Only the geniculate ganglion and tympanic and mastoid segments of the facial nerve can normally enhance owing to the presence of a venous plexus.

DISCLOSURES

The authors have nothing to disclose.

REFERENCES

1. Laine FJ, Smoker WR. Anatomy of the cranial nerves. Neuroimaging Clin N Am 1998;8(1):69–100.
2. Klimaj Z, Klein JP, Szatmary G. Cranial Nerve Imaging and Pathology. Neurol Clin 2020;38(1):115–47.
3. Sheth S, Branstetter BF, Escott EJ. Appearance of normal cranial nerves on steady-state free precession MR images. Radiographics 2009;29(4):1045–55.
4. Casselman J, Mermuys K, Delanote J, et al. MRI of the cranial nerves–more than meets the eye: technical considerations and advanced anatomy. Neuroimaging Clin N Am 2008;18(2):197–231.
5. Figueiredo EG, Soga Y, Amorim RL, et al. The puzzling olfactory groove schwannoma: a systematic review. Skull Base 2011;21(1):31–6.
6. Romano N, Federici M, Castaldi A. Imaging of cranial nerves: a pictorial overview. *Insights Imaging* 2019;10(1):33.
7. Selhorst JB, Chen Y. The optic nerve. Semin Neurol 2009;29(1):29–35.
8. Brazis PW. Isolated palsies of cranial nerves III, IV, and VI. Semin Neurol 2009;29(1):14–28.
9. Pavone P, Cho SY, Praticò AD, et al. Ptosis in childhood: A clinical sign of several disorders: Case series reports and literature review. Medicine (Baltimore) 2018;97(36):e12124.
10. Joo W, Rhoton AL. Microsurgical anatomy of the trochlear nerve. Clin Anat 2015;28(7):857–64.
11. Hughes MA, Frederickson AM, Branstetter BF, et al. MRI of the Trigeminal Nerve in Patients With Trigeminal Neuralgia Secondary to Vascular Compression. AJR Am J Roentgenol 2016;206(3):595–600.
12. Baidoo EA, Tubbs RS. Anatomy of the Abducens Nerve. In: Tubbs RS, Rizk E, Shoia MM, et al, editors. Nerves and nerve Injuries. Academic Press; 2015. p. 351-355, chap 23.
13. Tubbs RS, Radcliff V, Shoja MM, et al. Dorello canal revisited: an observation that potentially explains the frequency of abducens nerve injury after head injury. World Neurosurg 2012;77(1):119–21.
14. Soldatos T, Batra K, Blitz AM, et al. Lower cranial nerves. Neuroimaging Clin N Am 2014;24(1):35–47.
15. Traylor KS, Sekula RF, Eubanks K, et al. Prevalence and severity of neurovascular compression in hemifacial spasm patients. Brain 2021;144(5):1482–7.
16. Gilchrist JM. Seventh cranial neuropathy. Semin Neurol 2009;29(1):5–13.
17. Landau ME, Barner KC. Vestibulocochlear nerve. Semin Neurol 2009;29(1):66–73.
18. Casselman JW, Offeciers EF, De Foer B, et al. CT and MR imaging of congential abnormalities of the inner ear and internal auditory canal. Eur J Radiol 2001;40(2):94–104.
19. Casselman JW, Kuhweide R, Deimling M, et al. Constructive interference in steady state-3DFT MR imaging of the inner ear and cerebellopontine angle. AJNR Am J Neuroradiol 1993;14(1):47–57.
20. Erman AB, Kejner AE, Hogikyan ND, et al. Disorders of cranial nerves IX and X. Semin Neurol 2009;29(1):85–92.

Anatomy of the Ventricles, Subarachnoid Spaces, and Meninges

John A. Morris, DO[a], Bruce C. Gilbert, MD[b], William T. Parker, MD[b], Scott E. Forseen, MD[a,*]

KEYWORDS

• Anatomy • Ventricles • Subarachnoid spaces • Meninges • Neuroanatomy • Radiology

KEY POINTS

- The ventricular system is an intricate series of cerebrospinal fluid (CSF)-filled intracranial chambers with complex anatomic boundaries.
- The subarachnoid space is an interval between the arachnoid mater and pia mater with free multi-directional flow of CSF. Regions of dilated subarachnoid space are termed "cisterns."
- The meninges support and protect the structures of the central nervous system (CNS) with an elaborate triple-layered membranous framework.

INTRODUCTION

The ventricular system is a series of interconnected cavities, derived from the central canal of the embryonic neural tube, in which cerebrospinal fluid (CSF) is produced and freely flows. In conjunction with the meninges, a triple-layered concentric membranous covering, a framework is formed to maintain, support, and protect the structures of the CNS. This article will focus on normal imaging anatomy of the ventricles, meninges, and communicating subarachnoid spaces within the intracranial compartment. Owing to space constraints, limited attention is given to anatomic variants and pathologic processes.

ANATOMY OF THE VENTRICULAR SYSTEM

The ventricular system is composed of 4 discrete cavities consisting of the paired lateral ventricles and unpaired midline third and fourth ventricles (**Fig. 1**). The ventricular system is continuous with the subarachnoid spaces through the fourth ventricle outlet foramina of Luschka (lateral apertures) and Magendie (median aperture) and continuous with the central canal of the spinal cord caudal to the obex (caudal apex). The central canal terminates in the ventriculus terminalis (the "fifth ventricle," a variably persistent embryologic structure) in the conus medullaris of the spinal cord.[1,2]

Lateral Ventricles

The lateral ventricles are paired C-shaped chambers contained deep within the substance of the cerebral hemispheres, consisting of a body and atrium along with 3 projections into the frontal, temporal, and occipital lobes, termed "horns." Each lateral ventricle has a capacity of 7 to 10 mL.[3,4]

The foramen of Monro marks the boundary between the body of the lateral ventricle and the frontal horn, with the frontal horn extending anteriorly. The anterior wall and roof of the frontal horn are formed by the genu of the corpus callosum, with the floor formed by the rostrum. The head of the caudate nucleus forms the lateral wall, whereas the columns of the fornix form the inferomedial wall (**Fig. 2**A–C).

[a] Department of Radiology and Imaging, Medical College of Georgia at Augusta University, 1120 15th Street, Augusta, GA 30912, USA; [b] Neuroradiology, Neuroradiology Section, Department of Radiology and Imaging, Medical College of Georgia at Augusta University, 1120 15th Street, Augusta, GA 30912, USA
* Corresponding author.
E-mail address: sforseen@augusta.edu

Neuroimag Clin N Am 32 (2022) 577–601
https://doi.org/10.1016/j.nic.2022.04.005

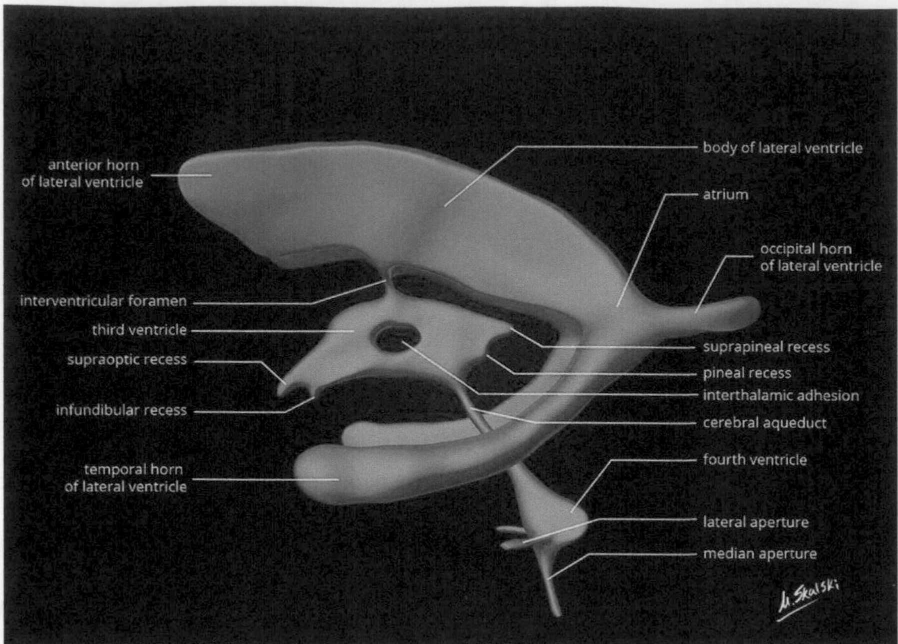

Fig. 1. Volumetric illustration of the ventricular system. (*Courtesy of* M. Skalski, DC, San Jose, California.)

The body of the lateral ventricle projects posteriorly from the foramen of Monro to the splenium of the corpus callosum where it communicates openly with the atrium. The roof of the ventricular body is formed by the body of the corpus callosum with the floor formed by the thalamus. The superomedial and inferomedial walls are, respectively, formed by the septum pellucidum and body of the fornix. The lateral wall is formed by the caudate nucleus and thalamus. The stria terminalis, a main outlet pathway of the amygdala, sits within the caudothalamic groove along with the thalamostriate vein.[5]

The *cavum septi pellucidi* (**Fig. 3**A) is a potential cavity between the laminae of the septum pellucidum bounded anteriorly by the genu of the corpus callosum, superiorly by the body of the corpus callosum, and posteriorly by the forniceal pillars. The cavum is a normal fetal structure with typical fusion of the septum pellucidum laminae by 3 to 6 months after birth.[6]

The *cavum vergae* (**Fig. 3**B) is a potential cavity between the laminae of the septum pellucidum persisting posterior to the forniceal pillars and is thus the caudal continuation of a cavum septi pellucidi. The posterior border is formed by the splenium of the corpus callosum with the superior border formed by the body of the corpus callosum. The inferior border is formed by the transverse portion of the fornix. The septum pellucidum leaflets begin fusing from posterior to anterior in utero with the cavum vergae closed in approximately 97% of term infants.[7] Owing to the progressive fusion of the septum pellucidum leaflets, a cavum vergae is essentially always accompanied by a cavum septum pellucidum and termed a *cavum septi pellucidi et vergae*.

The atrium or trigone is a triangular cavity where the ventricular body communicates with the occipital and temporal horns (see **Fig. 2**A, D; **Fig. 4**). The body and splenium of the corpus callosum form the roof. The tapetum (Latin for "carpet" or "tapestry") is a sheetlike bundle of decussating fibers in the splenium of the corpus callosum that arches over the atrium. The tapetum continues laterally and comprises the lateral wall with the caudate body. The floor is created by the collateral trigone, a flattened triangular area overlying the collateral sulcus. The sloping contour of the medial wall is formed by the calcar avis—the prominence that overlies the deep end of the calcarine sulcus—and bulb of the corpus callosum, which is a bulging created by the forceps major.[3,5]

The temporal horn is the longest and largest horn, extending anteriorly from the atrium and terminating at the amygdala (**Fig. 5**). The medial floor is formed by a prominence overlying the hippocampus and separated by a thin layer of white matter called the alveus. The collateral eminence forms the lateral part of the floor. The roof is created by the caudate nucleus and tapetum. The tapetum also runs inferiorly to comprise the lateral wall and separates the lateral wall from the optic radiations. The medial wall is a small cleft

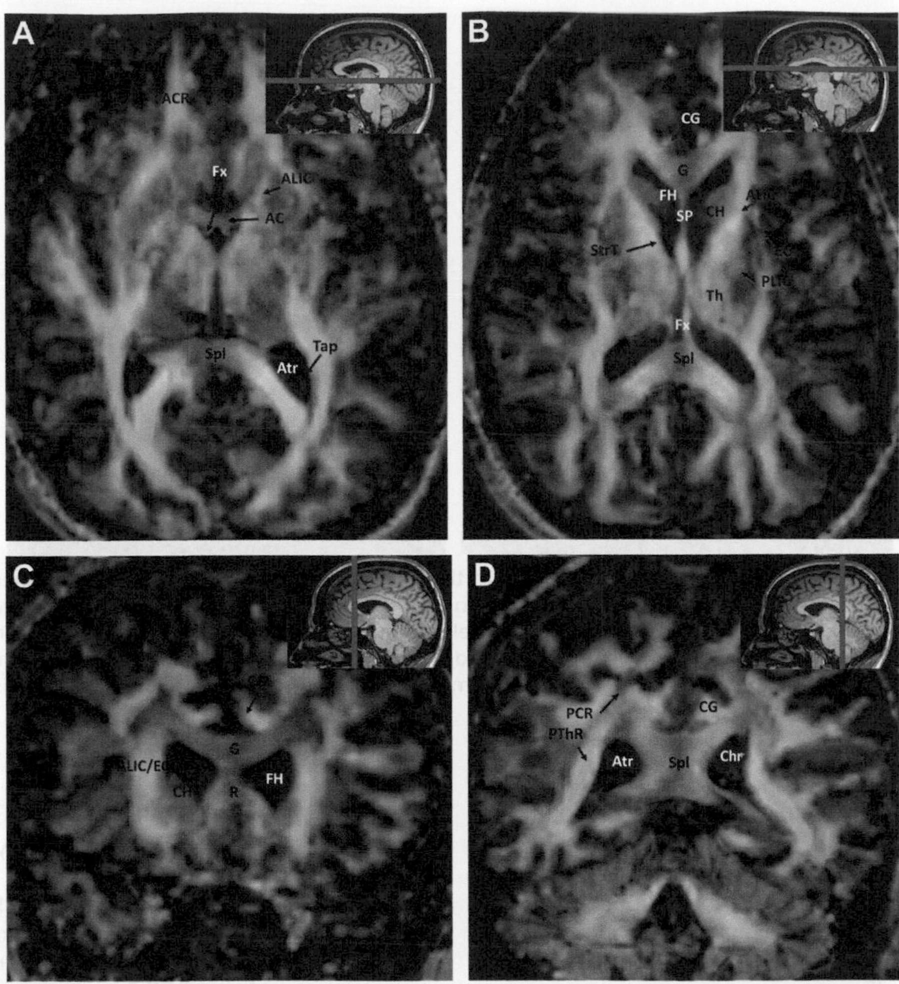

Fig. 2. Axial (*A, B*) and coronal (*C, D*) T1 images coregistered with a color-coded fractional anisotropy map at the level of the lateral ventricle floor (*A*), frontal horns (*B, C*), and atrium (*D*). AC, anterior commissure; ACR, anterior corona radiata; ALIC, anterior limb internal capsule; Atr, ventricular atrium; CG, cingulate gyrus; CH, caudate head; Chr, choroid plexus; EC, external capsule; FH, frontal horn of the lateral ventricle; Fx, fornix; G, genu of the corpus callosum; PCR, posterior corona radiata; PLIC, posterior limb of the internal capsule; PThR, posterior thalamic radiations; R, rostrum of the corpus callosum; SP, septum pellucidum; Spl, splenium of the corpus callosum; StrT, stria terminalis; Tap, tapetum; Th, thalamus.

between the fimbria of the fornix and the inferolateral thalamus.[3,5]

The occipital horn curves posteriorly and medially from the atrium and varies in size; it may be absent or may extend deep into the occipital lobe. The tapetum forms the roof and lateral wall and separates it from the optic radiations. The collateral trigone forms the floor. Similar to the atrium, the bulb of the corpus callosum and calcar avis form the medial wall (Fig. 6).[3,5]

Normal Anatomic Variants

Anatomic variations of the lateral ventricles are common findings in healthy individuals and, though not frequently a diagnostic dilemma, may mimic pathologic conditions. Several variants, including coarctation, asymmetry, and ependymitis granularis, are important for the radiologist to be aware of in order to prevent misinterpreting these findings as pathology. For a detailed description, we recommend reviewing Scelsi, and colleagues.[3]

Coarctation refers to close apposition or fusion of 2 ventricular walls, most commonly seen in the occipital and frontal horns.[8] The cause is likely developmental in nature because there is no histologic evidence of an underlying inflammatory or gliotic reaction.[9] When focal, a portion of the ventricle can be isolated creating an ependyma-lined cyst referred to as a "connatal cyst." These may be multiple and, when seen in infants, may regress.[10]

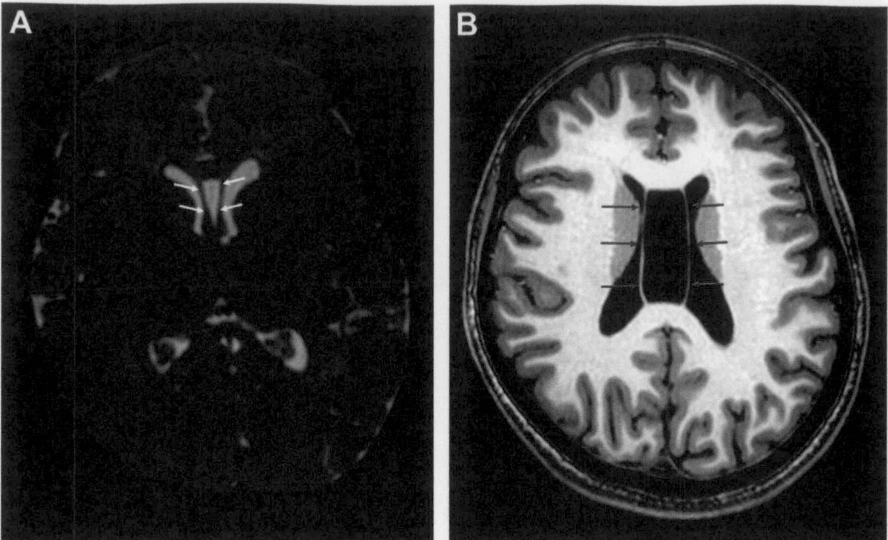

Fig. 3. (*A*) A cavity is present between the laminae of the septum pellucidum (*white arrows*) confined between the genu of the corpus callosum anteriorly and columns of the fornix posteriorly, consistent with a *cavum septi pellucidi*. (*B*) When the cavity between the septum pellucidum leaflets persists caudally to the columns of the fornix, it is termed a *cavum vergae*. Due to the ordered fusion of the septum pellucidum leaflets from posterior to anterior, a cavum vergae is essentially always accompanied by a cavum septum pellucidum and is termed a *cavum septi pellucidi et vergae* (*red arrows*).

Size and morphologic asymmetry of the lateral ventricles is common, particularly of the occipital and temporal horns.[11,12] Clinical significance of asymmetric lateral ventricles is controversial, although small volumetric or morphologic differences, in the absence of obstructing lesion or adjacent parenchymal disease, are likely of no clinical significance.[13]

Ependymitis granularis is a normal anatomic finding referring to symmetric foci of high T2 signal anterolateral to the frontal horns, typically less than 10 mm in extent and demonstrating a triangular morphology. This imaging finding is thought to relate to a loose network of axons with decreased tissue myelin content. This porous ependyma allows transependymal CSF flow. Despite the name

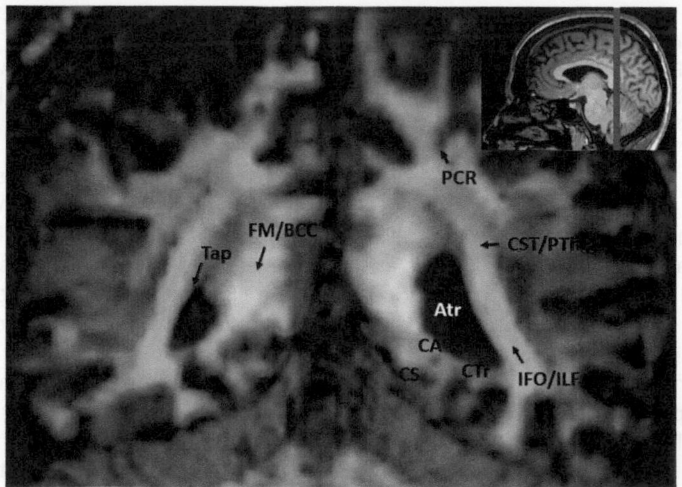

Fig. 4. Coronal T1 image coregistered with color-coded fractional anisotropy map at the level of the lateral ventricle atrium. Atr, atrium of the lateral ventricle; CA, calcar avis; CS, calcarine sulcus; CST/PThR, corticospinal tract/posterior thalamic radiations; CTr, collateral trigone; FM/BCC, forceps major/bulb of the corpus callosum; IFO/ILF, inferior fronto-occipital fasciculus/inferior longitudinal fasciculus; PCR, posterior corona radiata; Tap, tapetum.

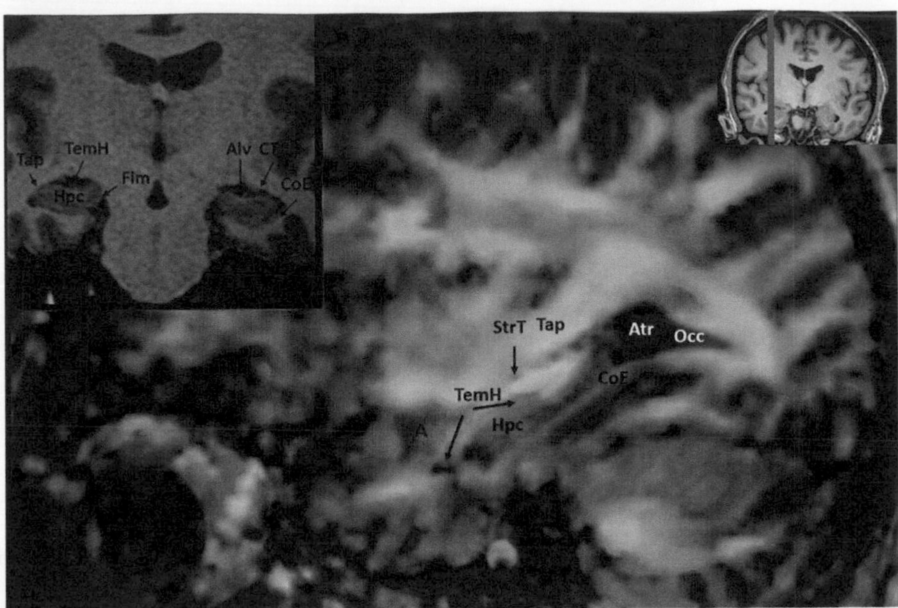

Fig. 5. Sagittal T1 image coregistered with color-coded fractional anisotropy map at the level of the lateral ventricle atrium and temporal horn. Inset: coronal T1 image through the anterior temporal horns. A, amygdala; Alv, alveus; Atr, atrium of the lateral ventricle; CoE, collateral eminence; CS, collateral sulcus; CT, caudate tail; Fim, fimbria of the fornix; Hpc, hippocampus; Occ, occipital horn of the lateral ventricle; StrT, stria terminalis; Tap, tapetum; TemH, temporal horn of the lateral ventricle.

implicating an inflammatory process, there is no histologic evidence that this is the case.[14] This finding may mimic pathologic condition including transependymal edema relating to obstruction (typically not confined to the frontal horns and ventricles would be enlarged), demyelinating lesions (rarely symmetric or triangular in morphology), or chronic microvascular ischemic changes (usually not symmetric or abutting the ventricles).

Foramina of Monro

The 2 interventricular foramina of Monro (Fig. 7) are bilateral channels that connect the lateral ventricles to the third ventricle. They are cylindrical conduits with a crescentic-to-oval cross section that flare out at their proximal and distal ends and slope caudally from lateral to medial and anterior to posterior with a cross-sectional area of approximately 5 mm^2. The left foramen is typically slightly larger than the right.[15] The foramina and are bounded by the forniceal pillars anteriorly and anterior pole of the thalamus posteriorly.[16] The structures that pass through include choroid plexus, branches of the choroidal artery, and internal cerebral, thalamostriate, superior choroidal, and septal veins.[17] Matys and colleagues[18] have recently described in detail the age-related neuroimaging anatomic features of foramen of Monro and also suggested renaming each structure as the *interventricular canalicilus*.

Third Ventricle

The third ventricle (Fig. 8) is a funnel or slit-shaped midline cavity with an estimated capacity of 1 mL, varying by age and gender.[4] The third ventricle communicates with the lateral ventricles anterosuperiorly through the foramina of Munro and with the fourth ventricle posteroinferiorly through the cerebral aqueduct of Sylvius.

The anterior wall of the third ventricle extends from the foramina of Monro superiorly to the optic chiasm inferiorly. From superior to inferior, it is made up of the foramina of Monro, anterior commissure, lamina terminalis, optic recess, and optic chiasm. The optic chiasm is positioned at the junction of the anterior wall and floor of the third ventricle.[19,20]

The posterior wall of the third ventricle extends from the suprapineal recess superiorly to the aqueduct of Sylvius inferiorly. From superior to inferior, the posterior wall of the third ventricle is formed by the suprapineal recess, habenular commissure, pineal body, pineal recess, posterior commissure, and aqueduct of Sylvius.[19,20]

The roof of the third ventricle extends from the foramina of Monro anteriorly to the suprapineal recess posteriorly. It is made up of 4 layers (superior to inferior): fornix, superior layer of the tela choroidea, vascular layer, and inferior layer of the tela choroidea. The body of the fornix makes up the anterior portion of the superior layer and the

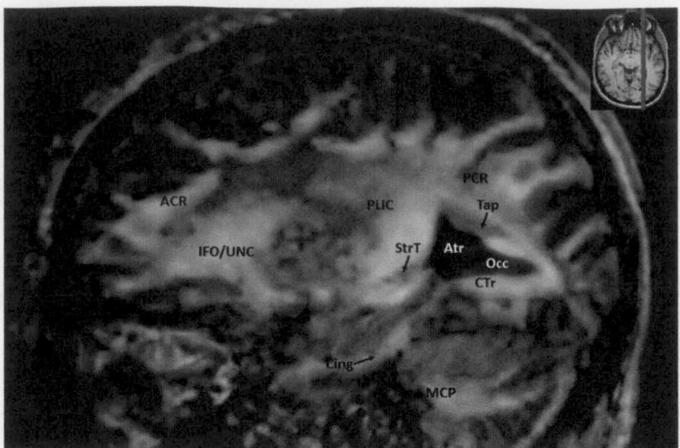

Fig. 6. Sagittal T1 image coregistered with color-coded fractional anisotropy map at the level of the lateral ventricle occipital horn. ACR, anterior corona radiata; Atr, atrium of the lateral ventricle; Cing, cingulum; CTr, collateral trigone; IFO/UNC, inferior fronto-occipital fasciculus/uncinate fasciculus; MCP, middle cerebellar peduncle; Occ, occipital horn of the lateral ventricle; PCR, posterior corona radiata; PLIC, posterior limb of the internal capsule; StrT, stria terminalis.

crura of the fornices and hippocampal commissure form the posterior portion of the superior layer.[19,20]

The tela choroidea is a loose trabecular pial tissue forming 2 layers above and below the vascular layer. The vascular layer is composed of the internal cerebral veins and medial posterior choroidal arteries. Choroid plexus projects inferiorly from the lower layer of the tela choroidea at the roof of the third ventricle and from components of the tela choroidea that project into the lateral ventricles.[19,20]

The velum interpositum is a subarachnoid space located between the layers of the tela choroidea. It has a triangular shape with apex located just behind the foramina of Monro and posterior inferior attachment just above the pineal body. The velum interpositum is typically a closed space but when it communicates with the quadrigeminal cistern, it is referred to as the *cavum veli interpositi* (**Fig. 9**).[21]

The floor of the third ventricle spans from the optic chiasm anteriorly to the margin of the aqueduct of Sylvius posteriorly. The anterior part of the third ventricular floor is made up of diencephalic

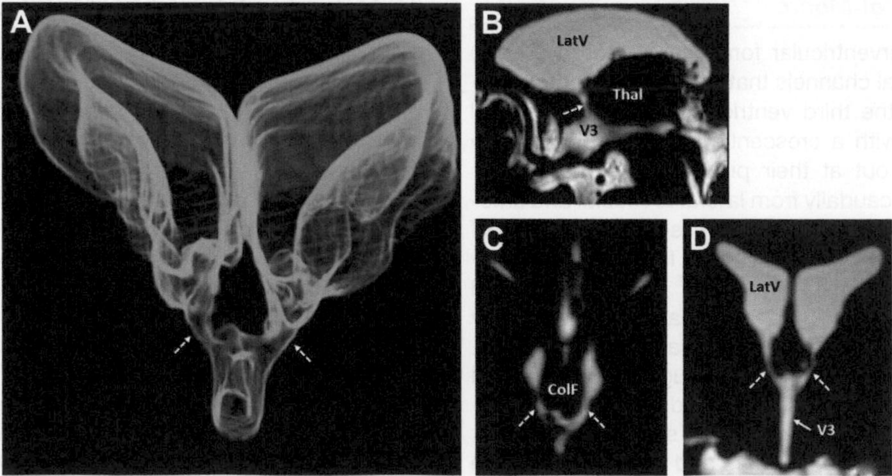

Fig. 7. Foramina of Monro (*dashed white arrows*) as viewed from a coronal perspective on a three-dimensional model (*A*) connecting the lateral ventricles superiorly to the third ventricle inferiorly. Foramina as viewed on oblique sagittal (*B*), axial (*C*), and coronal (*D*) constructive interference in steady state (CISS) magnetic resonance (MR) images. ColF, columns of the fornices; LatV, lateral ventricle; Thal, thalamus; V3, third ventricle.

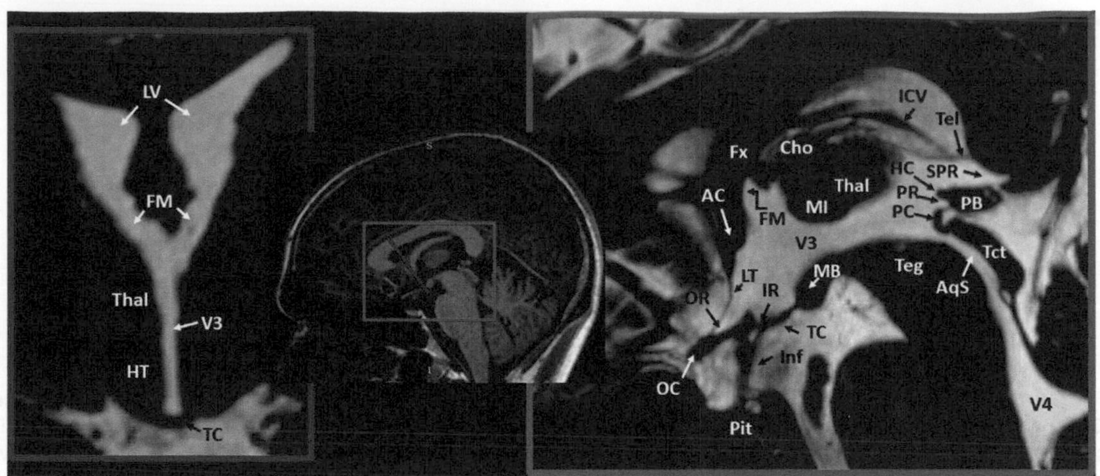

Fig. 8. Oblique coronal (*left*) and sagittal (*right*) CISS MR images of the third ventricle. AC, anterior commissure; Aqs, aqueduct of Sylvius; Cho, choroid plexus; ForM, foramen of Monro; Fx, fornix; HC, habenular commissure; HT, hypothalamus; ICV, internal cerebral vein; Inf, pituitary infundibulum; IR, infundibular recess; LV, lateral ventricle; MB, mammillary body; MI, massa intermedia; OC, optic chiasm; OR, optic recess; PB, pineal body; PC, posterior commissure; Pit, pituitary gland; PR, pineal recess; SPR, suprapineal recess; TC, tuber cinereum; Tec, tectum; Teg, tegmentum; Tel, tela choroidea, Thal, thalamus; V3, third ventricle; V4, fourth ventricle.

structures, and the posterior part of the floor is made up of mesencephalic structures. The floor of the third ventricle, from anterior to posterior, is made up of the inferior surface of the optic chiasm, pituitary infundibulum, tuber cinereum, mammillary bodies, posterior perforated substance, and midbrain tegmentum.[19,20]

The floor of the third ventricle is formed by hypothalamic structures. The hypothalamus is below the thalamus, forming the ventral part of the diencephalon, and is also a component of the limbic system. The hypothalamus is divided into 3 regions (supraoptic, tuberal, and mammillary) from anterior to posterior; and 3 areas (periventricular, medial, and lateral) from medial to lateral. These regions and areas contain the hypothalamic nuclei. The hypothalamus is highly interconnected with other parts of the brain, especially the brainstem and its reticular formation. In the limbic system, it has connections to other structures, including the amygdala and septal nuclei located rostral to the anterior commissure, and is also connected with areas of the autonomic nervous system.

The pituitary gland is composed of 2 lobes, anterior and posterior, with an intermediate lobe (pars intermedia) that joins the 2 regions but this is avascular and almost absent in humans. An intraglandular or hypophyseal cleft lies between the anterior and intermediate lobes. The portion of the anterior third ventricle floor forming the infundibulum ends in the posterior lobe of the pituitary gland (neurohypophysis [NH] or pars nervosa) via the pituitary (infundibular) stalk. The NH, originating from neuroectoderm, is therefore neuronally connected to the median eminence (ME) and tuber cinereum of the hypothalamus via the pituitary stalk. However, the glandular anterior pituitary (adenohypophysis or pars distalis plus the pars tuberalis, which wraps around the pituitary stalk) is distinct and arises from an invagination of the oral ectoderm (Rathke pouch).

The lateral walls of the third ventricle are formed by the hypothalamus inferiorly and thalamus superiorly. The hippocampal sulcus extends from the foramina of Monro to the aqueduct of Sylvius and separates the medial surfaces of the hypothalamus and thalamus. The massa intermedia (interthalamic adhesion, adhesio interthalamica) is a connection between the thalami that contains commissural fibers and neurons. It is present in 80% of people, is variable in size, and is typically located in the anterior superior quadrant of the third ventricle. Its precise function is unknown. The outline of the lateral walls has the appearance of a bird's head, with beak formed by the optic and infundibular recesses and the head formed by the lateral surface of the thalamus.[19,20]

Cerebral aqueduct (of Sylvius)

The cerebral aqueduct connects the third ventricle to the fourth ventricle and measures 15 to 18 mm in length with a highly variable cross-sectional area.[22] It is located within the midbrain and bounded circumferentially by a column of

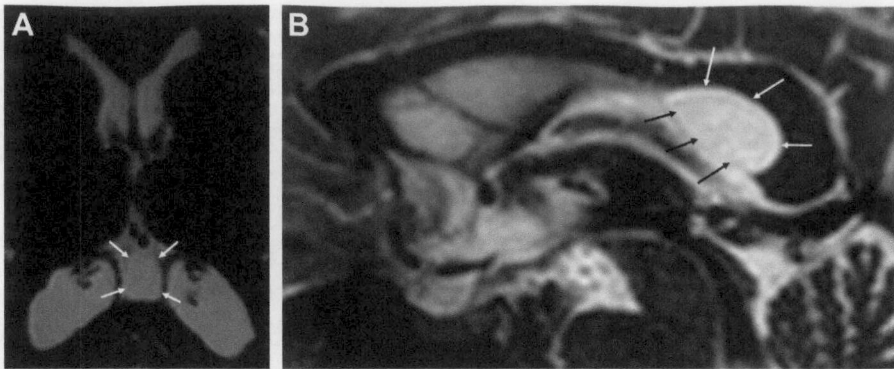

Fig. 9. Axial (*A*) and sagittal (*B*) T2 MR images of the lateral and third ventricles. (*A*) There is enlargement of the CSF space between the lateral ventricle atria (*arrows*) with splaying of the fornices. (*B*) On sagittal images this is confirmed to represent dilatation of the velum interpositum (*cavum veli interpositi, arrows*) as positioned below the splenium of the corpus callosum/columns of the fornices and above the internal cerebral veins. The apex points anteriorly but remains posterior to the foramina of Monro.

periaqueductal gray matter. The tegmentum sits anteriorly with the tectum posteriorly. The superior opening of the aqueduct (*aditus aquaeducti*) is triangular in shape with the base positioned dorsally and bounded by the posterior commissure. Two small, rounded bulges are visible at the ventral aditus separated by a median sulcus. They are likely caused by protrusion of the rubral nuclei into the aqueductal lumen and are thus identified as the rubral eminences. The median sulcus persists along the floor of the aqueduct and continues as the median sulcus in the rhomboid fossa of the fourth ventricle. There are 2 constrictions within the aqueduct corresponding to the superior and inferior colliculi with an intervening dilatation termed the ampulla that corresponds to the tegmental sulcus. Beyond the second constriction, the chamber dilates abruptly into the fourth ventricle.[23] Detailed neuroimaging anatomy and morphometry of the aqueduct is also available in Matys and colleagues.[24]

Fourth Ventricle

The fourth ventricle is the tent-shaped midline terminal compartment of the intracranial ventricular system with an estimated CSF capacity of 1 to 2 mL.[4] The fourth ventricle has a floor, a roof, and 2 lateral recesses.

The floor of the fourth ventricle, known as the rhomboid fossa, has a characteristic diamond shape with the rostral point at the cerebral aqueduct, the caudal point at the obex, and lateral points formed by 2 lateral recesses at the pontomedullary junction (Fig. 10). The dorsal surface of the pons forms the rostral two-thirds of the floor and the inferior one-third is formed by the dorsal surface of the medulla. The median sulcus is a longitudinally oriented vertical centerline that separates the floor into equal halves. The sulcus limitans is a discontinuous longitudinal sulcus that separates each half of the floor into the ME and the lateral vestibular area. The ME is a raised strip that borders the midline and contains, from cranial to caudal, the facial colliculus and 3 triangular areas that overly the nuclei of the hypoglossal and vagus nerves, as well as the area postrema. The stacked arrangement of these 3 paired triangular areas gives the caudal floor a feather or pen nib appearance on gross inspection and has been termed the calamus scriptorius.

The locus ceruleus is at the rostral tip of each sulcus limitans (see Fig. 10). The sulcus limitans is deepest at the pontine and medullary portions of the floor, forming 2 distinct dimples, the superior and inferior fovea, respectively. At the level of the superior fovea, there is an elongated swelling of the ME that is formed by the abducens nucleus and ascending portion of the facial nerve root, the facial colliculus. The hypoglossal triangle overlies the hypoglossal nucleus and is medial to the inferior fovea and the vagal triangle is caudal to the inferior fovea overlying the dorsal nucleus of the vagal nerve. The area postrema is a tongue-shaped projection from the lower aspect of the ME immediately rostral to the obex (see Fig. 10; Fig. 11).

The vestibular area of the floor of the fourth ventricle is lateral to the sulcus limitans at the level of the junction of caudal pons and rostral medulla, overlying the vestibular nuclei. The dorsal. cochlear nucleus, and cochlear portion of the vestibulocochlear nerve form the auditory tubercle. In the lateral part of the vestibular area.

The roof of the fourth ventricle resembles a rhomboid-based pyramid with the edges of the

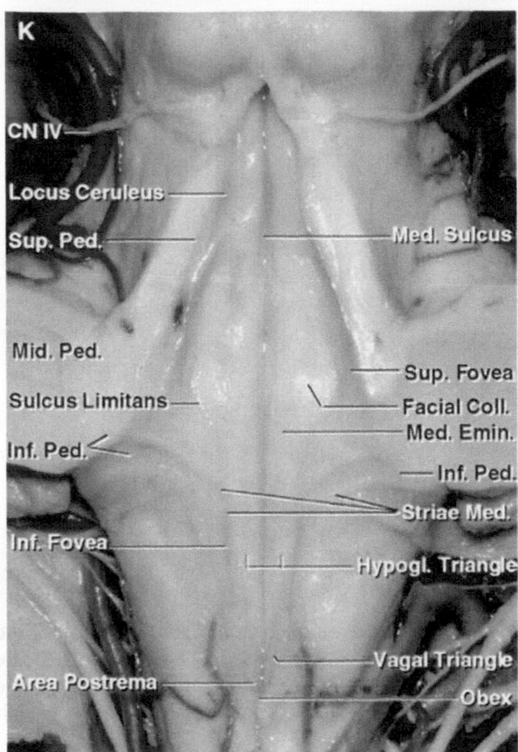

Fig. 10. Floor of the fourth ventricle. The cerebellar peduncles have been sectioned and the cerebellum removed in order to expose the floor of the fourth ventricle. (*Adapted from* Rhoton AL. Relationships of the Inferior Medullary Velum, Dentate Nucleus, Tonsil, and Cerebellomedullary and Cerebellomesencephalic Fissures. The Neurosurgical Atlas. Available at: https://www.neurosurgicalatlas.com/neuroanatomy/relationships-of-the-fourth-ventricular-floor-and-cerebellar-peduncles. Accessed April 7, 2022; with permission.)

pyramid base representing the ventricular borders and the cerebellar fastigium forming the apex and dividing the roof into superior and inferior parts[25] (see Fig. 11; Fig. 12). The superior part of the roof is formed at the midline by the superior medullary velum, a thin lamina of white matter between the superior cerebellar peduncles and rostral to the lingula of the cerebellum. The lateral wall of the superior part of the roof is formed by the superior cerebellar peduncle. The fibers of the superior cerebellar peduncle arise in the dentate nucleus and track along the medial surface of the middle cerebellar peduncle to form the superior part of the lateral wall. The inferior part of the lateral wall is formed by the fibers of the inferior cerebellar peduncle. The inferior part of the roof of the fourth ventricle projects ventral and slightly caudal from the fastigium to attach on the taeniae of the inferolateral floor. The inferior part of the roof adjacent to the fastigium is formed by the nodulus at the midline and inferior medullary velum laterally (Fig. 13). These structures blend inferiorly with the tela choroidea, which forms the most caudal part of the roof. The tela choroidea attaches to ridges on the inferolateral floor that meet at the obex called the taeniae.

The tela choroidea of the inferior fourth ventricle has 3 openings, the paired lateral foramina of Luschka and the midline caudal foramen of Magendie, which communicate with the subarachnoid spaces of the cerebellopontine angle cisterns and foramen magnum, respectively.[26,27]

The lateral recesses are lateral tunnel-like extensions of the fourth ventricle at the level of the pontomedullary junction (widest segment of the floor) that are formed by the junction of the roof and floor (Fig. 14). The floor and a sheetlike layer of neural tissue that extends laterally from the floor to join the tela choroidea, the rhomboid lip, forms the ventral wall of the lateral recess. The caudal margin of the cerebellar peduncles forms the rostral wall. The peduncle of the flocculus crosses the dorsal margin of the lateral recess and interconnects the inferior medullary velum and the flocculus. The tela choroidea extends from the taenia of the inferolateral floor to attach on the edge of the peduncle of the flocculus to form the caudal wall of the lateral recess. The biventral lobule of the cerebellum is dorsal to the lateral recess. The flocculus lies superior to the extreme lateral margin of the lateral recess. Several cranial nerves are also intimately associated with the lateral recess with the glossopharyngeal and vagus nerves arising ventral to the lateral recess (see Fig. 14 *inset*). The facial nerve arises rostral to the lateral recess and the vestibulocholear nerves runs across the lateral recess floor.[28–30]

Choroid Plexus

Choroid plexus is present within the lateral, third, and fourth ventricles and absent within the frontal and occipital horns of the lateral ventricles and cerebral aqueduct.

Choroid plexus is the primary source of CSF, producing 500 to 600 mL per day (0.4 mL/min). At any given time, there is approximately 150 mL total CSF volume, with 125 mL within the subarachnoid space and 25 mL within the ventricles[31] amounting to a turnover of 4 times per day. Other less prominent sources of CSF include brain interstitial fluid (up to 20% of CSF),[32] ventricular ependyma, and brain capillaries.[33]

Within the lateral ventricles, the choroid plexus runs along a cleft between the fornix and thalamus called the choroidal fissure. The choroidal fissure forms a C-shape extending from the foramina of

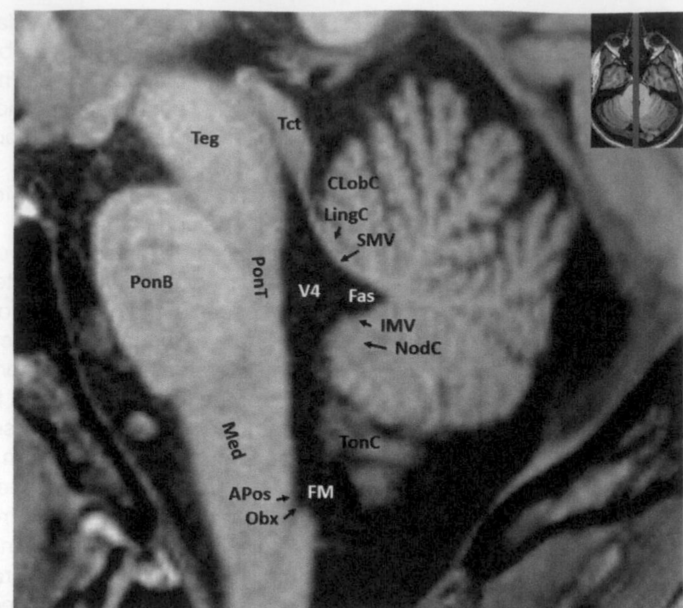

Fig. 11. Midsagittal T1-weighted image through the fourth ventricle. APos, area postrema; CLobC, central lobule of the cerebellum; Fas, fastigium; FM, foramen of Magendie; IMV, inferior medullary velum; LingC, lingula of the cerebellum; Med, medulla; NodC, nodule of the cerebellum; Obx, obex; PonB, basis pontis; PonT, pontine tegmentum; SMV, superior medullary velum; Tct, tectum; Teg, tegmentum; TonC, cerebellar tonsil; V4, fourth ventricle.

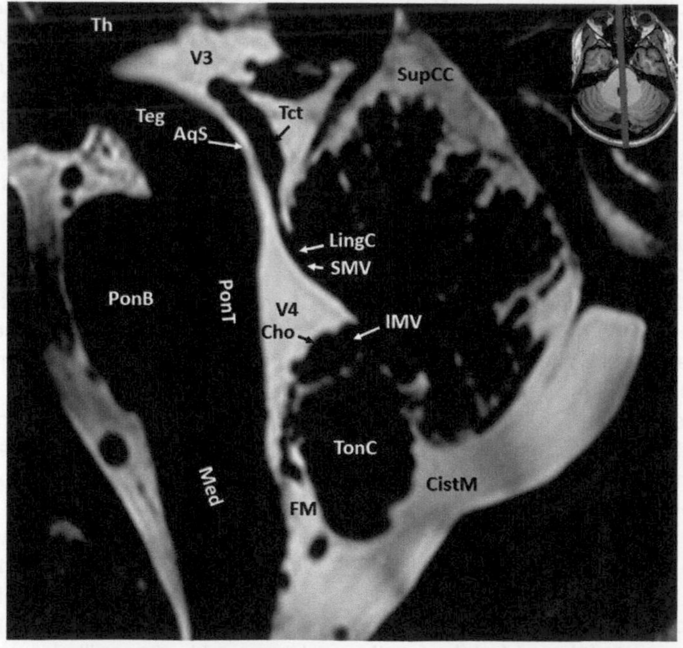

Fig. 12. Oblique sagittal CISS image through the fourth ventricle. AqS, aqueduct of Sylvius; Cho, choroid plexus; CistM, cisterna magna; FM, foramen of Magendie; IMV, inferior medullary velum; LingC, lingula of the cerebellum; Med, medulla; PonB, basis pontis; PonT, pontine tegmentum; SMV, superior medullary velum; SupCC, superior cerebellar cistern; Tct, tectum; Teg, tegmentum; Th, thalamus; TonC, cerebellar tonsil; V3, third ventricle; V4, fourth ventricle.

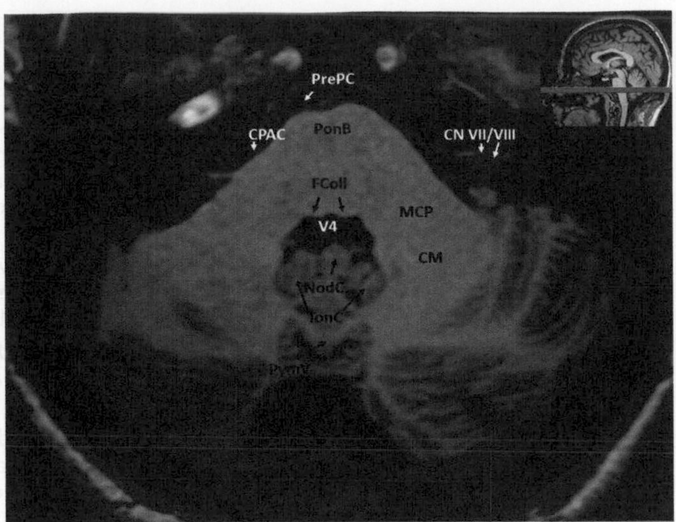

Fig. 13. Axial T1-weighted image through the fourth ventricle at the level of the pons. CM, corpus medullare; CN VII/VIII, cranial nerves VII and VIII; CPAC, cerebellopontine angle cistern; FColl, facial colliculi; MCP, middle cerebellar peduncle; NodC, nodule of the cerebellum; PonB, basis pontis; PrePC, prepontine cistern; PymV, pyramid of the vermis; TonC, cerebellar tonsil; V4, fourth ventricle.

Monro to its inferior terminal point, which is termed the "inferior choroidal point." Within the atria, there is a prominent triangular tuft called the glomus.

The tela choroidea is an invagination of the pia mater and ependyma, which gives rise to the choroid plexus within the choroidal fissure and along the roof of the third ventricle.[3] Choroid plexus within the third ventricle is often hypoplastic and not apparent on imaging studies. Within the fourth ventricle, there are 2 prominent inverted L-shaped tufts of choroid along the roof. These typically protrude prominently from the foramina of Luschka into the cerebellopontine angle cisterns to form the flower baskets of Bochdalek.[16,34]

Circumventricular Organs of the Brain

There are 7 described midline circumventricular organs (CVOs) that are neuroendocrine structures

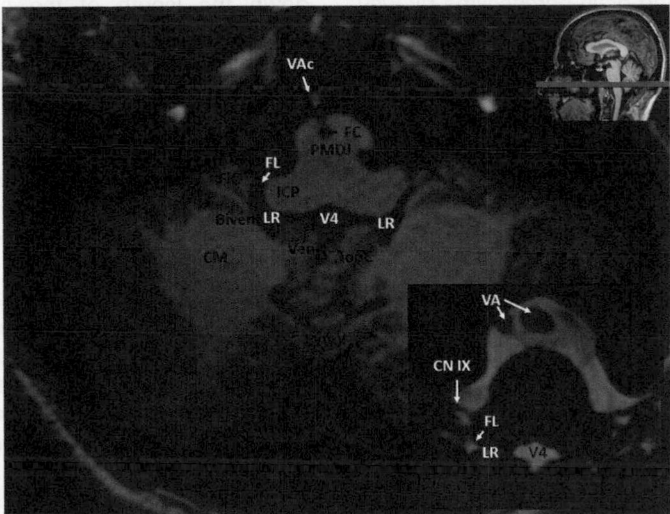

Fig. 14. Axial T1-weighted image through the PMDJ at the foramen of Luschka. Inset: axial CISS through the superior medulla at the foramen of Luschka. Biven, biventral lobule of the cerebellum; CM, corpus medullare; CN IX, cranial nerve IX; FC, foramen cecum of the medulla; FL, foramen of Luschka; FlC, cerebellar flocculus; ICP, inferior cerebellar peduncle; LR, lateral recess of the fourth ventricle; PMDJ, pontomedullary junction; PymV, pyramid of the vermis; TonC, cerebellar tonsil; V4, fourth ventricle; VA, vertebral artery; Vac, confluence of the vertebral arteries into the basilar; VenA, ventricular aperture of the lateral recess.

Table 1
Characteristics of circumventricular organs of the brain

	Type	Location	Primary Functions
AP	Sensory	Floor of the distal fourth ventricle at the level of the obex (only paired CVO)	Chemoreceptor trigger zone for vomiting. Autonomic cardiorespiratory control
OVLT	Sensory	Anterior wall of third ventricle	Osmoregulation via angiotensin and vasopressin pathways. Possible mediator of inflammatory reactions to plasma molecules
SFO	Sensory	Underside of the fornix at the confluence of the foramina of Monro	Osmoregulation and fluid balance via angiotensin and vasopressin pathways
SCO	Secretory	Ventral surface of the posterior commissure adjacent to the cerebral aqueduct	Not well understood; likely plays a role in water homeostasis and electrolyte balance via aldosterone
NH	Secretory	Posterior portion of the pituitary (originating from the floor of the third ventricle)	Release of vasopressin and oxytocin
ME	Secretory	Small protuberance on the tuber cinereum posterior to the infundibular stalk	Collection of releasing and inhibiting regulatory hypothalamic hormones (CRF, GnRH, TRH, GHRH, DA)
PG	Secretory	Posterior wall of third ventricle	Regulation of circadian rhythms via melatonin

Abbreviations: AP, area postrema; CRF, corticotropin-releasing factor; DA, dopamine; GHRH, growth hormone-releasing factor; GnRH, gonadotropin-releasing hormone; ME, median eminence; NH, neurohypophysis; OVLT, organum vasculosum of the lamina terminalis; PG, pineal gland; SCO, subcommissural organ; SFO, subforniceal organ; TRH, thyrotropin-releasing hormone.

characterized by a rich network of permeable capillaries with an incomplete blood–brain barrier.[35] These organs serve a homeostatic function between blood, CSF, and brain parenchyma by way of sensory and secretory functions. The CVOs include the organum vasculosum of the lamina terminalis (OVLT), subforniceal organ (SFO), area postrema (AP), NH, ME, and pineal gland (PG). The subcommissural organ (SCO) is inconsistently listed as a CVO because it lacks a high concentration of fenestrated capillaries making its blood–brain barrier less permeable than other CVOs; however, its function as a secretory neuroendocrine structure has been used as an argument for classification as a CVO. The CVOs are commonly classified as being sensory (AP, OVLT, SFO) or secretory (SCO, NH, ME, PG) in nature. See **Table 1** for an overview of CVO characteristics. A more detailed discussion of imaging features by Horsburgh and Massoud[36] is recommended for further reading.

SUBARACHNOID SPACES AND CISTERNS

The subarachnoid space is an interval between the arachnoid mater and pia mater with free multidirectional flow of CSF that allows for equalization of composition. Additionally, cranial nerves and intracranial vasculature are transmitted through the subarachnoid space. Within the subarachnoid space, CSF flows over the surface of the brain and down the length of the spinal cord. CSF is resorbed via arachnoid granulations (Pacchionian bodies), projections of the arachnoid membrane into the dural sinuses that allow CSF to pass from the subarachnoid space into the venous system, accounting for most CSF resorption. A small amount of CSF may also enter the lymphatic system via the nasal cribriform plate in association with olfactory nerve roots[37,38] or in association with spinal nerve roots.[38]

The subarachnoid cisterns are compartments within the subarachnoid space where there is a pool of CSF within an expanded pia-arachnoid interval. Although described as distinct compartments, in reality, they are continuous or separated by porous membranes, trabeculae, and septa[39]; major partitions are discussed in the meninges section of this article. For ease of organization, the major named subarachnoid cisterns presented below are organized in a roughly anatomic fashion from inferior to superior divided by infratentorial and supratentorial compartments (**Table 2**). Major contents of the subarachnoid cisterns are detailed in **Table 3**.

Table 2
Subarachnoid cisterns by intracranial compartment

Infratentorial	At the Level of the Tentorium	Supratentorial
Cisterna magna	Interpeduncular	Crural (paired)
Cerebellomedullary (paired)	Quadrigeminal	Suprasellar
Premedullary	Ambient (paired)	Carotid (paired)
Prepontine		Oculomotor (paired)
Cerebellopontine angle (paired)		Sylvian (paired)
Superior cerebellar		Lamina terminalis
Subdiaphragmatic		Pericallosal

INFRATENTORIAL

Cisterna Magna

The largest of the subarachnoid cisterns is the cisterna magna (**Figs. 15** and **16**), bounded superiorly by the cerebellar vermis, anteriorly by the dorsal surface of the medulla, posteriorly by the inner table of the occipital bone, and inferiorly by the foramen magnum where it communicates freely with the posterior spinal cistern. CSF drains into the inferior aspect of the cisterna magna from foramen of Magendie. The posterior inferior cerebellar arteries (PICAs) enter the cisterna magna and commonly divide into lateral and medial trunks supplying the cerebellar hemispheres and vermis, respectively. The cisterna magna communicates superiorly with the superior cerebellar cistern and laterally with the cerebellomedullary cisterns via the cerebellomedullary fissure.[39,40]

Cerebellomedullary Cisterns

The cerebellomedullary cisterns (see **Fig. 16**) are occasionally included under the umbrella of the cisterna magna or referred to as the inferior cerebellopontine angle cisterns. The cisterns are limited superiorly by the lateral pontomedullary membrane that crosses the subarachnoid space between CN VIII and CN IX just caudal to the pontomedullary junction. The inferior border is formed by the foramen magnum. The premedullary cistern lies anteriorly and is separated by arachnoid trabeculations anterior to CN IX, CN X, and CN XI. As well as CN IX, X, and XI, the PICA is contained within the cerebellomedullary cisterns. The cisterns are continuous with the cisterna magna posteroinferiorly via the cerebellomedullary fissure.[39,40]

Premedullary Cistern

The premedullary cistern (see **Figs. 15** and **16**) lies between the lower aspect of the clivus and the anterior surface of the medulla. The cranial boundary is at the pontomedullary junction (at the level of the foramina of Luschka) and is separated from the prepontine cistern by the medial pontomedullary membrane. The cistern communicates freely with the anterior spinal cistern inferiorly. The lateral extent is defined by dense arachnoid trabeculae crossing the subarachnoid space anterior to the CN IX–X–XI complex. The premedullary cistern contains the distal vertebral arteries terminating as the basilar origin, PICA, and CN XII.[39,40]

Prepontine Cistern

The prepontine cistern (see **Fig. 15**; **Fig. 17**) is located ventral to the pons and dorsal to the clivus. The superior boundary is formed by the mesencephalic leaf of the Liliequist membrane, inferiorly by the medial pontomedullary membrane (at the origin of the basilar artery), and laterally by the anterior pontine membranes. The basilar artery is found within the prepontine cistern and gives rise to the anterior inferior cerebellar artery (AICA), whereas CN VI traverses in the anterior pontine membrane.[39,40]

Cerebellopontine Angle Cisterns

The cerebellopontine angle cisterns (see **Fig. 17**) are triangular in shape on axial images and bounded superiorly by the tentorium cerebelli, posteriorly by the anterior surface of the cerebellum, anteriorly by the anterior pontine membrane (separating from the prepontine cistern and containing CN VI), laterally by the petrous temporal bone (including the internal acoustic meatus), and inferiorly by the lateral pontomedullary membrane, which serves as a boundary between the cerebellopontine angle and cerebellomedullary cisterns. CN V, CN VII, CN VIII, portions of the AICA, the superior cerebellar

Table 3
Major contents of the subarachnoid cisterns

Cistern	Common Major Contents
Ambient	Nerves: CN IV Arteries: Posterior cerebral artery (PCA) P2p segment, lateral posterior choroidal, medial posterior choroidal, short and long circumflex, thalamogeniculate, inferior temporal, parieto-occipital
Carotid	Arteries: Internal carotid, ophthalmic, anterior choroidal, posterior cerebral, posterior communicating, middle cerebral, anterior cerebral
Cerebellomedullary	Nerves: CN IX, CN X, CN XI Arteries: Vertebral, PICA
Cerebellopontine	Nerves: CN V, CN VI, CN VII, CN VIII Arteries: SCA and AICA, both commonly bifurcating into rostral and caudal trunks Veins: tributary veins converge to form the superior petrosal vein
Cisterna magna	Arteries: PICA, commonly dividing into medial and lateral trunks
Crural	Arteries: PCA P2a segment, peduncular perforating, anterior choroidal, medial posterior choroidal, short and long circumflex, thalamogeniculate, inferior temporal
Interpeduncular	Nerves: CN III (in lateral wall) Arteries: Posterior thalamoperforating, basilar bifurcation, PCA origin, PComm, SCA, medial posterior choroidal, short and long circumflex Veins: Peduncular, posterior communicating, median anterior pontomesencephalic
Lamina terminalis	Arteries: ACA A1 and A2 segments, recurrent artery, anterior communicating, orbitofrontal; perforators supplying the chiasm, anterior third ventricle, and anterior hypothalamic area
Oculomotor	Nerves: CN III
Pericallosal	Arteries: ACA A2–A5 segments, callosomarginal, frontopolar, internal frontal, paracentral, parietal
Premedullary	Nerves: CN XII rootlets (in posterior wall) Arteries: Vertebral, anterior spinal
Prepontine	Arteries: Basilar, AICA origin
Quadrigeminal	Nerves: CN IV Arteries: Trunks and branches of PCA (P3 segment) and SCA Veins: Convergence of internal cerebral, basal veins, and other tributaries of the vein of Galen
Subdiaphragmatic	Pituitary gland
Superior cerebellar	Arteries: Median and paramedian branches of the SCA Veins: Superior vermian
Suprasellar	Nerves: CN II, optic chiasm Arteries: Carotid perforating branches including superior hypophyseal and infundibular
Sylvian	Arteries: MCA branches, lenticulostriate, distal recurrent artery branches Veins: Superficial Sylvian

artery (SCA), the vein of the cerebellopontine fissure as it ascends to reach the superior petrosal vein, and Bochdalek's flower basket are contained in this space. The cerebellopontine angle cisterns are continuous with the fourth ventricle via the foramina of Luschka.[39,40]

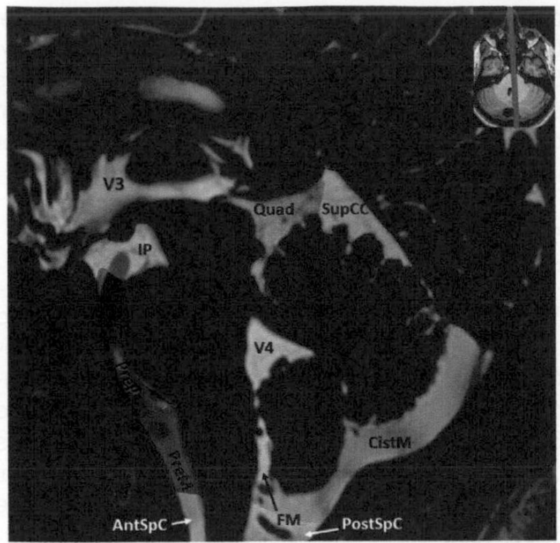

Fig. 15. Sagittal CISS image through the posterior fossa. AntSpC, anterior spinal cistern; CistM, cisterna magna; FM, foramen of Magendie; IP, interpeduncular cistern; PostSpC, posterior spinal cistern; PreM, premedullary cistern; PreP, prepontine cistern; Quad, quadrigeminal cistern; SupCC, superior cerebellar cistern; V3, third ventricle; V4, fourth ventricle.

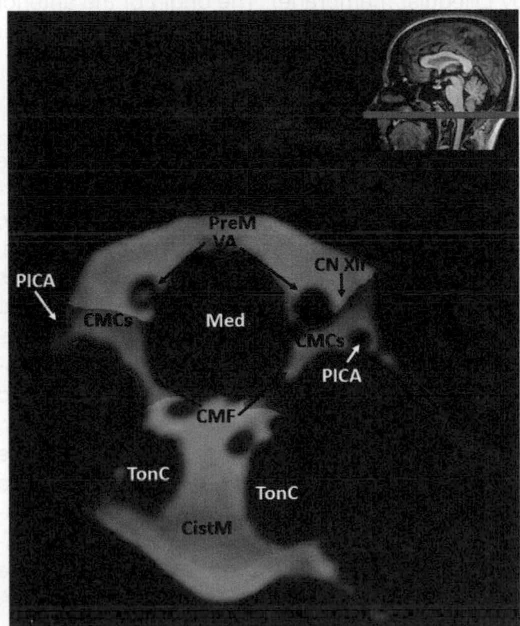

Fig. 16. Axial CISS image through the posterior fossa at the level of the medulla. CistM, cisterna magna; CMCs, cerebellomedullary cistern; CMF, cerebellomedullary fissure; CN XII, cranial nerve XII; Med, medulla; PICA, posterior inferior cerebellar artery; PreM, premedullary cistern; TonC, cerebellar tonsils; VA, vertebral artery.

Superior Cerebellar Cistern

The superior cerebellar cistern (see **Fig. 15**) is located between the superior surface of the cerebellum and the tentorium and communicates anteriorly with the quadrigeminal cistern and posteriorly with the cisterna magna below the confluence of the dural venous sinuses. The cistern tapers laterally and blends into the subarachnoid space over the cerebellar hemispheres. Terminal branches of the SCA are found within the superior cerebellar cistern.[39,40]

Subdiaphragmatic Cistern

The subdiaphragmatic cistern (see **Fig. 19**) is a variably present (seen on MR imaging in approximately 70% of patients) small but distinct subarachnoid space with considerable variability in structure. The roof of the cistern is formed by the diaphragma sellae, the floor by the superior aspect of the pituitary gland, the lateral walls by the arachnoid extending laterally through the medial walls of the cavernous sinus, and the medial walls by the infundibular stem. The cistern communicates with the suprasellar cistern by way of the ostium of the diaphragma.[41]

COMMUNICATING THROUGH THE TENTORIAL INCISURA

Interpeduncular Cistern

The interpeduncular cistern (see **Fig. 15**; **Figs. 18–19**) is conical in shape on axial images. Located between the cerebral peduncles and the posterior perforated substance, the interpeduncular cistern serves as the confluence of the supratentorial and infratentorial subarachnoid space and straddles the tentorial incisura. Boundaries are formed by the Liliequist membrane superiorly (diencephalic leaf) and inferiorly (mesencephalic leaf), which separates the interpeduncular cistern from the suprasellar and prepontine cisterns, respectively. Anteriorly the cistern is limited by the origin of the Liliequist membrane and posteriorly by the posterior perforated substance. It communicates with the crural and ambient cisterns laterally beyond the medial borders of the cerebral peduncles. The cistern contains the bifurcation of the basilar artery, proximal (peduncular) segments of the posterior cerebral and superior cerebellar arteries, and posterior communicating arteries. CN III courses within the lateral wall of the cistern and projects between the posterior cerebral and superior cerebellar arteries.[39,40,42]

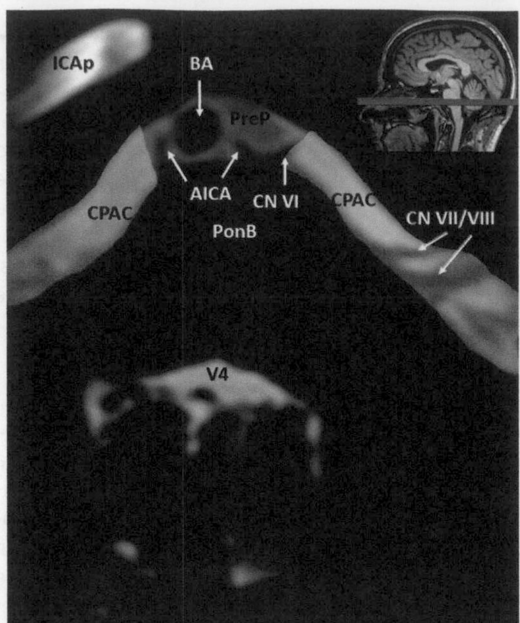

Fig. 17. Axial CISS image through the posterior fossa at the level of the cerebellopontine angle. AICA, anterior inferior cerebellar artery; BA, basilar artery; CN VI, cranial nerve VI; CN VII/VIII, cranial nerves VII and VIII; CPAC, cerebellopontine angle cistern; ICAp, petrous portion of the internal carotid artery; PonB, basis pontis; PreP, prepontine cistern; V4, fourth ventricle.

Quadrageminal Cistern

The midline quadrigeminal cistern (see **Figs. 15, 18, and 19**) is located between the colliculi rostrally, the splenium of the corpus callosum superiorly, the superior surface of the cerebellum inferiorly, and the great cerebral vein of Galen caudally, roughly encompassing the pineal region. The lateral walls are formed by the pulvinar anteriorly and infrasplenial occipital cortex posteriorly. The cistern communicates with the posterior aspect of the pericallosal cistern superiorly, the ambient cisterns inferolaterally, and posteriorly with the superior cerebellar cistern. The quadrigeminal cistern contains posterior cerebral, posterior choroidal, and superior cerebellar arteries as well as CN IV. The confluence of the vein of Galen and inferior sagittal sinus into the straight sinus is contained within the cistern.[39,40]

Ambient Cisterns

The ambient cisterns (see **Figs. 18** and **19**) are found posterolateral to the midbrain. In conjunction with the crural cisterns, they act as a connection between the quadrigeminal cistern and the interpeduncular cistern and are considered to have supratentorial and infratentorial components divided by the superior cerebellar membrane. Contents include the posterior cerebral artery, SCA, the basal vein, and CN IV. The crural cisterns are occasionally labeled as the *anterior* ambient cistern in which case the ambient cistern proper is labeled as the *posterior* ambient cistern.[40,42]

SUPRATENTORIAL

Crural Cisterns

The crural cisterns (see **Fig. 18**) are situated around the ventrolateral aspect of the midbrain between the cerebral crus and the uncus of the temporal lobe. They communicate dorsally with the Sylvian cistern and ambient cistern. Contents include the anterior choroidal artery, the medial portion of the posterior choroidal artery, and the basal vein.[40,42]

Suprasellar Cistern (Chiasmatic Cistern)

The suprasellar cistern (see **Figs. 18** and **19**) is a midline cistern anterior to the interpeduncular cistern that surrounds the pituitary infundibulum and optic chiasm. The cistern communicates with the cistern of the lamina terminalis superiorly, the middle cerebral artery cisterns leading to the Sylvian cisterns anterolaterally, and the interpeduncular cistern posteriorly (partially separated by Liliequist membrane). The origin of the anterior cerebral arteries is contained in the suprasellar cistern.[40,42]

Carotid Cisterns

The carotid cisterns (see **Figs. 18** and **19**) are bounded by the anterior portion of the uncus laterally, the lateral edge of the optic chiasm medially, superiorly by the anterior perforated substance, and inferiorly by the posterior clinoid process and cavernous sinus. The cistern is separated from the suprasellar cistern medially by the medial carotid membrane. The middle cerebral artery cisterns leading to the Sylvian cisterns are found laterally, interpeduncular cistern posteromedially, lamina terminalis cistern superomedially, and the crural cisterns posteriorly. There is commonly a confluent area between the carotid, interpeduncular, and crural cisterns without membranous separation. The carotid cisterns primarily contain the internal carotid arteries (ICA) and proximal ICA branches.[40,42]

Oculomotor Cisterns

The oculomotor nerve arises from the ventral midbrain and has a “free” portion, a segment within the oculomotor cistern, and a segment where it is incorporated into the fibrous lateral

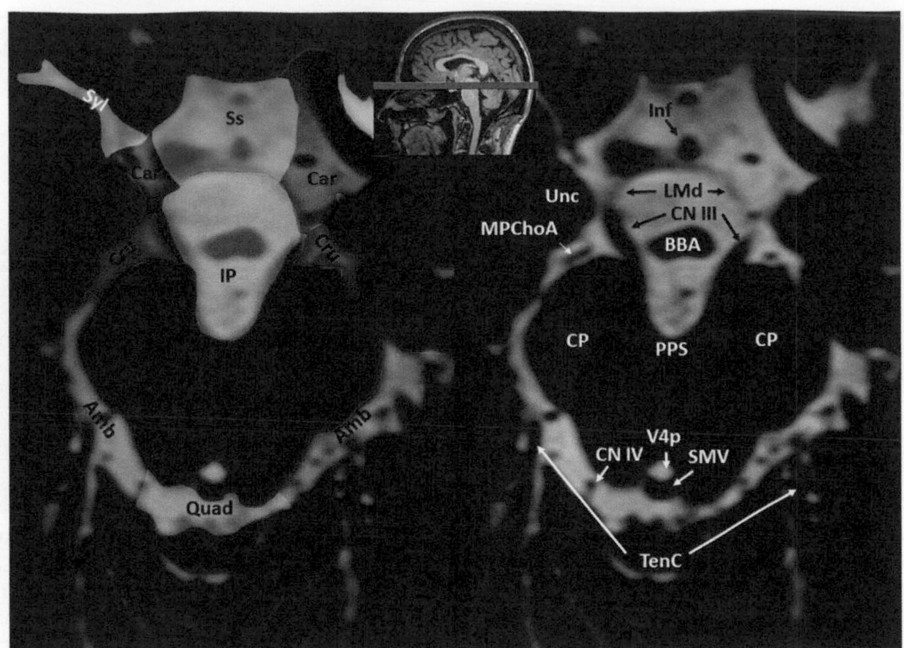

Fig. 18. Axial CISS images at the level of the basal cisterns with (left) and without (right) color overlays. Amb, ambient cistern; BBA, bifurcation of the basilar artery; Car, carotid cistern; CN IV, cranial nerve IV; CP, cerebral peduncle; Cru, crural cistern; Inf, pituitary infundibulum; IP, interpeduncular cistern; LMd, diencephalic leaf of the Liliequist membrane; MPChoA, medial posterior choroidal artery; PPS, posterior perforated substance; Quad, quadrigeminal cistern; SMV, superior medullary velum; SS, suprasellar cistern; Syl, Sylvian cistern; TenC, tentorium cerebelli; Unc, uncus; V4p, proximal fourth ventricle.

wall of the cavernous sinus (see Fig. 20). The free portion of the oculomotor nerve courses in an intersection of arachnoid membranes at the junction of the carotid, suprasellar, prepontine, interpeduncular, and cerebellopontine cisterns. The opening of the oculomotor cistern is located at the roof of the cavernous sinus and is termed the "porus," formed by a complex network of subarachnoid membranes and a dural cuff. The oculomotor cistern surrounds the nerve for a variable distance then gradually tapers and terminates below the tip of the anterior clinoid process as the nerve enters the orbit through the superior orbital fissure.[40,42,43]

Sylvian Cisterns (Insular Cisterns)

The middle cerebral artery cisterns lead to the "T" shaped Sylvian cisterns (see Figs. 18 and 19), considered the transitional subarachnoid space between the basal cisterns and the hemispheric subarachnoid space. The cistern is bounded by the optic tract medially with other boundaries formed by the anterior cerebral and anterior choroidal membranes, insular cortex, and opercular cortices. Contents include the M1 segment of the middle cerebral artery and its proximal branches as well as the middle cerebral vein, fronto-orbital veins, and collaterals to the basal vein.[40,42]

Cistern of the Lamina Terminalis

The "tent-shaped" midline cistern of the lamina terminalis (see Fig. 19) communicates inferiorly with the suprasellar cistern and superiorly with the pericallosal cistern. The anterior boundary is formed by the union of pia mater rostral to the anterior communicating arteries. The lamina terminalis of the third ventricle forms the posterior wall with the inferior wall formed by the optic chiasm. Lateral boundaries are formed by the gyri recti and septal areas of the frontal lobes. Important structures traversing the cistern of the lamina terminalis include major components of the anterior circulation with the A1 and proximal A2 segments of the anterior cerebral arteries, the anterior communicating artery, the recurrent artery of Heubner, the hypothalamic arteries, the origin of the fronto-orbital arteries, and venous structures of the lamina terminalis.[40,42]

Pericallosal cistern

The pericallosal cistern (see Fig. 19) extends under the falx cerebri between the cerebral hemispheres

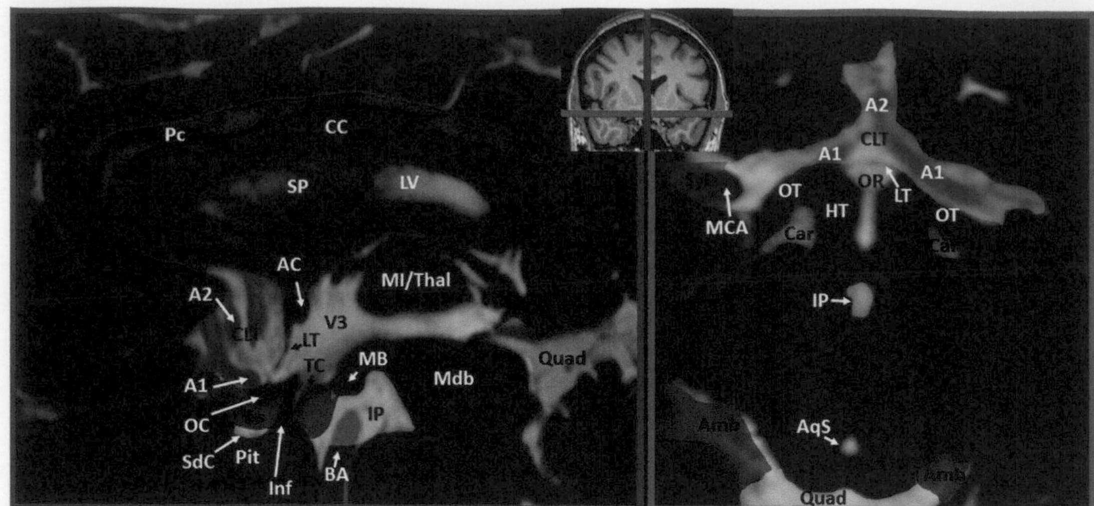

Fig. 19. Sagittal and axial CISS images centered on the supratentorial cisterns. A1, A1 segment of the ACA; A2, A2 segment of the ACA; AC, anterior commissure; Amb, ambient cistern; Aqs, aqueduct of Sylvius; Car, carotid cistern; CC, corpus callosum; CLT, cistern of the lamina terminalis; HT, hypothalamus; Inf, pituitary infundibulum; IP, interpeduncular cistern; LT, lamina terminalis; LV, lateral ventricle; MB, mammillary body; MCA, middle cerebral artery; Mdb, midbrain; MI/Thal, massa intermedia/thalamus; OC, optic chiasm; OR, optic recess; OT, optic tract; Pc, pericallosal cistern; Pit, pituitary; Quad, quadrigeminal cistern; SdC, subdiaphragmatic cistern; SP, septum pellucidum; Syl, Sylvian cistern; TC, tuber cinereum; V3, third ventricle.

and above the corpus callosum from the rostrum to the splenium. It communicates inferiorly with the cistern of the lamina terminalis. Contents include the pericallosal artery.[40,42]

THE MENINGES

The meninges are an intricate covering of the central nervous system, composed of 3 distinct concentric outermost-to-innermost layers: dura mater (pachymeninges), arachnoid mater, and pia mater that together form the leptomeninges. The pia mater (tender mother) is firmly adherent to the surface of the brain and loosely connected to the arachnoid layer; it is generally not visualized on imaging studies under normal physiologic circumstances and will not be discussed further.

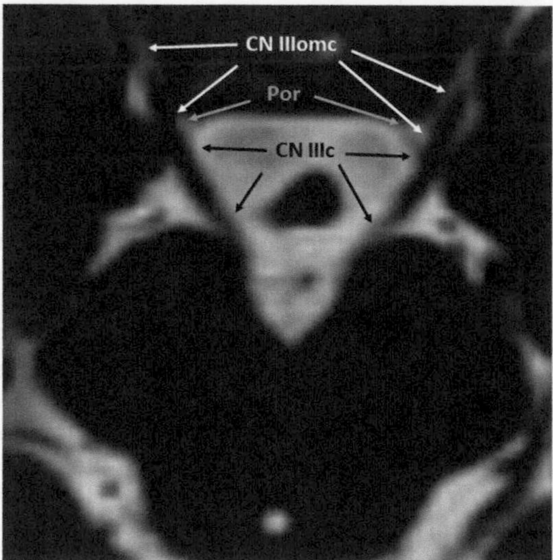

Fig. 20. Oblique axial CISS image of the oculomotor nerves. CN IIIc, cisternal segment of cranial nerve III; CN IIIomc, segment of cranial nerve III within the oculomotor cistern; Por, oculomotor porus.

Dura Mater

The dura mater (hard mother) is the outermost layer of the meninges and is primarily composed of fibroblasts and extracellular collagen. The dura mater arises from a sheath of somitic mesoderm, the *meninx primitiva*, that forms around the rostral neural tube after closure and ultimately forms the scalp, skull, and meninges. The dura mater is composed of 3 layers, the periosteal layer, the meningeal layer, and the dural border cell layer. The dural border cell layer is only visible microscopically.

The periosteal layer is tightly adherent to the calvarium, particularly around the foramen magnum. It is continuous with the pericranium (external periosteum covering the outer surface of the skull) through the cranial sutures. The periosteal layer creates sheathes that surround the cranial nerves as they course through the skull base foramina, transitioning to epineurium as they exit. It is also continuous with the periorbita (orbital periosteum) through the superior orbital fissure.

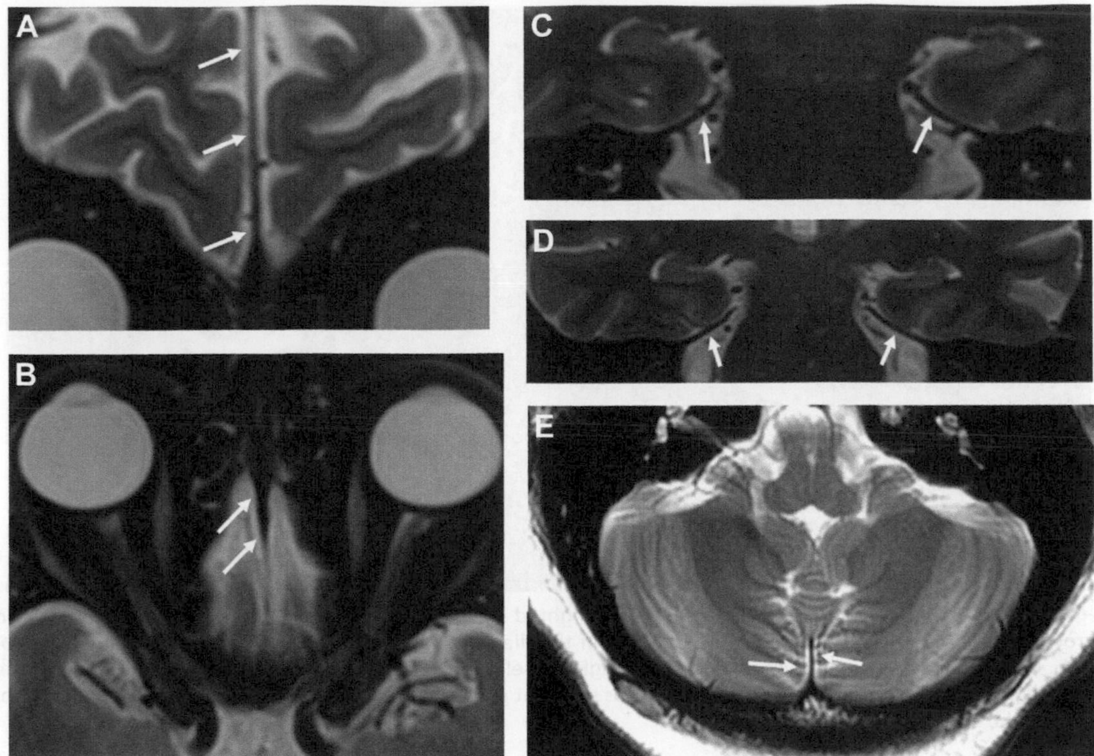

Fig. 21. Coronal (*A, C, D*) and axial (*B, E*) T2-weighted MR images. The falx cerebri is a vertically oriented dural reflection (*arrows A*) and extends rostrally from the internal frontal crest and crista galli (*arrows B*) to the tentorium cerebelli. The tentorium cerebelli has fixed and free edges with the free edge (*arrows C, D*) forming a U-shaped opening that is the sole connection between the supratentorial and infratentorial compartments. The falx cerebelli is a vertically oriented dural fold that separates the cerebellar hemispheres (*arrows E*).

The inner meningeal layer extends through the foramen magnum and is contiguous with the spinal dura mater. The periosteal and meningeal layers of the dura mater are adherent to one another throughout most of their intracranial expanse, with the exception of the dural reflections and the dural venous sinuses.

Dural Reflections

The dural reflections are folds of the meningeal layer that compartmentalize the cranium and assist in dampening motion of the brain. The major dural reflections are the falx cerebri and tentorium cerebelli (Fig. 21A–D). The minor dural reflections are the falx cerebelli (Fig. 21E) and diaphragma sellae (Fig. 22).[44]

The falx cerebri is the largest dural reflection that is oriented vertically and separates the 2 cerebral hemispheres in the interhemispheric fissure. It has a sickle shape and extends from the internal frontal crest and crista galli to the internal occipital protuberance. Posteriorly, the falx cerebri blends with the tentorium cerebelli. The superior margin of the falx cerebri is attached to the groove for the superior sagittal sinus. The free edge of the falx cerebri is closely associated with the superior margin of the corpus callosum and contains the inferior sagittal sinus.

The tentorium cerebelli is the second largest dural reflection that forms superior and inferior compartments within the cranial cavity. It has both fixed and free edges. The fixed edges attach to the anterior and posterior clinoid process anteriorly, the superior margin of the petrous temporal bones laterally, and the grooves for the transverse sinuses and internal occipital protuberance posteriorly. The free edge of the tentorium cerebelli forms a roughly U-shaped opening that is the sole connection between the supratentorial and infratentorial compartments, the *tentorial incisura* or *tentorial notch*. The anterior margin of the tentorial incisura is the dorsum sella and the apex is located just posterior to the PG. The anatomic interrelationships with the tentorial incisura are displayed in Fig. 21 panels C and D.

The falx cerebelli (see Fig. 21E) is a vertically oriented dural fold that extends along the internal

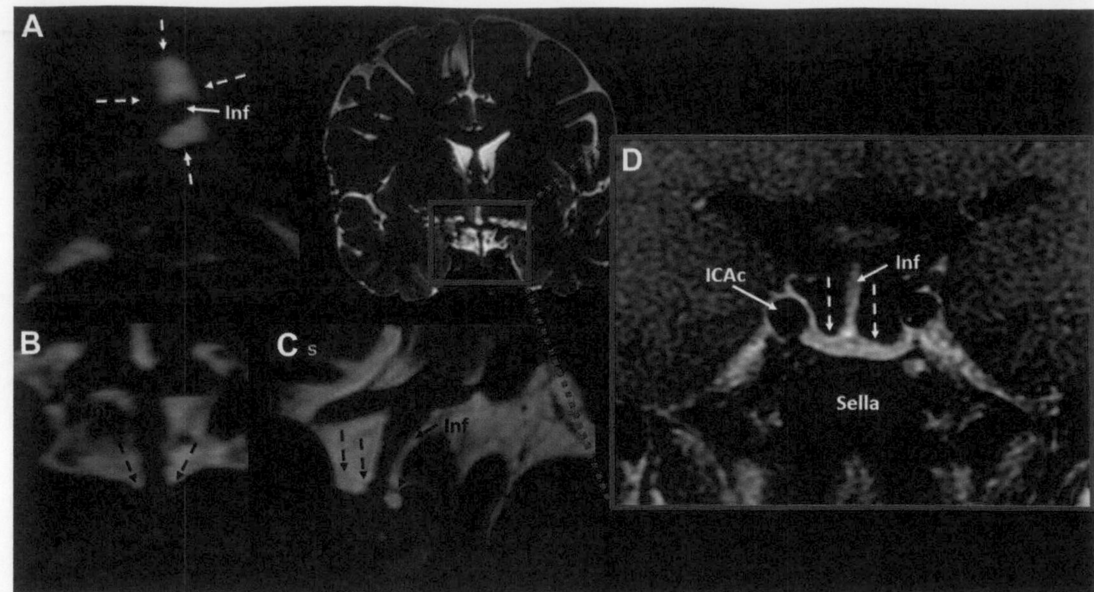

Fig. 22. Axial (*A*), coronal (*B*), and sagittal (*C*) T2-weighted ZOOM MR images of the diaphragma sella (*dashed arrows*). Axial image A demonstrates the opening of the diaphragma allowing for the passage of the infundibulum. Coronal postcontrast T1 MR image (*D*) through the sella turcica demonstrates normal enhancement of the diaphragma sella (*dashed arrows*). ICAc, cavernous segment of the internal carotid artery; Inf, pituitary infundibulum; Sella, sella turcica.

occipital crest anteriorly into the posterior cerebellar notch, partially separating the cerebellar hemispheres. It extends from the inferior margin of the posterior falx cerebri superiorly to the foramen magnum inferiorly. The falx cerebelli contains the occipital sinus and occasionally splits in 2 near the foramen magnum.

The *diaphragma sellae* is the smallest dural reflection. It extends from the tuberculum sellae anteriorly to the posterior clinoid processes posteriorly, covering the sella turcica (see **Fig. 22**). There is a small opening in the diaphragma sellae through which the pituitary infundibulum projects (see **Fig. 22**A).

Dural Venous Sinuses

The dural venous sinuses are formed by separation of the periosteal and meningeal layers of the dura mater, are lined by endothelium, and are valveless. They drain portions of the scalp (via emissary veins), calvarium, dura, and brain ultimately into the internal jugular veins. CSF also drains into the dural venous sinuses via the arachnoid granulations.

The *superior sagittal sinus* courses along the midline from the foramen cecum to the occipital protuberance (**Figs. 23** and **24**A,B). It is located within the falx cerebri along its convex superior margin and drains the cortical veins, meningeal veins, veins of the falx cerebri, emissary veins, and diploic veins. The superior sagittal sinus typically drains into the sinus confluence (torcular Herophili) or into one of the transverse sinuses.

The *inferior sagittal sinus* is located within the falx cerebri along its free edge (see **Figs. 23**A and **24A**). It begins at the crista galli and drains to the straight sinus. It drains the medial frontal lobes, corpus callosum, falx cerebri, and cingulate gyri.

The inferior sagittal sinus and the vein of Galen join to form the *straight sinus* (see **Figs. 23**A and **24A**). The straight sinus is a midline structure that is found at the junction of the falx cerebri and tentorium cerebelli that most commonly drains into the sinus confluence, less commonly the transverse sinuses. Occasionally, a *falcine sinu*s may be encountered, most commonly a communication between the superior and inferior sagittal sinuses within the posterior aspect of the falx cerebri (see **Fig. 23**H).[45] The falcine sinus may be persistent or recanalized and the straight sinus may or may not be present.

The *occipital sinus* extends from the marginal sinus (see **Fig. 23**G) of the foramen magnum to the sinus confluence along the internal occipital crest (see **Fig. 23**B). It is the smallest of the dural venous sinuses and is most commonly a single vessel located at the midline. The occipital sinus is much less commonly duplicated or absent and

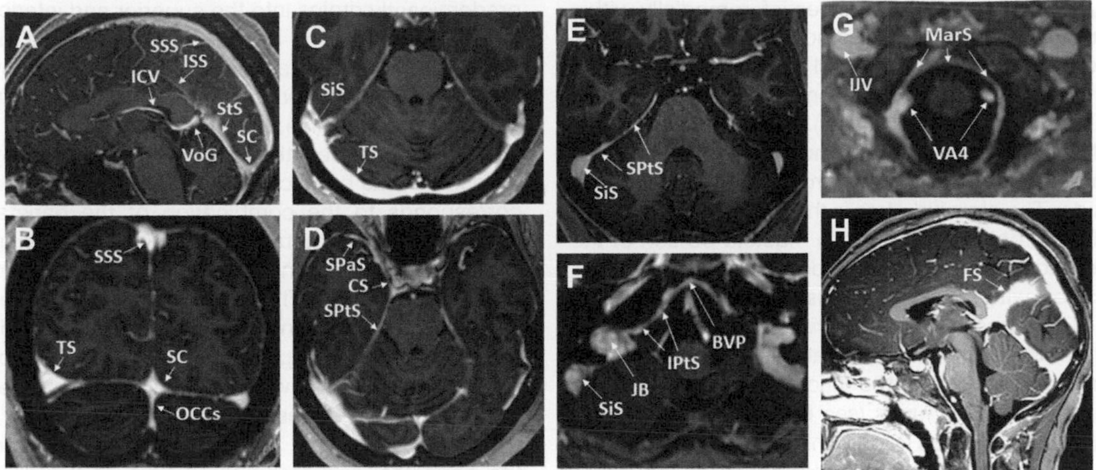

Fig. 23. Sagittal (*A, H*), coronal (*B*), and axial (*C, D, E, F,* G) post-contrast T1 images of the dural venous sinuses. BVP, basilar venous plexus; CS, cavernous sinus; FS, falcine sinus; ICV, internal cerebral vein; IJV, internal jugular vein; IPtS, inferior petrosal sinus; ISS, inferior sagittal sinus; JB, jugular bulb; MarS, marginal sinus; OCCs, occipital sinus; SC, sinus confluence; SiS, sigmoid sinus; SPaS, sphenoparietal sinus; SPtS, superior petrosal sinus; SSS, superior sagittal sinus; StS, straight sinus; TS, transverse sinus; VA4, V4 segment of the vertebral arteries; VoG, vein of Galen.

positioned just off the midline, varying in size with age. The variability in the morphology of the occipital sinus and inconsistent demonstration on imaging studies can create problems in posterior fossa surgical approaches.[46,47]

The *transverse (lateral) sinus* is a paired dural venous sinus that is contained within the folds of the tentorium cerebelli along the inner surface of the occipital bone, within a groove at the margin of the cruciform eminence (see **Figs. 23**B, C and **24**A, B). There is significant variability in the configuration of the transverse sinus. Most commonly, the left transverse sinus is hypoplastic or aplastic and the right transverse sinus is dominant. The transverse sinus may arise from the sinus confluence, straight sinus, or directly from the superior sagittal sinus and drain into the sigmoid sinus.[48] The transverse sinus transitions to the *sigmoid sinus* as it exits the tentorium cerebelli and receives venous drainage from the inferior anastomotic vein of Labbe and superior petrosal sinus.

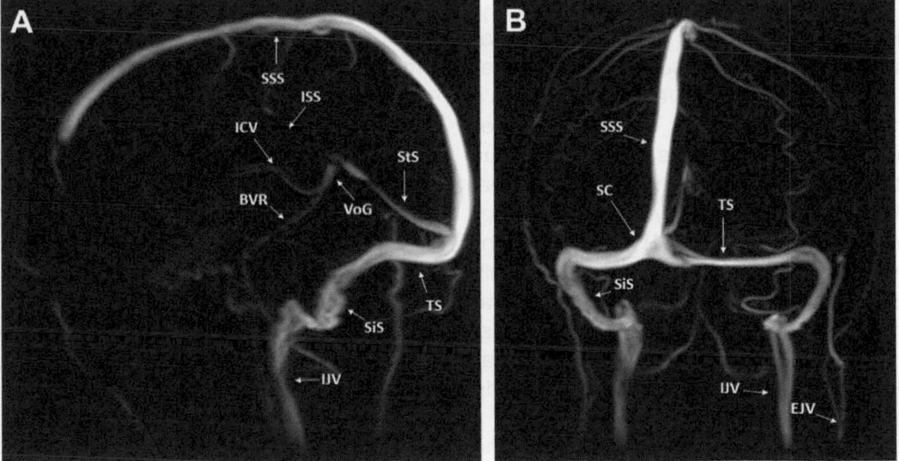

Fig. 24. Sagittal (*A*) and oblique coronal (*B*) maximum intensity projection time-of-flight magnetic resonance venography (MRV) images. BVR, basal vein of Rosenthal; EJV, external jugular vein; ICV, internal cerebral vein; IJV, internal jugular vein; ISS, inferior sagittal sinus; SC, sinus confluence; SiS, sigmoid sinus; StS, straight sinus; SSS, superior sagittal sinus; TS, transverse sinus; VoG, vein of Galen.

The *sigmoid sinus* courses inferomedially within an S-shaped groove (sigmoid sulcus) in the mastoid portion of the temporal bone, ultimately draining to the jugular bulb and internal jugular vein (see Figs. 23C, E, F and 24A, B). The relative depths of the sigmoid sulci give an indication of sinus dominance, with the deeper groove on the dominant side. The sigmoid plate is thin bone that separates the sigmoid sinus from the mastoid portion of the temporal bone that, when dehiscent, can be associated with pulsatile tinnitus of venous origin.

The *superior petrosal sinus* is a paired dural venous channel that originates in the cavernous sinus and drains to the junction of the transverse and sigmoid sinuses (see Fig. 23D, E). It travels along the petrous ridge within the superior petrosal sulcus within the attached margins of the tentorium cerebelli and receives venous drainage from the cerebellum, inferior cerebral vein, and labyrinthine vein. The superior petrosal sinus is closely associated with the trigeminal nerve, typically traveling along the superior margin of the porus trigeminus.

The *inferior petrosal sinus* is a paired dural venous channel that originates from the cavernous sinus along the posteroinferior margin and drains to the junction of the sigmoid sinus and the jugular bulb (see Fig. 23F). It travels in the inferior petrosal sulcus, a groove in the petrous temporal bone and basiocciput, and receives venous blood from the internal auditory canal, pons, medulla, and inferior cerebellar peduncle.

The *cavernous sinus* is unlike the other dural venous sinuses in that it communicates with the spinal epidural space, is extradural, and can contain fat (see Fig. 23D). It is a paired structure that is located on either side of the sella turcica along the lateral margins of the sphenoid body. The cavernous sinus extends from the superior orbital fissure anteriorly to the petrous apex posteriorly. The medial wall of the cavernous sinus has a single periosteal layer of dura. The lateral, superior, anterior, and posterior walls of the cavernous sinus contain 2 layers of dura, the inner periosteal layer and the outer meningeal layer. The oculomotor, trochlear, and ophthalmic (V1) nerves are contained within the layers of dura in the lateral wall. The maxillary (V2) nerve is located just inferior to the junction of the medial and lateral dural walls. The cavernous segment of the ICA, the sympathetic plexus, and the abducens nerve reside within the cavernous sinus.

The cavernous sinus receives drainage from the superior and inferior ophthalmic veins, central retinal vein, the pterygoid venous plexus, sphenoparietal sinus, superficial middle cerebral vein, and middle meningeal vein. The cavernous sinus predominantly drains into the superior and inferior petrosal sinuses. The left and right cavernous sinuses are connected anteriorly and posteriorly by the *intercavernous sinuses* that are located within the diaphragma sellae.[49]

What was termed the *sphenoparietal sinus* by Breschet[50] has been considered a misnomer and corresponds to the combination of the parietal portion of the frontal ramus of the middle meningeal vein and the sinus of the lesser sphenoid wing (see Fig. 23D). The sinus of the lesser sphenoid wing receives venous drainage from the middle meningeal vein, diploic veins of the orbital roof and greater sphenoid wing and the ophthalmomeningeal vein and drains to the cavernous sinus.[51]

The *basilar venous plexus* is located between the periosteal and meningeal layers of the dura along the posterior surface of the clivus (see Fig. 23F). It extends from the cavernous sinus superiorly to the foramen magnum inferiorly. It has extensive and variable communications with the cavernous sinuses, intercavernous sinuses, superior petrosal sinuses, inferior petrosal sinuses, marginal sinus, and internal vertebral venous plexus.[52]

Arachnoid Mater

The arachnoid mater is the delicate and avascular middle layer of the meninges that lies in direct contact with the dura (easily separated along a potential space, the *subdural space*). Between the arachnoid mater and pia mater is the CSF-filled *subarachnoid space*, traversed by porous membranes, trabeculae, and septa. These septations play an important role in CSF flow dynamics and provide support for transiting neurovascular structures. The arachnoid has widely variable structure, and detailed anatomic aspects of the arachnoid membranes have been debated in the neurosurgical literature for over a century. Although not frequently discussed in the radiology literature, the development of high-resolution MR imaging techniques now allows some arachnoid membranes to be visualized on routine imaging; some of the more frequently encountered membranes are discussed below.

The medial carotid membranes (Fig. 25A) separate the suprasellar and carotid cisterns. They extend from the lower part of the optic chiasm and attach to the lateral margin of the sella.[42]

The Liliequist membrane is a thin arachnoid membrane that separates the suprasellar, interpeduncular, and prepontine cisterns. It arises from the basal arachnoid membrane at the dorsum sellae and extends posteriorly while separating into 2 sheets. The diencephalic membrane

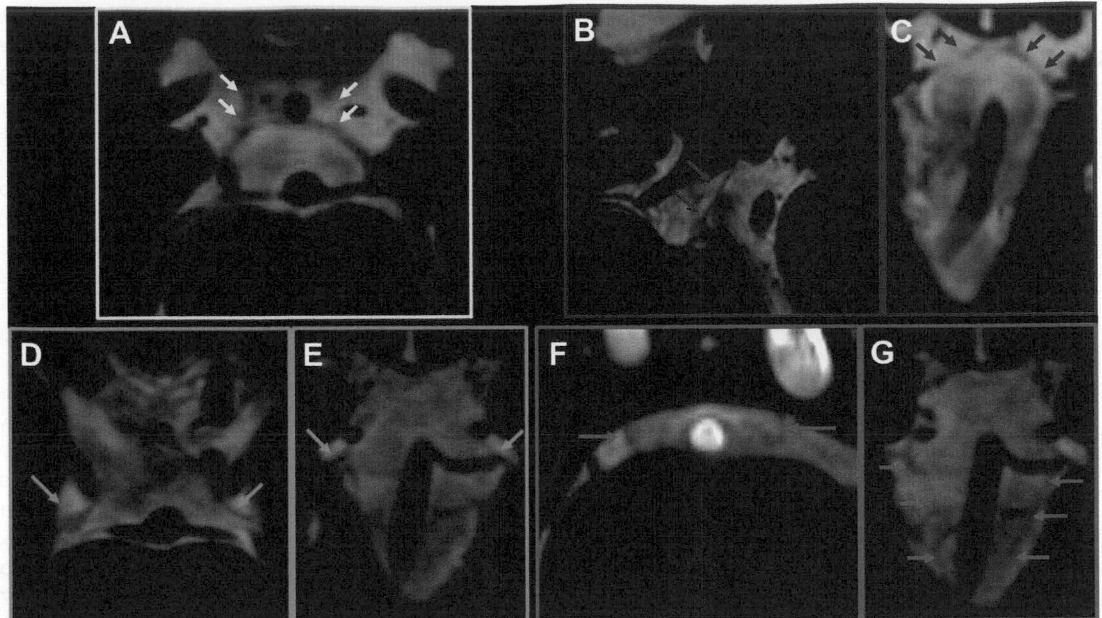

Fig. 25. T2-weighted axial (*A, D, F*), sagittal (*B*), and coronal (*C, E, G*) MR images. The medial carotid membranes (*arrows A*) separate the suprasellar and carotid cisterns. The diencephalic leaf of the Liliequist membrane (*arrows B, C*) extends from the diaphragma sella to the mammillary bodies and separates the suprasellar and interpeduncular cisterns. The lateral pontomesencephalic membranes (*arrows D, E*) separate the ambient and cerebellopontine cisterns. The anterior pontine membranes (*arrows F, G*) separate the prepontine and cerebellopontine cisterns.

(Fig. 25B, C) extends posterosuperiorly to the floor of the third ventricle at the mammillary bodies and separates the suprasellar and interpeduncular cisterns. The mesencephalic membrane extends posteroinferiorly to the pontomesencephalic junction and separates the interpeduncular and prepontine cisterns. The membranes extend laterally to the oculomotor nerve. The diencephalic membrane is thicker and more readily seen on MR imaging while the mesencephalic leaf is typically thinner or incomplete and infrequently visualized on MRI.[42,53,54]

The lateral pontomesencephalic membranes (Fig. 25D, E) separate the ambient and cerebellopontine cisterns and are lateral extensions of the mesencephalic leaf of the Liliequist membrane extending from the oculomotor nerve.[55]

The medial pontomedullary membrane is transversely oriented at the pontomedullary sulcus and separates the premedullary and prepontine cisterns. The lateral pontomedullary membrane separates the cerebellopontine and cerebellomedullary cisterns. They are not typically seen on imaging.[53]

The anterior pontine membranes (Fig. 25F, G) are oriented in a roughly craniocaudal direction lateral to the basilar artery and medial to the abducens nerve. They separate the prepontine and cerebellopontine angle cisterns.[53]

SUMMARY

The ventricular system, subarachnoid spaces, and meninges lend structure, support, and protection to the brain and spinal cord parenchyma. This article provides a detailed look at the imaging anatomy of the intracranial portions of these structures.

CLINICS CARE POINTS

- The anatomy of the ventricular system is complex and variable. A broad understanding of normal and variant anatomy is important for diagnostic accuracy.
- The intracranial subarachnoid space contains numerous important subdivisions and structures with broad clinical implications.

DISCLOSURE

The authors have nothing to disclose.

REFERENCES

1. Coleman LT, Zimmerman RA, Rorke LB. Ventriculus terminalis of the conus medullaris: MR findings in children. AJNR Am J Neuroradiol 1995;16(7): 1421–6.
2. Unsinn KM, Geley T, Freund MC, et al. US of the spinal cord in newborns: spectrum of normal findings, variants, congenital anomalies, and acquired diseases. Radiographics 2000;20(4):923–38.
3. Scelsi C, Rahim T, Morris J, et al. The lateral ventricles: a detailed review of anatomy, development, and anatomic variations. AJNR Am J Neuroradiol 2020;41(4):566–72.
4. Lamers MJ, Klein WM, Goraj B. Normal values of ventricular volume and cerebrospinal fluid (CSF) circulation in healthy subjects. Scientific exhibit presented Eur Soc Radiol 2010. https://doi.org/10.1594/ecr2010/C-2729.
5. Borden N, Forseen S, Stefan C. Imaging anatomy of the human brain: a comprehensive atlas including adjacent structures. New York, NY: Springer Publishing Company; 2015.
6. Shaw CM, Alvord EC Jr. Cava septi pellucidi et vergae: their normal and pathogical states. Brain 1969; 92(1):213–23.
7. Farruggia S, Babcock DS. The cavum septi pellucidi: its appearance and incidence with cranial ultrasonography in infancy. Radiology 1981;139(1): 147–50.
8. Epstein JA. Coarctation of the walls of the lateral angles of the lateral cerebral ventricles; a comparative anatomical study. J Neuropathol Exp Neurol 1953; 12(3):302–9.
9. Bates JI, Netsky MG. Developmental anomalies of the horns of the lateral ventricles. J Neuropathol Exp Neurol 1955;14(3):316–25.
10. Cooper S, Bar-Yosef O, Berkenstadt M, et al. Prenatal Evaluation, Imaging Features, and Neurodevelopmental Outcome of Prenatally Diagnosed Periventricular Pseudocysts. AJNR Am J Neuroradiol 2016;37(12):2382–8.
11. Hori A, Bardosi A, Tsuboi K, et al. Accessory cerebral ventricle of the occipital lobe. Morphogenesis and clinical and pathological appearance. J Neurosurg 1984;61(4):767–71.
12. Vandewalle G, Beuls E, Vanormelingen L, et al. Accessory intraventricular prominence of the occipital horn of the lateral ventricle. J Neurosurg 2003; 99(1):151–5.
13. Shapiro R, Galloway SJ, Shapiro MD. Minimal asymmetry of the brain: a normal variant. AJR Am J Roentgenol 1986;147(4):753–6.
14. Sze G, De Armond SJ, Brant-Zawadzki M, et al. Foci of MRI signal (pseudo lesions) anterior to the frontal horns: histologic correlations of a normal finding. AJR Am J Roentgenol 1986;147(2):331–7.
15. Jean WC, Tai AX, Hogan E, et al. An anatomical study of the foramen of Monro: implications in management of pineal tumors presenting with hydrocephalus. Acta Neurochir (Wien) 2019;161(5): 975–83.
16. Tubbs RS, Shoja MM, Aggarwal A, et al. Choroid plexus of the fourth ventricle: Review and anatomic study highlighting anatomical variations. J Clin Neurosci 2016;26:79–83.
17. Yamamoto I, Rhoton AL Jr, Peace DA. Microsurgery of the third ventricle: Part I. Microsurgical anatomy. Neurosurgery 1981;8(3):334–56.
18. Matys T, Brown FS, Zaccagna F, et al. A critical appraisal of Monro's erroneous description of the cerebral interventricular foramina: Age-related magnetic resonance imaging spatial morphometry and a proposed new terminology. Clin Anat 2020;33(3):446–57.
19. Patel T, Gould G, Baehring J, Piepmeier, J. Chapter 27 - Surgical Approaches to Lateral and Third Ventricular Tumors. In: Quiñones-Hinojosa A. Schmidek & Sweet operative neurosurgical techniques: indications, methods, and results. 2012.
20. Chaichana K, Quiñones-Hinojosa A. Comprehensive overview of modern surgical approaches to intrinsic brain tumors. San Diego, CA: Elsevier; 2019.
21. Kier. The evolutionary and embryologic basis for the development and anatomy of the cavum veli interpositi. AJNR Am J Neuroradiol 1999;20(7):1383–4.
22. Flyger G, Hjelmquist U. Normal variations in the caliber of the human cerebral aqueduct. Anat Rec 1957;127(2):151–62.
23. Longatti P, Fiorindi A, Perin A, et al. Endoscopic anatomy of the cerebral aqueduct. Neurosurgery 2007;61(3 Suppl):1–6.
24. Matys T, Horsburgh A, Kirollos RW, et al. The aqueduct of Sylvius: applied 3-T magnetic resonance imaging anatomy and morphometry with neuroendoscopic relevance. Neurosurgery 2013; 73(2 Suppl Operative):ons132–40.
25. Salma A, Yeremeyeva E, Baidya NB, et al. An endoscopic, cadaveric analysis of the roof of the fourth ventricle. J Clin Neurosci 2013;20(5):710–4.
26. Mortazavi M, Adeeb N, Griessenauer C, et al. The ventricular system of the brain: a comprehensive review of its history, anatomy, histology, embryology, and surgical considerations. Childs Nerv Syst 2014;30(1):19–35.
27. Mercier P, Bernard F, Delion M. Microsurgical anatomy of the fourth ventricle. Neurochirurgie 2021; 67(1):14–22.
28. Matsushima T, Rhoton A, Lenkey C. Microsurgery of the fourth ventricle: Part 1 Microsurgical anatomy. Neurosurgery 1982;11(5):631–67.

29. Mussi A, Rhotgon R. Telovelar approach to the fourth ventricle: microsurgical anatomy. J Neurosurg 2000; 92(5):812–23.
30. Rhoton A. Rhoton's cranial anatomy and surgical approaches. Oxford, UK: Oxford University Press; 2019.
31. Sakka L, Coll G, Chazal J. Anatomy and physiology of cerebrospinal fluid. Eur Ann Otorhinolaryngol Head Neck Dis 2011;128(6):309–16.
32. Edsbagge M, Tisell M, Jacobsson L, et al. Spinal CSF absorption in healthy individuals. Am J Physiol Regul Integr Comp Physiol 2004;287(6):R1450–5.
33. Hall JE. Guyton and Hall textbook of medical physiology. Philadelphia (PA): Elsevier; 2016.
34. Horsburgh A, Kirollos RW, Massoud TF. Bochdalek's flower basket: applied neuroimaging morphometry and variants of choroid plexus in the cerebellopontine angles. Neuroradiology 2012;54(12):1341–6.
35. Noback C, Strominger N, Demarest R, et al. The human nervous system: structure and function. 6th edition 2005. https://doi.org/10.1007/978-1-59259-730-7.
36. Horsburgh A, Massoud TF. The circumventricular organs of the brain: conspicuity on clinical 3T MRI and a review of functional anatomy. Surg Radiol Anat 2013;35(4):343–9.
37. Kida S, Pantazis A, Weller RO. CSF drains directly from the subarachnoid space into nasal lymphatics in the rat. Anatomy, histology and immunological significance. Neuropathol Appl Neurobiol 1993; 19(6):480–8.
38. Zakharov A, Papaiconomou C, Djenic J, et al. Lymphatic cerebrospinal fluid absorption pathways in neonatal sheep revealed by subarachnoid injection of Microfil. Neuropathol Appl Neurobiol 2003; 29(6):563–73.
39. Rhoton AL Jr. The posterior fossa cisterns. Neurosurgery 2000;47(3 Suppl):S287–97.
40. Altafulla J, Bordes S, Jenkins S, et al. The basal subarachnoid cisterns: surgical and anatomical considerations. World Neurosurg 2019;129:190–9.
41. Di Ieva A, Tschabitscher M, Matula C, et al. The subdiaphragmatic cistern: historic and radioanatomic findings. Acta Neurochir (Wien) 2012;154(4): 667–74.
42. Inoue K, Seker A, Osawa S, et al. Microsurgical and endoscopic anatomy of the supratentorial arachnoidal membranes and cisterns. Neurosurgery 2009;65(4):644–65.
43. Everton K, Rassner U, Osborn A, et al. The oculomotor cistern: anatomy and high-resolution imaging. AJNR Am J Neuroradiol 2008;29(7):1344–8.
44. Patel N, Kirmi O. Anatomy and imaging of the normal meninges. Semin Ultrasound CT MR 2009; 30(6):559–64.
45. Ryu C. Persistent falcine sinus: Is it really rare? Am J Neuroradiol 2010;31:367–9.
46. Gaumont-Darcissac M, Viart L, Foulon VP, et al. The occipital sinus: a radioanatomic study. Morphologie 2015;99(324):18–22.
47. Balak N. Inconsistencies between radiologic and cadaveric studies of the occipital sinus. Am J Neuroradiol 2021;42:E27.
48. Alper F, Kantarci M, Dane S, et al. Importance of anatomical asymmetries of transverse sinuses: an MR venographic study. Cerebrovasc Dis 2004; 18(3):236–9.
49. Mahalingam H, Mani S, Patel B, et al. Imaging spectrum of cavernous sinus lesions with histopathologic correlation. Radiographics 2019;39:795–819.
50. Breschet G. Research of the anatomy, physiology, and pathology of the venous system with special emphasis on the veins of bones [in French]. Paris (France): Villeret et Rouen; 1829.
51. Ruiz D, Fasel J, Rufenacht D, et al. The sphenoparietal sinus of Breschet: does it exist? An anatomic study. Am J Neuroradiol 2004;25:112–20.
52. Tubbs R, Hansasuta A, Loukas M, et al. The basilar venous plexus. Clin Anat 2007;20(7):755–9.
53. Lu S, Brusic A, Gaillard F. Arachnoid Membranes: Crawling Back into Radiologic Consciousness [published online ahead of print, 2021 Oct 28]. AJNR Am J Neuroradiol 2021. https://doi.org/10.3174/ajnr.A7309.
54. Dias DA, Castro FL, Yared JH, et al. Liliequist membrane: radiological evaluation, clinical and therapeutic implications. Radiol Bras 2014;47(3):182–5.
55. Anik I, Ceylan S, Koc K, et al. Microsurgical and endoscopic anatomy of Liliequist's membrane and the prepontine membranes: cadaveric study and clinical implications. Acta Neurochir (Wien) 2011; 153(8):1701–11.

Anatomy of the Intracranial Arteries

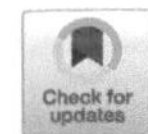

The Internal Carotid Artery

Dylan N. Wolman, MD[a], Adrienne M. Moraff, MD[b], Jeremy J. Heit, MD, PhD[a,*]

KEYWORDS

• Artery • Intracranial • Cerebral • Internal carotid artery • Ophthalmic artery
• Posterior communicating artery • Anterior choroidal artery • Superior hypophyseal artery

KEY POINTS

- The internal carotid artery is defined segmentally by anatomic landmarks and branch vasculature into the cervical, petrous, cavernous, ophthalmic, superior hypophyseal, posterior communicating, anterior choroidal, and terminal segments.
- The ophthalmic through terminal segments are together grouped under the supraclinoid segment of the internal carotid artery and are named for each eponymous segmental vessel origin.
- The caroticotympanic and mandibulovidian arteries arise from the petrous segment, and the meningohypophyseal and inferolateral trunks arise from the cavernous segment and form a rich anastomotic network through remnant fetal connections to the dura and the external carotid circulation.

INTRODUCTION

The cerebral arteries provide blood flow to the brain through perhaps the most elegant vascular anatomy bed in the body. The arterial supply to the brain is separated into the anterior circulation, which is composed of arteries that arise from the bilateral internal carotid arteries, and the posterior circulation, which is composed of arteries that arise from the paired vertebral arteries. A detailed understanding of normal and variant cerebral arterial anatomy is important to understanding common cerebrovascular diseases, such as ischemic stroke, steno-occlusive disease, cerebral aneurysms, cerebral arteriovenous malformations, and pial and dural arteriovenous fistulae.

In this article, we will discuss the internal carotid artery and its complex branch vasculature, anastomotic pathways, and touch on portions of its embryologic development as they relate to persistent fetal anastomoses and arterial variants. Cerebrovascular diseases are discussed as examples in this article, with a particular focus on characteristic aneurysms of the internal carotid artery but all are considered in the context of the underlying anatomy. A discussion of the remainder of the anterior circulation and of the posterior circulation follows in the subsequent article.

INTERNAL CAROTID ARTERY

The internal carotid arteries provide the dominant arterial supply to the right and left cerebral hemispheres, and they are generally the largest intracranial arteries. Each internal carotid artery arises from the bifurcation of the common carotid artery

[a] Department of Radiology, Department of NeuroImaging and NeuroIntervention, Stanford School of Medicine, Center for Academic Medicine, 453 Quarry Road, Palo Alto, CA 94304, USA; [b] Division of Neurosurgery, Howard University School of Medicine, 2041 Georgia Avenue Northwest, Suite 4000, Washington, DC 20060, USA
* Corresponding author. Stanford School of Medicine, 453 Quarry Road, Palo Alto, CA 94304.
E-mail address: jheit@stanford.edu
Twitter: @JeremyHeitMDPHD (J.J.H.)

Neuroimag Clin N Am 32 (2022) 603–615
https://doi.org/10.1016/j.nic.2022.04.006
1052-5149/22/

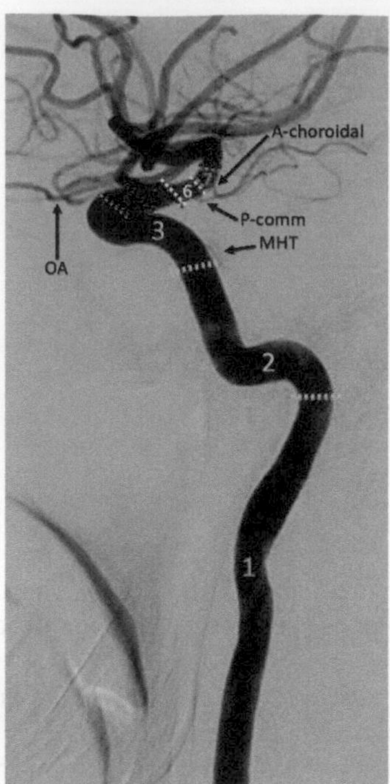

Fig. 1. Lateral angiographic view of a normal internal carotid artery. Each segment of the internal carotid artery is color labeled as follows: (1) Cervical segment in light blue; (2) petrous segment in light green; (3) cavernous segment in orange; (4) ophthalmic segment in light red; (5) superior hypophyseal segment in purple; (6) posterior communicating segment in yellow; (7) anterior choroidal segment in dark green; and (8) the carotid terminus in crimson. The anterior choroidal artery (A-choroidal), posterior communicating artery (P-comm), ophthalmic artery (OA), and meningohypophyseal trunk (MHT) are labeled in black and marked by arrows.

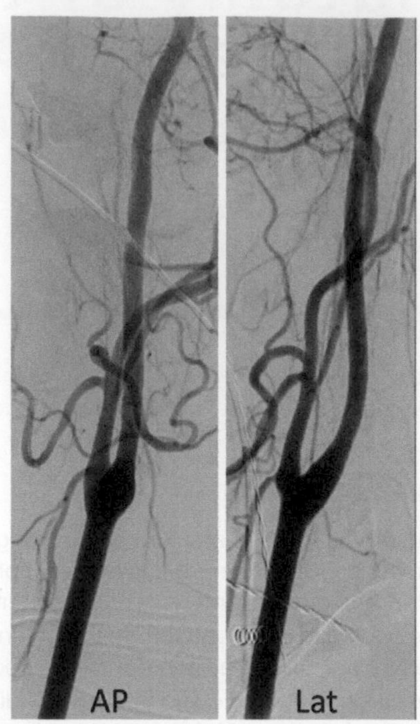

Fig. 2. Normal anteroposterior (AP) and lateral (Lat) angiographic views of the carotid bifurcation demonstrating a normal course and caliber of the distal common carotid artery, the proximal external carotid artery trunk, and the carotid bulb and cervical segment of the internal carotid artery with a normal posterolateral origin of the internal carotid artery. Note slight dilation of the normal carotid bulb.

into the external and internal carotid arteries. This bifurcation is located in the cervical soft tissues, most commonly at the C3–C5 vertebral body levels, although it has been reported as high as the C1 or as low as the T2 vertebral level.[1] There are multiple proposed systems of subdivision to classify the segments of the internal carotid artery based on the embryologic origins of each segment as they arise from segmental regression and anastomoses of the third fetal aortic arches and extensions of the dorsal aortae,[2] or based on anatomically distinct subdivisions of the internal carotid artery from cadaveric dissections.[3,4] However, although anatomically accurate, the segments defined by these systems can be difficult to apply to cross-sectional or angiographic images, which are used frequently in modern medical practice. Therefore, a descriptive and practical naming scheme is used here to account for angiographically visible anatomic landmarks, definable branch vessels, and typical sites of pathologic condition.[5] The internal carotid artery may be considered as having 8 separate segments[1]: the cervical segment, which includes the carotid bulb[2]; the petrous segment, which includes the origins of the caroticotympanic and mandibulovidian arteries[3]; the cavernous segment, which includes the origins of the inferolateral trunk and the meningohypophyseal trunk[4]; the ophthalmic segment at the origin of the ophthalmic artery[5]; the superior hypophyseal segment from which the superior hypophyseal arteries arise[6]; the posterior communicating segment from which the posterior communicating artery arises[7]; the anterior choroidal segment from which the anterior choroidal artery arises; and[8] the carotid terminus (Fig. 1). In the following paragraphs, we briefly discuss each segment and the relevant arteries that arise from each segment.

The origin of the cervical segment of the internal carotid artery is termed the carotid bulb and is often broad and bell-shaped before smoothly tapering into the true cervical segment, which typically has no branches. Rare variant branches from the cervical segment may be encountered, which

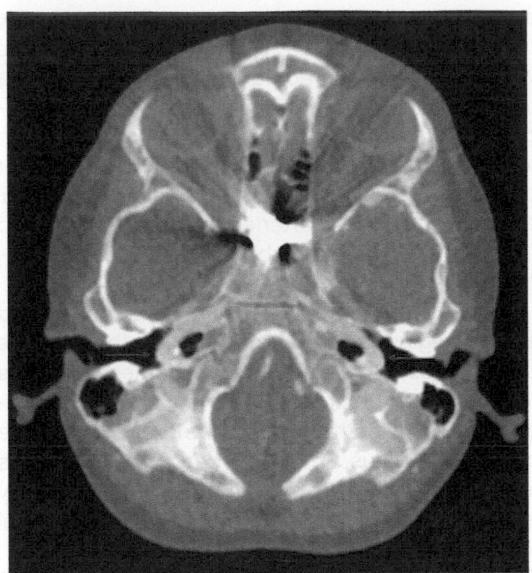

Fig. 3. Axial computed tomography image through the skull base demonstrating incidental bilateral aberrant internal carotid arteries extending within the middle ear (*red arrows*), formed by reconstitution of the caroticotympanic artery as a continuation of the internal carotid artery in the setting of aplasia of the petrous segment. Hyperattenuating material within the anterior clivus is an unrelated shrapnel fragment from a prior injury.

includes the origins of the ascending pharyngeal, occipital, or superior thyroidal arteries, or persistent carotico-basilar anastomotic arteries, such as the persistent hypoglossal or proatlantal segmental arteries.[1,2] The cervical internal carotid usually arises posterolateral relative to the origin of the external carotid artery at the common carotid bifurcation but approximately 15% of patients demonstrate a reverse orientation.[1,6]

Approximately 70% of the inflow from the common carotid artery is drawn into the internal carotid artery, and there are complex flow dynamics within the bulb owing to the sharp divergence from the common carotid. Slipstreams of laminar blood flow at the acute angle of the carotid artery bifurcation and recirculatory eddies within the posterior bulb may result in temporary stagnation of flow within the posterior carotid bulb predisposing this segment to significant atherosclerotic plaque formation, thrombus formation in the setting of carotid webs, or significant tortuosity owing to predominantly helical rather than laminar downstream flow dynamics in chronic hypertension or with age, including a predisposition to the development of cervical loops (Fig. 2).[1,6] The cervical segment terminates at the skull base where the artery enters the bony petrous canal and courses anteromedially.

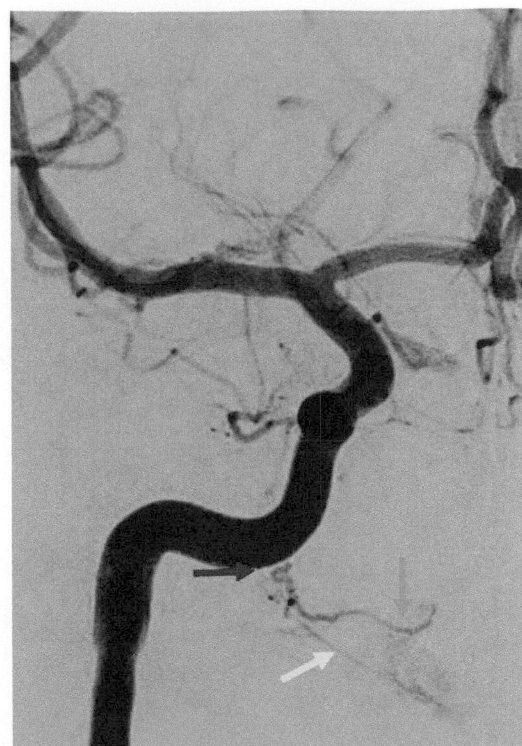

Fig. 4. Single AP magnified angiographic projection of the right internal carotid artery demonstrating a prominent mandibulovidian artery (*red arrow*) arising from the petrous segment. There is a prominent artery of the pterygoid canal/Vidian artery (*blue arrow*) extending superiorly and a pterygovaginal artery extending inferiorly (*yellow arrow*) with supply to the fossa of Rosenmüller and the Eustachian tube.

The petrous segment of the internal carotid artery courses through the carotid canal within the petrous bone and is anatomically defined by 3 separate segments: a vertical segment that ascends into the bone from the carotid sheath within the neck, an anteromedial genu as the artery is deflected along the course of the canal, and a longer horizontal segment toward the petrous apex. There are 2 normal branches that arise from the petrous segment: the caroticotympanic artery and the mandibulovidian artery.

The caroticotympanic artery is often small and angiographically obscured by the skull base but it may be enlarged in vascular tumors of the skull base or middle ear that derive blood supply from this vessel. A remnant of the embryologic hyoid artery, the caroticotympanic artery arises from the posterior vertical petrous segment and courses posterolaterally to the middle ear where it passes through the stapes and anastomoses with the inferior tympanic branch of the ascending pharyngeal artery. This normal anastomosis forms the basis of

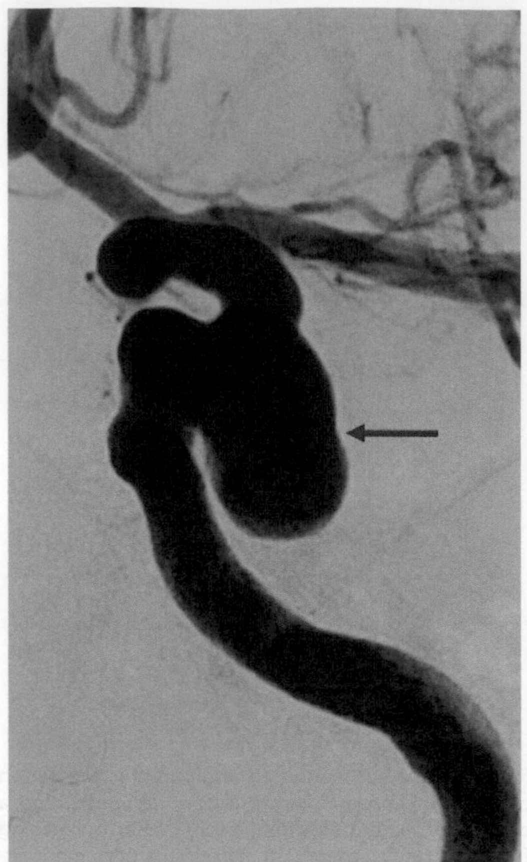

Fig. 5. Single magnified oblique projection of the left internal carotid artery demonstrating a laterally and inferiorly directed aneurysm (*red arrow*) of the cavernous segment of the internal carotid artery. The anterior and posterior genua of the cavernous segment are seen as double densities in plane and medial to the aneurysm dome.

the course of the aberrant internal carotid artery, an uncommon variant in which there is regression or agenesis of the petrous segment of the internal carotid artery, which subsequently reconstitutes through hypertrophy of the caroticotympanic branch resulting in a sharply angulated and retrotympanic course of the petrous internal carotid artery through the middle ear. This aberrant internal carotid artery often demonstrates a focal stenosis as the vessel courses through the bony ostium of the inferior tympanic canaliculus (Fig. 3).[7]

The mandibulovidian artery is a variable branch that arises from the anterior horizontal petrous segment and courses anteromedially toward the pterygopalatine fossa. This artery is often hypertrophied in vascular nasopharyngeal tumors, such as juvenile nasopharyngeal angiofibromas.[8] There are 2 common subdivisions of the mandibulovidian artery. First, the Vidian artery (or artery of the pterygoid canal), which courses superiorly through the pterygoid canal and anastomoses with a posteriorly directed branch of the distal internal maxillary artery (Fig. 4). Second, the pterygovaginal artery, which courses inferiorly through foramen lacerum to anastomose with the superior pharyngeal branch of the ascending pharyngeal artery. Both of these arteries provide arterial blood flow to the Eustachian tube and the fossa of Rosenmüller (see Fig. 4).

The cavernous segment of the internal carotid artery begins as the artery exits the petrous bone, crosses the petrolingual ligament, which is the periosteal reflection of the sphenoid bone lingula and the petrous apex, before entering the cavernous sinus. The cavernous segment is located lateral to the sella turcica and formed by apposition of the dural leaflets of the middle cranial fossa and the endosteum of the sphenoid bone.[9] The cavernous segment is often divided into 3 subsegments[1]: a posterior vertical segment,[2] a horizontal segment, and[3] an anterior vertical segment, which are separated by the characteristic posterior and anterior genua, respectively. Within the cavernous sinus, cranial nerves III, IV, and the first and second divisions of cranial nerve V are located lateral to the cavernous sinus, whereas cranial nerve VI is located medial to the cavernous sinus. Laterally directed aneurysms of the cavernous internal carotid artery classically result in a third cranial nerve palsy owing to mass effect or a water hammer effect on the immediately adjacent nerve (Fig. 5).

The relationship of the dura to the distal cavernous segment is critical to understanding the risk of subarachnoid hemorrhage posed by aneurysms that arise from this segment. The dural leaflets of the cavernous sinus and of the tentorium form 2 dural rings that envelop the cavernous carotid artery: a proximal and a distal dural rings that attach to the anterior clinoid process. The distal dural ring, which is typically located at the level of the clinoid process, demarcates the transition between the extradural segment of the cavernous carotid artery. Aneurysms that arise distal to the dural ring incur a risk of subarachnoid hemorrhage, whereas aneurysms below this point present a risk of direct carotid-cavernous fistula but not subarachnoid hemorrhage in most cases. There is a potential space between the distal cavernous carotid artery and the distal dural ring, which is termed the carotid cave. The carotid cave is located immediately inferior to the distal ring, and an aneurysm in this location may extend superiorly into the intradural compartment, and the indentation of the dural ring may be visible on the aneurysm wall at angiography (Fig. 6).[10]

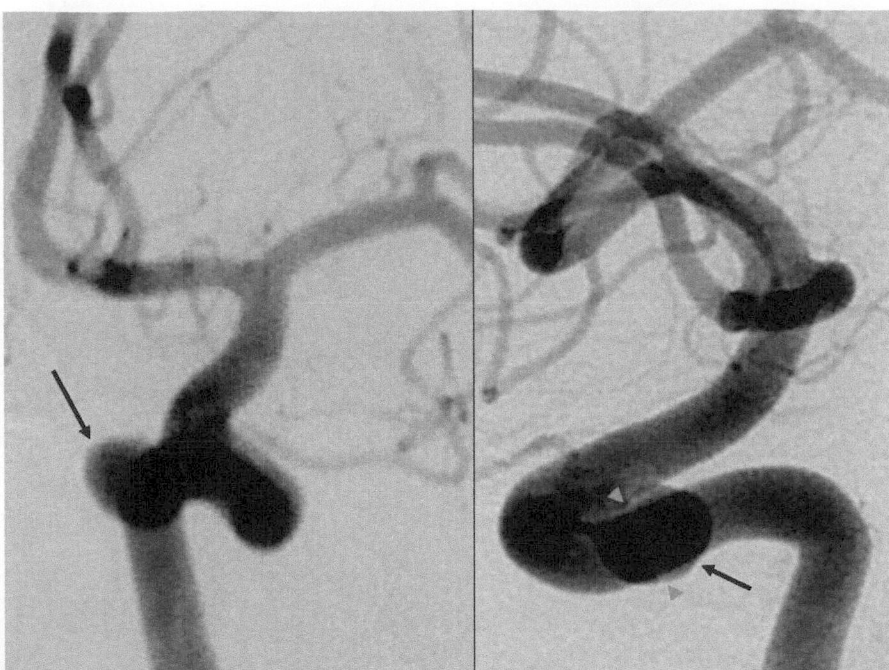

Fig. 6. Anteroposterior and lateral magnified views of the right internal carotid artery demonstrating a laterally and superiorly oriented aneurysm (*red arrows*) arising from the distal cavernous segment of the internal carotid artery adjacent to the anterior genu at the expected location of the clinoid process. There is a linear indentation (*blue arrowheads*) on the aneurysm dome seen on the lateral projection due to impingement by the distal dural ring, therefore confirming location of the aneurysm within the carotid cave.

There are 2 major visible branches that arise from the cavernous segment of the carotid artery: the meningohypophyseal trunk and the inferolateral trunk. There is an inconsistent third group of arteries that may be seldom observed on angiography, which represent the capsular arteries of McConnell.[6] These small arteries supply the adenohypophysis and extend medially from the horizontal cavernous segment before penetrating the diaphragma sellae and becoming intradural. Therefore, aneurysms that arise in this arterial group may pose a risk of subarachnoid hemorrhage.

The meningohypophyseal trunk originates from the posteromedial surface of the posterior genu of the cavernous segment and gives rise to the inferior hypophyseal artery that supplies the neurohypophysis. In addition, there are multiple dural branches that arise from the meningohypophyseal trunk, such as the basal tentorial artery, the dorsal and medial clival branches, and the marginal tentorial artery, which may be referred to as the artery of Bernasconi and Cassinari.[6,11] The marginal tentorial artery describes a posterior course and follows the medial tentorial incisura toward the midline posteriorly, and this vessel is often hypertrophied in dural arteriovenous fistulae or hypervascular tentorial tumors (Fig. 7).

The inferolateral trunk originates from the anterolateral surface of the horizontal segment just proximal to the anterior genu and courses inferolaterally along the inferior aspect of the cavernous sinus, where it courses deep to the sixth cranial nerve and provides vasa nervorum supply to the third, fourth, and sixth nerves, and to the Gasserian ganglion of the fifth cranial nerve and the dura of the cavernous sinus. There are 3 significant anastomotic branches that arise from the inferolateral trunk[1]: the deep recurrent meningeal artery, which is a vestige of the primitive dorsal ophthalmic artery. This artery passes through the superior orbital fissure and provides a potential anastomotic pathway to the ophthalmic artery and vasa nervorum supply to the first division of the fifth cranial nerve[2]; the tentorial branch, which provides dural supply and may anastomose with the middle meningeal artery at foramen spinosum and the accessory meningeal artery; and[3] the artery of the foramen rotundum, which is a commonly seen persistent anastomosis between the distal internal maxillary artery and the internal carotid artery; this vessel is often seen in cases of proximal arterial steno-occlusive disease as a pathway of collateral reconstitution of the distal internal carotid (Fig. 8).

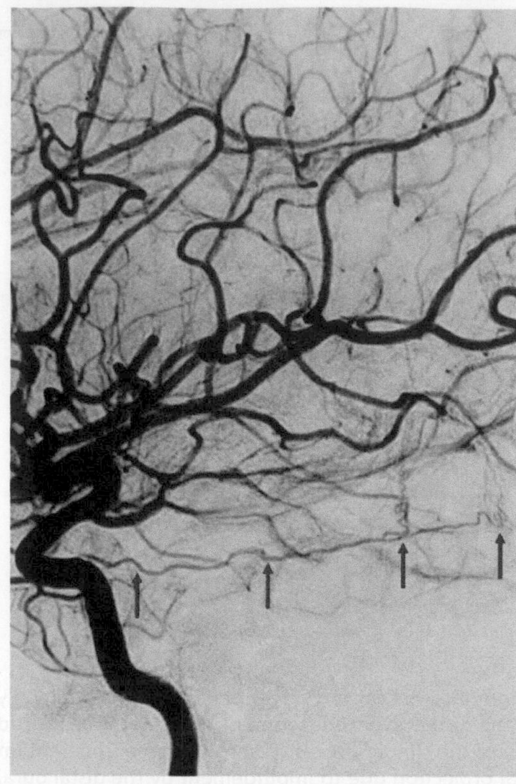

Fig. 7. Lateral magnified view of the internal carotid artery demonstrating a hypertrophied and tortuous marginal tentorial artery of Bernasconi and Cassinari (*red arrows*) arising from the MHT, which had previously provided arterial supply to a now treated dural arteriovenous fistula.

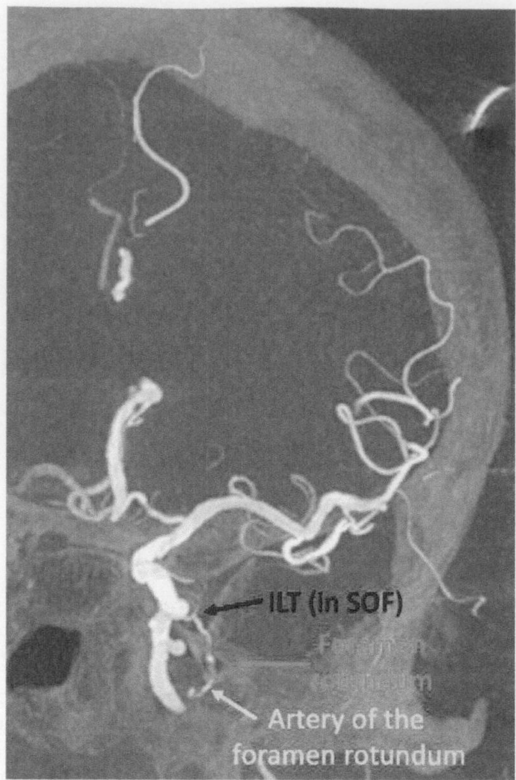

Fig. 8. Coronal maximum intensity projection of an unsubtracted 3 dimensional rotational angiogram of the left internal carotid artery demonstrating a hypertrophied inferolateral trunk (ILT) with a branch extending through the superior orbital fissure with supply to the artery of the foramen rotundum (*yellow arrow*, with the bony foramen marked by a *blue arrow*). Note the incidental caroticotympanic artery pseudoaneurysm medial to the foramen rotundum on this projection, which was the result of a surgical injury following resection of a hypervascular skull base tumor.

The persistent trigeminal artery is an additional uncommon variant that arises from the cavernous segment of the internal carotid artery, seen in only 0.2% of patients. The persistent trigeminal artery is a remnant fetal carotico-basilar anastomosis derived from incomplete or absent regression of the fetal trigeminal artery. The persistent trigeminal artery may be classified into 4 general subtypes defined by the degree of supply to the posterior circulation[1]: type 1: supplies the distal basilar artery and anastomoses to the basilar artery between the superior cerebellar and anterior inferior cerebellar arteries[2]; type 2: supplies the ipsilateral superior cerebellar artery territory and anastomoses distal to the superior cerebellar artery (seen with an ipsilateral fetal posterior cerebral artery)[3]; type 3: similar to type 2, except with additional supply to the contralateral posterior cerebral artery; and[4] a persistent trigeminal artery variant, a rare subtype in which the trigeminal artery does not join the basilar trunk and instead directly supplies one or multiple cerebellar arteries (such as the superior cerebellar, anterior inferior, or posterior inferior cerebellar arteries; **Fig. 9**).[1,2]

The supraclinoid segment of the internal carotid artery begins just above the distal dural ring, and it courses anteroposteriorly between the optic nerve medially and the anterior clinoid process laterally. This segment is often considered as a single segment until its terminal division into the anterior cerebral and middle cerebral arteries just below the anterior perforating substance. However, the supraclinoid segment may be practically subdivided into the ophthalmic, hypophyseal, posterior communicating, choroidal, and terminal segments, and each segment is named for the arteries arising from each division. These segments are also common sites of eponymous aneurysm formation (**Fig. 10**).

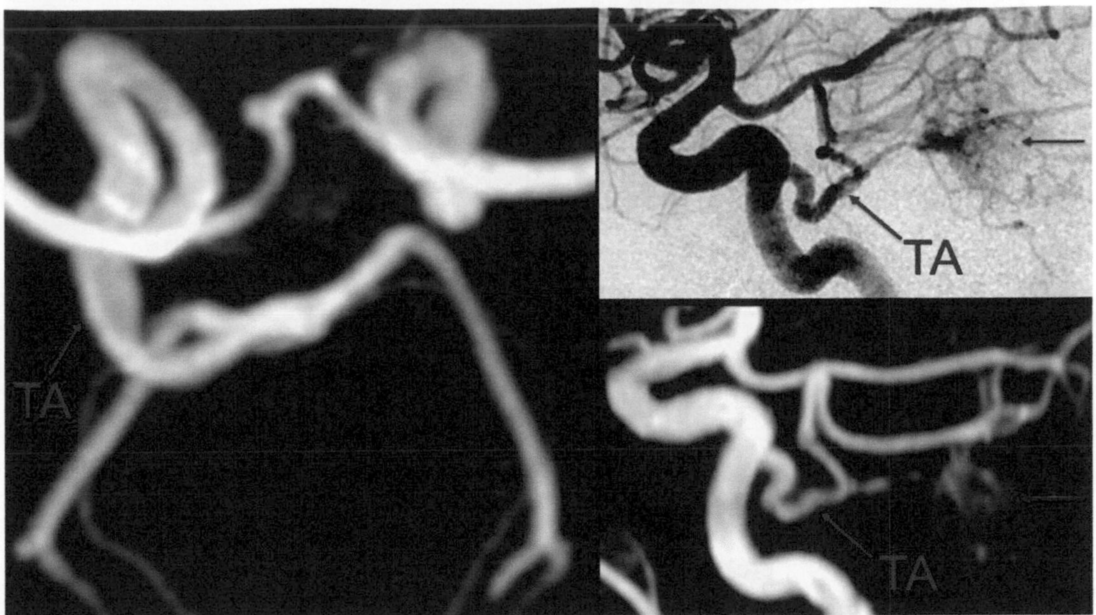

Fig. 9. Left panel: Axial maximum intensity projection MRA demonstrating a persistent trigeminal artery (type 1; *red arrow*) arising from the cavernous segment of the right internal carotid artery to supply the distal basilar artery. Right upper and lower panels: Lateral angiogram of the right internal carotid artery (upper panel) and sagittal maximum intensity projection MRA (lower panel) demonstrating a persistent trigeminal artery variant arising from the cavernous segment of the internal carotid artery with supply to a posterior fossa arteriovenous malformation (*purple arrow*). MRA, Magnetic resonance angiogram.

The ophthalmic division is the first short horizontal intradural segment from which the normal ventral ophthalmic artery arises, typically just inferior and slightly medial to the internal carotid artery. The embryology of the ophthalmic artery is complex but in simplified form, a fetal orbital arterial complex is formed between the primitive dorsal ophthalmic artery (arising from the fetal cavernous internal carotid artery), the primitive ventral ophthalmic artery (arising from the fetal anterior cerebral artery), and the stapedial artery (arising from the fetal hyoid artery), which provides an orbital branch through the superior orbital fissure and an extracranial segment to the middle cranial fossa dura. Through segmental regression of the primitive dorsal ophthalmic artery and the stapedial artery, the stapedial artery gives rise to the definitive caroticotympanic artery and variable persistence of the extracranial segment leads to meningeal variants, such as a recurrent meningeal artery that arises from the ophthalmic artery (Fig. 11) or persistent meningolacrimal branches, which may provide an anastomotic pathway between the middle meningeal and ophthalmic arteries (Fig. 12). Variable ophthalmic artery regression may lead to additional variant origins of the ophthalmic artery from the middle meningeal artery (Fig. 13). The primitive ventral ophthalmic artery originates at the anterior cerebral artery and segmentally regresses and reanastomoses to its final position as the definitive ophthalmic artery at the superomedial aspect of the supraclinoid internal carotid artery. However, variants of persistence of the dorsal ophthalmic artery, both dorsal and ventral ophthalmic arteries, or of a deep recurrent ophthalmic artery arising from the cavernous internal carotid artery owing to persistent anastomosis between the definitive ophthalmic artery and the inferolateral trunk may be rarely identified (Figs. 14–16).

The normal ophthalmic artery has 3 defined segments[1]: the ocular segment, which usually courses below the optic nerve and provides the origins of the central retinal and ciliary arteries immediately before coursing laterally and superiorly to round the nerve within the orbit[2]; the orbital segment, which is the straight segment along the optic nerve that provides arterial supply to the lacrimal gland, the extraocular muscles, and the site of origin of the recurrent meningeal artery (if present); and[3] the extraorbital segment, which provides multiple anastomotic branches to the distal facial artery, and is the origin of the ethmoidal and anterior falcine arteries. The anterior and posterior ethmoidal branches may anastomose with the sphenopalatine arteries of the

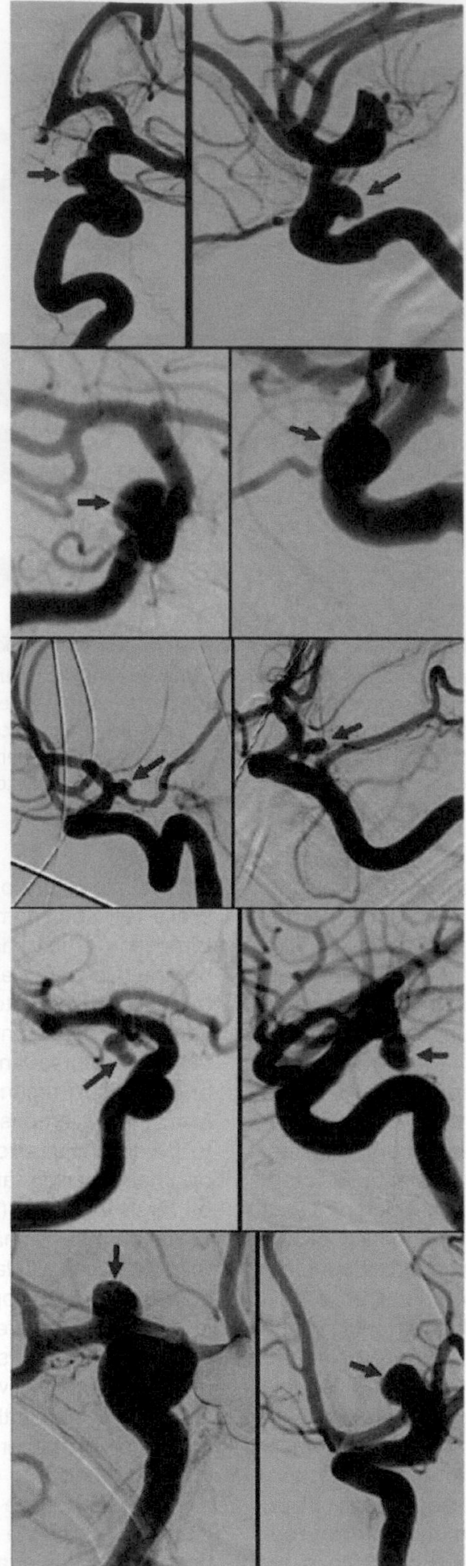

Fig. 10. Anteroposterior and lateral magnified oblique internal carotid angiograms demonstrating example superior hypophyseal (first row), paraophthalmic (second row), posterior communicating (third row), anterior choroidal (fourth row), and carotid terminus (fifth row) aneurysms, each respectively arranged by row with

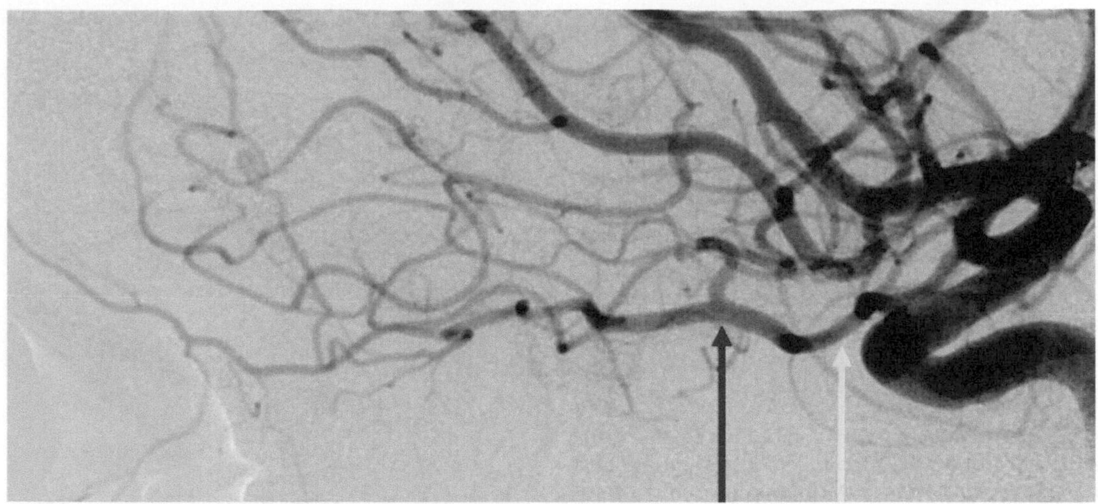

Fig. 11. Lateral magnified internal carotid angiogram demonstrating the course of a normal ophthalmic artery (*yellow arrow*) with origination of a robust recurrent meningeal artery (*red arrow*) from the midophthalmic artery.

internal maxillary artery and provide a pathway of collateral reconstitution of the internal carotid artery (Fig. 17). The anterior falcine artery is a distal dural branch supplying the anterior cerebral falx, and it is frequently hypertrophied in frontal dural arteriovenous fistulae (see Fig. 17).

The hypophyseal segment of the internal carotid artery is a short segment distal to the ophthalmic artery origin just superior and lateral to the sella turcica, from which the grouped superior hypophyseal arteries arise. These arteries are typically angiographically invisible and are variable in number, and they course medially toward the pituitary infundibulum to supply the adenohypophysis. The origin of the superior hypophyseal arteries may serve as a common site of inferomedially oriented aneurysms that arise from the internal carotid artery in this segment.

The posterior communicating and choroidal segments, respectively, refer to the short portions of the mid-to-distal supraclinoid segment from which the posterior communicating and anterior choroidal arteries originate (Fig. 18). The posterior communicating artery is a common but variable branch that connects the internal carotid artery to the P1 segment of the posterior cerebral artery, and this vessel forms the basis of the circle of Willis in concert with the anterior communicating artery. Arising from the posteroinferior surface of the distal supraclinoid segment of the internal carotid artery, the posterior communicating artery is typically medial to the cisternal segment of the third cranial nerve, and in its normal configuration is smaller than the posterior cerebral artery to which it anastomoses. A fetal-type configuration of this vessel is seen when the posterior communicating artery is larger than the ipsilateral P1 segment of the posterior cerebral artery, and a true fetal configuration is seen with an aplastic ipsilateral P1 segment of the posterior cerebral artery, which indicates failed regression of the early fetal origin of the posterior cerebral artery from the embryonic internal carotid artery (Fig. 19).[6]

the aneurysm labeled with a red arrow. First row: Left internal carotid angiogram demonstrating a broad-based saccular inferomedially oriented superior hypophyseal aneurysm extending from the ventromedial internal carotid artery surface. Second row: Right internal carotid angiogram demonstrating a broad-based superolaterally oriented paraophthalmic artery saccular aneurysm without the involvement of the origin of the ophthalmic artery, with the aneurysm dome seen as a double density on the lateral projection. Third row: Left internal carotid angiogram demonstrating a narrow necked saccular aneurysm with involvement of the origin of a large fetal-type left posterior communicating artery at the aneurysm neck. Fourth row: Right internal carotid angiogram demonstrated a wide-necked, bilobed saccular and posteroinferiorly oriented aneurysm of the anterior choroidal artery with involvement of the anterior choroidal artery origin from the aneurysm neck. Fifth row: Right internal carotid angiogram demonstrating a wide-necked anterosuperiorly oriented saccular aneurysm of the carotid terminus at the bifurcation of the supraclinoid segment into the right middle and anterior cerebral arteries.

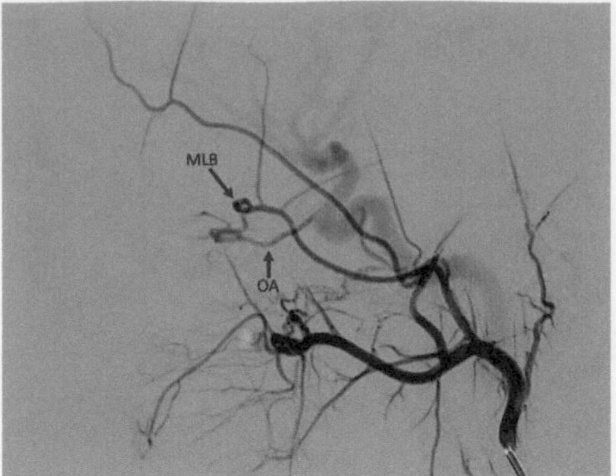

Fig. 12. Lateral magnified angiogram of the distal external carotid artery trunk demonstrating a robust meningolacrimal branch (MLB) arising from the frontal division of the middle meningeal artery, which takes a recurrent course through the Foramen of Hyrtl to enter the orbit, subsequently retrogradely opacifying the proximal OA trunk. Note flash reflux into the internal carotid artery that faintly opacifies the petrous through supraclinoid segments and clearly demonstrates the normal origin of the OA from the proximal supraclinoid internal carotid artery.

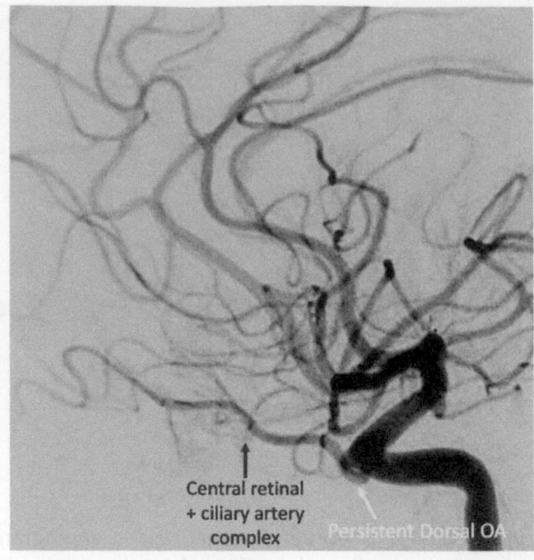

Fig. 14. Lateral magnified angiogram of the internal carotid artery demonstrates variant origin of the OA from the undersurface of the distal cavernous segment consistent with a persistent dorsal (persistent dorsal OA; yellow *arrow*), with an otherwise normal course and caliber of the OA and normal origination of the central retinal arteries and ciliary arterial complex (red *arrow* and text).

Throughout the embryologic development, the arterial supply between the anterior choroidal and posterior cerebral arteries remains in balance, and there is a rich anastomotic network through thalamic arterial supply that allows each artery to share or trade their supplied territories. However, in a normal configuration, the anterior choroidal artery arises just distal to the origin of the posterior communicating artery and is divided into cisternal and plexal segments. The cisternal segment courses around the lateral aspect of the midbrain within the circumpeduncular cistern before entering the choroidal fissure, with grouped perforator supply along this course to the optic tract, posterior lentiform nucleus, posterior limb of the

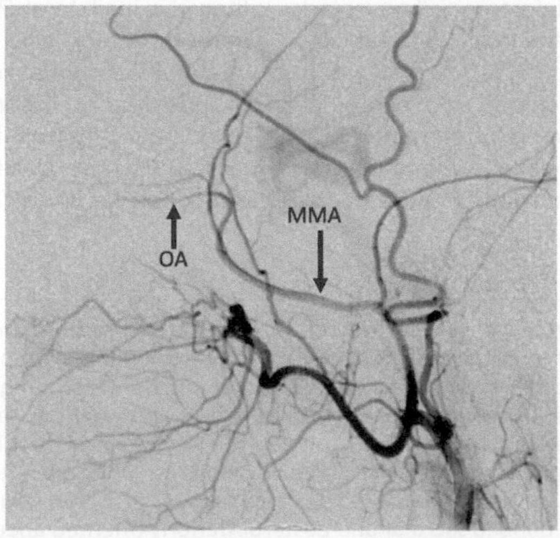

Fig. 13. Lateral magnified angiogram of the distal external carotid artery trunk demonstrating the origin of the OA proper from the hypertrophied frontal division of the MMA. Selective angiography of the ipsilateral internal carotid artery (not shown) demonstrated no associated OA branch or anastomotic vessel.

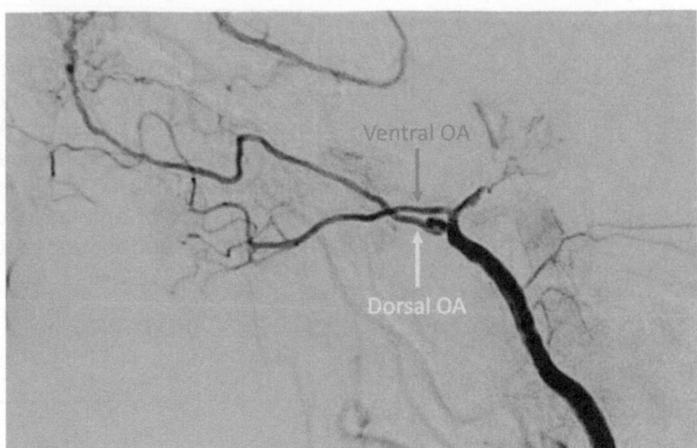

Fig. 15. Lateral magnified angiogram of the internal carotid artery in a patient with Moyamoya disease resulting in steno-occlusive disease of the supraclinoid segment of the internal carotid artery. Variant persistent of both the ventral and dorsal ophthalmic arteries (green and yellow *arrows*, respectively), with retinal and ciliary arterial supply arising from the distal ventral OA with the ethmoidal, supratrochlear, and anterior falcine arteries seem to arise from the dorsal OA.

internal capsule (superior perforator group), the uncus, amygdala and hippocampus (lateral perforator group), and the anterolateral midbrain and lateral geniculate nucleus (medial perforator group).[9] The plexal segment of the anterior choroidal artery extends posteriorly and superiorly from the choroidal fissure to the atrium of the lateral ventricle and supplies a portion of the ipsilateral choroid plexus, where it anastomoses with the lateral posterior choroidal artery from the posterior cerebral artery. It is common to see infundibular origins of either the posterior communicating or anterior choroidal arteries, and these structures

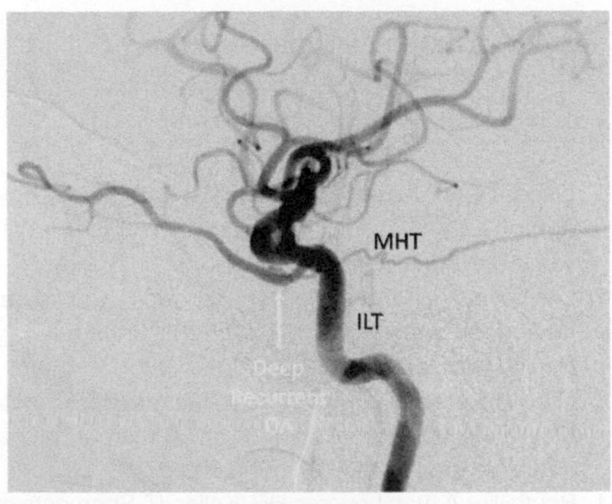

Fig. 16. Lateral magnified angiogram of the internal carotid artery demonstrating origination of the ophthalmic artery from the proximal horizontal cavernous segment consistent with a deep recurrent (OA; *yellow arrow*). A prominent MHT and ILT are additionally annotated in black text.

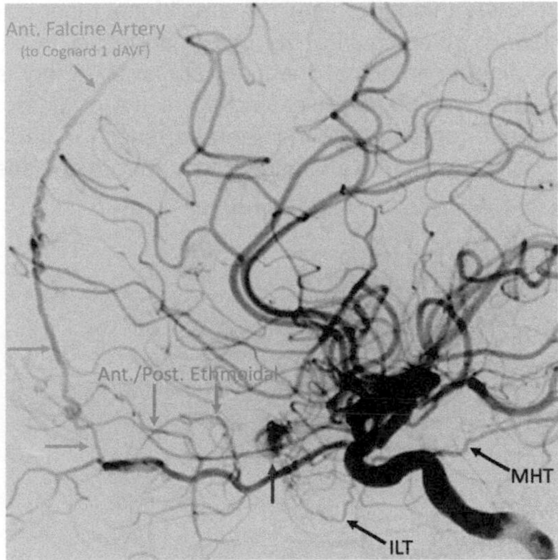

Fig. 17. Lateral magnified angiogram of the internal carotid artery demonstrating a normal ventral ophthalmic artery with robust anterior and posterior ethmoidal arteries (*green arrows*) and a tortuous hypertrophied anterior falcine artery arising from the distal ophthalmic artery, which provides arterial supply to a Cognard grade I dural arteriovenous fistula of the anterior superior sagittal sinus (*blue arrows*). There are multiple hypertrophied deep recurrent and clival meningeal branches arising from the inferolateral trunk (ILT), which supply an incidental intraorbital vascular malformation (*red arrow*). A prominent marginal tentorial artery of the meningohypophyseal trunk (MHT) is also present.

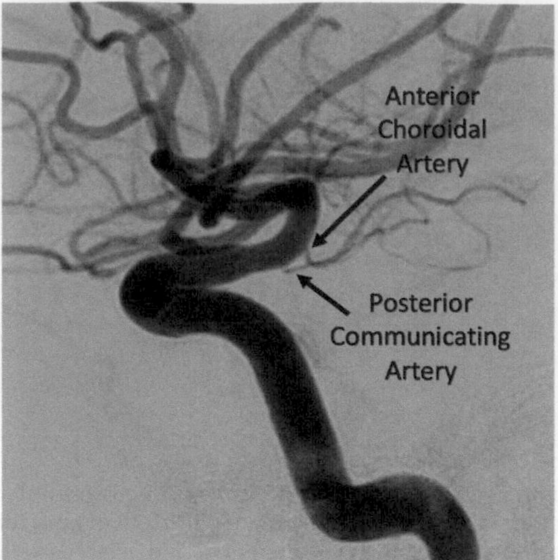

Fig. 18. Lateral magnified angiogram of the internal carotid artery demonstrating a normal origin of the posterior communicating and anterior choroidal arteries from the distal embryologically termed "ventral" but anatomically posterior surface of the supraclinoid internal carotid artery.

are seen angiographically as small focal triangular dilations, leading into the proximal vessel trunk. The final segment of the internal carotid artery is the terminal segment extending to the origins of the anterior and middle cerebral arteries, an additional potential site of aneurysm formation (see Fig. 10).

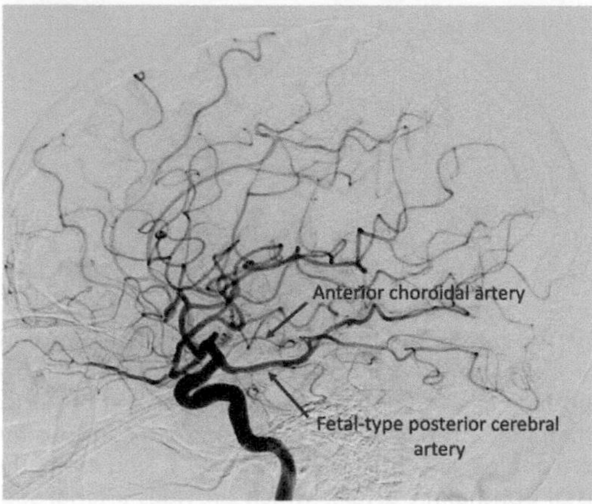

Fig. 19. Lateral magnified angiogram of the internal carotid artery demonstrating a normal origin of the anterior choroidal artery from the distal embryologically termed "ventral" but anatomically posterior surface of the supraclinoid internal carotid artery and a large, fetal-type posterior communicating artery with supply to the entirety of the ipsilateral posterior cerebral artery.

SUMMARY

The internal carotid artery is an elegant and complex vessel that serves as the dominant pathway to the anterior circulation. An understanding of the underlying development and branch anatomy of the internal carotid artery is critical to the accurate diagnosis of anterior circulation cerebrovascular disease and for subsequent treatment.

CLINICS CARE POINTS

1. Segmental anatomy of the internal carotid artery is anatomically defined by the course of the vessel through the skull base and in relationship to definable branch vessels.
2. Defined branch vessels arising from the internal carotid artery provide pathways of collateral reconstitution, meningeal and cranial nerve arterial supply, and additionally provide a framework for understanding common pathologic condition of the internal carotid artery, such as aneurysm development and treatment.
3. Variant arterial anatomy is common and is frequently owing to remnant embryonic arteries or incomplete regression of fetal arteries, which additionally form the basis of a rich network of anastomotic pathways among multiple circulations.

DISCLOSURE

The authors have nothing to disclose.

REFERENCES

1. Osborn AG, Jacobs JM. Diagnostic cerebral angiography. 2nd edition. Philadelphia: Lippincott Williams & Wilkins; 1999. p. 1999.
2. Lasjaunias P, Berenstein A, ter Brugge KG. Surgical neuroangiography, 2001. New York: Spring-Verlag Berlin Heidelberg; 2001. p. 789.
3. Gibo H, Lenkey C, Rhoton AL Jr. Microsurgical anatomy of the supraclinoid portion of the internal carotid artery. J Neurosurg 1981;55(4):560–74.
4. Bouthillier A, van Loveren HR, Keller JT. Segments of the internal carotid artery: a new classification. Neurosurgery 1996;38(3):425–32 [discussion: 32-3].
5. Shapiro M, Becske T, Riina HA, et al. Toward an endovascular internal carotid artery classification system. AJNR Am J Neuroradiol 2014;35(2):230–6.

6. Bradac GB, Boccardi E. Applied cerebral angiography. 3rd edition. Germany: Springer-Verlag GmbH; 2017. p. 2017.
7. Sullivan AM, Curtin HD, Moonis G. Arterial anomalies of the middle ear: a pictorial review with clinical-embryologic and imaging correlation. Neuroimaging Clin N Am 2019;29(1):93–102.
8. Overdevest JB, Amans MR, Zaki P, et al. Patterns of vascularization and surgical morbidity in juvenile nasopharyngeal angiofibroma: a case series, systematic review, and meta-analysis. Head Neck 2018;40(2):428–43.
9. Peris-Celda MM-S F, Rhoton AL. Rhoton's atlas of head, neck, and brain. 1st edition. Stuttgart, New York, Delhi, Rio: Thieme Verlagsgruppe; 2018.
10. Joo W, Funaki T, Yoshioka F, et al. Microsurgical anatomy of the carotid cave. Neurosurgery 2012; 70(2 Suppl Operative):300–11. ; discussion 11-2.
11. Bernasconi V, Cassinari V, Gori G. Diagnostic Value of the Tentorial Arteries of the Carotid Siphon. (Angiographic Study of a Case of Falcotentorial Angioma). Neurochirurgia (Stuttg) 1965; 8:67–72.

Anatomy of the Intracranial Arteries

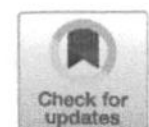

The Anterior Intracranial and Vertebrobasilar Circulations

Dylan N. Wolman, MD[a,b], Adrienne M. Moraff, MD[c], Jeremy J. Heit, MD PhD[b,*]

KEYWORDS

• Artery • Intracranial • Cerebral • Middle cerebral artery • Anterior cerebral artery • Posterior cerebral artery • Vertebral artery

KEY POINTS

- The middle cerebral artery is segmented into M1 through M4 segments, each of which is anatomically defined by location, not by branch order.
- The middle cerebral artery is classically divided into anterior and posterior divisions, with the anterior division supplying the frontal lobe and the posterior division supplying the temporal lobe, whereas supply to the parietal lobe is provided through whichever division is larger and therefore dominant.
- The anterior cerebral artery is segmented into the A1 through A5 segments, each of which is anatomically defined primarily in relation to the corpus callosum.
- The pericallosal artery is the dominant anterior cerebral artery segment from which each cortical branch arises, whereas the callosomarginal artery is often a secondary branch supplying a portion of the frontal lobe but is variable and is not defined in all patients.
- The posterior cerebral artery is segmented into P1 through P4 segments, each of which is anatomically defined primarily in relation to the brainstem and basal cisterns, with multiple branch vessels forming a complex thalamic arterial network in addition to providing primary supply to the occipital lobes.

INTRODUCTION

The cerebral arteries provide blood flow to the brain through perhaps the most elegant vascular anatomy bed in the body. The arterial supply to the brain is separated into the anterior circulation, which is composed of arteries that arise from the bilateral internal carotid arteries, and the posterior circulation, which is composed of arteries that arise from the paired vertebral arteries. A detailed understanding of normal and variant cerebral arterial anatomy is important to understanding common cerebrovascular diseases, such as ischemic stroke, steno-occlusive disease, cerebral aneurysms, cerebral arteriovenous malformations, and pial and dural arteriovenous fistulae.

In this article, the authors discuss common and variant cerebral arterial anatomy, and they have

[a] Department of Neuroimaging and Neurointervention, Stanford School of Medicine, Center for Academic Medicine, 453 Quarry Road, Palo Alto, CA 94304, USA; [b] Department of Radiology, Stanford University School of Medicine, Stanford, CA 94304, USA; [c] Division of Neurosurgery, Howard University School of Medicine, 2041 Georgia Avenue NW, Suite 4000, Washington, DC, USA
* Corresponding author. Stanford School of Medicine, 453 Quarry Road, Palo Alto, CA 94304.
E-mail address: jheit@stanford.edu
Twitter: @JeremyHeitMDPHD (J.J.H.)

Neuroimag Clin N Am 32 (2022) 617–636
https://doi.org/10.1016/j.nic.2022.04.007
1052-5149/22/

organized this discussion by arterial circulation, which includes the anterior, middle, and posterior cerebral arteries, and the vertebrobasilar system, but excludes the internal carotid artery that is discussed separately. Cerebrovascular diseases are discussed as examples in this article, but they are considered in the context of cerebral arterial anatomy. A more detailed discussion of cerebrovascular disease is beyond the scope of this article.

ANTERIOR CIRCULATION

Anterior Cerebral Artery

The paired anterior cerebral arteries originate from the primitive olfactory arteries, which are themselves branches of the fetal internal carotid arteries. The anterior cerebral arteries eventually develop toward the midline and are joined by a plexiform anastomotic network that becomes the adult anterior communicating artery complex. In its adult form, the anterior cerebral artery is commonly divided into 5 ordered segments: A1 to A5. The A1 segment is the horizontal or precommunicating segment, and it extends medially from the carotid terminus to the anterior communicating artery complex, which overlies the optic chiasm (**Fig. 1**). Two groups of perforating medial lenticulostriate arteries arise from the A1 segment: a superiorly oriented group that enters the anterior perforating substance and supplies the anterior hypothalamus, the septum pellucidum, the forniceal pillars, the anterior striatum, and the medial aspect of the anterior commissure, and an additional inferiorly oriented group arising from the distal A1 segment that supplies the optic chiasm and proximal cisternal segments of the optic nerves.[1,2] The largest perforator is the recurrent artery of Heubner, which has a variable origin from the distal A1 segment, the proximal A2 segment, or the anterior communicating artery complex. The recurrent artery of Heubner describes a characteristic recurrent course back parallel to the A1 and M1 segments of the anterior and middle cerebral arteries before extending posterosuperiorly to supply the head of caudate, the anterior limb of the internal capsule, and the adjacent anterior lentiform nucleus (**Figs. 2** and **3**). The relationship between the anterior communicating artery complex, a common site of aneurysm

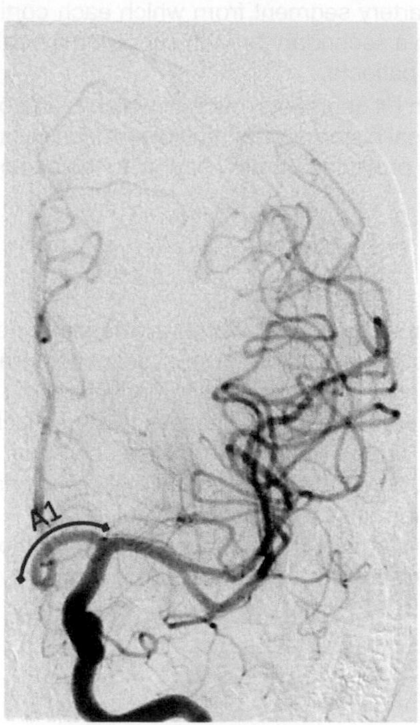

Fig. 1. Anteroposterior angiogram of the left internal carotid artery demonstrating the normal course of the horizontal A1 segment of the left anterior cerebral artery, extending medially from the carotid terminus to the anterior communicating artery complex and extending over the optic nerve.

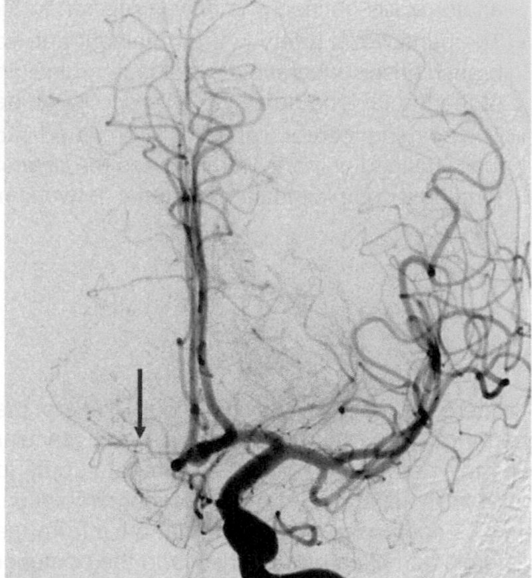

Fig. 2. Anteroposterior angiogram of the left internal carotid artery demonstrating the normal course of the contralateral recurrent artery of Heubner (*red arrow*), which is typically best seen on contrast opacification of the contralateral internal carotid artery owing to potential obscuration by angiographic overlap of the horizontal segment of the middle and anterior cerebral arteries. Inferior-to-superior hairpin of the distal portion of the recurrent artery of Heubner reflects the recurrent nature of the artery in its normal course. Note an incidental anterior communicating artery aneurysm in plane on this projection.

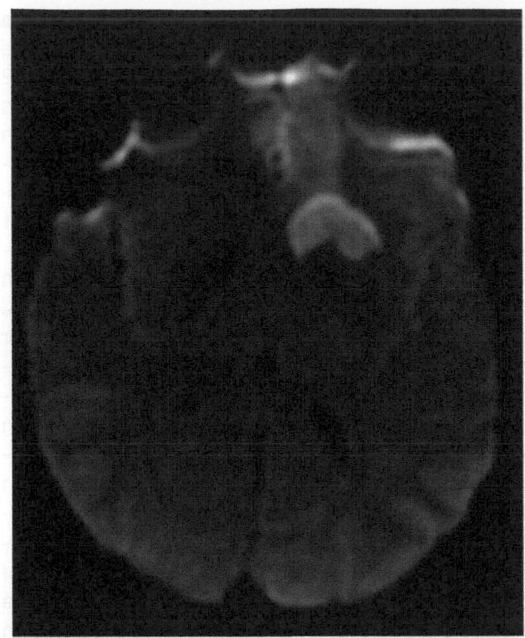

Fig. 3. Axial DWI image of the brain at the level of the basal ganglia demonstrating acute infarction of the left recurrent artery of Heubner territory involving the head of caudate, anterior genu of the internal capsule, and the anterior lentiform nucleus following microsurgical clipping of a ruptured anterior communicating artery aneurysm from a right pterional approach. Bifrontal susceptibility artifact related to postsurgical pneumocephalus. DWI, diffusion-weighted imaging.

development, and the recurrent artery of Heubner is critical to identify before surgical aneurysm clipping, given a high risk for inadvertent clipping of this critical perforator.[3]

Asymmetry between the A1 segments is common, and a unilaterally hypoplastic or aplastic A1 segment is seen in approximately 10% of patients,[4] which results in supply to the distal bilateral anterior cerebral arteries from the contralateral dominant A1 segment across a patent anterior communicating artery. The A2 segment of the anterior cerebral artery is the vertical or postcommunicating segment that turns sharply superiorly within the interhemispheric fissure and courses anterior to the rostrum of the corpus callosum, with an anatomically defined transition to the A3 segment at the genu of the corpus callosum. Bihemispheric supply from the A2 segment of the anterior cerebral artery is a common variant, with variable origination of bilateral cortical branches from a single A2 in the setting of a hypoplastic or aplastic contralateral A2 segment.[5,6] The A3 segment is termed the precallosal segment, and it is short and confined only to the segment that overlies the anterior callosal genu. The A3 segment is classically where the callosomarginal artery originates. The A4 segment is the supracallosal segment that courses over the callosal body, and it is often the segment that is termed the pericallosal artery. The A5 or postcallosal segment extends posterior to the callosal body and beyond the splenium, beyond the plane of the coronal suture (**Fig. 4**).

The first 2 major cortical branches that arise from the anterior communicating artery are the orbitofrontal and frontopolar arteries, which typically arise separately but may share a common origin from the proximal A2 segment. These arteries supply the inferior frontal lobe, including the gyrus rectus, medial orbital gyrus, the olfactory bulb, and the anteromedial aspect of the superior frontal gyrus. The next 2 major branches are the pericallosal and callosomarginal arteries, from which the remainder of the defined but variable cortical branches arise. The pericallosal artery is

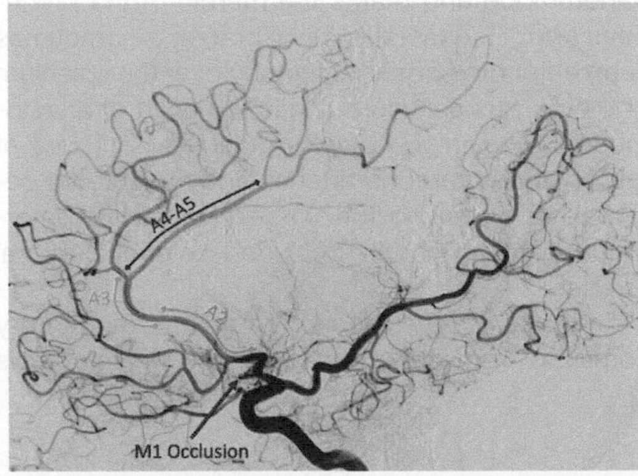

Fig. 4. Lateral internal carotid angiogram performed in the setting of a chronic occlusion of the proximal M1 segment of the middle cerebral artery (*red arrow*), highlighting the anterior cerebral artery segments. Note the fetal-type origin of the posterior cerebral artery. The A2 segment of the anterior cerebral artery (*green*) is seen coursing superiorly from the anterior communicating artery complex within the interhemispheric fissure and anterior to the rostrum of the corpus callosum. The A3 segment (*blue*) of the anterior cerebral artery then courses anteriorly over the genu of the corpus callosum before becoming the A4 segment (*purple*) after it turns sharply posteriorly. On this angiographic image, a typical origin of the callosomarginal artery is seen between the labeled A3 and A4 segments, which extends posterosuperiorly within the cingulate sulcus. The A4 and A5 segments (*purple*) of the anterior cerebral artery then course over the body of the corpus callosum. The entire trunk of the A2 through A5 segments of the anterior cerebral artery is often referred to as the pericallosal artery.

constant and may be defined as the entire segment distal to the anterior communicating artery, whereas others may define its origin at the junction with the callosomarginal artery, if present. The callosomarginal artery may variably originate from the proximal A2 to distal A3 segments of the anterior cerebral artery and take a posterosuperior course within the cingulate sulcus, giving rise to a variable degree of frontal lobe supply. The callosomarginal artery is not definable in approximately 18% of hemispheres[2] with its vascular territory supplanted by the pericallosal artery in these cases (Fig. 5).

The remaining cortical branches of the anterior cerebral artery are variable and are typically subdivided as follows (from anterior to posterior): frontal branch group (anterior, middle, and posterior internal frontal arteries), which supplies the superior frontal gyrus; the precentral or paracentral artery, which supplies the paracentral lobule and the medial aspect of the precentral and postcentral gyri, and the parietal branch group (superior and inferior parietal arteries), which supplies the medial parietal lobe and marks the margin of the precuneus (Fig. 6). A distal splenial branch is sometimes seen extending posteroinferiorly over the splenium of the corpus callosum and is the point of anastomosis between the parieto-occipital branches of the posterior cerebral arteries and the anterior cerebral artery, a common site of retrograde collateralization of proximally occluded anterior cerebral arteries.

The origin of the anterior communicating artery complex from the fetal plexiform anastomosis between the anterior cerebral arteries has great anatomic variability. Classically, there is a single anterior communicating artery joining the A1-A2 junctions of the bilateral anterior cerebral arteries (Fig. 7). However, there is a wide array of variation seen in the anterior communicating artery complex, including single or multiple fenestrations, duplications, or aplasia, asymmetry of the A1 segments of the anterior cerebral arteries, persistence of the median artery of the corpus callosum or of the primitive olfactory artery, or failed midline cleavage with persistence of an azygos anterior cerebral artery (Fig. 8). Approximately 80% of aneurysms developing from the anterior communicating artery complex are associated with asymmetry of the A1 segments and are subsequently directed along the pathway of flow from the dominant segment (Fig. 9).[2,4,6] Complex fenestrations are additionally associated with aneurysm formation, given the greater number of branch points (Fig. 10). The median artery of the corpus callosum is an uncommon variant in which there is a persistent third branch arising from the anterior communicating artery complex and extending superiorly, parallel to the A2 segments of the anterior cerebral arteries. This branch may supply only the corpus callosum at the midline, extending along the lamina terminalis, in which case it is a true persistent median artery of the corpus callosum, or it may provide additional variable cortical supply, making it a duplicated pericallosal artery or pericallosal triplex (Fig. 11).

The persistent primitive olfactory artery represents failed regression of the embryonic olfactory

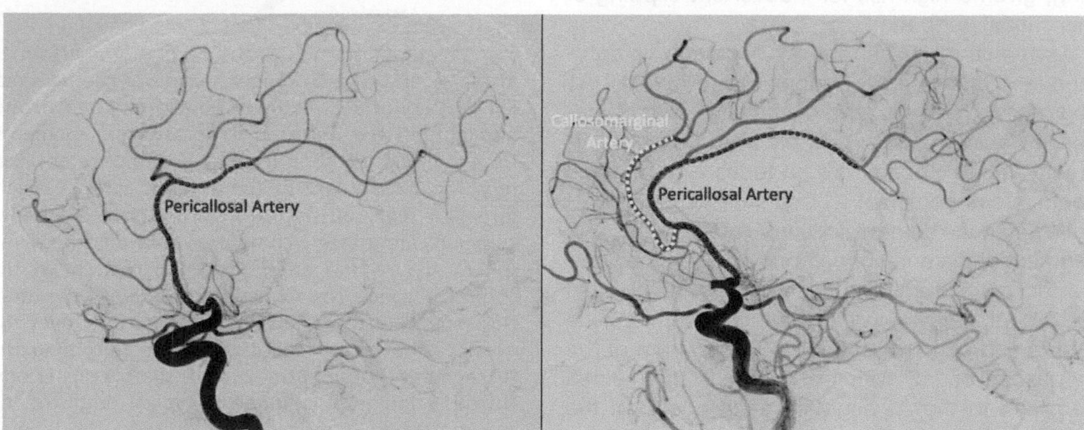

Fig. 5. Two separate lateral angiograms of the internal carotid artery in patients with occluded proximal M1 segments of the middle cerebral arteries to highlight the anterior cerebral artery anatomy. The left image demonstrates a typical pericallosal artery without a clearly defined callosomarginal artery, but rather a short common trunk at the origin of the middle and posterior internal frontal arteries at a common site of origination of the callosomarginal artery. The right image demonstrates a typical origin of a defined callosomarginal artery from the distal A2 segment of the anterior cerebral artery that provides supply to the frontopolar, anterior, middle, and posterior internal frontal arteries. Please refer to Fig. 6 for mapping of each named cortical branch.

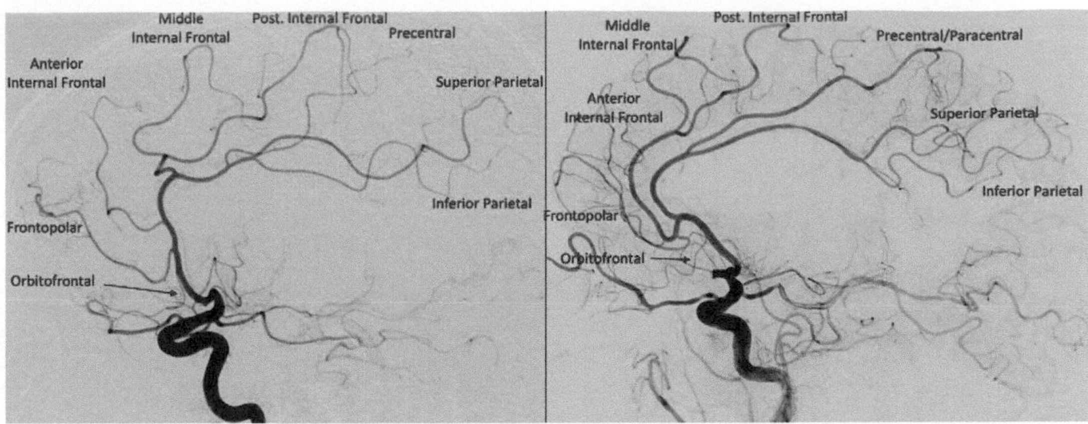

Fig. 6. Two separate lateral angiograms of the internal carotid artery of the same patients shown in Fig. 5 with occluded proximal M1 segments of the middle cerebral arteries to highlight the anterior cerebral artery anatomy. The left image demonstrates a typical pericallosal artery without a clearly defined callosomarginal artery, whereas the right image demonstrates a typical origin of a defined callosomarginal artery from the distal A2 segment of the anterior cerebral artery. Each image labels the most common cortical branches of the anterior cerebral artery, listed in clockwise order as follows: the orbitofrontal, frontopolar, anterior internal frontal, middle internal frontal, posterior internal frontal, precentral (or paracentral), superior parietal, and inferior parietal arteries. A small inferiorly oriented branch arising from the distal A5 segment of the pericallosal artery is the splenial artery (not labeled).

artery extending along the olfactory tract, which describes a characteristic anteriorly oriented and elongated anterior cerebral artery appearance or anterior communicating artery with a hairpin turn extending along the olfactory bulb. The ipsilateral recurrent artery of Heubner is typically absent with this variant, and there is an increased risk of aneurysm formation and additional anterior cerebral artery anomalies (Fig. 12). A rare anomalous

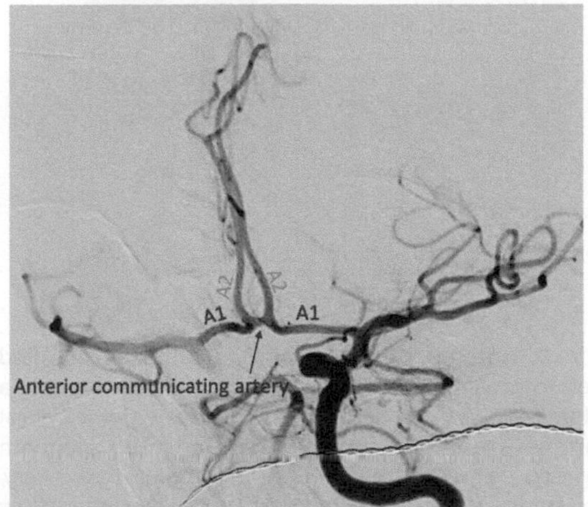

Fig. 7. Anteroposterior transorbital oblique view of a left internal carotid angiogram demonstrating a normal patent anterior communicating artery (*red arrow*) with robust opacification of the bilateral A1 (*red text*) and A2 (*green text*) segments of the anterior cerebral arteries.

infraoptic origin of the A1 segment of the anterior cerebral artery is seen when the A1 segment originates proximal to the origin of the M1 segment of the middle cerebral artery and extends inferior and medial to the optic nerve (Fig. 13). The infraoptic anterior cerebral artery is additionally associated with aneurysm formation, ipsilateral agenesis of the internal carotid artery, and agenesis or hypoplasia of the contralateral A1 segment of the anterior cerebral artery.[1,7]

Middle Cerebral Artery

The middle cerebral arteries develop as second-order branches of the primitive anterior cerebral arteries, which in turn arise from the fetal internal carotid arteries. The middle cerebral arteries initially lay over the surface of the primitive telencephalon during development, and they arborize along the developing insula amid progressive infolding of the developing frontal and temporal lobes to form the Sylvian fissure.[4] The mature and tortuous anatomy of the middle cerebral artery reflects this embryologic infolding with the developing brain, as the middle cerebral artery overlies and supplies most of the right and left cerebral hemispheres.

The ordered segments of the middle cerebral artery are anatomically defined and numbered M1 through M4. The M1 segment is the horizontal segment that extends from the internal carotid artery terminus within the middle cerebral artery cistern below the anterior perforating substance

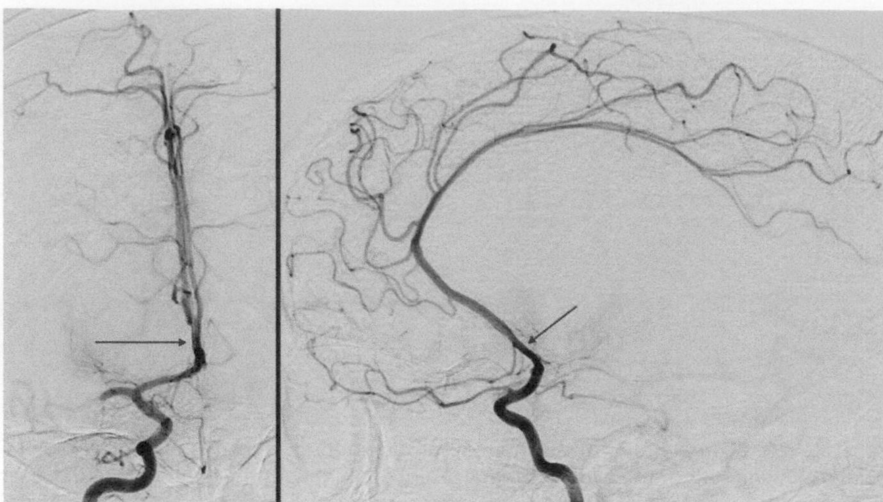

Fig. 8. Anteroposterior (*left*) and lateral (*right*) right internal carotid angiograms demonstrating an acute occlusion of the proximal M1 segment of the right middle cerebral artery, highlighting an incidental azygous anterior cerebral artery with robust opacification of the bilateral A2 segments of the anterior cerebral arteries. Note elevation of the A3, A4, and A5 segments of the pericallosal artery on the lateral projection consistent with hydrocephalus.

until the limen insulae (Fig. 14). Notably, the termination of the M1 segment is not defined by the site of branch divisions, and prebifurcation and postbifurcation M1 segments can exist with variable lengths of the proximal prebifurcation M1 trunk (see Fig. 14). The M2 segments, called the insular or vertical segments, begin as the vessels take a sharp superior turn along the insula until they reach their superior-most extent within the circular sulcus. The M2 segments terminate at the point of lateral deflection to exit along the margin off the circular sulcus (see Fig. 14). The M3 or opercular segments course under the margins of the frontal and temporal opercula until the exit of the Sylvian fissure, which demarcates the start of the M4 segments. The M4 segments of the middle cerebral artery begin as the distal branches course over the cortical surface that deliver arterial supply to the cerebral cortex (see Fig. 14).

The middle cerebral artery typically either bi- or trifurcates near the distal M1 or proximal M2 segments. The classic middle cerebral artery bifurcation creates the anterior division that supplies the frontal lobe and the posterior division that supplies the temporal lobe. The dominant division (or middle division in cases of a middle cerebral artery trifurcation) is defined as the one that supplies the parietal lobe. The territorial supply patterns are reflected in perfusion imaging patterns in cases of large vessel ischemic stroke, therefore allowing accurate prediction of the anatomic pattern and site of occlusion by perfusion alone.[8] The most common configuration is that of a

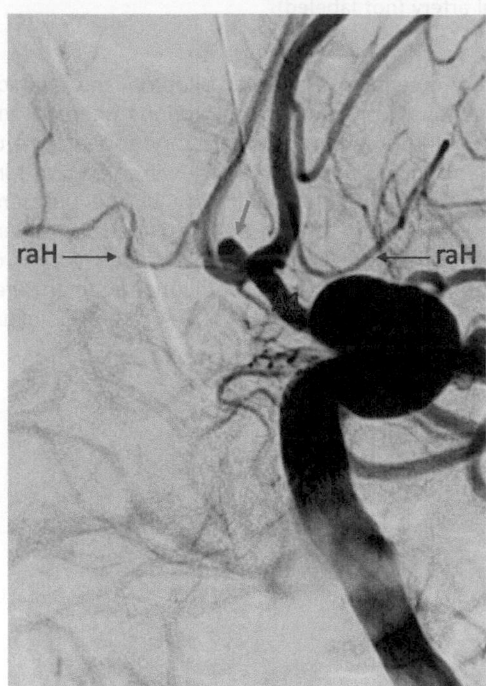

Fig. 9. Anteroposterior transorbital oblique magnified left internal carotid artery angiogram demonstrating a dominant A1 segment of the left anterior cerebral artery with a right superolaterally oriented aneurysm (*green arrow*) of the anterior communicating artery, oriented along the plane of the expected inflow pathway from the dominant anterior cerebral artery. Note inflow of unopacified blood from the contralateral circulation washing out the contrast stream within the A2 segment of the right anterior cerebral artery. The bilateral recurrent arteries of Heubner are well opacified (rAH; *red arrows*).

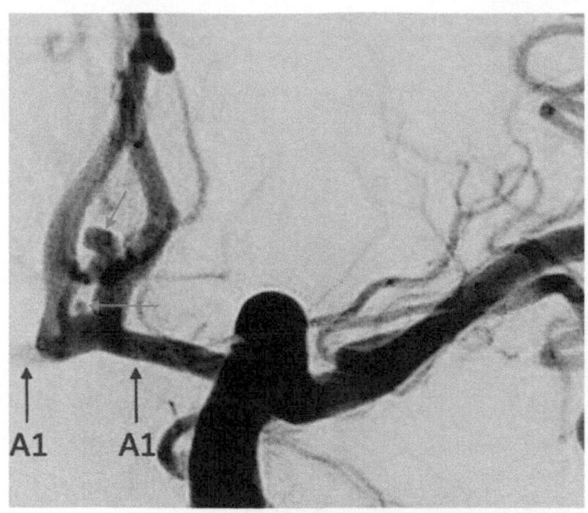

Fig. 10. Anteroposterior transorbital oblique magnified left internal carotid angiogram demonstrating a multiply fenestrated anterior communicating artery complex that is opacified through the A1 segment of the left anterior cerebral artery (*red arrow*; with the faintly opacified contralateral A1 segment similarly marked). There are 2 small and irregular aneurysms arising from each fenestration limb (*green arrows*).

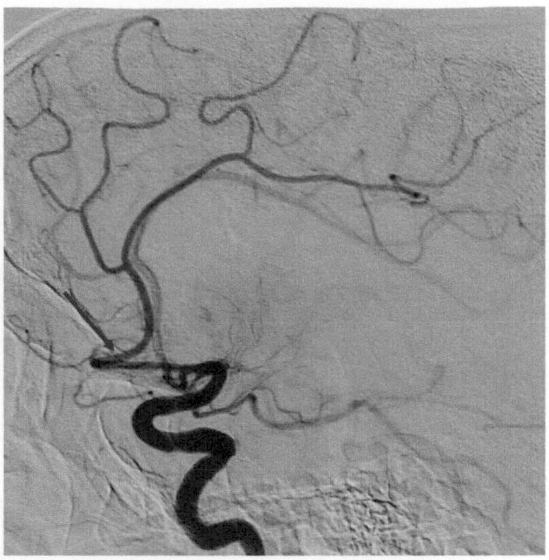

Fig. 12. Lateral magnified internal carotid angiogram demonstrating an anomalous anteriorly oriented and elongated ipsilateral proximal anterior cerebral artery with a characteristic anterior hairpin turn extending over the floor of the anterior cranial fossa along the olfactory bulb, consistent with a persistent primitive olfactory artery (*red arrow*).

bifurcation with a dominant posterior division and a nondominant anterior division, seen in just more than one-third of patients, whereas a codominant pattern is seen in just less than one-fifth of patients in which supply to the parietal lobe is split between each division.[6] Middle cerebral artery trifurcations are common and are present in approximately one-quarter of patients (Fig. 15). On cross-sectional imaging, the anterior division typically describes an acute and superiorly directed origin from the distal M1 segment of the middle cerebral artery, coursing superiorly along the anterolateral aspect of the insula within the circular sulcus, whereas the posterior division describes a more posterosuperior course along the posterolateral aspect of the insula.

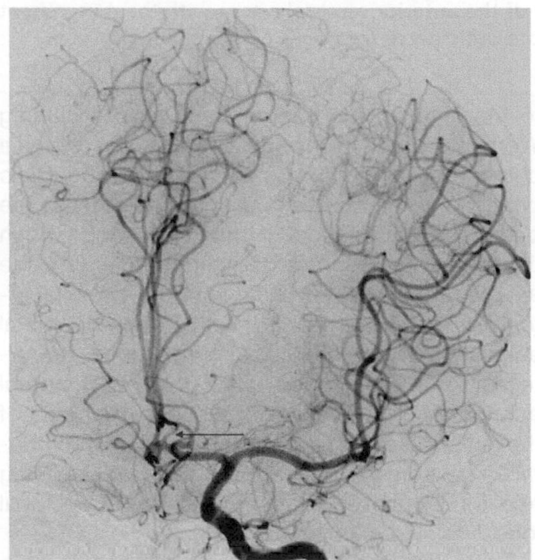

Fig. 11. Anteroposterior left internal carotid angiogram demonstrating a separate vessel arising from the center of the anterior communicating artery complex and coursing superiorly between the A2 segments of the anterior cerebral arteries consistent with a median artery of the corpus callosum (*red arrow*).

There are approximately 12 M4 segment cortical branches of the middle cerebral artery that have wide variability in the supplied territories and possible common origination from proximal trunks. When viewed on a lateral angiographic projection from anterior to posterior in a clockwise direction, commonly identified cortical branches include the polar, orbitofrontal, prefrontal, precentral, central, anterior parietal, posterior parietal, angular, parieto-occipital, anterior temporal, middle temporal, and posterior temporal arteries (Fig. 16).

The most common pattern of cortical branch supply is described later, and several larger branches, such as the polar and angular arteries, are frequently identifiable and may be used as angiographic signposts for subsequent vessel identification. The polar artery, which is commonly

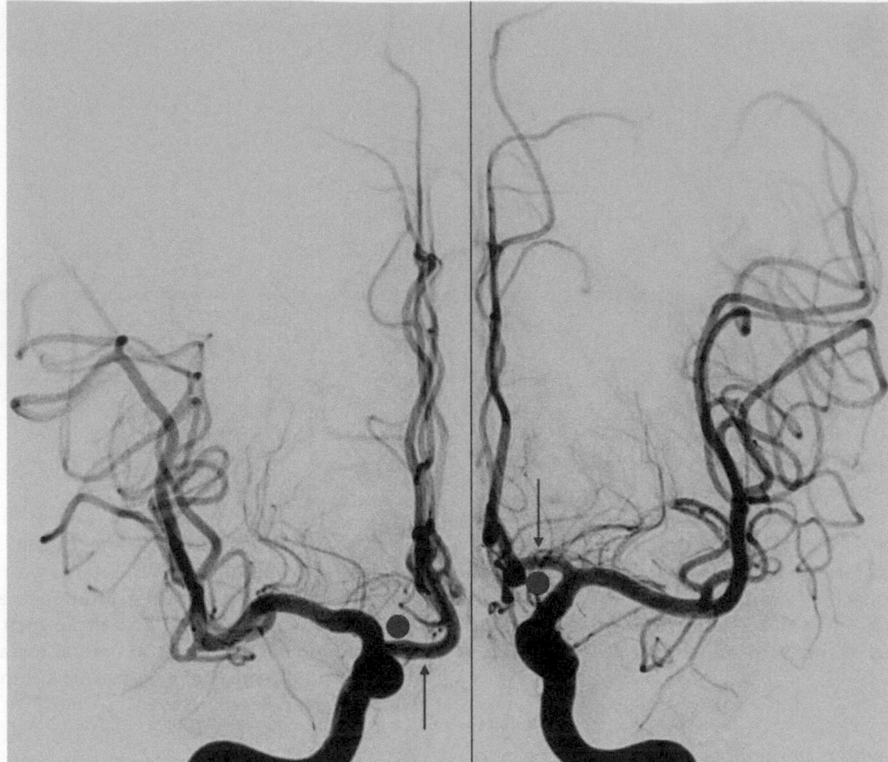

Fig. 13. Anteroposterior right and left internal carotid angiograms demonstrating a right-sided infraoptic origin of the anterior cerebral artery. (*Left*) Anteroposterior right internal carotid angiogram demonstrating proximal bifurcation of the carotid terminus into the anterior and middle cerebral arteries. The A1 segment of the right anterior cerebral artery (*red arrow*) takes an inferior and flattened course under the expected location of the optic nerve (*red dot*) consistent with an infraoptic origin of the anterior cerebral artery. (*Right*) Anteroposterior left internal carotid angiogram demonstrating a normal course of the anterior cerebral artery, with the A1 segment (*red arrow*) coursing superior to the expected location of the optic nerve (*red dot*).

referred to as the anterior temporal artery, typically arises from the horizontal M1 segment of the middle cerebral artery and courses anteroinferiorly to supply the anterior temporal pole (Fig. 17). The orbitofrontal branches supply the inferior frontal lobe and the pars triangularis of the inferior frontal gyrus including Broca area, respectively. These arteries typically arise from the proximal anterior division. The precentral and central arteries are the most posteriorly located of the ascending frontal branches and may share a common trunk. These arteries course to the posterior aspect of the frontal lobe to supply the lateral portions of the precentral and postcentral gyri (primary motor and sensory cortices, respectively). The anterior and posterior parietal arteries usually arise from the inferior division of the middle cerebral artery in a typical inferior dominant pattern, with the posterior parietal branch coursing along and marking the anterior aspect of the supramarginal gyrus. The angular artery is the most frequently recognizable terminal middle cerebral artery branch with supply to the angular and supramarginal gyri, including Wernicke area. The angular artery describes a characteristic “bump” on the lateral angiographic projection as it courses over Heschl gyrus at the posterosuperior aspect of the temporal lobe within the Sylvian fissure. A variable branch inferior to the angular artery is termed the temporo-occipital artery, which may arise directly from the distal angular artery. A variable group of temporal arteries, the anterior, middle, and posterior temporal arteries, course over their respective portions of the temporal operculum, with the posterior temporal artery typically being the largest and providing additional variable supply to the lateral occipital lobe.

Anomalies of the middle cerebral artery include rare proximal fenestrations of the M1 segment (Fig. 18) and the 3 middle cerebral artery variants codified by Manelfe.[9] A type 1 duplicated middle cerebral artery is often described as an origin of a large temporal branch from the distal supraclinoid segment immediately proximal to the origin

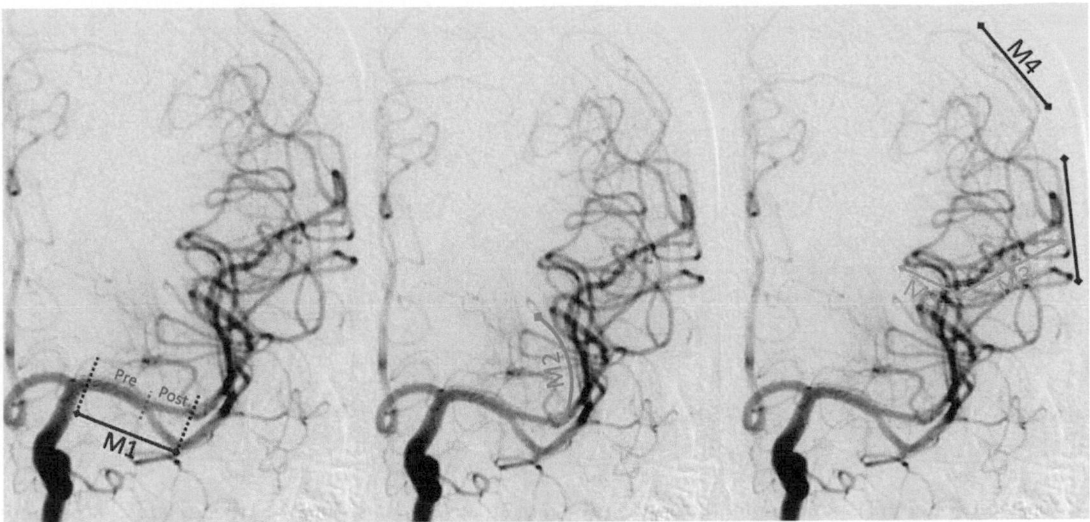

Fig. 14. Anteroposterior left internal carotid artery angiograms schematizing the normal segmental anatomy of the middle cerebral artery. (*Left*) Annotation of the horizontal M1 segment of the left middle cerebral artery (*red line and text*) with hashed lines marking the beginning and end of the M1 segment, transitioning to the M2 segment of the middle cerebral artery as the vessel takes a superior or posterosuperior turn within the circular sulcus. Blue text and hashed lines denote a typical prebifurcation and postbifurcation division of the M1 segment of the middle cerebral artery, demonstrating that the superior and inferior divisions of the middle cerebral artery may begin within the M1 segment. (*Middle*) Green text and line demonstrating the typical course of the M2 segments of the middle cerebral artery as they course within the circular sulcus over the insula. (*Left*) Blue text and lines demonstrate the course of the opercular M3 segments of the middle cerebral artery as they exit the circular sulcus and course under the frontal operculum and over the temporal operculum. Purple text and lines demonstrate the terminal M4 cortical segments of the middle cerebral artery as they exit the Sylvian fissure and extend over the cortical surface of the hemisphere.

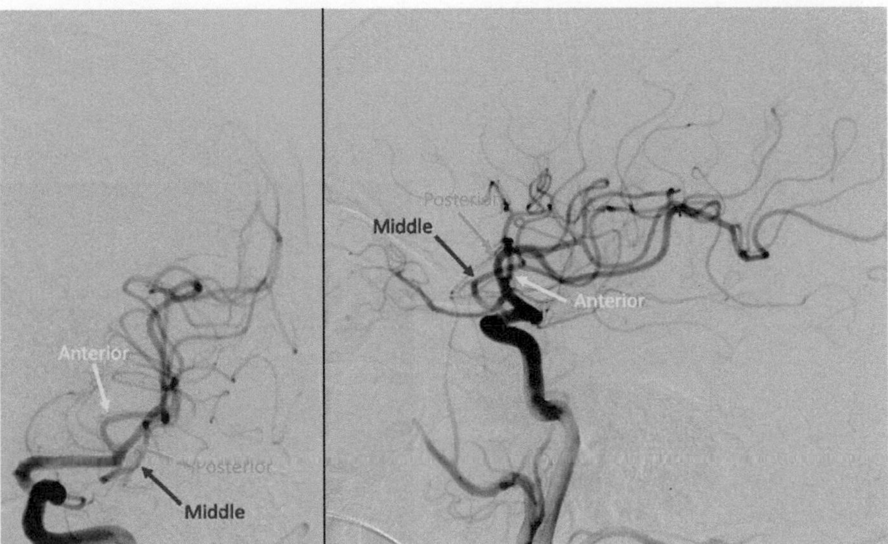

Fig. 15. Anteroposterior and lateral left internal carotid angiograms in the setting of an aplastic A1 segment of the ipsilateral anterior cerebral artery demonstrating a typical trifurcation of the left middle cerebral artery, with each division labeled and color coded as follows: anterior division (*yellow*) supplying the frontal lobe, middle division (*red*) supplying the parietal lobe, and the posterior division (*blue*) supplying the temporal lobe.

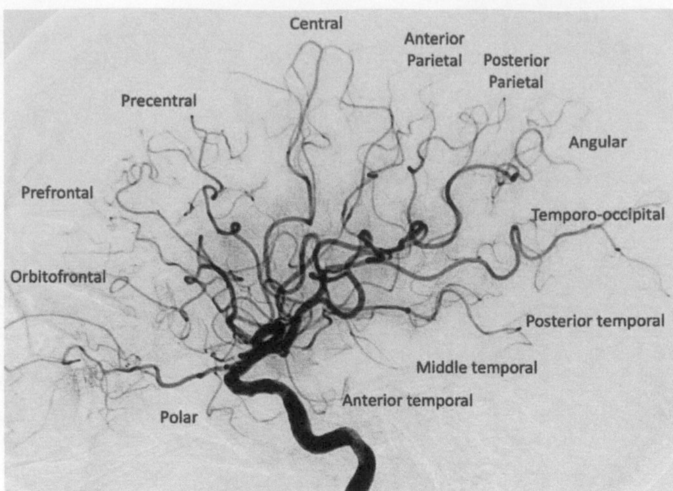

Fig. 16. Lateral internal carotid angiogram in the setting of an aplastic A1 segment of the ipsilateral anterior cerebral artery, highlighting the cortical branches of the middle cerebral artery. Each typical cortical branch of the middle cerebral artery is labeled in clockwise fashion from the ophthalmic artery as follows: the orbitofrontal artery; the prefrontal and precentral arteries or operculofrontal artery if combined (which supplies the pars triangularis and Broca area); the central or Rolandic artery that supplies the primary motor and sensory cortices; the anterior and posterior parietal arteries; the angular artery (with a characteristic posterior bump extending over Heschl gyrus); and the temporal artery group, including posterior, middle, anterior, and polar arteries.

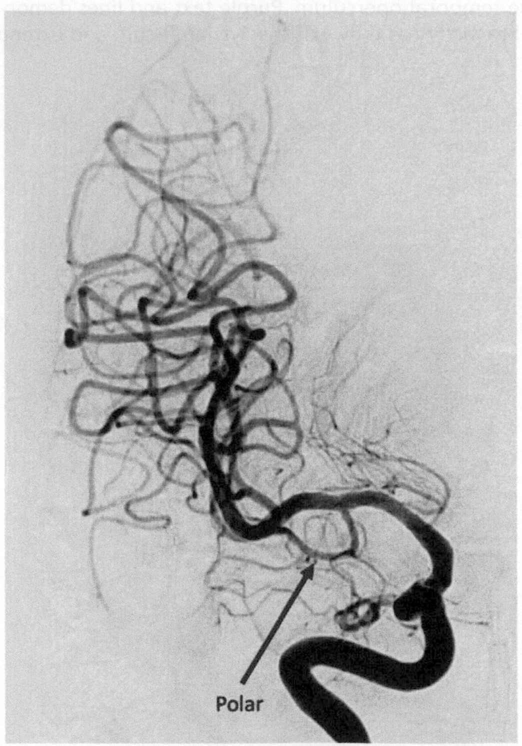

Fig. 17. Anteroposterior right internal carotid angiogram demonstrating the polar artery (*red arrow*) that most frequently arises from the proximal anteroinferior surface of the M1 segment of the middle cerebral artery to supply the anterior temporal pole.

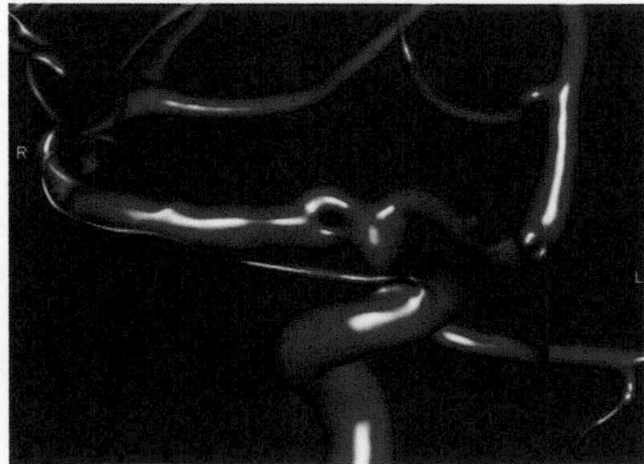

Fig. 18. Three-dimensional reconstruction of a right internal carotid angiogram demonstrating a fenestration of the proximal M1 segment of the right middle cerebral artery.

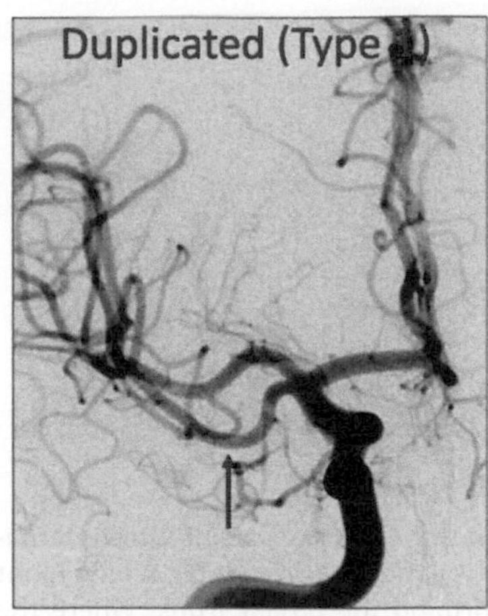

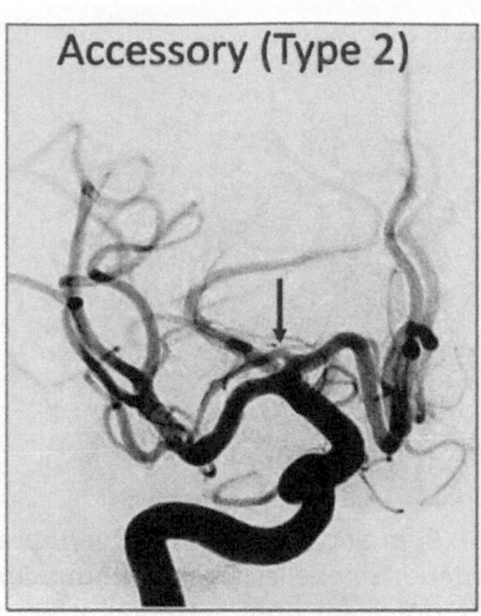

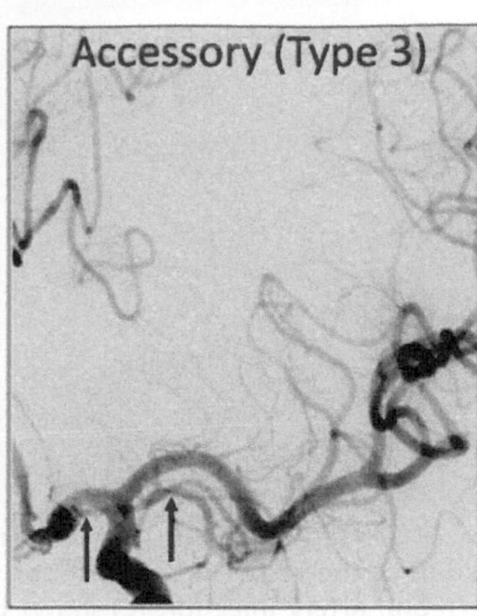

Fig. 19. Three separate anteroposterior internal carotid angiograms demonstrating the 3 Manelfe variants of the middle cerebral artery. (*Left*) A duplicated (type 1) M1 segment of the right middle cerebral artery present (*red arrow*), seen as a large branch proximal to the carotid terminus that includes cortical branches but no lenticulostriate arteries. (*Middle*) An accessory (type 2) right middle cerebral artery (*red arrow*) is seen as a smaller branch arising from the proximal A1 segment of the ipsilateral anterior cerebral artery with a parallel course to the M1 segment of the middle cerebral artery and that includes several small lenticulostriate perforating arteries. (*Right*) An accessory (type 3) left middle cerebral artery is seen as a smaller branch arising from the distal A1 (*red arrows*) with a recurrent course parallel to the ipsilateral middle cerebral artery and that similarly provides supply to multiple lenticulostriate arteries.

of the true M1 segment, and it is differentiated from the true middle cerebral artery by an absence of lenticulostriate arteries. This vessel may seem angiographically similar to an M1 segment with a very short prebifurcation portion, and the distinction is typically of no consequence (**Fig. 19**). Type 2 and type 3 accessory middle cerebral arteries are larger branches that respectively arise

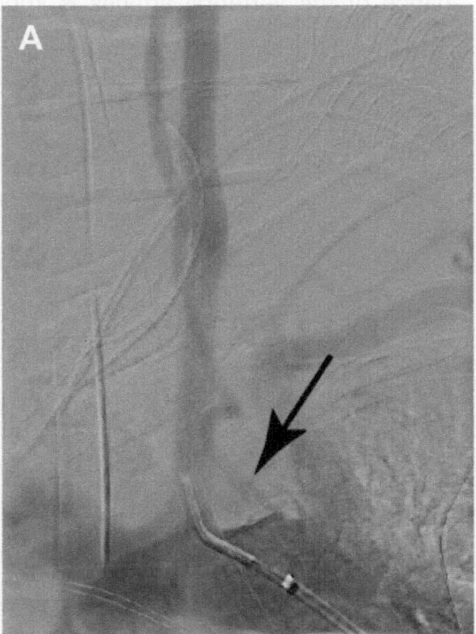

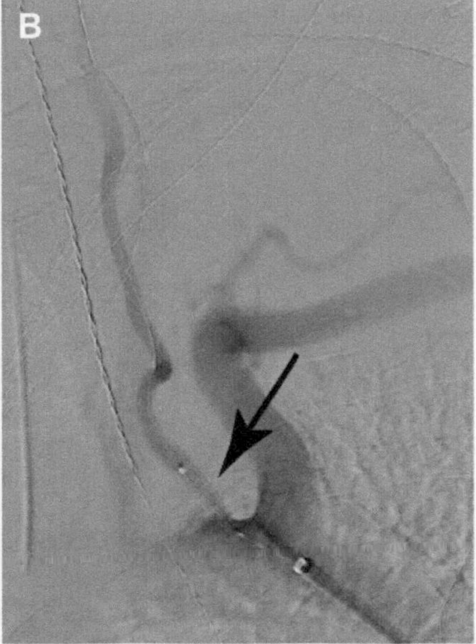

Fig. 20. Oblique anteroposterior projection of left common carotid artery with reflux into the aorta demonstrating origin of the left vertebral artery directly from the aortic arch (*black arrow*) with a flow-limiting vertebral artery origin stenosis (*A*). After angioplasty and stenting of the left vertebral artery origin there is improved contrast opacification of the left vertebral artery, indicating resolution of flow limitation in the vessel (*B*).

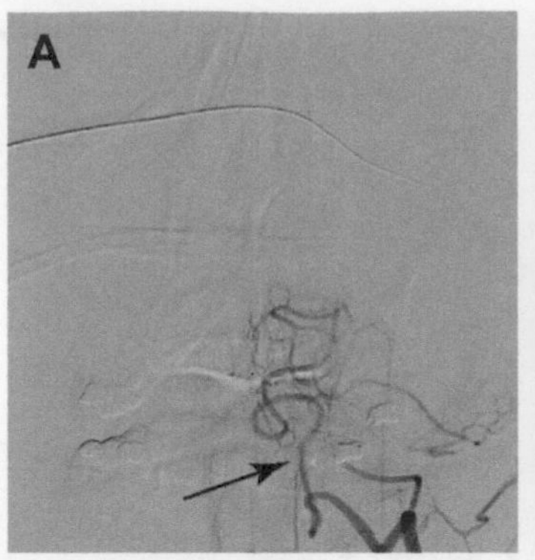

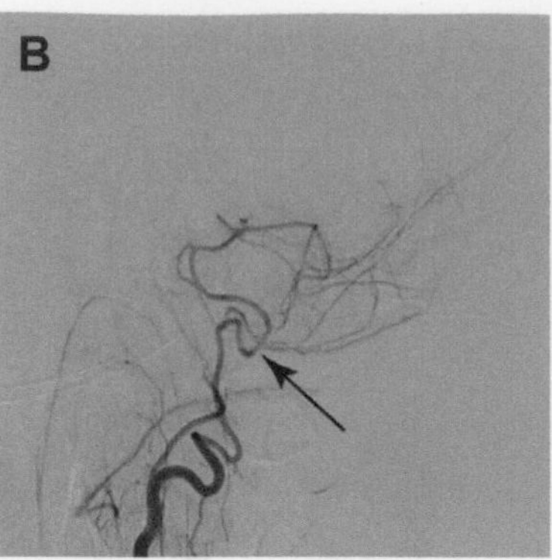

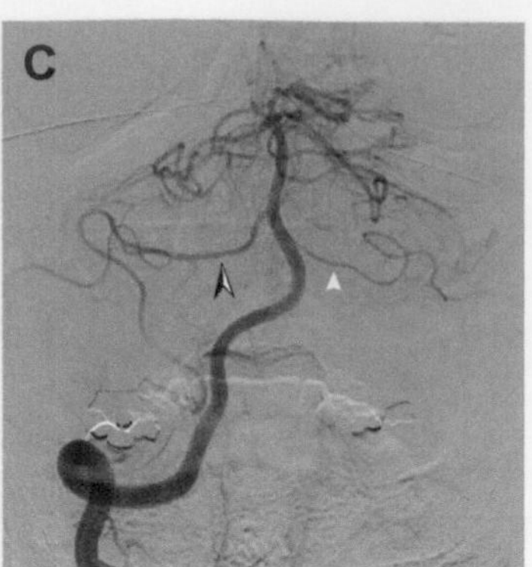

Fig. 21. Anteroposterior (*A*) and lateral (*B*) projections of the left vertebral artery injections demonstrate termination of the vessel in the posterior inferior cerebellar artery without continuation to the basilar artery. Right vertebral artery injection (*C*) shows the dominant right vertebral artery forming the basilar trunk, where the left anterior inferior cerebellar artery originates. The separation of the anterograde flow into the left posterior inferior and left anterior inferior cerebellar arteries demonstrates their relative supply to the inferior cerebellum. In contrast, the right inferior cerebellum is supplied by a single artery from the basilar trunk, termed an anterior inferior cerebellar artery-posterior inferior cerebellar artery complex.

from the proximal or distal A1 segment of the ipsilateral anterior cerebral artery. The accessory middle cerebral arteries supply a variable but typically small portion of the middle cerebral artery territory (see **Fig. 19**).

POSTERIOR CIRCULATION

Vertebrobasilar System

The vertebrobasilar system refers to the vascular territories of the right and left vertebral arteries and the midline basilar artery, and these vessels are the largest vessels of the posterior circulation. The vertebral and basilar arteries supply the craniocervical junction, medulla, pons, midbrain, and cerebellum. The paired vertebral arteries typically originate from the right and left subclavian arteries, but there are common variants such as origination directly from the aortic arch (**Fig. 20**). The left vertebral artery is slightly more likely to be larger or dominant.[1,7] In cases with one strongly dominant vertebral artery, the smaller contralateral vertebral artery may terminate in the posterior inferior cerebellar artery (**Fig. 21**). The relative dominance of the vertebral arteries is important and

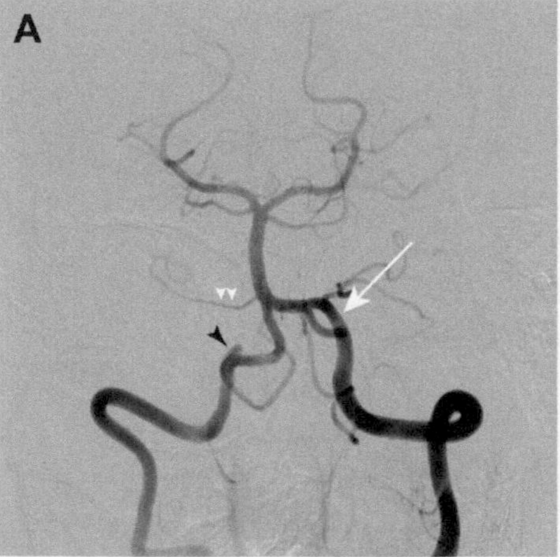

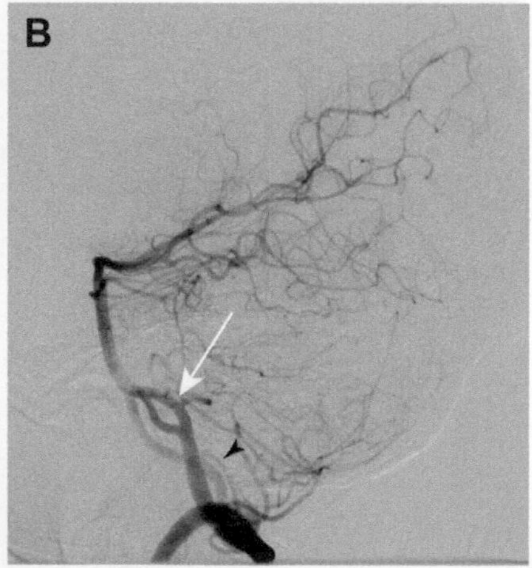

Fig. 22. Left vertebral artery injection, transfacial (*A*) and lateral (*B*) projections, showing a left vertebral artery fenestration within the V4 segment (*white arrow*). The most common origins of the posterior and anterior inferior cerebellar arteries are demonstrated. Reflux down the right vertebral artery shows the right posterior inferior cerebellar artery (black *arrowhead*) originates from the V4 segment, as seen on anteroposterior and lateral projections. The right anterior inferior cerebellar artery (*double white arrowheads*) takes off from the basilar trunk, best appreciated on the anteroposterior view.

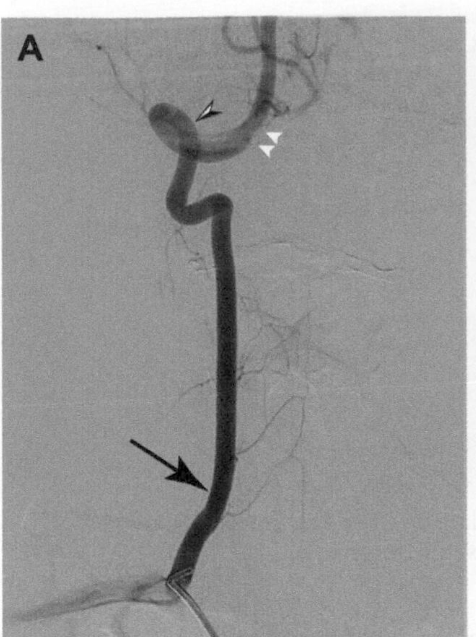

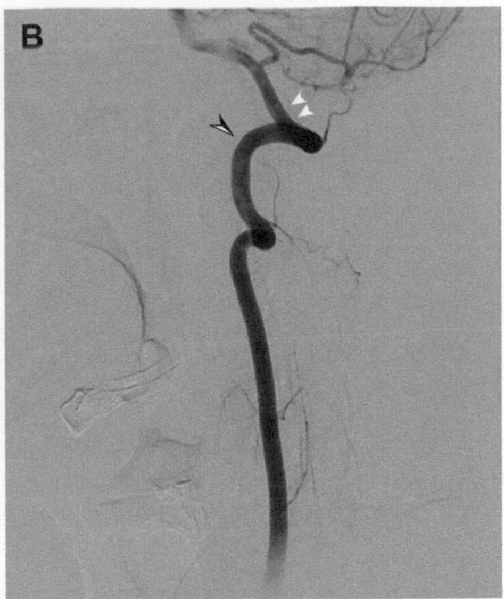

Fig. 23. Right vertebral artery injection, anteroposterior (*A*) and lateral (*B*) cervical views, showing the segments of the right vertebral artery. The V1 segment runs from the origin of the vessel from the right subclavian artery (catheter) to the entry of the artery into the bony foramen transversarium (*black arrow*), beginning the V2 segment. The V3 segment begins as the artery emerges from the transverse process of the atlas (*black and white arrowhead*) and continues until the artery pierces the dura of the posterior fossa (*double white arrowheads*), starting the V4 segment. The V4 segment continues until the pair vertebral arteries converge to form the basilar artery.

may explain patterns of injury or ischemia in the posterior circulation, as well as for planning cranial and spinal interventions. Fenestration of the vertebral arteries is a normal variant in which the artery divides into 2 distinct channels before rejoining back into the same single vessel, resulting in a "window" (fenestration) between the 2 channels (Fig. 22). Duplications, an anatomic variant in which there are distinct origins for an ipsilateral vertebral artery, are quite rare.

The vertebral arteries are divided into 4 anatomic segments, V1 through V4 (Fig. 23). The first vertebral artery segment (V1) begins at the artery origin from the subclavian artery and terminates as the artery enters the foramen transversarium of the cervical spine, usually at the C6 level. There is often an abrupt turn in the vessel just distal to its origin, which should be noted to avoid vessel dissection and injury during angiographic catheterization of the vertebral artery. The V2 segment comprises most of the length of the vertebral artery, and it extends from the foramen transversarium segment (at the C6 level in most patients) until the exit of the artery from the C2 foramen transversarium. The V3 segment continues from this point until the artery pierces the dura of the posterior fossa. Thus, the V3 segment courses posteriorly and medially along the posterior arch of C1, where it creates a groove in the

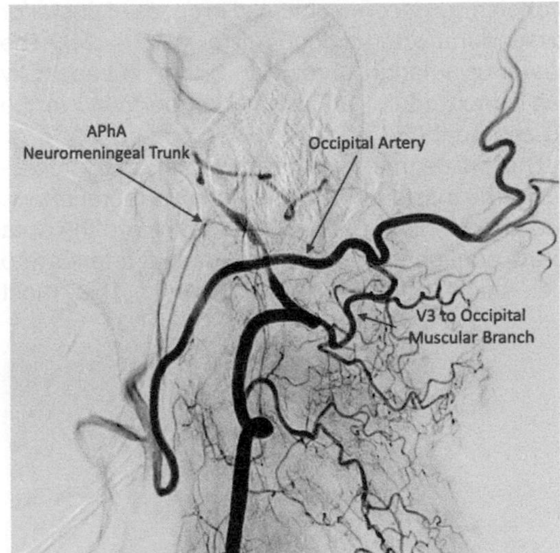

Fig. 24. Lateral left vertebral artery angiogram demonstrating multifocal and tapering critical stenoses of the proximal through distal V4 segments of the left vertebral artery resulting in robust reflux through a large muscular collateral artery to the left occipital artery (*arrows*), with retrograde opacification of the occipital trunk to the proximal external carotid artery. There is additional separate collateral opacification of the hypoglossal division of the neuromeningeal trunk of the ascending pharyngeal artery (*arrow*) through similar small muscular collaterals to the odontoid arcade.

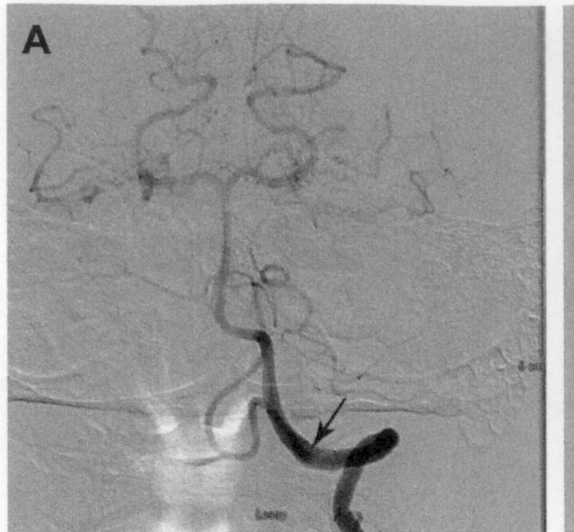

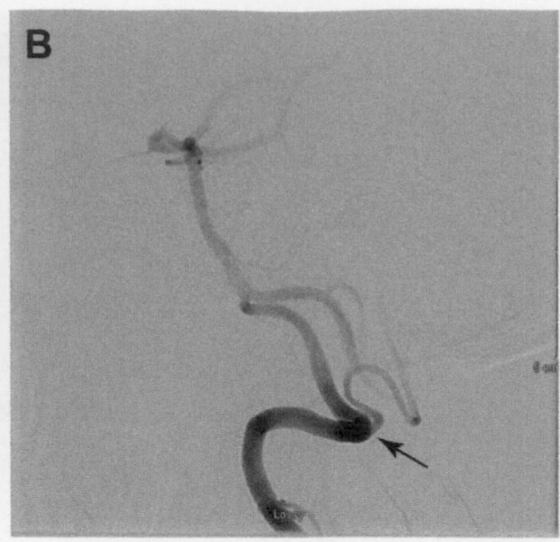

Fig. 25. Left vertebral artery injection, transfacial (*A*) and lateral (*B*) views, demonstrates the origin of the left posterior inferior cerebellar artery from the extradural V3 segment (*arrow*).

bony arch that is termed the sulcus arteriosus. Posterior approaches to the cervicomedullary junction can injure V3 during lateral exposure of the C1 arch. There is typically an extracranial muscular branch that originates from V3, and this branch represents an important potential anastomosis with the occipital artery, with the largest of these collateral branches termed the artery of Salmon or artery of Pendahar. This muscular branch may become enlarged in cases of posterior fossa dural arteriovenous fistulae (Fig. 24). The posterior inferior cerebellar artery occasionally has an extradural origin and can be found in the V3 segment (Fig. 25).

The V4 segment of the vertebral artery represents the intradural portion of the vertebral artery, and it extends from the arterial entry into the dura to the confluence of bilateral vertebral arteries into the single midline basilar artery. The most prominent branch of the V4 segment is the posterior inferior cerebellar artery (Fig. 26). The proximal posterior inferior cerebellar artery lies along the lateral medulla. Small perforating vessels arise from the posterior inferior cerebellar artery that supply the descending tract of the ipsilateral trigeminal nucleus, the spinothalamic tract of the contralateral hemibody, and the ipsilateral nuclei of cranial nerves IX, X, and XII. Injury or infarction of this medullary loop of posterior inferior cerebellar artery results in a lateral medullary or Wallenberg syndrome. The posterior inferior cerebellar artery then continues posteriorly along the medulla and courses superiorly between the cerebellar hemispheres. The distal posterior inferior cerebellar artery courses from medial to lateral along the inferior margin of the ipsilateral cerebellar hemisphere. Common variants of the posterior inferior cerebellar artery include an extradural

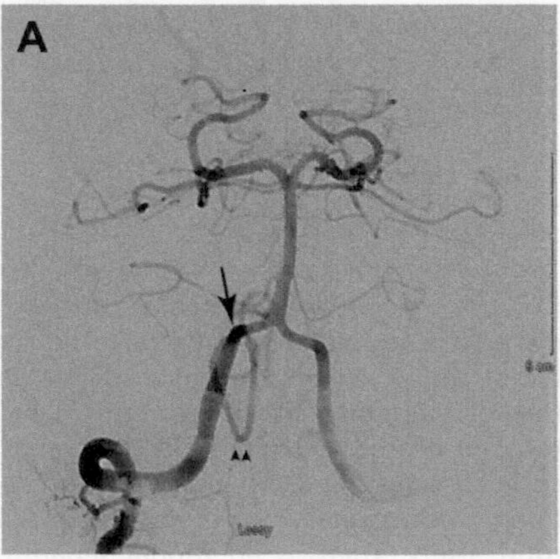

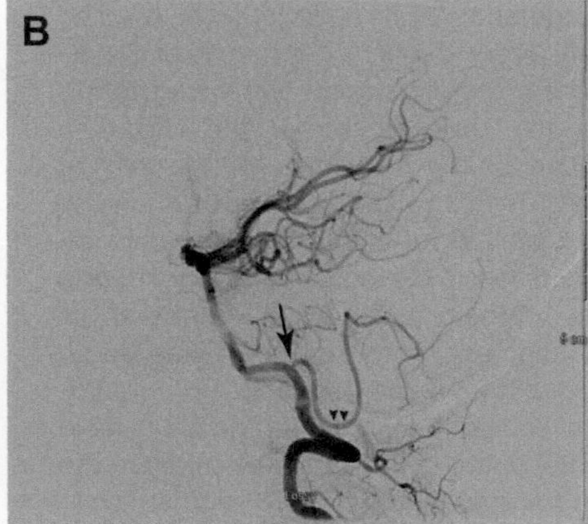

Fig. 26. Left vertebral artery injection, transfacial (*A*) and lateral (*B*) views, shows the classic posterior inferior cerebellar artery course from its origin at the V4 segment (*black arrow*). The artery travels inferiorly along the lateral medulla, then turns upward along the posteromedial medulla, forming a medullary loop (double *arrowheads*).

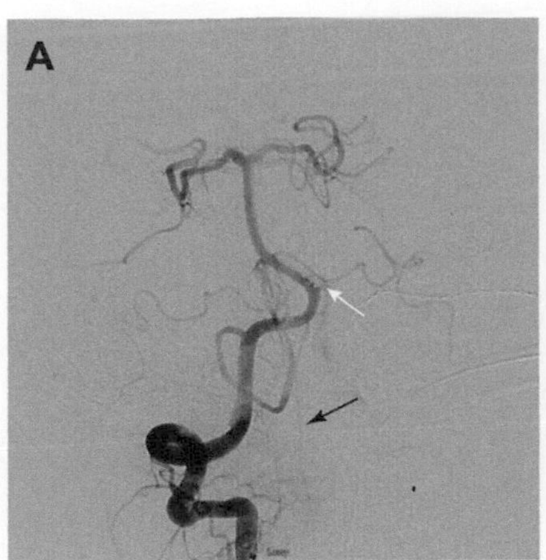

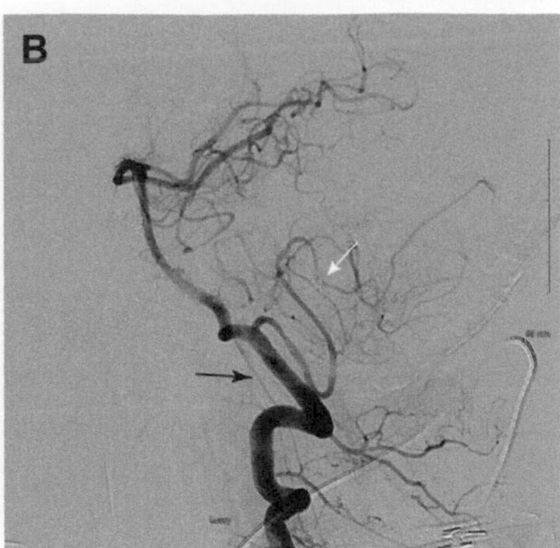

Fig. 27. Right vertebral artery injection, transfacial (*A*) and lateral (*B*) views, demonstrating origin of the anterior spinal artery from the distal V4 segment of the right vertebral artery (*black arrow*). The patient's status postcoiling of a distal right PICA aneurysm (*white arrow*).

(V3) origin, a single origin supplying the bilateral cerebellar hemispheres, and an origin from the posterior meningeal artery. In cases of a hypoplastic vertebral artery, the vertebral artery may terminate in the ipsilateral posterior inferior cerebellar artery without reaching the basilar artery.

The anterior spinal artery is a small artery that commonly arises from the distal V4 segment of the vertebral artery or the vertebrobasilar junction. The anterior spinal artery supplies the anterior two-thirds of the cervical spinal cord and is reinforced inferiorly by radiculomedullary arteries at multiple levels throughout the axis of the spinal cord (Fig. 27). The anterior spinal artery origin can occur on dominant, nondominant, or hypoplastic vertebral arteries ending in posterior inferior cerebellar artery. Failure to preserve this vessel during planned interventions of the distal V4 or vertebrobasilar junction risks anterior spinal cord infarction and resultant quadriplegia. The posterior spinal artery is a separate vessel that supplies a portion of the posterior medulla and is seldom seen on a normal cerebral angiogram, although it may be seen more inferiorly on dedicated spinal angiography. The posterior spinal artery may be more prominent in cases of high-flow arteriovenous shunting lesions or tumors.[2]

The basilar artery is formed by the confluence of the vertebral arteries, and it courses in the midline along the anterior margin of the brainstem. The distal V4 segments and the trunk of the basilar artery give rise to numerous perforating branches, most of which are too small to be appreciated on standard angiography. These are end arteries that supply the midbrain, pons, and medulla, and occlusion of the basilar artery and these perforating vessels may result in brainstem infarction and a catastrophic outcome. The location of the vertebrobasilar junction and basilar apex relative to the midbrain, pons, and medulla is variable and dictates the pattern of perforator vessel origination. Fenestration of the basilar artery is not infrequently encountered, but true duplication of the basilar artery is extremely rare.

The anterior inferior cerebellar artery arises from the midportion of the basilar artery and courses from medial to lateral along the pons and cerebellar convexity to supply the pons and midcerebellum. The inferior two-thirds of the cerebellar hemispheres are supplied by posterior and anterior inferior cerebellar arteries, and there is significant variation in the relative dominance of these 2 arteries, analogous to the variation in the relative supply of the posterior and anterior divisions of the middle cerebral artery to the cerebral hemisphere. In cases where there is a single common trunk supplying the entire territory of the mid-to-inferior cerebellum, the configuration is termed an anterior inferior cerebellar artery—posterior inferior cerebellar artery complex.

The superior cerebellar artery is the last branch of the basilar artery before its termination at the basilar apex. The paired superior cerebellar arteries supply the ipsilateral craniodorsal pons, midbrain, superior cerebellar hemisphere, and the cerebellar vermis (Fig. 28). The superior cerebellar artery courses along the superolateral aspect of the pons toward the quadrigeminal cistern, where it divides into cranial and caudal branches. Duplication of the superior cerebellar arteries is frequently identified, which represents separate origins for the cranial and caudal branches. In distinguishing branches of the superior cerebellar artery from those of the posterior cerebral artery on angiographic views, it is worth noting that the structures supplied by the superior

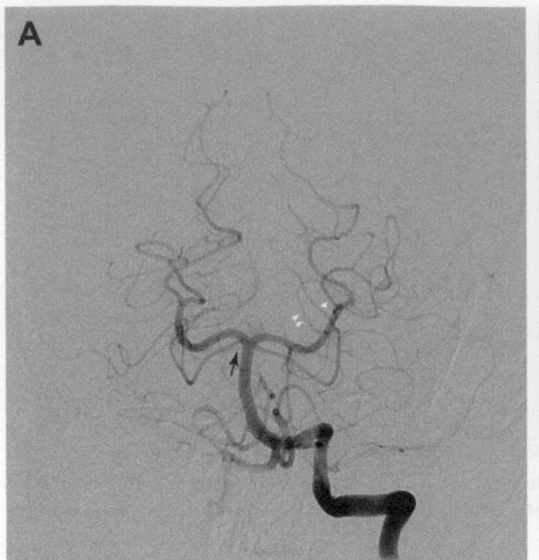

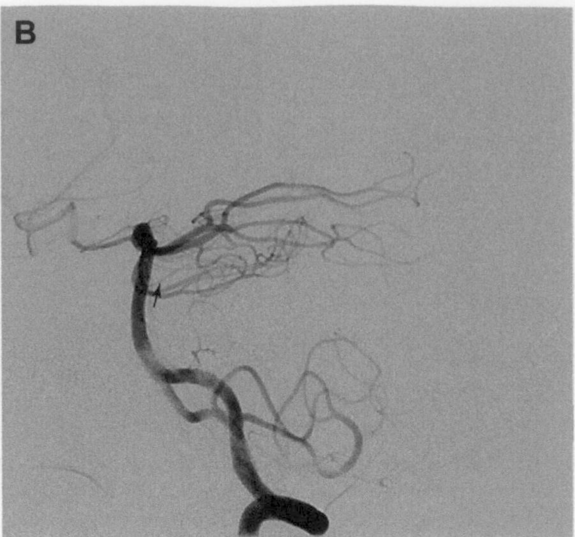

Fig. 28. Left vertebral artery injection, transfacial (*A*) and lateral (*B*) views, shows branching of the left superior cerebellar artery into lateral (*double white arrow*) and medial (*white arrowhead*) on the transfacial view. There is a perforator to the right superior pons and midbrain with origin distinct from the right SCA (*black arrow*).

cerebellar artery are infratentorial and that the tentorium is angled superomedially toward midline.

Posterior Cerebral Artery

The posterior cerebral artery arises from the basilar apex and is divided into 4 segments[1]: the precommunicating P1 segment[2]; the ambient P2 segment[3]; the quadrigeminal P3 segment; and[4] the terminal P4 branches. The P1 segment extends from the basilar apex to the site of anastomosis with the posterior communicating artery within the interpeduncular fossa, and it crosses just superior to the cisternal segment of the third cranial nerve. Aneurysms of the P1 segment are rare, but they may present with a cranial nerve III palsy owing to compression of the nerve by the aneurysm (similar to the presentation of some posterior communicating artery aneurysms). The P2 segment courses posterolaterally around the lateral aspect of the midbrain within the ambient cistern before extending slightly toward midline at the quadrigeminal plate cistern. The P3 segment extends posterosuperiorly along the surface of the quadrigeminal plate, and the terminal P4 branches arborize into the calcarine, parieto-occipital, and splenial branches supplying the distal cortical and subcortical territories (Fig. 29).

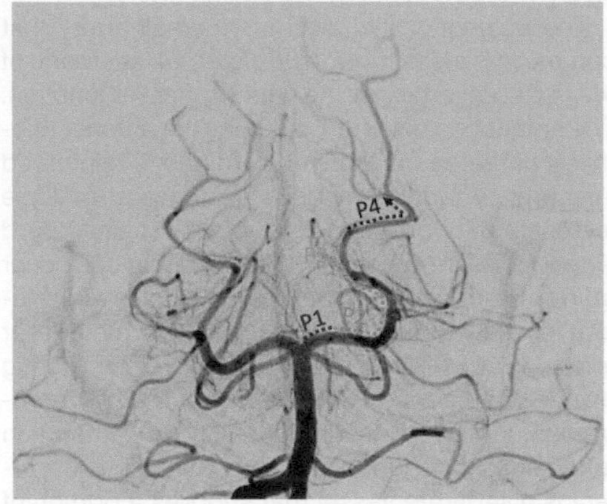

Fig. 29. Anteroposterior magnified Waters projection of a left vertebral artery angiogram demonstrating a normal posterior circulation with annotation of the segmental anatomy of the posterior cerebral arteries. The P1 or precommunicating segment of the posterior cerebral artery (*red hashed line and text*) is seen extending from the basilar apex to the point of inflow from the posterior communicating arteries, which are retrogradely opacified on this image (*orange arrows*). The P2 or ambient segment courses from the posterior communicating artery inflow posterolaterally around the midbrain within the ambient cistern before taking a recurrent inflection and extending superiorly at the origin of the P3 or quadrigeminal segment. The P4 segment of the posterior cerebral artery arises as the P3 segment exits the quadrigeminal cistern and divides into the calcarine, parieto-occipital, and splenial cortical and subcortical branches.

Cortical branches arising from the posterior cerebral arteries begin with the temporal arteries, which typically supply the inferomedial temporal lobe and arise from the P2 segment. These vessels frequently overlap angiographically with branches of the superior cerebellar artery, which makes them difficult to identify on cerebral angiography. The most readily identified cortical branches are the calcarine and parieto-occipital branches that arise from the P4 segment. The calcarine artery is the most medially oriented branch and demonstrates a characteristic lateral hairpin turn where it courses over the cortical surface to supply primary visual cortex in most patients. The parieto-occipital artery courses more laterally within the parieto-occipital fissure and supplies the medial portions of the posterior parietal lobe and the occipital lobe and is a common source of pial collateral supply to the middle cerebral artery territory in cases of arterial steno-occlusive disease. The splenial artery typically arises from the P3 segment of the posterior cerebral artery and takes a medial course over the splenium, where it anastomoses with the splenial branch of the distal pericallosal artery. This anastomosis forms an additional connection between the anterior and posterior circulations that may be important in cases of arterial steno-occlusive disease, such as Moyamoya disease.

There is a rich network of small and variable arteries that arise throughout the course of the posterior cerebral artery to supply portions of the midbrain, the thalamus and choroid plexi, the deep posterior falcotentorial dura, and the occipital lobes (Fig. 30). The collicular arteries arise from the distal P1 or proximal P2 segments of the posterior cerebral arteries and take a parallel course around the midbrain to supply the posterolateral midbrain and the colliculi. The artery of Davidoff and Schechter is a meningeal branch that arises from the distal P1 or proximal P2 segment of the posterior cerebral artery and is usually too small to be seen at angiography in patients without arteriovenous shunting diseases, and this vessel courses posteriorly within the ambient cistern deep to the posterior cerebral artery to the junction of the tentorium with the falx to supply the deep falcotentorial dura. In the setting of hypervascular falcotentorial tumors or posterior dural arteriovenous fistulae, this artery is frequently enlarged (Fig. 31).

The arterial supply to the thalamus is similarly intricate and arises from small perforating vessels of the posterior circulation. There are 4 major categories of arteries that supply distinct thalamic territories. First, the tuberothalamic arteries (anterior thalamoperforators) arise from the posterior communicating arteries and supply the anterior thalamus. Second, the paramedian thalamoperforators arise from the P1 segment and supply the anteromedial midbrain and medial thalamus. Third, the thalamogeniculate arteries arise from the P2 (or rarely the P3) segment and supply the lateral thalamus and posterior limb of the internal capsule. Last, the medial and lateral posterior choroidal arteries typically arise from the P2 segment and supply the respective medial and lateral portions of the posterior thalamus and the pulvinar and portions of the posterior limb of the internal capsule (Fig. 32). Classic thalamic infarct

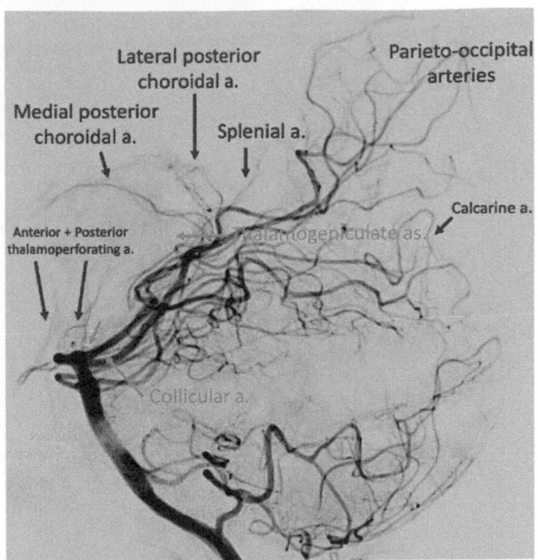

Fig. 30. Lateral magnified left vertebral artery angiogram demonstrating the major cortical and subcortical branches of the posterior cerebral artery, listed from image left to right as follows: the anterior thalamoperforating arteries (or tuberothalamic arteries; *red arrows and text*) arise from the posterior communicating arteries (*orange arrow and text*) and supply the anterior thalamus. The posterior or paramedian thalamoperforating arteries (*red arrows and text*) arise from the P1 segment of the posterior cerebral artery and predominantly supply the medial thalamus. The quadrigeminal or collicular arteries (*green arrows and text*) arise from the P1 or proximal P2 segment of the posterior cerebral artery course around the midbrain and provide posterolateral midbrain and collicular perforator supply. The thalamogeniculate arteries (*green arrows and text*) arise from the P2 segment of the posterior cerebral artery and are a small group of arteries that are faintly opacified on this angiographic image and provide arterial supply to the lateral thalamus. The medial and lateral posterior choroidal arteries (*red arrows and text*) arise from the P2 segment of the posterior cerebral artery and provide supply to the posteromedial and posterolateral thalamus, respectively, and the medial posterior choroidal arteries are typically angiographically recognizable by their more "S" shaped course. The parieto-occipital arteries are distal P4 branches of the posterior cerebral artery and supply the posterior parietal lobe and the occipital lobe, whereas the calcarine artery (*red arrows and text*) is an additional P4 branch that demonstrates a characteristic hairpin turn on the lateral projection and supplies primary visual cortex.

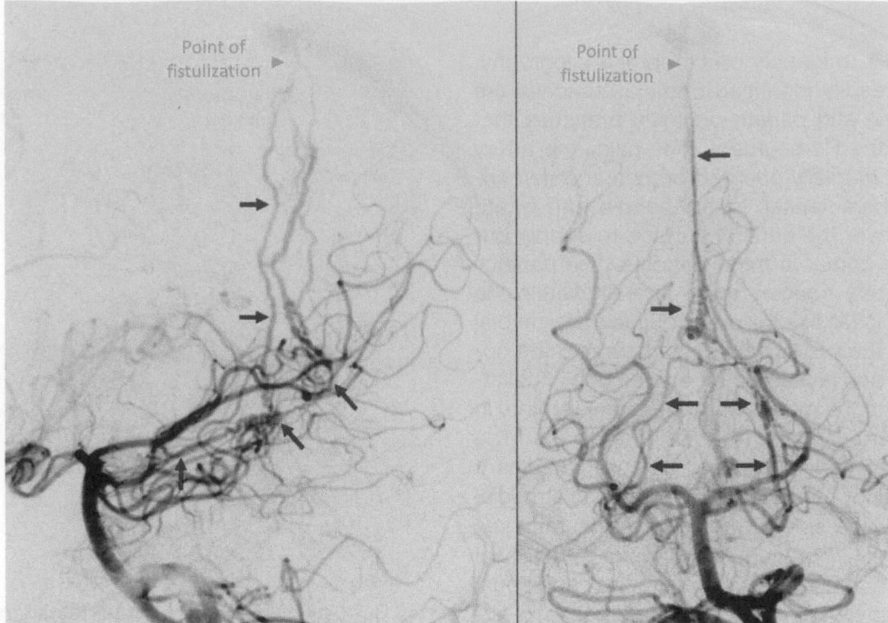

Fig. 31. Lateral and anteroposterior left vertebral artery angiograms demonstrating a Cognard grade 1 falcotentorial dural arteriovenous fistula supplied by tortuous and hypertrophied left greater than right arteries of Davidoff and Schechter (*red arrows*) that arise from the P2 segments of the posterior cerebral artery. These arteries course toward midline at the falcotentorial junction before extending superiorly toward the point of fistulization (*blue arrowheads*) at the superior sagittal sinus.

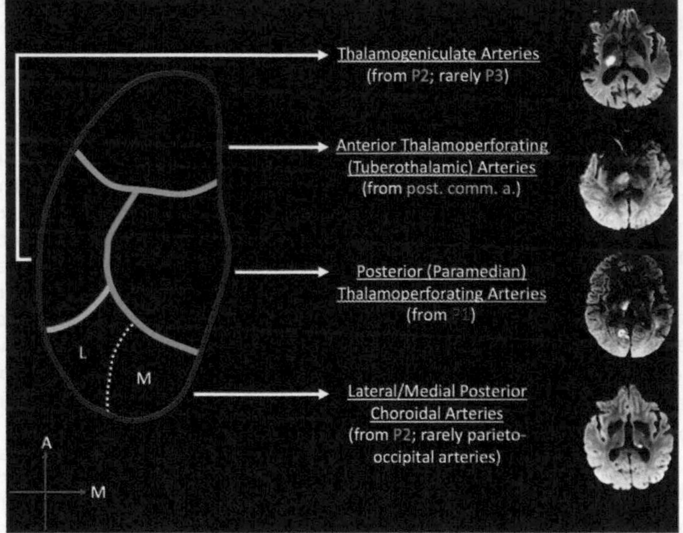

Fig. 32. The arterial supply to the thalamus with example axial DWI images through the thalamus of classic infarct patterns seen following occlusion of each supplying artery. The anterior thalamus is supplied by the anterior thalamoperforating or tuberothalamic arteries, which arise from the posterior communicating arteries. Anterior thalamic infarcts cause a syndrome of fluctuating consciousness, apathy, disorientation, abulia, and perseveration. The thalamogeniculate arteries, which typically arise from the P2 or P3 segments of the posterior cerebral artery, provide supply to the lateral thalamus. Infarction of the lateral thalamus causes a lateral thalamic syndrome of Dejerine-Roussy, defined as a homonymous hemianopsia, a contralateral sensory deficit with hyperesthesia, and contralateral hypotonic hemiplegia with ataxia. The posterior paramedian thalamoperforators arise from the P1 segment of the posterior cerebral artery and supply the medial thalamus. Unilateral infarction of the medial thalamus may cause a syndrome of confabulatory amnesia, asterixis, and aphasia. The lateral and medial posterior choroidal arteries supply the posterior thalamus and arise from the P2 segment of the posterior cerebral artery, with infarcts of the medial posterior thalamus resulting in aphasia, hand weakness, and dystonia and infarcts of the lateral thalamus causing a hemi- or quadrantanopsia. Note that only a lateral posterior thalamic infarct pattern is pictured.

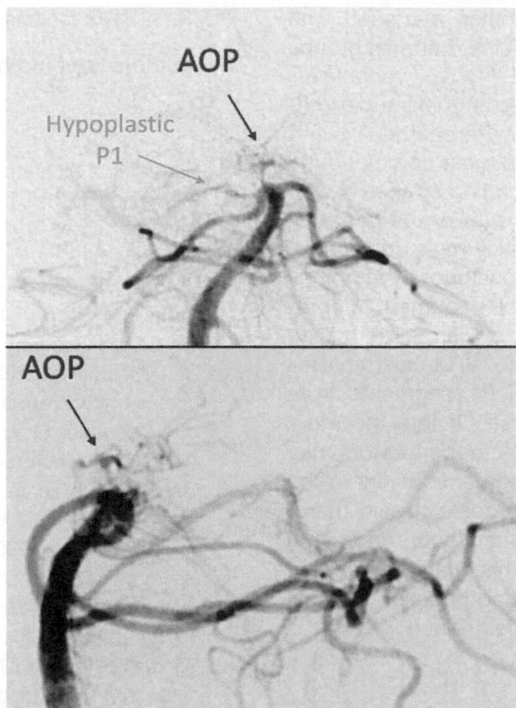

Fig. 33. Anteroposterior (*top*) and lateral (*bottom*) magnified left vertebral artery angiograms demonstrating a prominent artery of Percheron (*red arrow*, AOP) arising from the junction of the basilar tip with a hypoplastic P1 segment (*blue arrow*) of the right posterior cerebral artery, with perforator arborization through the bilateral medial thalamic nuclei.

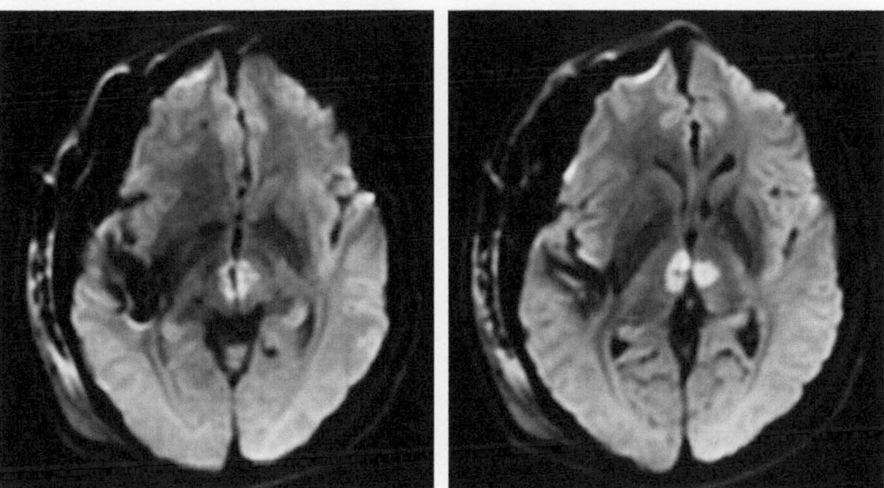

Fig. 34. Axial DWI images through the thalamus demonstrating a classic artery of Percheron infarct pattern with diffusion restriction in the bilateral medial thalami and the medial rostral midbrain. Infarcts of this territory cause a classic triad of altered mental status, vertical gaze palsy, and memory impairment. Note susceptibility artifact over the right hemisphere and within the right scalp related to prior right pterional craniotomy with small underlying subdural fluid and gas causing mass effect on the right hemisphere.

patterns and clinical syndromes are seen with injury or occlusion of each of the 4 arterial groups supplying the thalamus (see Fig. 32).[10] Variable origins of the posterior paramedian thalamoperforators have been described by Percheron[11,12] in 4 patterns, with the classic and most common type of paired equal thalamoperforating arteries arising from the ipsilateral P1 segments of the posterior cerebral arteries. However, they have additionally been described as separate posterior thalamoperforators arising from a single P1 segment, a common trunk termed the artery of Percheron arising from a single P1 segment (Fig. 33) or an arterial arcade spanning the bilateral P1 segments from which the perforators may arise. Of note, the artery of Percheron or posterior thalamoperforators may arise from hypoplastic P1 segments. Injury to the artery of Percheron demonstrates a classic infarct of the bilateral medial thalami and the rostral midbrain, and patients with this infarction present with a classic clinical triad of obtundation, vertical gaze palsy, and memory impairment (Fig. 34).[13]

SUMMARY

The arterial supply to the brain is complex, variable, and elegant. An understanding of how the arterial anatomy relates to the underlying brain parenchyma is essential for a more complete understanding of cerebrovascular disease and its consequences.

CLINICS CARE POINTS

- Segmental anatomy of the intracranial arteries is anatomically defined by the course and location of the vessel, not by branch order and location, which can demonstrate considerable variability.
- Named cortical branches of each major intracranial artery are variable but follow general territorial supply patterns, and knowledge of these general rules are critical for safe endovascular and surgical arterial manipulation.
- Variant arterial anatomy is common and is frequently owing to remnant embryonic arteries or incomplete regression of fetal arteries, which additionally form the basis of a rich network of anastomotic pathways between multiple circulations.

DISCLOSURE

The authors have nothing to disclose.

REFERENCES

1. Peris-Celda MM, Francisco S, Rhoton Albert L. Rhoton's atlas of head, Neck, and brain. 1st edition. Stuttgart, New York, Delhi, Rio: Thieme Verlagsgruppe; 2018.
2. Bradac GB, Boccardi E. Applied cerebral angiography. 3rd edition. Cham, Switzerland: Springer-Verlag GmbH Germany; 2017.
3. Heit JJ, Ball RL, Telischak NA, et al. Patient Outcomes and Cerebral Infarction after Ruptured Anterior Communicating Artery Aneurysm Treatment. AJNR Am J Neuroradiol 2017;38(11):2119–25.
4. Osborn AG, Jacobs JM. Diagnostic cerebral angiography. 2nd edition. Philadelphia: Lippincott Williams & Wilkins; 1999. p. 1999.
5. Perlmutter D, Rhoton AL Jr. Microsurgical anatomy of the distal anterior cerebral artery. J Neurosurg 1978;49(2):204–28.
6.. Morris PP. Practical Neuroangiography. 2nd edition. New York: Lippincott Williams & Wilkins, Wolters Kluwer; 2007.
7. Lasjaunias P, Berenstein A, ter Brugge KG. Surgical Neuroangiography. New York: Spring-Verlag Berlin Heidelberg; 2001. p. 789.
8. Wolman DN, Iv M, Wintermark M, et al. Can diffusion- and perfusion-weighted imaging alone accurately triage anterior circulation acute ischemic stroke patients to endovascular therapy? J Neurointerv Surg 2018;10:1132–6.
9. Komiyama M, Nakajima H, Nishikawa M, et al. Middle cerebral artery variations: duplicated and accessory arteries. AJNR Am J Neuroradiol 1998;19(1): 45–9.
10. Schmahmann JD. Vascular syndromes of the thalamus. Stroke 2003;34(9):2264–78.
11. Percheron G. [Arteries of the human thalamus. II. Arteries and paramedian thalamic territory of the communicating basilar artery]. Rev Neurol (Paris) 1976;132(5):309–24.
12. Percheron G. [Arteries of the human thalamus. I. Artery and polar thalamic territory of the posterior communicating artery]. Rev Neurol (Paris) 1976; 132(5):297–307.
13. Lazzaro NA, Wright B, Castillo M, et al. Artery of percheron infarction: imaging patterns and clinical spectrum. AJNR Am J Neuroradiol 2010;31(7): 1283–9.

Anatomy of Intracranial Veins

Michiya Kubo, MD, PhD[a,b], Naoya Kuwayama, MD, PhD[b,c], Tarik F. Massoud, MD, PhD[d], Lotfi Hacein-Bey, MD[e,*]

KEYWORDS

• Veins • Cerebral • Dural sinuses • Deep venous system • Emissary veins

KEY POINTS

- The cranial venous system is complex and extensive.
- Familiarity with cerebral embryology helps understand cerebral venous anatomy.
- Significant redundancy exists regarding cerebral venous pathways.
- Several pathophysiological processes may result from alterations in cerebral venous integrity.

INTRODUCTION

The intracranial venous system drains the cerebrum, brainstem, eyes, meninges, and part of the face. In addition, the cerebrospinal fluid (CSF), which is reabsorbed in part by the arachnoid granulations, is returned to the bloodstream via the cerebral dural sinuses that drain extracranially into the internal jugular veins primarily.[1,2] Therefore, the integrity of the cerebral venous system plays a crucial role in brain homeostasis by eliminating metabolic waste and deoxygenated blood, and contributes directly to the healthy perfusion of cerebral tissue.

Unlike dural sinuses that are contained by the 2 dural layers (periosteal and meningeal), cerebral veins are valveless and have thin walls that do not contain muscular tissue. While cortical veins are mostly located within the subarachnoid space, deep medullary and transmedullary veins lie within the cerebral white matter and its contained CSF spaces.[3] Intracranial veins are primarily categorized as superficial or deep. Superficial venous structures mainly include the superior sagittal sinus and the cortical veins, with major superficial interconnecting anastomosing veins, that is, the veins of Trolard and Labbé. The deep venous system drains primarily into the paired internal cerebral veins and the basal veins of Rosenthal, which join into the midline vein of Galen and drain into the straight sinus, then the transverse and sigmoid sinuses, and eventually into the internal jugular veins. Although considered separately in some textbooks, the veins of the posterior fossa are intimately related to the remainder of the cerebral venous system, and are also generally categorized as superficial and deep veins of the cerebellum and the brainstem. The general arrangement of the cerebral venous system is overall established and predictable; however, numerous variations exist, some of which can lead to clinical consequences.

Embryology of the Cerebral Venous System

Most of the current understanding of human brain embryology may be derived from the works of George Linius Streeter and Dorcas Hager Padget

[a] Department of Neurosurgery, Stroke Center, Saiseikai Toyama Hospital, 33-1 Kusunoki, Toyama 931-8533, Japan; [b] Department of Neurosurgery, University of Toyama, 3190 Gofuku, Toyama 930-8555, Japan; [c] Toyama Red Cross Hospital, 2 Chome-1-58 Ushijimahonmachi, Toyama 930-0859, Japan; [d] Division of Neuroimaging and Neurointervention, Department of Radiology, Stanford University School of Medicine, Center for Academic Medicine, Radiology, MC: 5659, 453 Quarry Road, Palo Alto, CA 94304, USA; [e] Division of Neuroradiology, Radiology Department, University of California, Davis Medical School of Medicine, 4860 Y Street, Sacramento, CA 95817, USA
* Corresponding author.
E-mail address: lhaceinbey@yahoo.com

Neuroimag Clin N Am 32 (2022) 637–661
https://doi.org/10.1016/j.nic.2022.05.002
1052-5149/22/

who studied large numbers of human embryos ranging in size between 4 mm and 80 mm at the Carnegie Institution of Washington, in Washington, DC and in Baltimore, MD (at the Johns Hopkins Carnegie department of Embryology). Between 1917 and 1940, Streeter, a physician, and anatomist, directed the department of Embryology at the Carnegie Institution of Washington. Later, Padget, who started her career as a medical illustrator in Walter Dandy's Neurosurgery department at Johns Hopkins University, Baltimore, became a scientific researcher at the Carnegie Institution whereby she made remarkable contributions.[4] The enormous work of those 2 pioneers laid the ground for modern embryologic concepts of cerebral vasculature (and many cerebrovascular anomalies).

The first identifiable cerebral venous structure is the primary head vein (Fig. 1), identified in the early embryo (5–8 mm) as a cephalad continuation of the cardinal vein (the anterior portion of which will become the internal jugular vein), which consists of a single layer of endothelial cells.[5] The head vein (the combination of the vena capitis medialis, the vena capitis lateralis and the posttrigeminal vein) gives rise to a continuous primitive meningeal venous plexus that drains the brain through three stems (anterior, middle and posterior).[6] The ventral pharyngeal vein (the sole ventral projection of the head vein) later gives rise to the primitive maxillary vein, which lies medial to the primitive trigeminal ganglion and later contributes to the cavernous sinus (Fig. 2).

Around the 11 to 14 mm stage, lateral dural sinuses develop, which drain the brain through primitive pia-arachnoid vessels as the mesenchyme around the brain gives off the lateral and basal dural coverings and the chondrocranium at the skull base (see Fig. 2). The anterior and middle venous plexi merge to form the embryonic "tentorial plexus" while the posterior plexus becomes the occipital plexus. The choroid plexus then develops fast—faster than the cortical mantle—and drains first into the inferior choroidal vein, then into the superior choroidal vein after the primitive internal cerebral vein develops in relation to small midline thalamus. Later, the thalami become paired, as do both internal cerebral veins, which then fuse posteriorly to form the vein of Galen and the straight sinus.

By the 17 to 20 mm stage, posterior (sigmoid, tentorial, and marginal) sinuses are formed (Fig. 3), while the 2 anterior components of the primitive venous plexus start to involute and form the pro-otic sinus (a stem of the middle dural plexus that connects to the posterior plexus via the sigmoid sinus).[5,7,8]

At the 40 mm stage, the cavernous sinuses form as medial extensions of the pro-otic sinus, which is continuous with the inferior petrosal sinus;

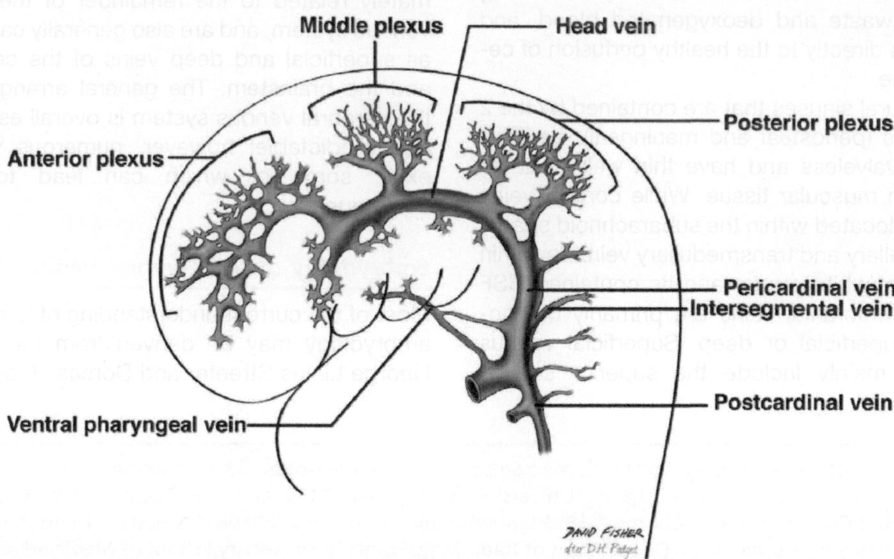

Fig. 1. Dural venous sinus development at day 28, approximately 4–6 mm. The head vein, the cephalad continuation of the cardinal vein, gives rise to a continuous venous plexus of the meninges, which drains all portions of the head. The anterior plexus relates to the diencephalon and mesencephalon, the middle plexus is related to the cerebellum and the posterior plexus is related to the occipital and upper neck regions. (*From* McBain L, Goren O, Tubbs RS. The Embryology of the Dural Venous Sinus: An Overview (Chapter 1), Anatomy, Imaging and Surgery of the Intracranial Dural Venous Sinuses. 2020, Pages 1-7.)

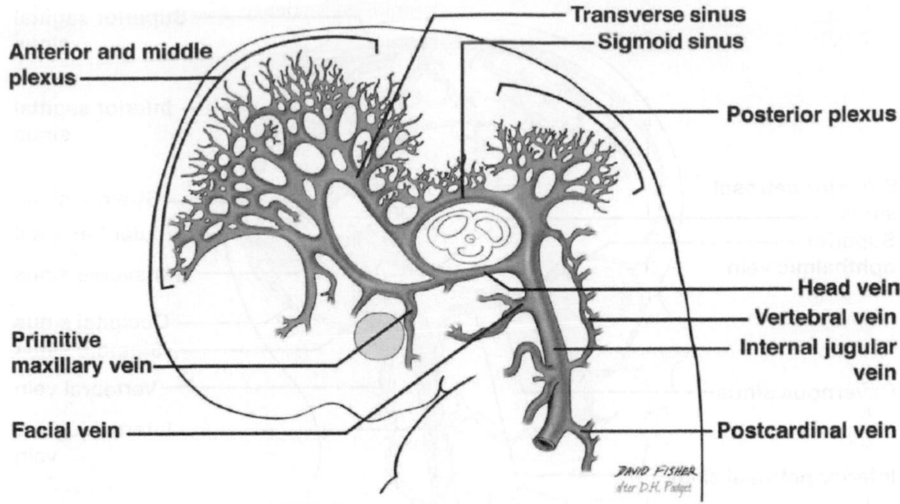

Fig. 2. In the 18 mm embryo, the middle and posterior plexi merge, resulting in forming the sigmoid sinuses posteriorly. The cerebellum and posterior midbrain drain into the posterior plexus. The cavernous sinuses and the pro-otic sinus start forming from the middle plexus. The drainage of the cavernous sinus is through a stalk of the middle plexus, which will give rise to the superior petrosal sinus. (*From* McBain L, Goren O, Tubbs RS. The Embryology of the Dural Venous Sinus: An Overview (Chapter 1), Anatomy, Imaging and Surgery of the Intracranial Dural Venous Sinuses. 2020, Pages 1-7.)

laterally, the pro-otic sinus anastomoses with a primitive temporal emissary vein to form the petrosquamous sinus. By the 60 to 80 mm embryonic stage, the superior and inferior sagittal sinuses are formed, while posterior (sigmoid, transverse, tentorial) sinuses move backward to their permanent configuration (Fig. 4). The otic capsule promotes the development of the superior petrosal sinus, while the pro-otic sinus remains continuous with the petrosquamous sinus.[7,8] Laterally, the petrosquamous sinus and pro-otic sinus remnants are later destined to involute as diploic veins that drain

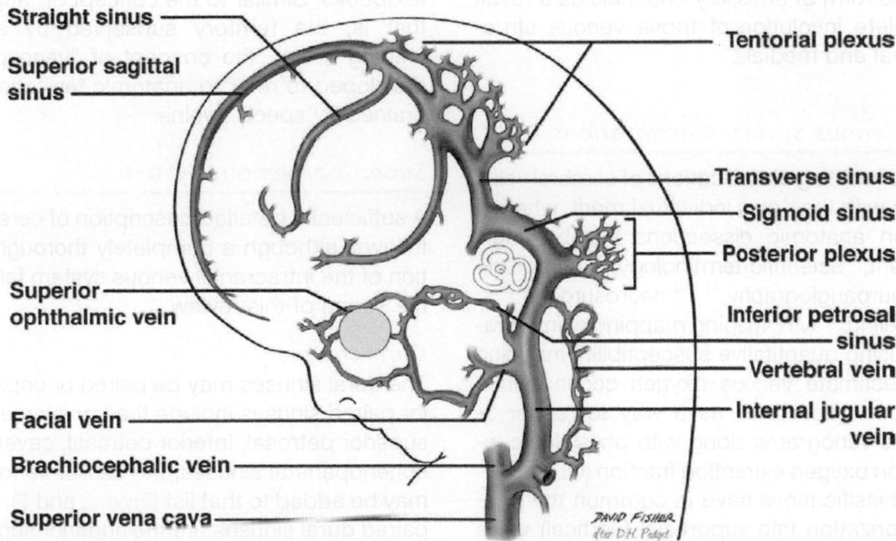

Fig. 3. In the 50 mm embryo, major supratentorial dural sinuses are formed. The growth of the cerebellum promotes the readjustment of the tentorial plexus and the neighboring superior petrosal sinus and posterior fossa veins. The dura mater becomes separated into 2 layers with intervening areolar tissue from which meningeal vessels form. (*From* McBain L, Goren O, Tubbs RS. The Embryology of the Dural Venous Sinus: An Overview (Chapter 1), Anatomy, Imaging and Surgery of the Intracranial Dural Venous Sinuses. 2020, Pages 1-7.)

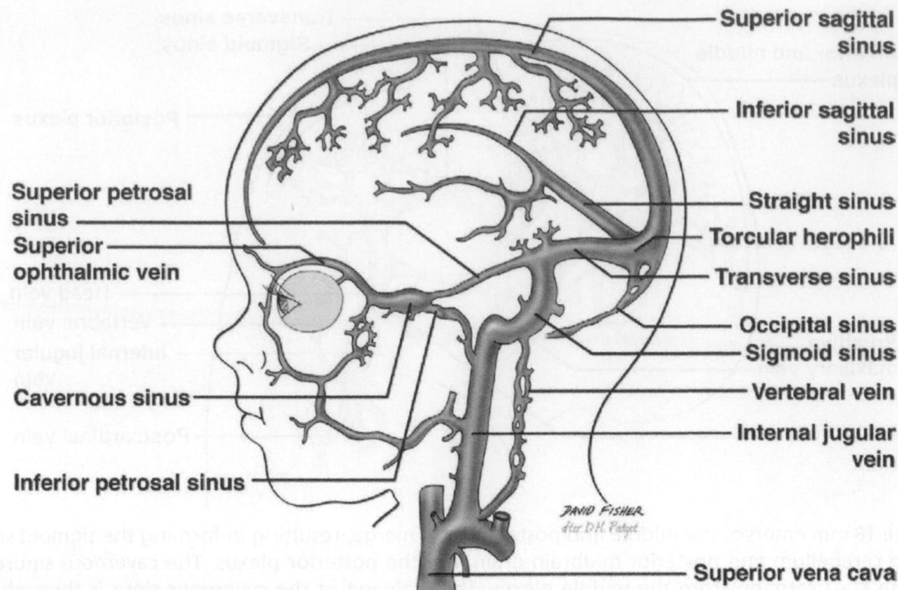

Fig. 4. In the 80 mm embryo (16th–20th weeks), the dural sinuses are formed. The torcular Herophili forms from a remnant of the embryonic tentorial plexus to connect the medial extensions of both transverse sinuses to the superior sagittal sinus. The deep venous (Galenic) system develops to increasingly drain the diencephalons instead of the primitive tentorial sinus. The cortical vein network is gradually formed. Of note, the superior and inferior anastomotic veins (veins of Trolard and Labbe) form beyond 3 months, as they are not primary venous structures. (*From* McBain L, Goren O, Tubbs RS. The Embryology of the Dural Venous Sinus: An Overview (Chapter 1), Anatomy, Imaging and Surgery of the Intracranial Dural Venous Sinuses. 2020, Pages 1-7.)

meningeal structures via the foramen ovale. Medially, the primitive tentorial sinus also involutes after the superior petrosal sinus has formed and is connected to the cavernous sinus.[5,7,8] Variations may occur in the form of emissary channels as a result of incomplete involution of those venous structures, lateral and medial.

Cerebral Venous System Classifications

A number of existing classifications of cerebral veins exist, each with their own individual merit, whether focused on anatomic dissections,[9] embryologic development,[7] scientific terminology,[10] neuroradiology,[11] neuroangiography,[12–14] neurosurgery,[15–19] or 3D modeling.[20] MR imaging mapping of intracranial veins using quantitative susceptibility mapping (QSM) to estimate venous oxygen concentration has also been described as a way to render 3-dimensional venograms along with physiologic information on oxygen extraction fraction (OEF).[21]

Those classifications have in common the general categorization into superficial (cortical) veins and dural sinuses, deep veins, and posterior fossa veins. The emissary veins and the diploic venous system, not commonly mentioned in most classifications, also have clinical and physiologic significance.

Considerable variations in cerebral venous anatomy exist between individuals, and between cerebral hemispheres within the same individuals. In addition, anatomic descriptions vary between textbooks. Similar to the concept of “angiosome,” that is, the territory subserved by a specific feeding artery, the concept of “venosome” was developed to refer to anatomic territories that are drained by specific veins.[22]

Superficial Venous System

A sufficiently detailed description of cerebral veins follows, although a completely thorough description of the intracranial venous system falls beyond the scope of this review.

Dural sinuses

The dural sinuses may be paired or unpaired. Major paired sinuses include the transverse, sigmoid, superior petrosal, inferior petrosal, cavernous and sphenoparietal sinuses; the basilar venous plexus may be added to that list (**Figs. 5** and **6**). Major unpaired dural sinuses are the superior sagittal sinus (SSS), the inferior sagittal sinus (ISS), the straight sinus, the occipital sinus, and the intercavernous sinus (**Fig. 7**). The dural sinuses are also discussed elsewhere in this issue (see Morris, et al), and Joseph and colleagues have provided a detailed

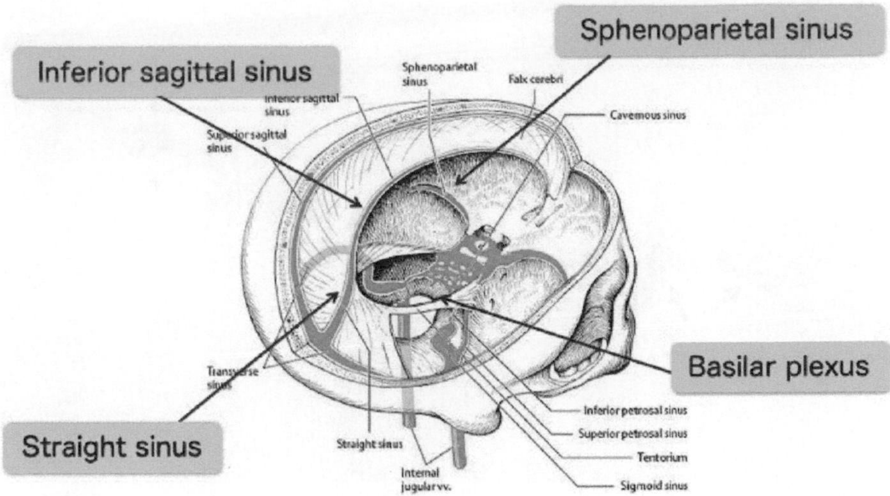

Fig. 5. Major dural sinuses. The superior and inferior sagittal sinuses run at the upper and lower edges of the falx cerebri. The cavernous sinuses are connected in the midline via intercavernous channels and connect laterally to the sphenoparietal sinuses. Note the basilar plexus lies on top of the clivus and connects posteriorly to the superior petrosal sinuses.

discussion of anatomic variants of the dural sinuses.[23]

The cavernous sinus receives blood from the superior and inferior ophthalmic veins, the sphenoparietal sinus, and the superficial middle cerebral vein (MCV). Numerous midline intercavernous communications are present normally (see Fig. 7). The cavernous sinus communicates posteriorly with the transverse/sigmoid sinus junction via the superior petrosal sinus, and inferiorly through the inferior petrosal sinus, which drains the auditory canal veins and ends in the internal jugular vein (IJV).

In case of sinus occlusion, numerous anastomotic channels may become functional to facilitate venous drainage (Fig. 8).

Superficial cerebral veins

Cortical veins drain the superficial subterritory of the brain which is supplied by cortical arteries and their perforating distal rami outside of the internal border zone that separates the deep cerebral territory, supplied by perforating lenticulostriate arteries.[24] Large eponymous anastomotic veins (veins of Trolard and Labbé) drain into the superficial middle cerebral vein (MCV), which

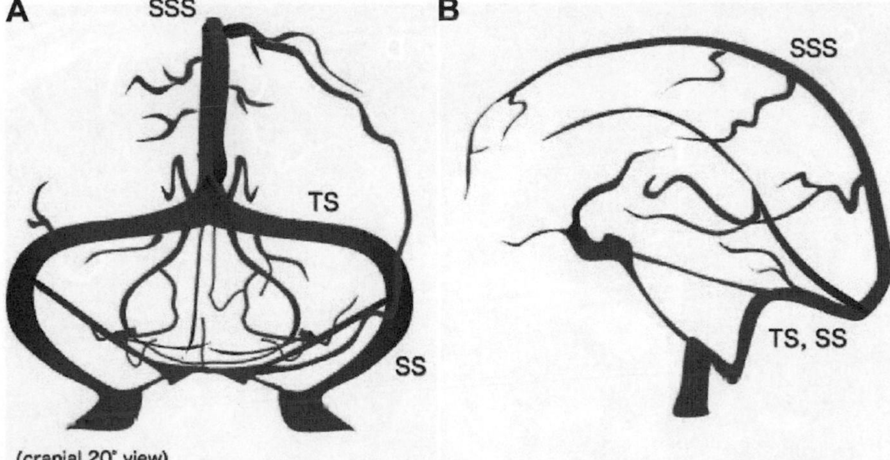

Fig. 6. Major dural sinuses anteroposterior (*A*) and lateral (*B*) views: the superior sagittal sinus (SSS) is midline, unpaired, and drains most of the blood of both hemispheres; the paired transverse (TS) and sigmoid (SS) sinuses drain cerebral venous blood into the paired internal jugular veins.

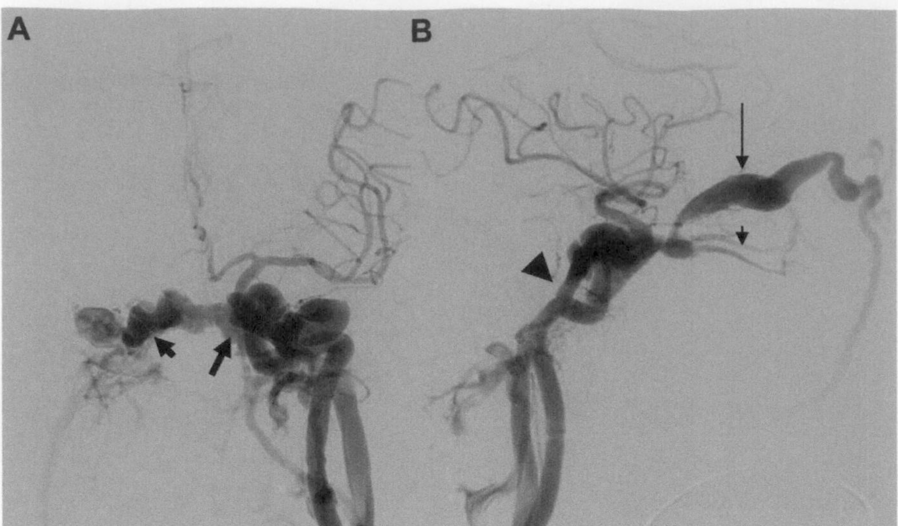

Fig. 7. (*A*, *B*) Early angiographic opacification of both cavernous sinuses in a patient with a carotid-cavernous fistula. Left internal carotid artery angiogram, antero-posterior view (*A*) shows early venous filling of the left cavernous sinus (*A*, *long thick arrow*) with near-immediate filling of the right cavernous sinus (*A*, short *thick arrow*) through midline intercavernous anastomoses. Lateral view of left carotid angiogram, early arterial view shows early filling of a massively dilated superior ophthalmic vein (*B*, *long thin arrow*) and duplicated inferior ophthalmic veins (*B*, *short thin arrow*), and dilated inferior petrosal sinus (*B*, *large arrowhead*).

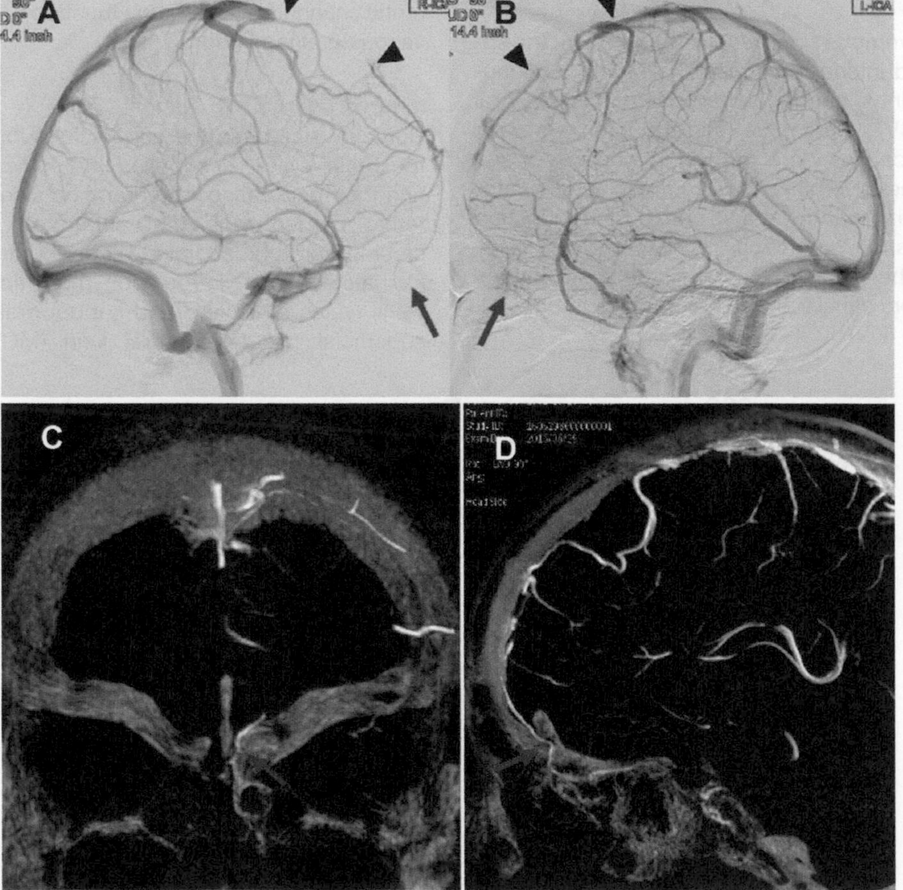

Fig. 8. (*A–D*) Superior sagittal sinus occlusion noted on the venous phase of right (*A*) and left (*B*) internal carotid artery angiograms (*blue arrowheads*); a small anterior skull base vein (*orange arrows*) is noted. CTA, coronal (*C*), and parasagittal (*D*) reconstructed images allow to characterize a bridging vein of the cribriform plate (*orange arrows*).

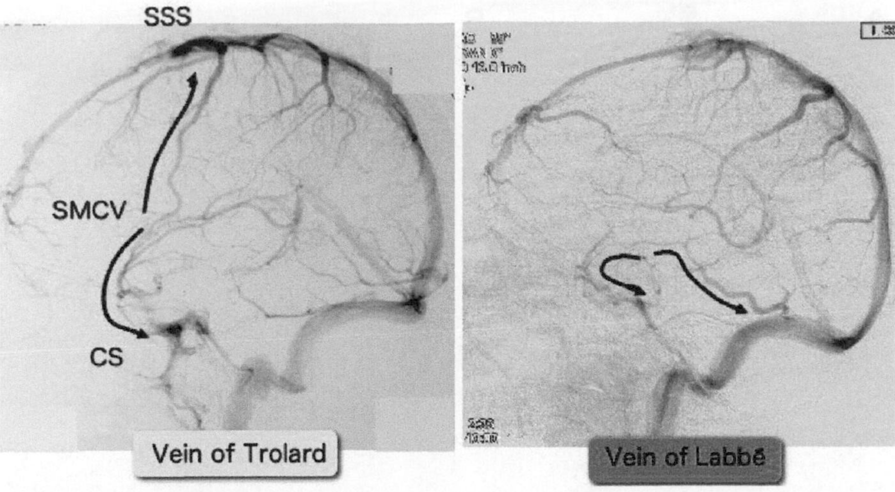

Fig. 9. (*A, B*) Lateral views of carotid artery angiograms, venous phase, show cortical veins and major anastomotic veins. The vein of Trolard (*A*) connects the superior sagittal sinus (SSS) to the superficial middle cerebral vein (SMCV) which eventually drains into the cavernous sinus (CS). The vein of Labbé (*B*) connects the posterior aspect of the SMCV to the sigmoid sinus.

drains into the cavernous sinus (Fig. 9). The vein of Labbé may originate from the posterior aspect of the MCV (Fig. 10).

All other hemispheric cortical veins are organized as several groups of cortical bridging veins that are fed by multiple small superficial veins of the surface of the medial and lateral surfaces of the frontal, parietal and occipital lobes, which eventually drain into the SSS at an acute angle[25] and with some degree of tortuosity (Fig. 11).[26] Large veins that course within the subarachnoid space are superficial to companion arteries, while subpial veins run under their corresponding arteries.[27] Although identical in terms of structure and function, cortical veins have been differentiated by Padget into a mediodorsal group that drains into the superior and inferior sagittal sinuses, and a posteroinferior and lateroventral group that drains into the transverse and cavernous sinuses.[7] Cortical veins are valveless, have thin walls with a minimal muscular layer and course through the subarachnoid space and the meningeal dural layer to reach dural sinuses (see Figs. 9–11).[25–27] Because of their thin walls and relationship to dural sinuses, large cortical veins may collapse when the intracranial pressure is elevated, leading to ischemia. Sadighi and colleagues have provided a detailed discussion of anatomic variants of the cerebral veins.[28]

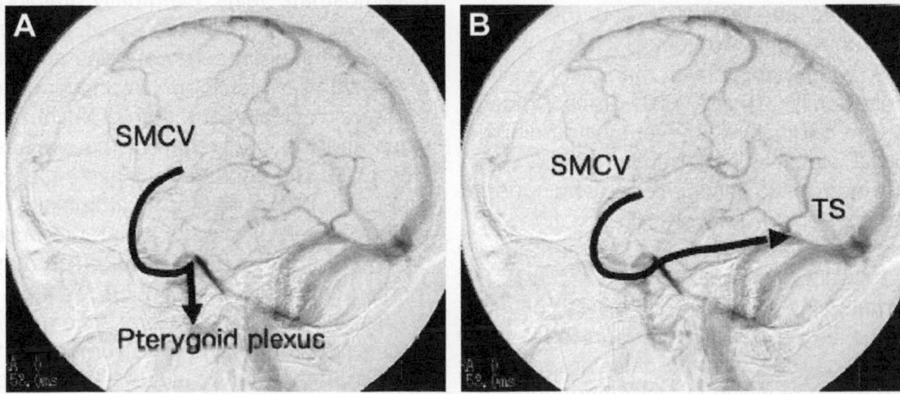

Fig. 10. (*A, B*) Lateral views of carotid artery angiograms, venous phase, show cortical veins. Alternate routes of SMCV extracranial drainage are seen whereby the SMCV drains inferiorly into the pterygoid plexus in a sphenobasal pattern (*A, blue arrow*), and whereby the SMCV drains posteriorly into the transverse sinus in a sphenopetrosal pattern (*B, blue arrow*).

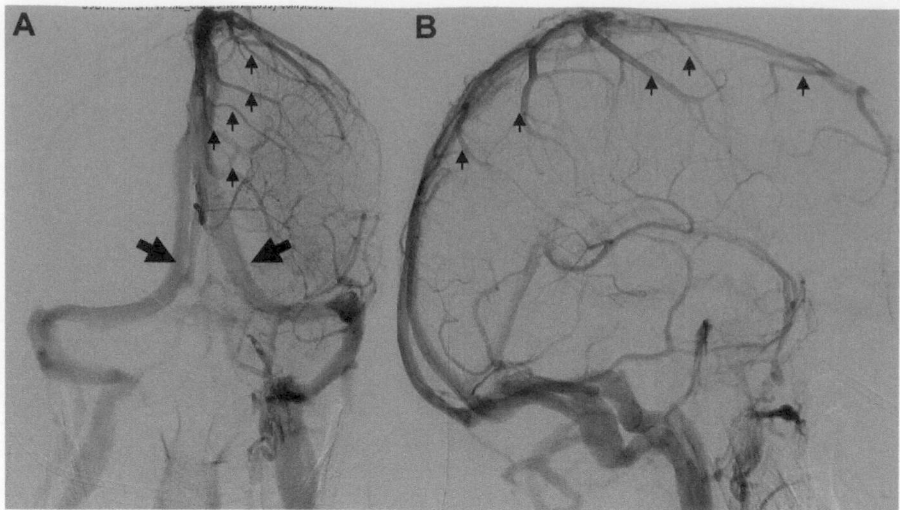

Fig. 11. (*A, B*) Cortical veins. Left internal carotid artery angiogram, anteroposterior (*A*) and lateral (*B*) views, late venous phase, show cortical veins draining into the superior sagittal sinus at an acute angle (*small arrows*). Note a duplicated posterior aspect of the superior sagittal sinus (*large arrows*). An incidental right mastoid emissary vein is also present.

Deep Venous System

In the early embryo, the venous drainage of deep cerebral structures is exclusively centrifugal in the direction of the maturing encephalon. Such deep drainage is via medullary veins, which have long been identified and well described by Duret in 1874.[29] As the diencephalon, telencephalon, and the ventricular system gradually develop, centripetal venous flow toward the increasingly structured deep venous system starts to develop (**Fig. 12**).[30] This leads to the dual configuration of a deep cerebral venous system which drains deep gray matter and deep and periventricular white matter blood through medullary veins in a centripetal fashion toward the subependymal veins, the internal cerebral veins and the basal vein of Rosenthal, then the vein of Galen, while venous flow within superficial medullary veins moves centrifugally toward pial (transcortical) veins, then into cortical veins, eventually draining into the dural sinuses. Importantly, connecting channels are interposed between deep and superficial medullary venous networks in the form of anastomotic medullary veins and transcerebral veins (**Fig. 13**).[31] Deep medullary veins may reach subependymal veins either directly or via collecting veins,[32] the largest and most recognized being the longitudinal caudate vein of Schlesinger,[33] the embryologic origin of which is the subependymal glial substance of the germinal matrix; this vein is continuous in the fetal brain and may remain so in the adult brain (**Fig. 14**).

The general arrangement of medullary veins, although related to deep perforating arteries, appears to primarily follow the organization of white matter tracts in their various directions, whether commissural, association, or projection fibers.[34]

Medullary vein flow disposition has clinical implications: for instance, various patterns of cerebral venous thrombosis, particularly in neonates and children result from this anatomic arrangement, especially as transmedullary venous flow remains bidirectional in infants (see **Fig. 13**).[35]

The main venous collector of the deep venous system is the vein of Galen, which may be likened to a "hub." Medullary veins radiate from the internal border zone to drain into subdependymal and thalamostriate veins, eventually draining via the 2 main components of the deep venous system: the paired internal cerebral veins and basal veins of Rosenthal, which join in a confluence at the level of the vein of Galen and then drain into the straight sinus and the confluence of the sinuses (torcular Herophili). The deep venous system also includes tributaries of the inferior sagittal sinus. Medullary veins may serve as major collaterals in case of occlusion of a major deep vein, which may result in marked enlargement (**Fig. 15**).

A - The internal cerebral vein (ICV) courses through the roof of the third ventricle in the velum interpositum. The ICV is a marker of midline shift, such that a deviation from the midline of 2 mm or more is considered abnormal.

The internal cerebral veins and their tributaries constitute the transcerebral venous system which

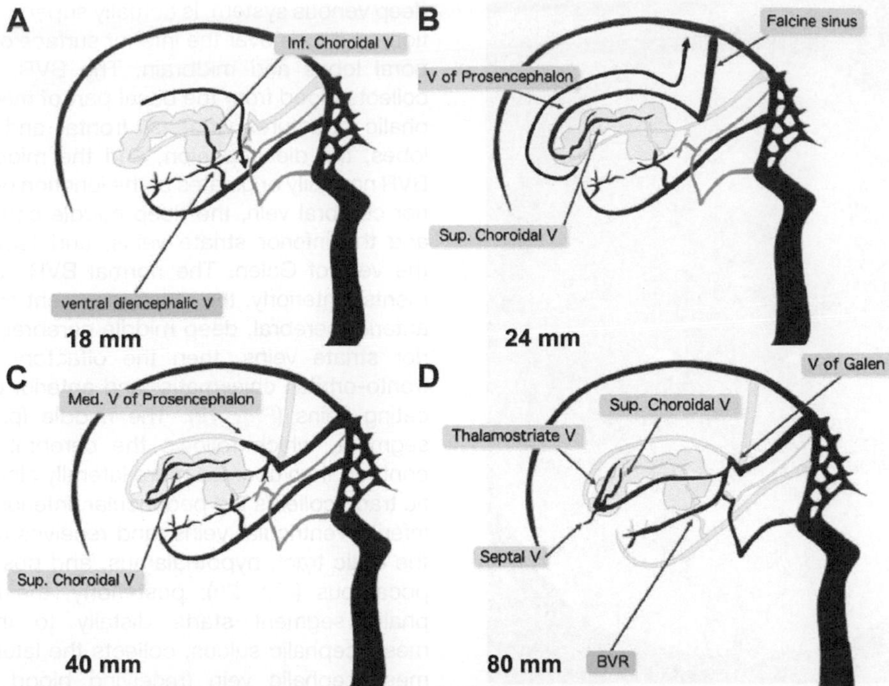

Fig. 12. (*A–D*) Embryologic development of the deep venous system. (*A*): in the 18 mm embryo, the ventral diencephalic vein and the inferior chroroidal vein drain into the tentorial sinus; (*B*): 24 mm embryo: superior choroidal vein continues as a vein of prosencephalon, drains into falcine sinus, while the tentorial sinus continues to drain diencephalic structures; (*C*): 40 mm embryo: regression of the vein of the prosencephalon, leaving the medial vein of the prosencephalon (vein of Markowski) which continues as falcine sinus; (*D*): 80 mm embryo: final configuration: septal and thalamostriate veins, and basal vein of Rosenthal are formed, join the vein of Galen and drain into the straight sinus; at this stage, both the falcine and tentorial sinuses should have regressed.

may be divided into 3 groups, the medial and lateral subependymal venous groups, and the choroidal and thalamo-callosal group. The medial subependymal group collects the septal, posterior septal, and medial atrial veins (Fig. 16), the lateral subependymal group collects the anterior caudate, longitudinal caudate (vein of Schlesinger), thalamostriate, transverse caudate, direct lateral, terminal, and the inferior ventricular veins (Fig. 17). Lastly, the choroidal and calloso-lateral

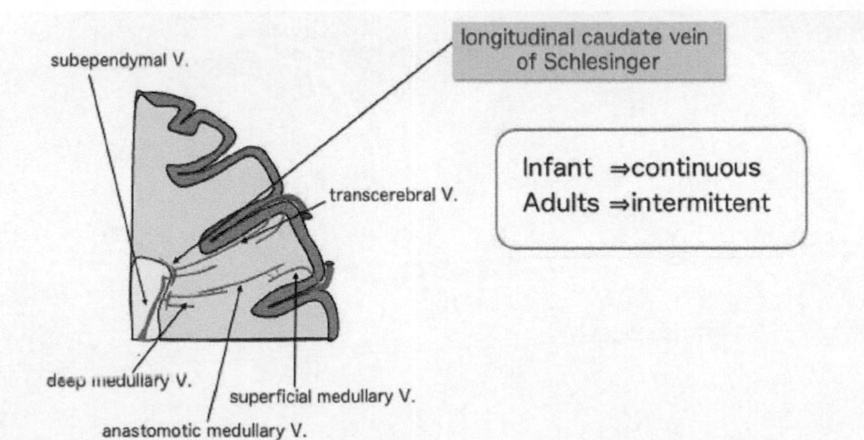

Fig. 13. Transcerebral venous system. Deep medullary and superficial medullary veins are connected by anastomotic medullary veins. Deep veins drain medially into subependymal (ventricular veins) while superficial veins drain into intracortical (transcerebral) veins. Note the longitudinal caudate vein of Schlesinger.

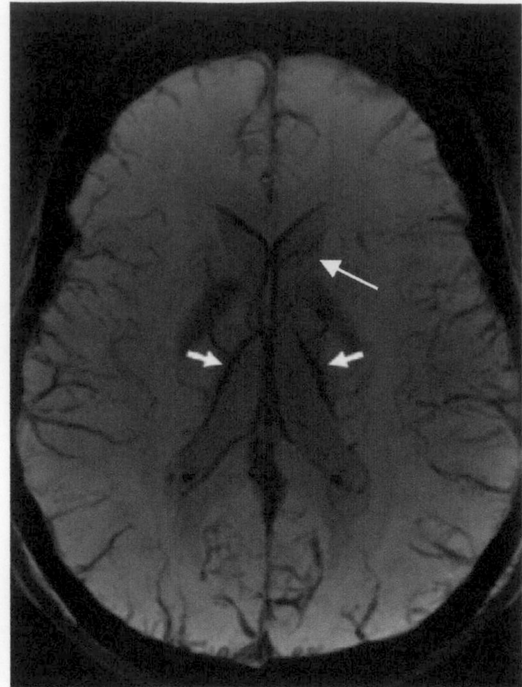

Fig. 14. Axial MR imaging SWAN MinIP (minimum intensity projection) shows dilated deep veins. Direct lateral veins (*short arrows*) and longitudinal caudate vein of Schlesinger (*thin long arrow*).

group collects the superior, inferior medial choroidal, third ventricular choroidal, direct lateral atrial, common atrial, superior thalamic, habenular, and the posterior pericallosal veins (Fig. 18).

B - The basal vein of Rosenthal (BVR), although considered one of the main components of the deep venous system, is actually superficial in location, as it runs over the inferior surface of the temporal lobes and midbrain. The BVR, therefore, collects blood from the basal part of medial encephalic structures, that is, frontal and temporal lobes, the diencephalon, and the midbrain. The BVR normally originates at the junction of the anterior cerebral vein, the deep middle cerebral vein, and the inferior striate veins, and terminates in the vein of Galen. The normal BVR has 3 segments: anteriorly, the striate segment collects the anterior cerebral, deep middle cerebral, and inferior striate veins, then the olfactory, posterior fronto-orbital, chiasmatic, and anterior communicating veins (Fig. 19). The middle (peduncular) segment, which follows the cerebral peduncle contour, then courses more laterally along the optic tract, collects the peduncular, inferior thalamic, inferior ventricular veins, and receives twigs from the optic tract, hypothalamus, and posterior hippocampus (Fig. 20); posteriorly, the mesencephalic segment starts distally to the lateral mesencephalic sulcus, collects the lateral pontomesencephalic vein (receiving blood from the anterior pontomesencephalic vein and the precentral cerebellar vein), tributaries from the atrial vein, the inferior temporo-occipital vein, then courses superiorly and posteriorly before joining to the ICV into the vein of Galen (Fig. 21). Although originally described in 1824 by the German anatomist Friedrich-Christian Rosenthal as a constant vein that terminates consistently into the vein of Galen,[14] it may occasionally be absent in case of incomplete regression of the tentorial sinus (Fig. 22),[36] and it has also been reported to drain into the superior petrosal sinus.[37]

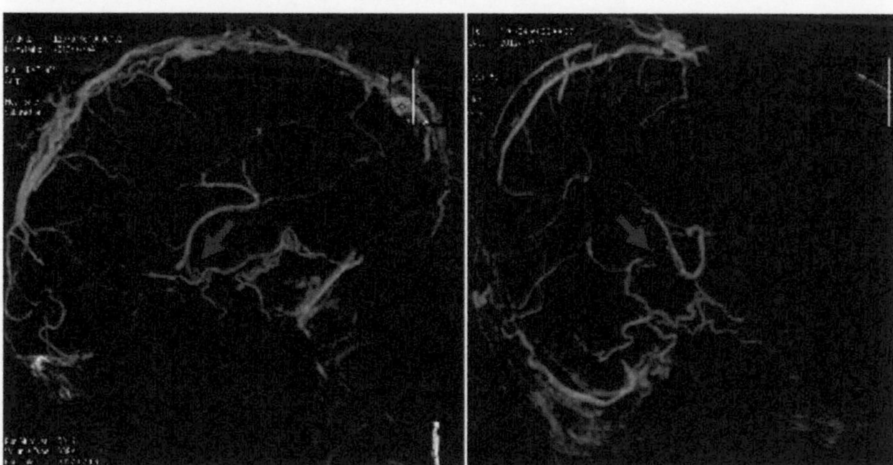

Fig. 15. Patient with an occluded Galenic system: deep venous drainage is via transcerebral veins into markedly dilated deep medullary veins (*red arrows*).

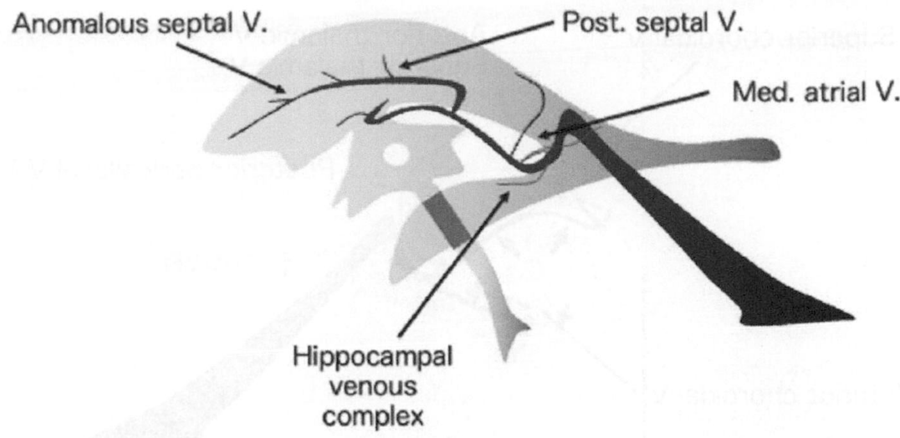

Fig. 16. Internal cerebral vein: Medial subependymal venous group mainly consists of anterior and posterior septal veins and medial atrial vein; note drainage of the posterior hippocampal veins into the posterior aspect of the vein.

Posterior Fossa Veins

Veins of the posterior fossa differ in their embryologic origin, as the brainstem derives directly from the neural tube while the cerebellum originates from the paired metencephalic plates. As a result, brainstem veins have a relatively simple geometric distribution, both longitudinal and transverse relative to the axis of the brainstem. Cerebellar veins, on the other hand, have a complex distribution that can be traced to the various stages of development of the vermis, the fourth ventricle, and the cerebellar hemispheres (Fig. 23).[38]

Veins of the Brainstem

The developing dura (meninx primitiva) is not organized, and only starts differentiating between various layers, that is, arachnoid, meningeal and parietal dura. In the 18 mm embryo (see Fig. 2), the meninx primitiva contains loose connective tissues that allow large vascular channels to develop. The paired ventral longitudinal veins, which run longitudinally on each side of the midline, are connected to each other by transverse veins that also connect to each other, more lateral longitudinal venous channels, that is, the anterior, middle,

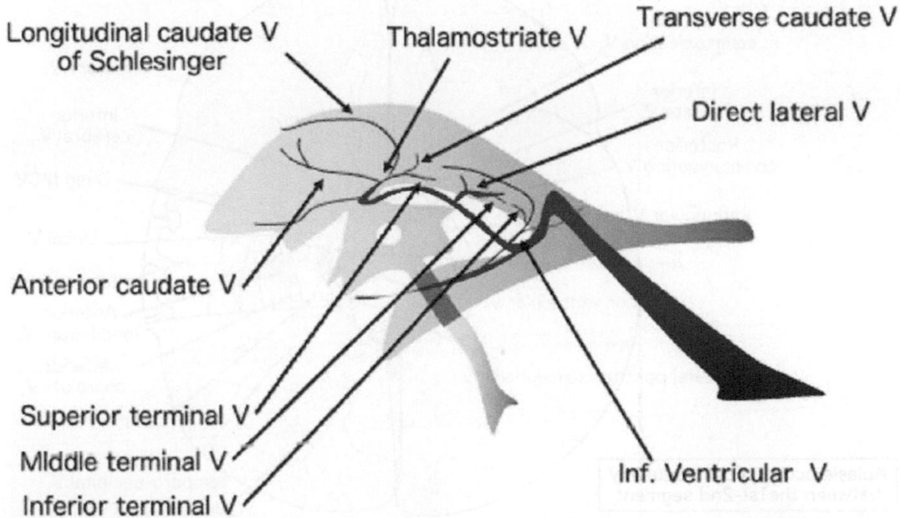

Fig. 17. Internal cerebral vein: Lateral subependymal venous group: Anterior caudate, longitudinal caudate (vein of Schlesinger), transverse caudate, thalamostriate, direct lateral, terminal (superior, middle, and inferior), and inferior ventricular veins.

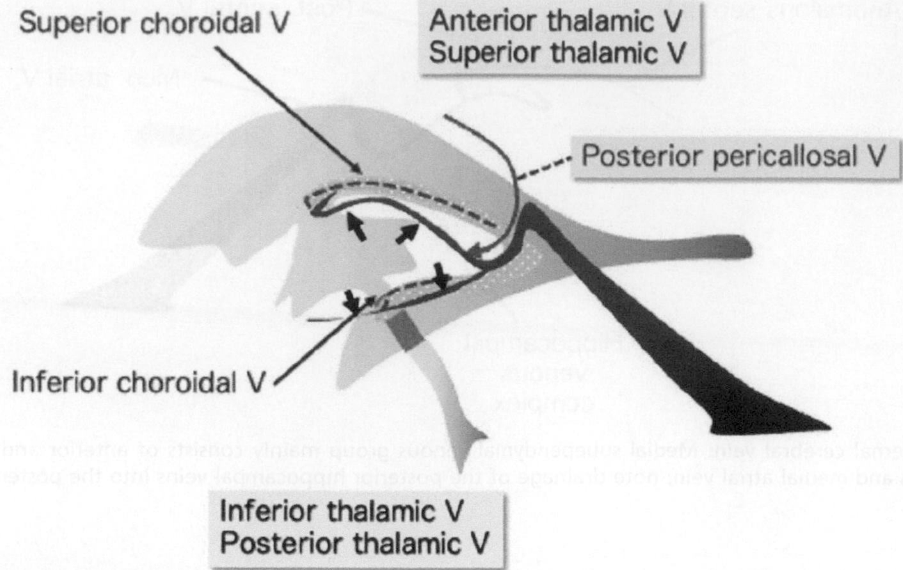

Fig. 18. Internal cerebral vein: Choroidal and calloso-lateral venous group: Superior and inferior medial choroidal veins, thalamic (anterior, posterior, superior, inferior) veins, third ventricular choroidal, direct lateral atrial, common atrial, habenular veins (not depicted), and posterior pericallosal veins.

and posterior dural plexi. The lateral longitudinal venous network demonstrates a distinct anatomic territorial distribution, that is, mesencephalic, metencephalic and myelencephalic. Blood flows always from transverse to longitudinal veins. The transverse veins drain major cranial nerve nuclei, that is, trigeminal, vagal, and hypoglossal (Fig. 24).

The main components of the longitudinal venous system are the anteromedian pontine vein, the anteromedian pontomedullary vein, and the anterolateral pontomedullary vein. Major transverse veins of the brainstem include the superior and inferior transverse pontine veins and the 3 transverse medullary veins (Fig. 25).

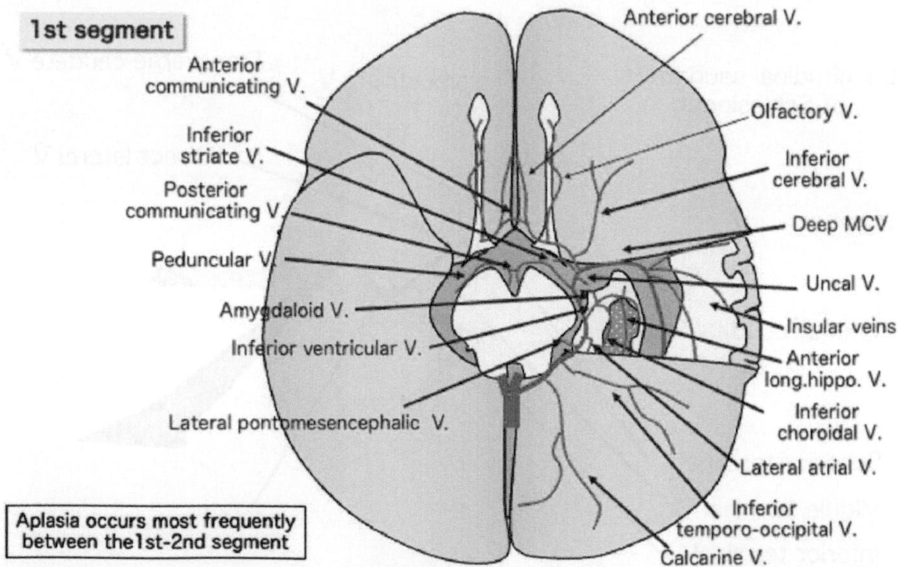

Fig. 19. Basal vein of Rosenthal: first segment. The striate segment collects the anterior cerebral, anterior communicating, inferior cerebral, deep middle cerebral and inferior striate veins, and the olfactory, posterior fronto-orbital, and chiasmatic veins.

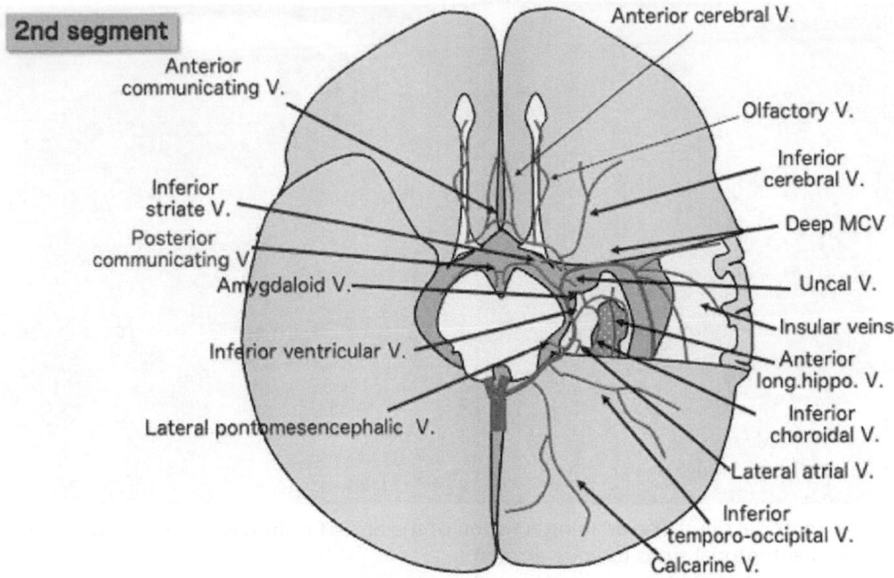

Fig. 20. Basal vein of Rosenthal: second segment. The peduncular segment drains the peduncular, inferior thalamic, inferior ventricular veins, and receives twigs from the optic tract, hypothalamus, and posterior hippocampus. The course of this middle segment of the BVR follows the cerebral peduncle contour before moving more laterally along the optic tract.

Other transverse oriented veins draining the posterior fossa are beyond the brainstem and include the peduncular vein, the posterior communicating vein, the vein of the pontomesencephalic sulcus, and the vein of the pontomedullary sulcus (Fig. 26).[38,39]

Deep transmedullary brainstem veins that reach the superficial transverse and longitudinal venous

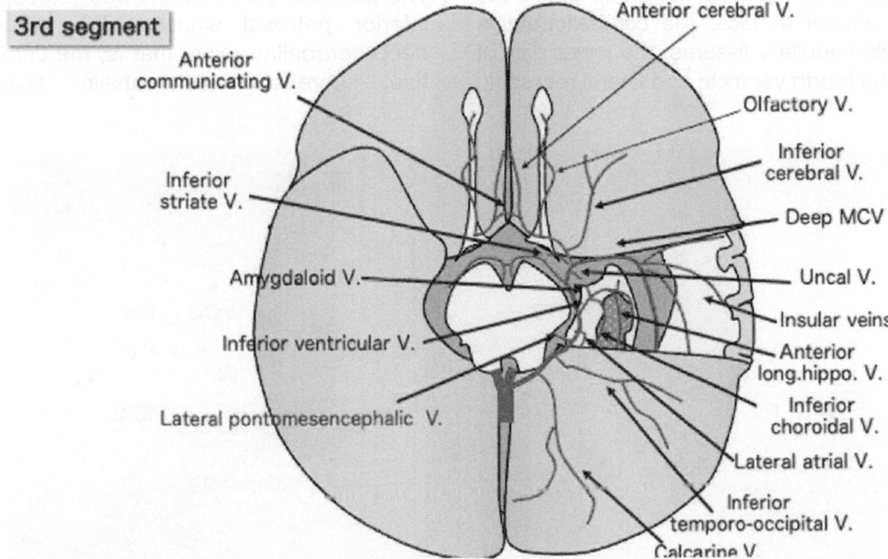

Fig. 21. Basal vein of Rosenthal: third segment. The mesencephalic segment collects the lateral pontomesencephalic vein (fed by both the anterior pontomesencephalic vein and the precentral cerebellar vein), tributaries from the atrial vein, and the inferior temporo-occipital vein before joining the ICV to empty into the vein of Galen.

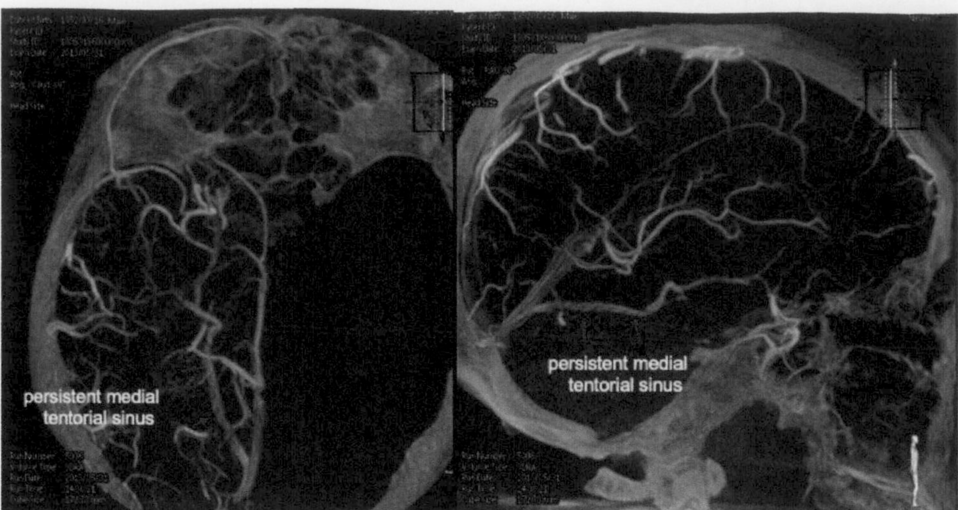

Fig. 22. Persistent tentorial sinus. The draining function of the absent right basal vein of Rosenthal is taken over by a persistent medial tentorial sinus (*orange arrows*).

systems drain in a centrifugal fashion (Fig. 27). Also, variability exists in the general configuration of brainstem venous drainage, as either the longitudinal or the transverse venous network may be dominant (Fig. 28).

Veins of the cerebellum

The veins of the cerebellum and the veins of the brainstem join into bridging veins which eventually drain into three collecting venous systems, petrosal, galenic, and tentorial that respectively drain into the petrosal sinuses, the vein of Galen, and the torcular/transverse sinuses. The petrosal group drains the cerebellar petrosal surface, the cerebellopontine and cerebellomedullary fissures, the lower part of the roof of the fourth ventricle and lateral recesses, and the lateral aspects of the pons and medulla. The galenic group drains the tentorial surface of the cerebellum, the upper part of the fourth ventricle, and the cerebellomesencephalic fissure. The tentorial group drains the infratentorial cerebellar surface. In addition to those major collecting systems, inconsistent direct bridging veins may be present which may connect to the cavernous sinuses, the basilar plexus, the marginal sinus, the sigmoid sinus, or the jugular bulb.[39]

Petrosal draining group

The petrosal group drains into the superior and inferior petrosal sinuses. This group drains deep cerebellar veins, that is, the cerebellopontine, cerebellomesencephalic fissure and

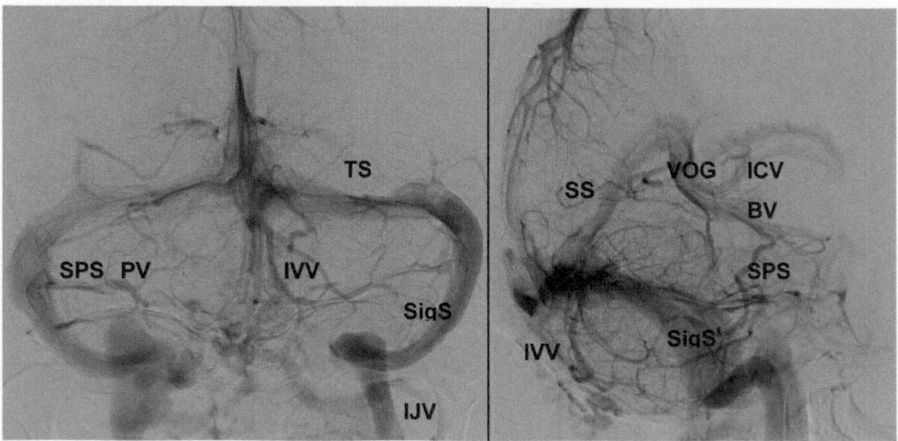

Fig. 23. Posterior fossa veins seen on left vertebral artery angiogram, venous phase. Few veins are reliably identified. BVR, basal vein of rosenthal; ICV, internal cerebral vein; IVV, inferior vermian vein; PV, Petrosal vein; SigS, sigmoid sinus; SPS, Superior petrosal sinus; SS, straight sinus; TS, transverse sinus; VOG, vein of galen.

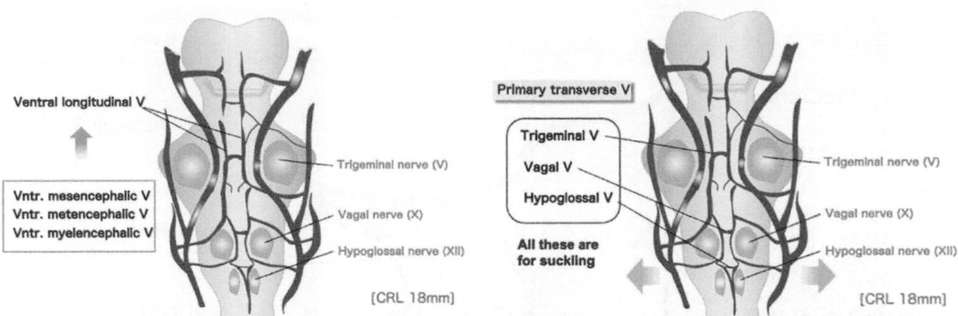

Fig. 24. Embryologic development of brainstem veins. Veins of the brainstem veins have a relatively simple geometric distribution, both longitudinal and transverse relative to the axis of the brainstem. This is because the brainstem derives directly from the neural tube. A prominent longitudinal and transverse venous network organizes throughout, prominent around major nuclei involved in the feeding function (trigeminal, vagus, and hypoglossal).

cerebellomedullary veins, the veins of the lower part and lateral wall of the fourth ventricle, superficial cerebellar veins, that is, superficial and lateral hemispheric cerebellar veins, and brainstem veins. The veins of the cerebellopontine fissure joining the transverse pontine vein to form the superior petrosal vein are the main culprits when causing neurovascular conflicts of venous origin with the cisternal segments of the trigeminal nerves (Fig 29).[40] The superior petrosal vein, which drains into the superior petrosal sinus, one of the largest and most constant posterior fossa veins, was named after Walter Dandy, a famous neurosurgeon who pointed out to the risk of major venous ischemia during surgery on the trigeminal nerve (Fig. 30), and is, therefore, referred to as Dandy's vein, or simply as the petrosal vein.[41]

Galenic draining group Posterior fossa veins that converge on the vein of Galen include deep cerebellar veins, that is, the paired veins of the

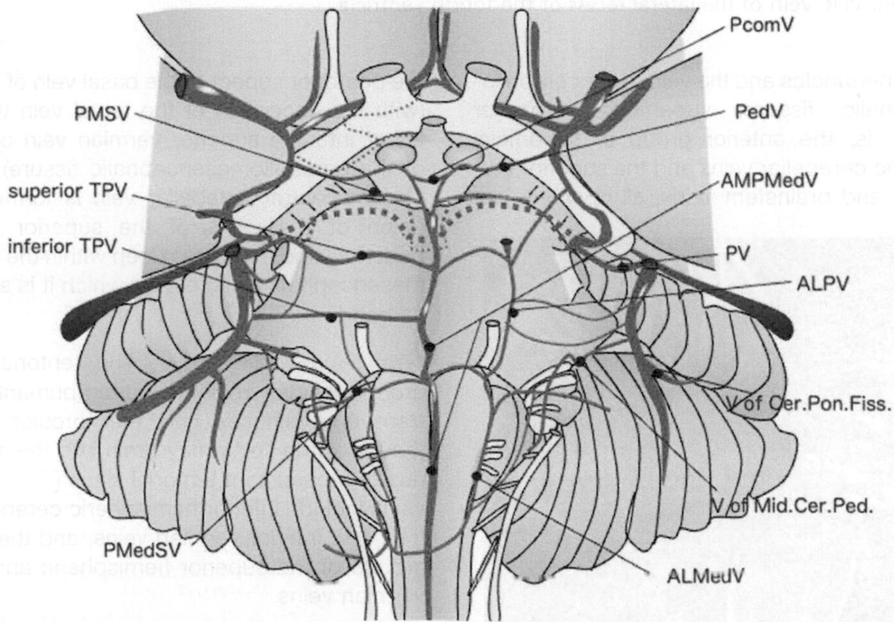

Fig. 25. Posterior fossa veins, anteroposterior view. Longitudinal brainstem venous system. ALMedV, anterolateral medullary vein; ALPV, anterolateral pontmesencephalic vein; AMPMedV, anteromedial pontomedullary vein; PcomV, posterior communicating vein; PmedSV, osterior medullary sulcus vein; PMSV, Pontomesencephalic vein Superior/inferior; TPV, transverse pontine vein; V of Cer.Pont.Fiss, Vein of the cerebellopontine fissure; V of Mid.Cer.Ped, Vein of the Middle cerebellar peduncle.

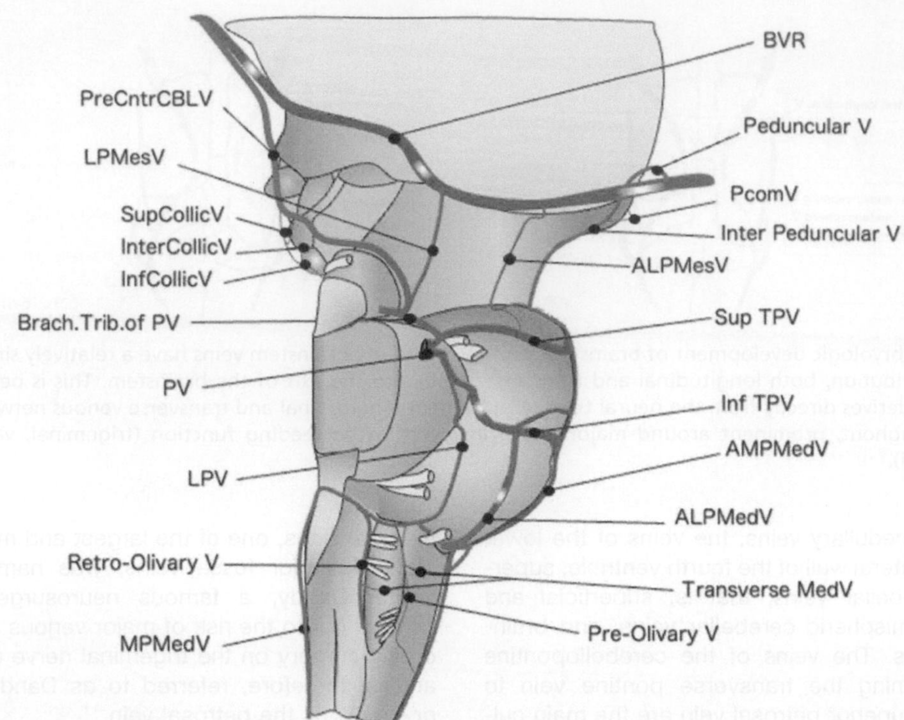

Fig. 26. Posterior fossa veins, lateral view. Transverse brainstem venous system. A Med V, anterior medullary vein; APMV, Anterior Pontine Mesencephalic Vein; Bra V, brachial vein; BVR, basal vein of rosenthal; CS, cavernous sinus; GHFV, greater horizontal fissure vein; ICV, internal cerebral vein; IJV, internal jugular vein; IPS, inferior petrosal sinus; IRTV, inferior retrotonsillar vein; IVV, inferior Vermian Vein; LPMV, lateral pontine mesencephalic vein; PedV, peduncular vein; PV, petrosal vein; Sgmd S, sigmoid sinus; SPS, superior petrosal sinus; SRTV, superior retrotonsillar vein; Strgt sinus, Straight sinus; SVV, superior Vermian Vein; Tento S, tentorial sinus; TPV, transverse pontine vein; VLR, vein of the lateral recess of the fourth ventricle.

cerebellar peduncles and the vein of the cerebellomesencephalic fissure, superficial cerebellar veins, that is, the anterior group of superficial hemispheric cerebellar veins and the superior vermian vein, and brainstem veins, all of which join the posterior aspect of the basal vein of Rosenthal (with the exception of the tectal vein that drains either into the superior vermian vein or the vein of the cerebellomesencephalic fissure) (**Fig. 31**). The precentral cerebellar vein is formed by the union of the veins of the superior cerebellar peduncle and originates deep within the cerebellomesencephalic fissure after which it is sometimes named (**Fig. 32**).[38,39,41]

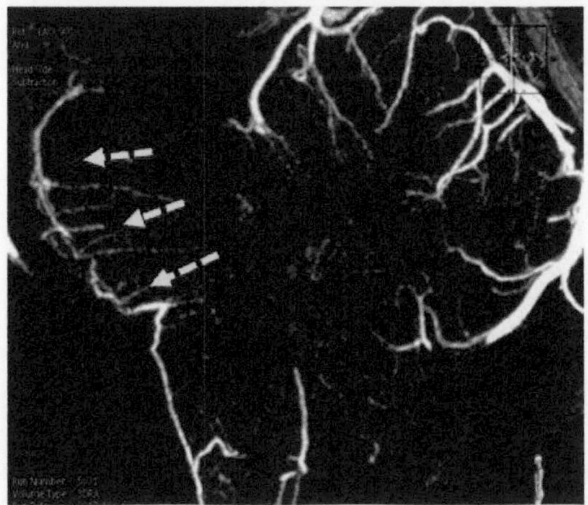

Fig. 27. CT angiogram, venous phase, shows brainstem veins draining into the pontmesencephalic venous system in a centrifugal pattern (*yellow arrows*).

Tentorial draining group The tentorial draining group includes veins that drain primarily into the transverse sinuses and the torcular Herophili, though some veins may drain into the straight sinus or a persistent tentorial sinus (**Fig. 33**). Those veins include inferior hemispheric cerebellar veins (**Fig. 34**), inferior vermian veins, and the posterior groups of the superior hemispheric and superior vermian veins.[38,39,41,42]

Emissary veins and persistent sinuses

Emissary veins are important pathways of extracranial venous drainage that become particularly relevant in cases of dural sinus stenosis or occlusion.

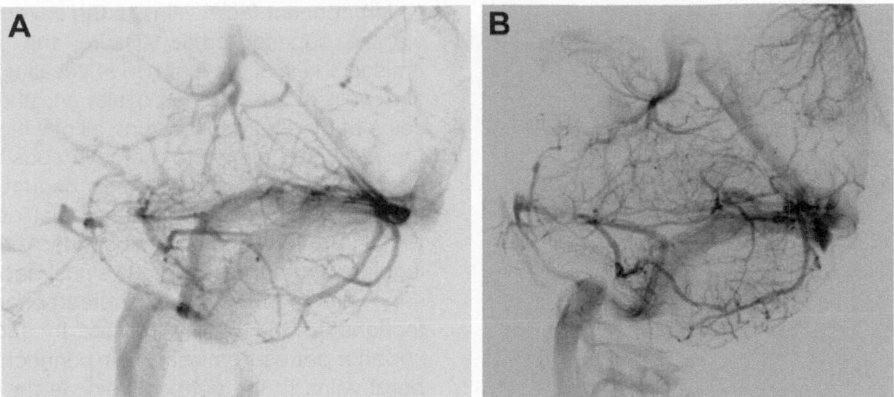

Fig. 28. Patterns of brainstem drainage. Dominant longitudinal brainstem venous drainage (*A*) manifests as paucity of venous opacification on lateral vertebral artery angiogram, venous phase. In contrast (*B*) significant venous brainstem venous opacification is seen with the dominant transverse drainage pattern.

Because they are valveless, emissary veins allow for bidirectional flow, which plays a role in maintaining stability in intracranial pressures, and in providing selective cooling of intracranial structures.[43–45] Emissary veins may propagate extracranial infections into the intracranial compartment, prompting Sir Frederick Treves (a prominent early 20th-century surgeon) to state that "If there were no emissary veins, injuries and diseases of the scalp would lose half their seriousness."[43]

Anterior and middle cranial fossa emissary veins include the superior and inferior ophthalmic veins,

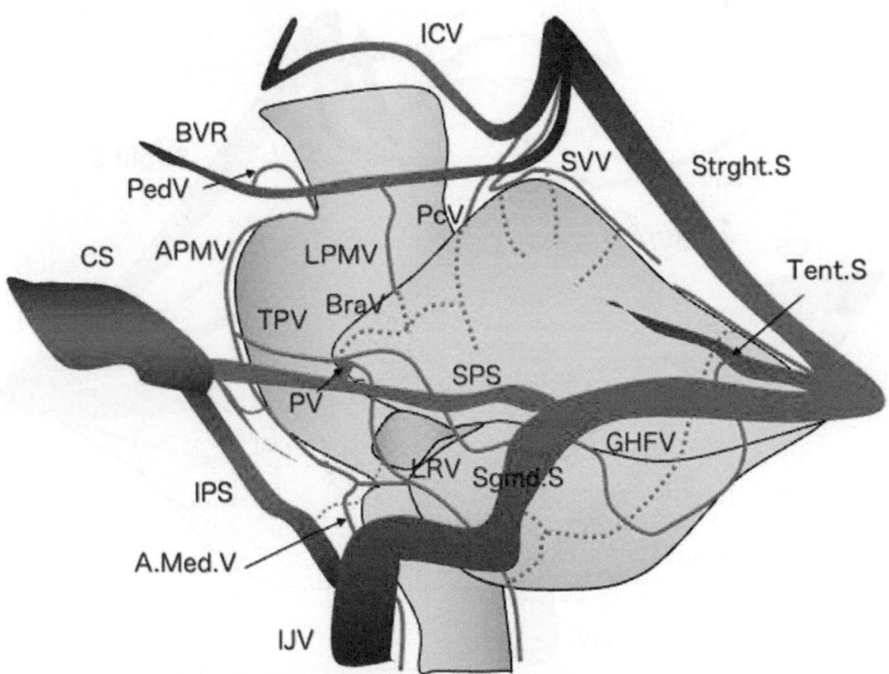

Fig. 29. Cerebellar veins, petrosal draining group. A Med V, anterior medullary vein; APMV, Anterior Pontine Mesencephalic Vein; Bra V, brachial vein; BVR, basal vein of rosenthal; CS, cavernous sinus; GHFV, greater horizontal fissure vein; ICV, internal cerebral vein; IJV, internal jugular vein; IPS, inferior petrosal sinus; IRTV, inferior retrotonsillar vein; IVV, inferior Vermian Vein; LPMV, lateral pontine mesencephalic vein; PedV, peduncular vein; PV, petrosal vein; Sgmd S, sigmoid sinus; SPS, superior petrosal sinus; SRTV, superior retrotonsillar vein; Strgt sinus, Straight sinus; SVV, superior Vermian Vein; Tento S, tentorial sinus; TPV, transverse pontine vein; VLR, vein of the lateral recess of the fourth ventricle.

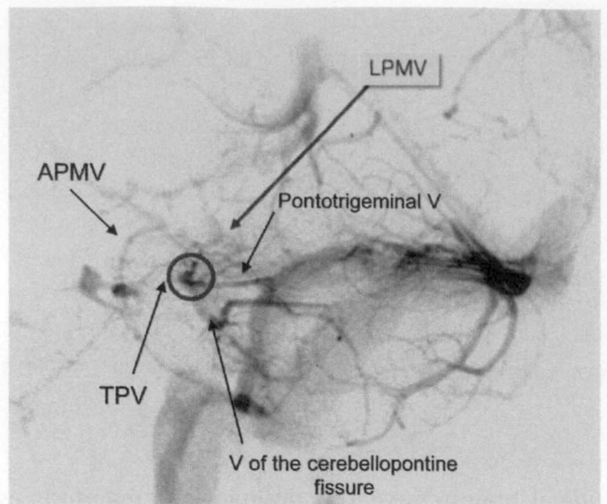

Fig. 30. Petrosal vein (vein of Dandy, also referred to as the superior petrosal vein) and tributaries. The petrosal vein (*red circle*) empties into the superior petrosal sinus, and normally receives between 3 and 5 tributaries, including: (1) the transverse pontine vein (TPV) from anterior pontine mesencephalic vein (APMV), (2) the vein of the cerebellopontine fissure, (3) the pontotrigeminal vein (from the posterior mesencephalic group), (4) the anterior lateral marginal vein, and (5) the vein of the middle cerebellar peduncle.

which connect facial veins to the cavernous sinus via the superior orbital fissure, the sphenoidal emissary vein of the foramen of Vesalius, the emissary vein of the foramen ovale, and the emissary veins of the foramen lacerum, all of which connect the pterygoid plexus to the cavernous sinus. The emissary vein of the foramen cecum connects the nasal cavity to the anterior cranial fossa, the internal carotid venous plexus connects the internal jugular vein to the cavernous sinus, and the emissary veins of the clivus may spread pharyngeal infections to the basilar plexus. In addition, the superior petrosal emissary vein connects infratemporal veins to the petrosal vein via the stylomastoid foramen (along with the facial nerve). The petrosquamosal sinus (which typically involutes before birth, but may persist) also connects the transverse-sigmoid junction to the antero-lateral temporal lobe, and the temporal emissary vein may connect the persistent petrosquamosal sinus to the deep temporal vein.[43,44]

Posterior fossa emissary veins include the posterior condylar emissary vein (which may connect occipital, marginal, and sigmoid sinuses), the anterior condylar vein within the hypoglossal canal, the

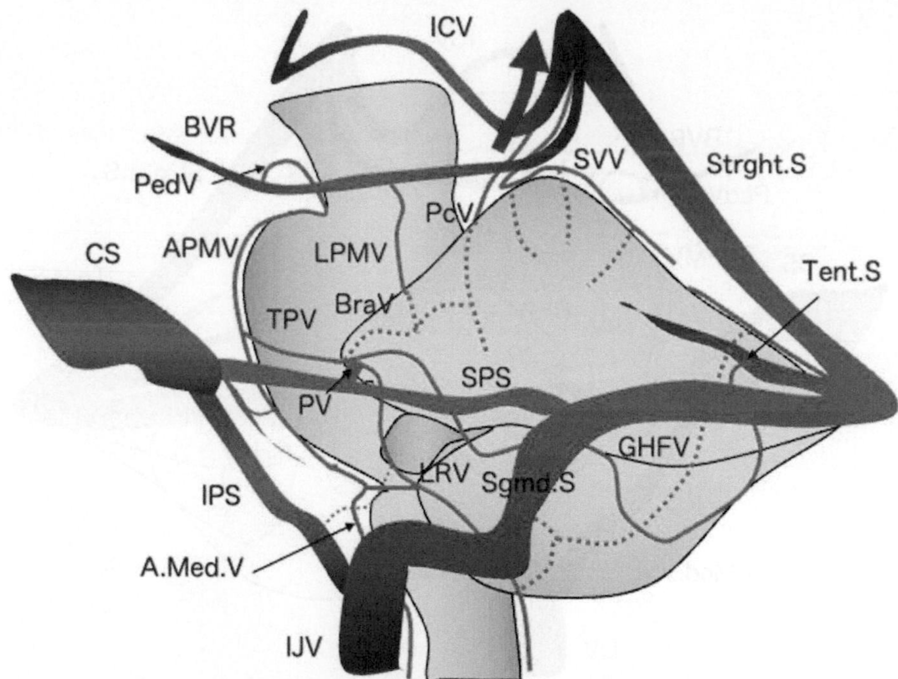

Fig. 31. Cerebellar veins, galenic draining group. A Med V, anterior medullary vein; APMV, Anterior Pontine Mesencephalic Vein; Bra V, brachial vein; BVR, basal vein of rosenthal; CS, cavernous sinus; GHFV, greater horizontal fissure vein; ICV, internal cerebral vein; IJV, internal jugular vein; IPS, inferior petrosal sinus; IRTV, inferior retrotonsillar vein; IVV, inferior Vermian Vein; LPMV, lateral pontine mesencephalic vein; PedV, peduncular vein; PV, petrosal vein; Sgmd S, sigmoid sinus; SPS, superior petrosal sinus; SRTV, superior retrotonsillar vein; Strgt sinus, Straight sinus; SVV, superior Vermian Vein; Tento S, tentorial sinus; TPV, transverse pontine vein; VLR, vein of the lateral recess of the fourth ventricle.

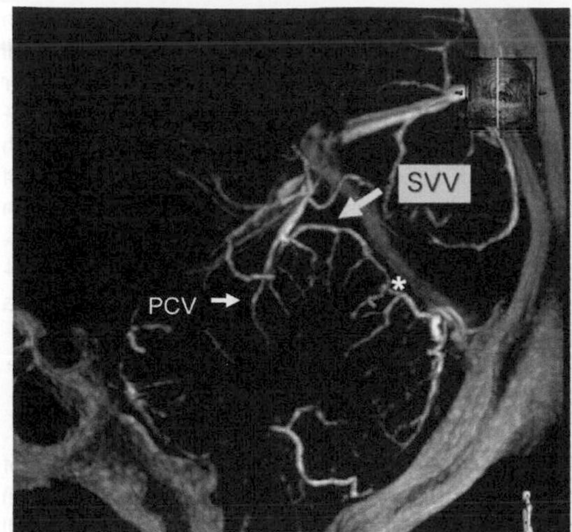

Fig. 32. Cerebellar veins, Galenic group. CT angiogram, sagittal view. PCV, precentral cerebellar vein (*white arrow*), which anastomoses with the petrosal group superiorly; SVV, superior vermian vein; Asterisk indicates anastomotic point between superior vermian vein and inferior vermian vein (tentorial draining group).

occipital emissary vein between the transverse sinus and the occipital vein, the parietal emissary vein that connects the superior sagittal sinus and the occipital vein, and the mastoid emissary vein that connects the sigmoid (or transverse) sinus to the posterior auricular or occipital veins and the vertebral plexus (Fig. 35).[43,45,46] The occipital emissary vein was found to be enlarged in patients with idiopathic intracranial hypertension (pseudotumor cerebri).[45] Also, enlarged posterior fossa emissary veins have been linked to benign pulsatile tinnitus.[46]

An occipital sinus is a persistent venous channel between the torcular Herophili and a draining venous system at the foramen magnum level, whether the marginal sinus or the vertebral plexus (Fig. 36). The occipital sinus, a remnant of the medial channel of the posterior dural plexus, is normally present at birth and destined to involute and close by 2 years of age.[47–49] Tubbs and colleagues have provided a detailed discussion of anatomic variants of the emissary veins.[50]

The falcine sinus, which is derived from the cranialmost portion of the sagittal plexus, is normally only present during the embryonic period and is

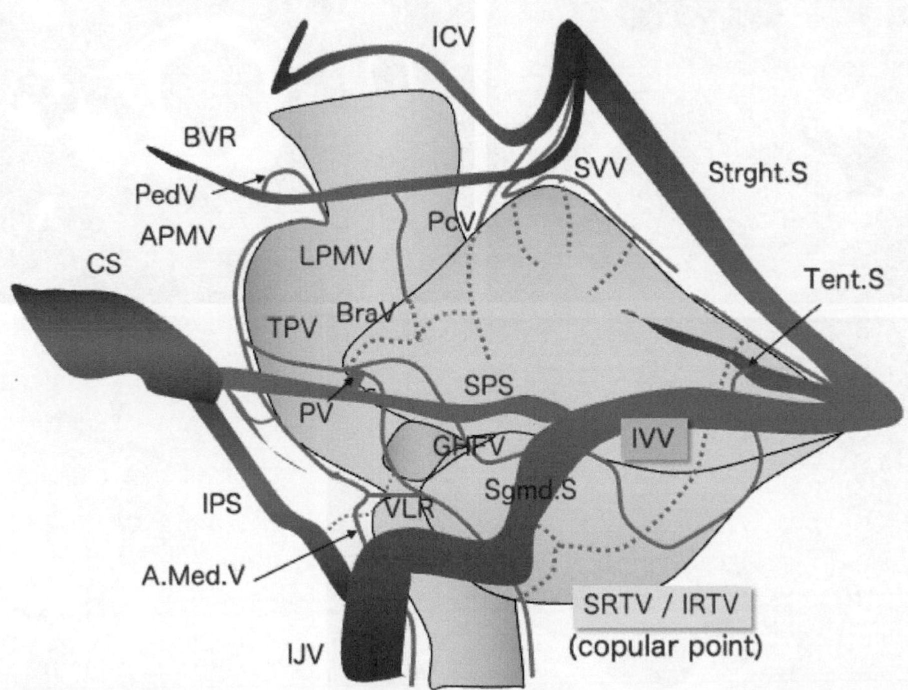

Fig. 33. Cerebellar veins, Tentorial group. A Med V, anterior medullary vein; APMV, Anterior Pontine Mesencephalic Vein; Bra V, brachial vein; BVR, basal vein of rosenthal; CS, cavernous sinus; GHFV, greater horizontal fissure vein; ICV, internal cerebral vein; IJV, internal jugular vein; IPS, inferior petrosal sinus; IRTV, inferior retrotonsillar vein; IVV, inferior Vermian Vein; LPMV, lateral pontine mesencephalic vein; PedV, peduncular vein; PV, petrosal vein; Sgmd S, sigmoid sinus; SPS, superior petrosal sinus; SRTV, superior retrotonsillar vein; Strgt sinus, Straight sinus; SVV, superior Vermian Vein; Tento S, tentorial sinus; TPV, transverse pontine vein; VLR, vein of the lateral recess of the fourth ventricle.

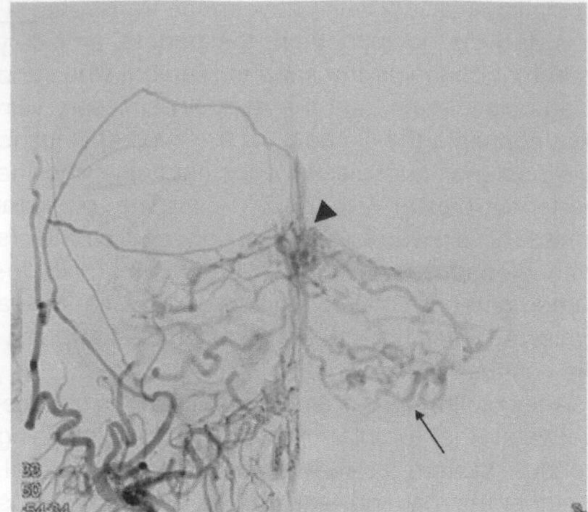

Fig. 34. Dilated tentorial veins (*arrow*) in a patient with a dural arteriovenous fistula (DAVF) of the torcular Herophili (*arrowhead*) seen on a right external carotid artery angiogram.

supposed to regress before birth.[51,52] The function of the falcine sinus is to connect the deep cerebral venous system to the posterior third of the superior straight sinus. The prevalence of a persistent falcine sinus is estimated at 1% to 2%.[51,52] Although commonly associated with other anomalies of development, that is, Chiari II malformations, vein of Galen aneurymal malformation, corpus callosum agenesis, encephalocele (**Fig. 37**), acrocephalosyndactyly or tentorial dysplasia, a persistent falcine sinus may be isolated.[51]

Diploic Veins

The diploic venous system is a complex network of veins enclosed within cancellous bone (the diploe) between the outer and inner tables of the skull made of compact bone. The French anatomist Gilbert Breschet is credited with the first anatomic description of the diploic venous system in 1829.

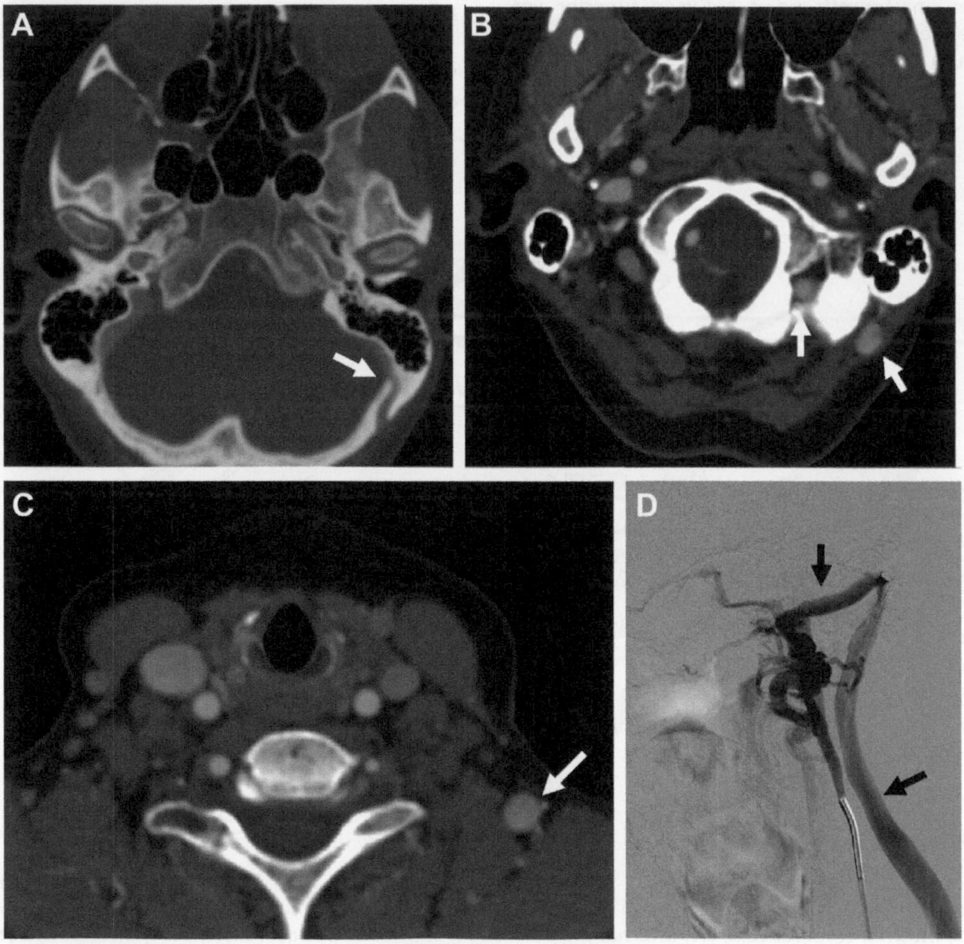

Fig. 35. (*A–D*) Mastoid (or retromastoid) emissary vein. CTA shows a large curved emissary foramen (remnant of the left occipitomastoid suture) in the left occipital bone (*A, white arrow*) which allows the passage of a mastoid emissary vein (*B, arrows*) that courses posteriorly and inferiorly to drain into the left subclavian vein (*C, arrow*). Angiographic view from left internal jugular vein injection demonstrates the lateral course of the mastoid emissary vein (*D, arrows*).

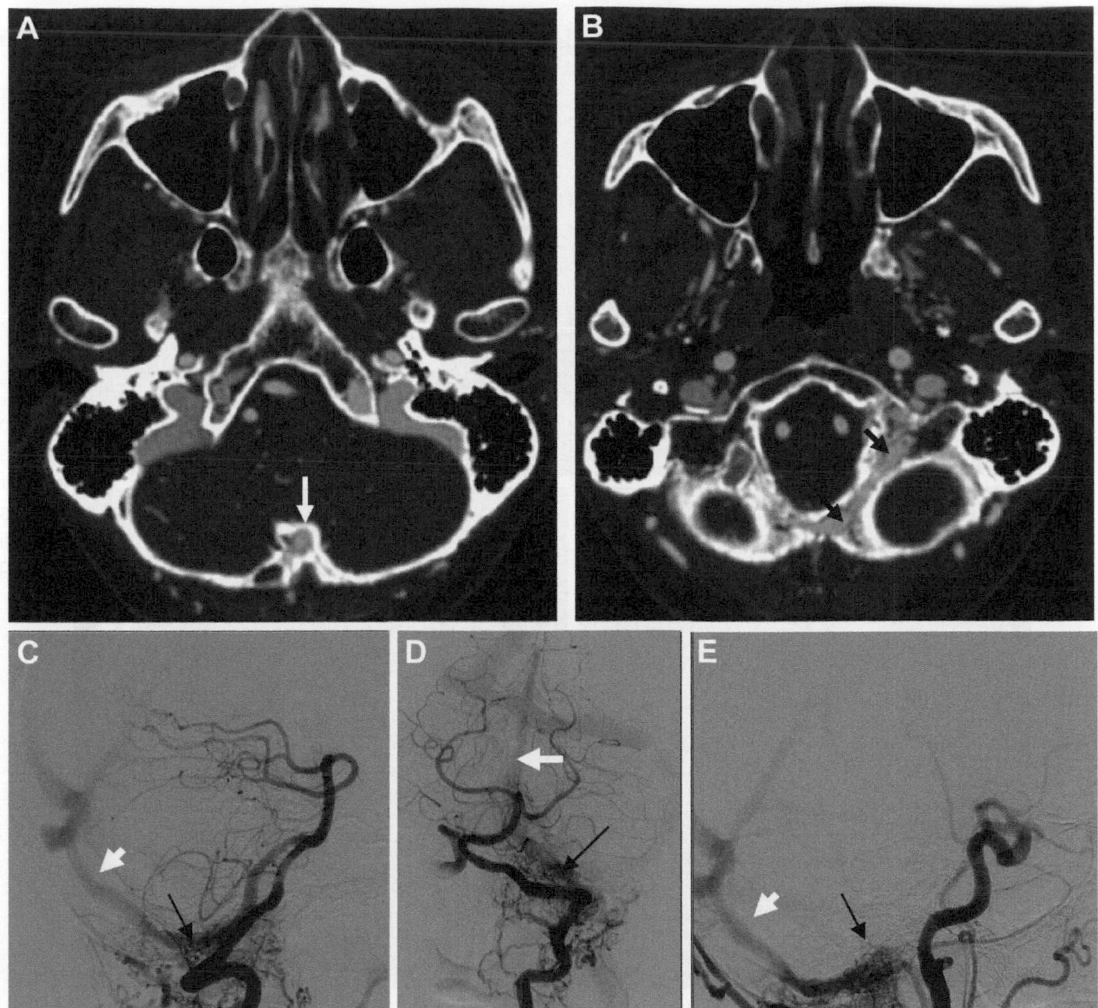

Fig. 36. (*A–E*) Occipital sinus. CTA obtained in an 82-year-old female patient who presents with tinnitus from a left posterior condylar foramen dural arteriovenous fistula (DAVF). An intraosseous occipital sinus is present (*A, arrow*), which connects to the left posterior condylar venous plexus (*B, arrows*). Left vertebral artery injection, lateral (*C*) and anteroposterior views (*D*) and left common carotid injection, lateral view (*E*) show occipital sinus (*short white arrows*) and posterior condylar foramen DAVF (*long black arrows*).

Although there is significant variability in the anatomic arrangement of diploic veins, the 3 main components of the diploic venous system are the frontal, the anterior temporal, and the posterior temporal diploic veins, with numerous focal areas of venous ectasia referred to as diploic lacunae or lakes.[53,54] Large main diploic veins anastomose extensively with each other, and with a network of microscopic venous channels. All those diploic veins, which are valveless and are lined by a layer of single endothelial cells, communicate freely with the large meningeal veins, the dural sinuses, and emissary veins. The diploic venous system, which is, therefore, in contact with the dural sinuses, the cerebral veins, and the CSF system, is considered to be an important communication pathway between the venous and CSF systems.[55] Tsutsumi has provided a detailed discussion of anatomic variants of the diploic veins.[56]

The clinical significance of diploic venous channels is multiple. They may serve as alternate drainage pathways in case of dural sinus stenosis, occlusion, congenital malformation, thrombosis, or trauma (see Fig. 37).[57,58] Arteriovenous fistulas with diploic venous drainage may develop spontaneously, that is, in patients with thrombophilia,[59] after meningioma resection[60] or trauma.[61] Diploic veins can also be a source of bleeding during neurosurgical procedures that require bone

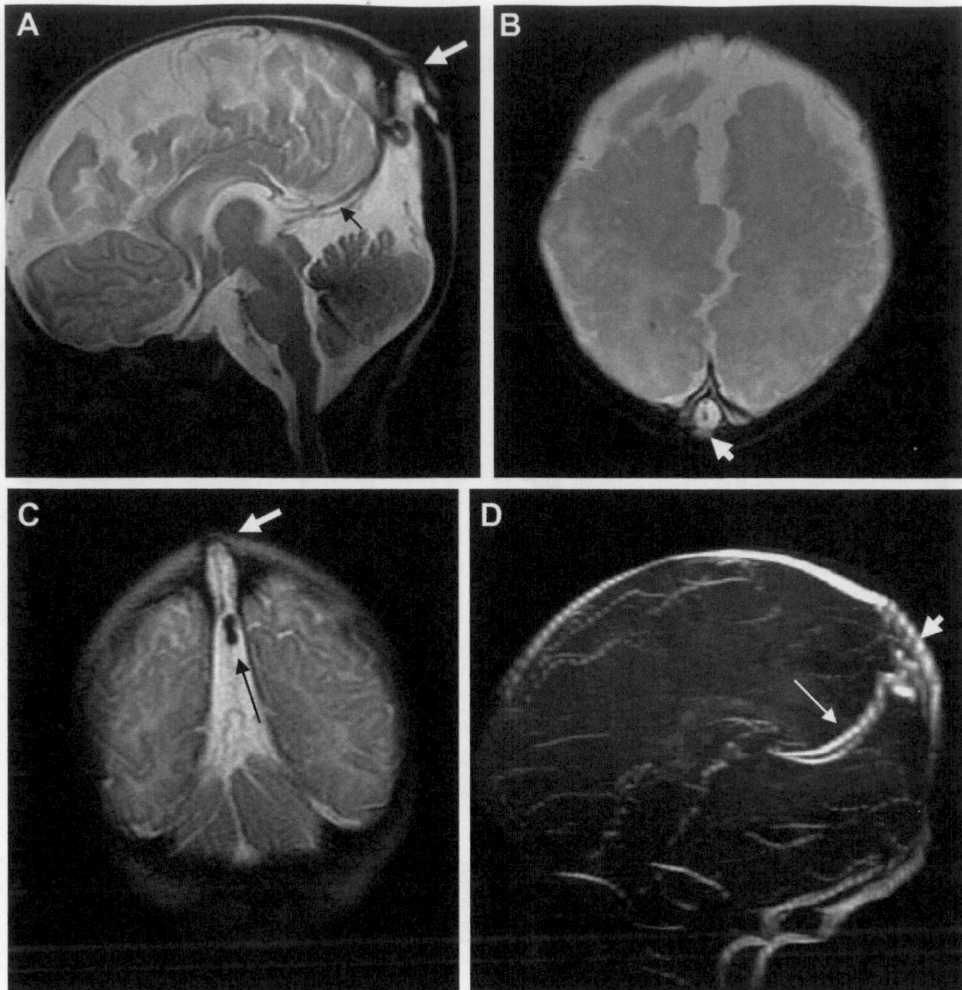

Fig. 37. *(A–D)* Persistent falcine sinus draining a hypoplastic deep venous system into a sinus pericranii continuous with the diploic venous system associated with atretic parietal cephalocele in a neonate (*thick arrow*). Sagittal (*A*), axial (*B*), and coronal (*C*) T2 MR imaging show sinus pericranii within parietal cephalocele (*short large arrows*) that drains extracranially a hypoplastic deep venous system (*thin long arrow*).

drilling, that is, craniotomies, burr holes, and pin placement. Epidural hematomas have been reported after head-holder pin placement.[62] Air emboli embolism can also occur after craniotomy or pin placement.[63,64] Diploic veins may promote the spread of infection[62,65] Spontaneous arteriovenous fistulas can occur between scalp arteries and diploic veins.[66]

CLINICS CARE POINTS

- Thrombosis of dural sinuses or cortical veins is an uncommon but significant cause of morbidity and mortality
- The understanding and management of intracranial arteriovenous and venous lesions requires a good understanding of the venous system
- The proximity of eloquent cerebral regions to intracranial veins, and technological advances in signal transmission through increasingly miniaturized transvenous devices will increasingly allow for therapeutic approaches, that is, neuromodulation for epilepsy, motor control of exoskeletons and robotic limbs in paralyzed patients, the enabling of speech paradigms in patients with poststroke and many more.

DISCLOSURE

The authors have no disclosures to declare in relation to this article.

REFERENCES

1. Hufnagle JJ, Tadi P. Neuroanatomy, brain veins. In: StatPearls [Internet]. Treasure Island (FL: StatPearls Publishing; 2021. PMID: 31536212.
2. Kiliç T, Akakin A. Anatomy of cerebral veins and sinuses. Front Neurol Neurosci 2008;23:4–15.
3. Stolz E. Cerebral veins and sinuses. In: Baumgartner RW. Handbook on neurovascular ultrasound. Front Neurol Neurosci Karger, Basel, Switzerland. 21:2006;182–93.
4. Kretzer RM, Crosby RW, Rini DA, et al. Dorcas Hager Padget: neuroembryologist and neurosurgical illustrator trained at Johns Hopkins. J Neurosurg 2004;100(4):719–30.
5. McBain L, Goren O, Tubbs RS. The embryology of the dural venous sinus: an overview (Chapter 1), anatomy, imaging and surgery of the intracranial dural venous sinuses. Elsevier Ed 2020;p. 1–7, 10.1016/B978-0-323-65377-0.00001-5.
6. Streeter GL. The development of the venous sinuses of the dura mater in the human embryo. Am J Anat 1915;18:145–78.
7. Padget DH. The cranial venous system in man in reference to development, adult configuration, and relation to the arteries. Am J Anat 1956;98:307–56.
8. Padget DH. The development of the cranial venous system in man from the viewpoint of comparative anatomy. Contrib Embryol 1957;36:81–139.
9. Kretschmann HJ, Weinrich W. Cranial neuroimaging and clinical neuroanatomy: magnetic resonance imaging and computed tomography. 3rd edition. Stuttgart (Germany): Georg Thieme Verlag; 2004. p. 451.
10. FCAT. Federative committee on anatomical terminology. terminologia anatomica. international anatomical terminology. 1st edition.292 Stuttgart (Germany): Thieme Medical Publishing; 1999. p. 1999.
11. Osborn AG. Diagnostic neuroradiology. Mosby; 1994. ISBN 0801674867, 9780801674860.
12. Huber P. Cerebral angiography. 2nd edition. Stuttgart (Germany): Georg Thieme Verlag; 1982.
13. Lasjaunias P, Berenstein A, ter Brugge KG. Surgical neuroangiography: clinical vascular anatomy and variations. 2nd edition. Berlin (Germany): Springer; 2001.
14. Huang YP, Wolf BS. The basal cerebral vein and its tributaries. In: Newton TH, Potts DG, editors. Radiology of the skull and brain, Vol. 2. Saint Louis (MO): Mosby; 1974. p. 2111–54.
15. Matsushima T, Rhoton AL Jr, de Oliveira E, et al. Microsurgical anatomy of the veins of the posterior fossa. J Neurosurg 1983;59:63–105.
16. Ono M, Rhoton AL Jr, Peace D, et al. Microsurgical anatomy of the deep venous system of the brain. Neurosurgery 1984;16:621–57.
17. Oka K, Rhoton AL Jr, Barry M, et al. Microsurgical anatomy of the superficial veins of the cerebrum. Neurosurgery 1985;17:711–48.
18. Yasargil MG. MicroneurosurgeryIIIA. Stuttgart (Germany): Thieme; 1987.
19. Macdonald RL. Neurosurgical operative atlas. vascular neurosurgery. 2nd edition. Rolling Meadows (IL): American Association of Neurological Surgeons; 2009.
20. Nowinski WL. Proposition of a new classification of the cerebral veins based on their termination. Surg Radiol Anat 2012;34(2):107–14.
21. Fan AP, Bilgic B, Gagnon L, et al. Quantitative oxygenation venography from MRI phase. Magn Reson Med 2014;72(1):149–59.
22. Available at: https://radiopaedia.org/cases/brain-venous-vascular-territories-diagram?lang=us.
23. Joseph SC, Rizk E, Tubbs RS. Dural venous sinuses. In: Tubbs RS, Shoja MM, Loukas M, editors. Bergman's Comprehensive encyclopedia of human anatomic variation. Hoboken (NJ): John Wiley & Sons; 2016. p. 775–99.
24. Yong SW, Bang OY, Lee PH, et al. Internal and cortical border-zone infarction: clinical and diffusion-weighted imaging features. Stroke 2006;37:841–6.
25. Yedavalli V, Telischak NA, Jain MS, et al. Three-dimensional angles of confluence of cortical bridging veins and the superior sagittal sinus on MR venography: does drainage of adjacent brain arteriovenous malformations alter this spatial configuration? Clin Anat 2020;33(2):293–9.
26. Telischak NA, Yedavalli V, Massoud TF. Tortuosity of superior cerebral veins: Comparative magnetic resonance imaging morphometrics in normal subjects and arteriovenous malformation patients. Clin Anat 2021;34(3):326–32.
27. Mortazavi MM, Denning M, Yalcin B, et al. The intracranial bridging veins: a comprehensive review of their history, anatomy, histology, pathology, and neurosurgical implications. Child's Nervous Syst 2013;29:1073–8.
28. Sadighi A, Cikla U, Kujoth GC, et al. Cerebral veins. In: Tubbs RS, Shoja MM, Loukas M, editors. Bergman's comprehensive encyclopedia of human anatomic variation. Hoboken (NJ): John Wiley & Sons; 2016. p. 800–16.
29. Duret H. Recherches anatomiques sur la circulation de l'encéphale. Arch Physiol Norm Pathol 1874;6: 316–53.
30. Jimenez JL, Lasjaunias P, Terbrugge K, et al. The transcerebral veins: normal and non-pathologic angiographic aspects. Surg Radiol Anat 1989;11: 63–72.
31. Okudera T, Huang YP, Fukusumi A, et al. Micro-angiographical studies of the medullary venous system of the cerebral hemisphere. Neuropathology 1999;19:93–111.

32. Huang YP, Wolf BS. Veins of the white matter of the cerebral hemispheres (the medullary veins). Am J Roentgenol Radium Ther Nucl Med 1964;92:739–55.
33. Schlesinger B. The venous drainage of the brain, with special reference to the Galenic system. Brain 1939;62(3):274–91.
34. Taoka T, Fukusumi A, Miyasaka T, et al. Structure of the medullary veins of the cerebral hemisphere and related disorders. Radiographics 2017;37(1): 281–97.
35. Khalatbari H, Wright JN, Ishak GE, et al. Deep medullary vein engorgement and superficial medullary vein engorgement: two patterns of perinatal venous stroke. Pediatr Radiol 2021;51:675–85.
36. Chung JI, Weon YC. Anatomic variations of the deep cerebral veins, tributaries of basal vein of rosenthal: embryologic aspects of the regressed embryonic tentorial sinus. Interv Neuroradiol 2005;11:123–30.
37. Gutierrez S, Iwanaga J, Dumont AS, et al. Direct drainage of the basal vein of Rosenthal into the superior petrosal sinus: a literature review. Anat Cell Biol 2020;53(4):379–84.
38. de Miquel MA. Posterior fossa venous drainage. Front Neurol 2021;12:680515.
39. Rhoton AL Jr. The posterior fossa veins. Neurosurgery 2000;47(3 Suppl):S69–92.
40. Dumot C, Sindou M. Trigeminal neuralgia due to neurovascular conflicts from venous origin: an anatomical-surgical study (consecutive series of 124 operated cases). Acta Neurochir (Wien) 2015; 157(3):455–66.
41. Bender B, Hauser TK, Korn A, et al. Depiction of the Superior petrosal vein complex by 3D contrast-enhanced MR angiography. AJNR Am J Neuroradiol 2018;39(12):2249–55.
42. Hu HH, Campeau NG, Huston J 3rd, et al. High-spatial-resolution contrast-enhanced MR angiography of the intracranial venous system with fourfold accelerated two-dimensional sensitivity encoding. Radiology 2007;243(3):853–61.
43. Mortazavi MM, Tubbs RS, Riech S, et al. Anatomy and pathology of the cranial emissary veins: a review with surgical implications. Neurosurgery 2012; 70(5):1312–8 [discussion: 1318-1319].
44. Ide S, Kiyosue H, Shimada R, et al. Petrobasal vein: a previously unrecognized vein directly connecting the superior petrosal sinus with the emissary vein of the foramen ovale. AJNR Am J Neuroradiol 2021. https://doi.org/10.3174/ajnr.A7345. Epub ahead of print. PMID: 34949590.
45. Hedjoudje A, Piveteau A, Gonzalez-Campo C, et al. The occipital emissary vein: a possible marker for pseudotumor cerebri. AJNR Am J Neuroradiol 2019;40(6):973–8.
46. Abdalkader M, Nguyen TN, Norbash AM, et al. State of the art: venous causes of pulsatile tinnitus and diagnostic considerations guiding endovascular therapy. Radiology 2021;300(1):2–16.
47. Mizutani K, Miwa T, Akiyama T, et al. Fate of the three embryonic dural sinuses in infants: the primitive tentorial sinus, occipital sinus, and falcine sinus. Neuroradiology 2018;60:325–33.
48. Sener RN. Association of persistent falcine sinus with different clinicoradiologic conditions: MR imaging and MR angiography. Comput Med Imaging Graph 2000;24:343–8.
49. Kobayashi K, Suzuki M, Ueda F, et al. Anatomical study of the occipital sinus using contrast-enhanced magnetic resonance venography. Neuroradiology 2006;48:373–9.
50. Tubbs RS, Watanabe K, Loukas M. Emissary veins. In: Tubbs RS, Shoja MM, Loukas M, editors. Bergman's comprehensive encyclopedia of human anatomic variation. Hoboken (NJ): John Wiley & Sons; 2016. p. 817–20.
51. Ryu CW. Persistent falcine sinus: Is it really rare? Am J Neuroradiol 2010;31:367–9.
52. Smith A, Choudhary AK. Prevalence of persistent falcine sinus as an incidental finding in the pediatric population. Am J Roentgenol 2014;203:424–5.
53. Segawa T, Shirai M, Izumikawa E. Contribution to the knowledge on the morphology of the diploic veins. Yokohama Med Bull 1960;11:158–62.
54. Jivraj K, Bhargava R, Aronyk K, et al. Diploic venous anatomy studied in-vivo by MRI. Clin Anat 2009;22: 296–301.
55. Krmpotić-Nemanić J, Vinter I, Kelović Z, et al. The fate of the arachnoid villi in humans. Coll Antropol 2003;27:611–6.
56. Tsutsumi S. Diploic veins. In: Tubbs RS, Shoja MM, Loukas M, editors. Bergman's comprehensive encyclopedia of human anatomic variation. Hoboken (NJ): John Wiley & Sons; 2016. p. 770–4.
57. Huang KL, Chang YJ, Chen CH. Dural sinus hypertension due to segmental stenosis. Eur J Radiol Extra 2005;53:91–3.
58. Habash AH, Sortland O, Zwetnow NN. Epidural haematoma: pathophysiological significance of extravasation and arteriovenous shunting. An analysis of 35 patients. Acta Neurochir (Wien) 1982;60:7–27.
59. Mironov A. Classification of spontaneous dural arteriovenous fistulas with regard to their pathogenesis. Acta Radiol 1995;36:582–92.
60. Sakuma I, Takahashi S, Ishiyama K, et al. Multiple dural arteriovenous fistulas developing after total removal of parasagittal meningioma: a case successfully treated with transvenous embolization. Clin Radiol Extra 2004;9(7).
61. Ishii R, Ueki K, Ito J. Traumatic fistula between a lacerated middle meningeal artery and a diploic vein: case report. J Neurosurg 1976;44:241–4.
62. García-González U, Cavalcanti DD, Agrawal A, et al. The diploic venous system: surgical anatomy and

neurosurgical implications. Neurosurg Focus 2009; 27(5):E2.
63. Wilkins RH, Albin MS. An unusual entrance site of venous air embolism during operations in the sitting position. Surg Neurol 1977;7:71–2.
64. Pang D. Air embolism associated with wounds from a pin-type head-holder. Case report. J Neurosurg 1982;57:710–3.
65. Ramos A, Rayo JI, Martín R, et al. Empiema epidural; una complicación de sinusitis frontal [Epidural empyema; a complication of frontal sinusitis]. Acta Otorrinolaringol Esp 1989;40(6):451–3.
66. Burger IM, Tamargo RJ, Broussard J, et al. Combined surgical and endovascular treatment of a spontaneous diploic arteriovenous fistula. Case report. J Neurosurg 2005;103:179–81.

Fetal Brain Anatomy

Carolina V.A. Guimaraes, MD[a,*], Hisham M. Dahmoush, MD[b]

KEYWORDS

• Fetal MRI • Fetal brain anatomy • Fetal brain development

KEY POINTS

- The fetal brain undergoes significant changes during development.
- Changes in the size, signal, and morphology of the fetal brain follow a predictable pattern of development during gestation, with only minor variations.
- MR has high sensitivity of detecting cerebral abnormalities during pregnancy and is considered the imaging modality of choice for the evaluation of fetal central nervous system abnormalities.
- Knowledge of the expected normal fetal brain development and anatomy is fundamental for accurate diagnosis of congenital anomalies.

INTRODUCTION

Fetal brain structural changes occur rapidly during pregnancy. Knowledge of the normal morphologic appearances, signal intensity, and expected changes with gestational age is important for accurate interpretation of imaging studies of the fetal central nervous system (CNS). Ultrasound (US) is a great screening modality for CNS abnormalities, and MRI is then performed for definitive evaluation when an abnormality is suspected on US.

The focus of this article is to delineate the normal anatomic landmarks of fetal brain development using fetal MRI at different stages of maturation. Normal brain parenchymal lamination, cortical formation, gyration, myelination, posterior fossa development, and anatomy of the ventricular system, as well of the septum pellucidum and corpus callosum are reviewed. In addition, cerebral biometry and anatomy of other important structures observed on brain imaging is discussed.

IMAGING CONSIDERATIONS

Normal fetal brain development can be evaluated in utero using both US and MRI.[1] MRI is the definitive modality for evaluation of the developing brain, given its superior soft tissue contrast and lack of artifact from bone. MRI is also less susceptible to limitations from maternal body habitus and abnormalities of amniotic fluid.[2] MRI has been shown to be an important tool for prenatal diagnosis of CNS abnormalities[1,2] with improved detection of brain abnormalities over conventional US.[3,4] Fetal MRI is not routinely performed during pregnancy. It is typically obtained after an abnormality is detected on routine US or if there is a known risk factor for CNS abnormality, such as family history of a genetic syndrome or history of traumatic, toxic, or infectious exposure.[2] Fetal MRI is commonly performed at around 20 weeks of gestation, typically after the performance of a routine morphologic US, when most fetal abnormalities are detected. Although fetal MRI can be performed at any stage of pregnancy [5] according to the current American College of Radiology guidelines,[6] it is preferably performed after 16 to 18 weeks of gestation, given the theoretic concern for teratogenesis related to the magnetic field exposure.[1,2,7,8] MRI can be safely performed on either 1.5 T or 3 T magnets.[2,9] There is less heat deposition and less artifacts from fetal motion and amniotic fluid dielectric effect on a 1.5 T magnet. On the other hand, imaging at 3 T has superior

[a] Division Chief of Pediatric Radiology, Department of Radiology, University of North Carolina, School of Medicine, 2006 Old Clinic Building, CB# 7510, Chapel Hill, NC 27599-7510, USA; [b] Department of Radiology, Stanford School of Medicine, Stanford University, 300 Pasteur Drive, Stanford, CA 94304, USA
* Corresponding author.
E-mail address: caroguimaraes55@gmail.com
Twitter: @cguimaraesMD (C.V.A.G.)

Neuroimag Clin N Am 32 (2022) 663–681
https://doi.org/10.1016/j.nic.2022.04.009

resolution and may aid detection of subtle brain parenchymal abnormalities.[2,9,10] The use of intravenous gadolinium contrast agents is contraindicated for fetal MRI evaluation[2,11] and in general is a relative contraindication during pregnancy as its crosses the placenta.[7,10] Contrast may be used during pregnancy for evaluation of maternal pathology if maternal benefits outweigh the fetal risks.[12]

Fast imaging sequences to minimize artifact from fetal motion are required for a good diagnostic quality fetal MRI. The main sequences used are T2-weighted sequences because of the high water and low fat contents of the fetal brain. These ultrafast MRI T2-weighted sequences are known as single-shot fast spin-echo (ssFSE) or half-Fourier acquired single-shot turbo spin echo sequences.[13] A 3-plane localizer of the maternal uterus is typically the first sequence performed and provides useful information such as fetal presentation, sidedness, and an overview of the uterus, placenta, umbilical cord, and amniotic fluid. Evaluation of fetal sidedness should be performed routinely on these first sequences of the maternal uterus, as these are the only true anatomic views where the left and right sides are clearly demarcated; this will determine if an abnormality is seen on the left or the right side of the fetal brain. Single-shot FSE sequences should be performed in all 3 planes and images repeated if they are not acquired in the intended plane or if fetal motion limits evaluation. Three-millimeter slice thickness with no gap is preferred. Fast steady-state free precession imaging is also routinely performed for CNS evaluation, at 3 to 4 mm slice thickness with no gap. This sequence is especially helpful when evaluating fluid structures or fluid-tissue interfaces.

Additional sequences commonly included in the evaluation of the fetal brain are diffusion-weighted imaging (DWI), fast multiplanar gradient recalled echo T1, and echo planar imaging (EPI). The use of EPI sequence is key for detection of intracranial hemorrhage. Although EPI sequences can also aid in the visualization of calcifications, intracranial calcification can be difficult to depict even on optimal EPI sequences. Advanced imaging such as diffusion tensor imaging, spectroscopy, and functional imaging may be performed when indicated or as part of research protocols. Cine images may be performed if evaluation of fetal motion and swallowing is desired.

Lastly, as many congenital anomalies may have associated abnormalities elsewhere, evaluation of the entire fetus and correlation with US findings is desirable, even when the focus is on CNS abnormalities.

PARENCHYMAL FORMATION/LAMINATION

The detailed description of the embryonic/fetal brain development before 16 to 18 weeks of gestation is beyond the scope of this article. It is, however, important to recognize that the primitive cerebral hemispheres develop at about 5 weeks of gestation and the cortical plate begins to appear after 7 weeks of gestation.[8] When fetal MRI is performed after 16 to 18 weeks of gestation, the immature cerebral parenchyma and ventricular system are already well delineated. Initially, the cerebral mantle is diffusely thin, and the ventricles seem relatively prominent (**Fig. 1**A). As gestation progresses, the cerebral mantle gets thicker, leading to a relative decrease in ventricular size[1] (see **Figs. 1**B–D).

Cortical development occurs in 3 phases: neuronal proliferation, neuronal migration, and neuronal organization. Cerebral cortical cells are generated and proliferate in the germinal matrix around the ventricles. Postmitotic cortical neurons then migrate from the germinal matrix to the cortical plate. Migration occurs along an infrastructure of specialized radial glial cells in successive waves to form the future 6-layer neocortex.[8] During these phases of cortical formation, complex histologic events occur in transient cerebral zones[14]; this is known as "cerebral lamination." Cerebral lamination changes with gestational age, mostly during the neuronal migration phase of cortical development. Histologically, the 7 layers of cerebral lamination can be distinguished after 15 weeks of gestation: the ventricular zone, the periventricular rich zone, the subventricular zone, the intermediate zone, the subplate zone, the cortical plate, and the marginal zone. The ventricular zone is the germinal matrix, possessing high neuron density. The periventricular zone is where the axons of the corpus callosum develop.[1] The intermediate zone is the central white matter that dramatically increases in size during gestation.

On MRI, these different layers corresponding to neuronal migration can be partially visible with changing patterns at different gestational ages.[8] High cellular areas, including the germinal matrix (ventricular zone) and cortex (cortical plate), demonstrate a lower T2 and higher DWI signal.[2] The early intermediate zone lacks myelination, is high in water content, and demonstrates high T2 signal. The periventricular and subplate zones also show high signal on T2-weighted images, because of the high extracellular matrix.[13] Therefore, between 16 and 20 weeks, MRI differentiates only 3 parenchymal layers on ssFSE[2,8]: the germinal matrix at the ventricular zone (low T2

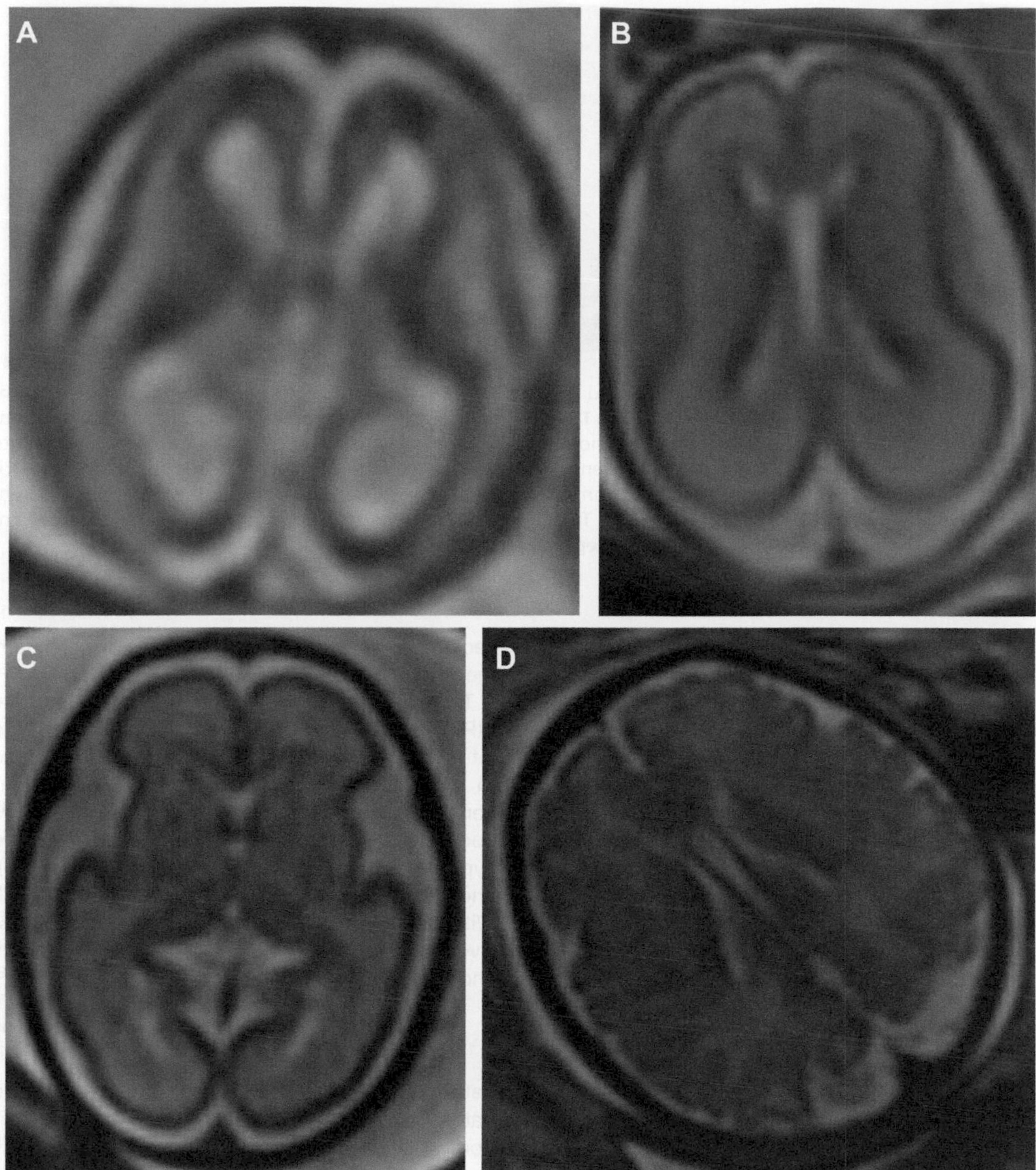

Fig. 1. Axial ssFSE sequences of 4 different normal fetuses demonstrating the expected changes in fetal brain parenchymal growth and formation during the second and third trimester of pregnancy. (*A*) A 16-week-old fetus, (*B*) 20-week-old fetus, (*C*) 26-week-old fetus, and (*D*) 35-week-old fetus.

signal), intermediate zone (high T2 signal) and the cortical plate (low T2 signal) (Fig. 2A). On DWI sequence, there will be also a 3-layer pattern with a thick high-intensity periventricular band, which is dark on apparent diffusion coefficient map, corresponding to a combination of the highly cellular ventricular zone, periventricular zone, subventricular zone, and intermediate zone all together[1,15](Fig. 3A). This band should not be mistaken for an ischemic insult. Between 20 and 28 weeks, MRI shows a 5-layer pattern on ssFSE: the germinal matrix at the ventricular zone (low T2 signal), periventricular rich zone (high T2 signal), the intermediate zone (ill-defined band of low T2 signal), the subplate zones (high T2 signal), and the cortical plate (low T2 signal) (see Fig. 2B). DWI will continue to show a 3-layer pattern throughout gestation with progressive decrease

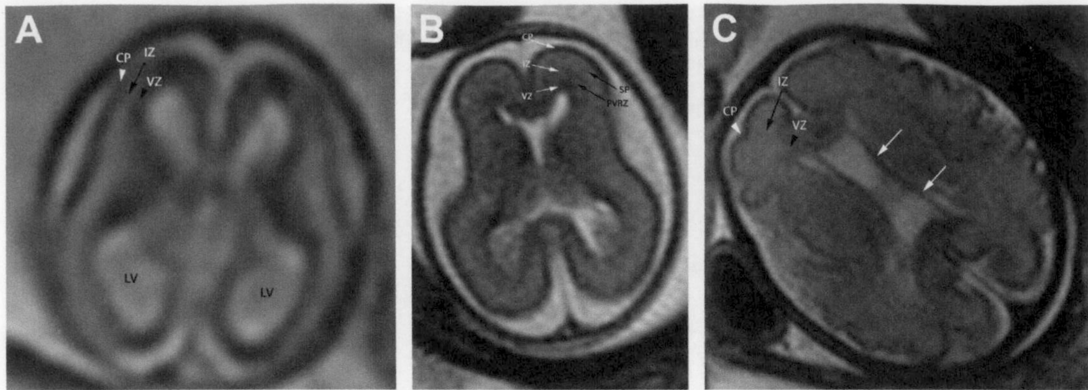

Fig. 2. Changes in cerebral lamination visualized on fetal MRI. (*A*) A 16-week-old fetus demonstrating 3 parenchymal layers: T2 hypointense cortical plate (CP), T2 hyperintense intermediate zone (IZ), and T2 hypointense ventricular zone (VZ). (*B*) A 22-week-old fetus demonstrating 5 parenchymal layers: T2 hypointense cortical plate (CP), T2 hyperintense subplate (SP), T2 hypointense intermediate zone (IZ), T2 hyperintense periventricular rich zone (PVRZ), and T2 hypointense ventricular zone (VZ). (*C*) A 33-week-old fetus demonstrating again 3 parenchymal layers: T2 hypointense cortical plate (CP), T2 hyperintense intermediate zone (IZ), and T2 hypointense ventricular zone (VZ). Incidentally noted is cavum septum pellucidum and vergae (*white arrows*).

in thickness of the periventricular high DWI signal (see Fig. 3B). After 28 weeks, the intermediate zone cannot be distinguished from the subplate zone on ssSFE sequence and again only 3 layers will be visualized on MRI[1,13](see Fig. 2C).

Another important fetal anatomic structure during cerebral formation is the ganglionic eminence. The ganglionic eminences are transient high cellular zones that give rise to the deep gray nuclei, thalami, and glial cells.[2] They are the germinal matrix of the basal forebrain and are located within the ventricular and subventricular zones, at the caudothalamic groove as well as adjacent to the atrium of the lateral ventricles. Given its high cell density, the ganglionic eminences are seen as prominent focal areas of dark T2 and high DWI signal and should not be mistaken for hemorrhage or ischemia[2] (Figs. 4A–B).

As neuronal migration progresses, the germinal matrix gradually regresses during the second trimester.[2,8,16] The germinal matrix is approximately half of its original size by 26 to 28 weeks.[2,17] Residual germinal matrix can be seen until about 33 weeks gestational age along the roof of the temporal horn and in the lateral wall of the occipital horns. Germinal matrix can be seen beyond 33 weeks in the caudothalamic grooves.[13]

The fetal white matter contains prominent hydrophilic extracellular matrix along the periventricular regions known as periventricular crossroads.[13,18] These zones are rich in axonal guidance cues, crossing fibers, and callosal fibers and can be visible on fetal MRI at about 20 weeks of gestation. These crossroads are slightly hyperintense on T2-weighted sequences when compared with the adjacent intermediate zone[13,14,18] (Fig. 5).

The appearance of the deep gray nuclei on fetal MRI also depends on the gestational age of the fetus. Early on, the deep gray nuclei are isointense to slightly hypointense compared with the adjacent white matter on T2-weighted images. At about 27 weeks of gestation, they seem more hypointense on T2-weighted images[19] (Fig. 6). The deep gray nuclei also change on fetal DWI. With increasing gestational age, there is a progressive decline in mean diffusivity in both the thalami and the basal ganglia.[13,20,21]

GYRATION

Fetal brain gyration occurs in a very predictable pattern during normal fetal development. The temporal pattern can help both date the pregnancy and identify abnormalities when gyration does not meet its expected normal developmental appearance. Initially, the fetal brain demonstrates a smooth surface resembling lissencephaly (see Fig. 1A). Progressive sulcation occurs during the second and third trimesters (see Figs. 1B–D). The primary sulci appear first as shallow indentations on the surface of the brain, which become progressively deeper and narrower. Secondary sulci are side branches of the primary sulci, and tertiary sulci are side branches of the secondary sulci.[13,22]

The first brain fissures seen are the interhemispheric fissures (14–15 weeks) and the Sylvian fissures (16–18 weeks) (Fig. 7A). These are followed

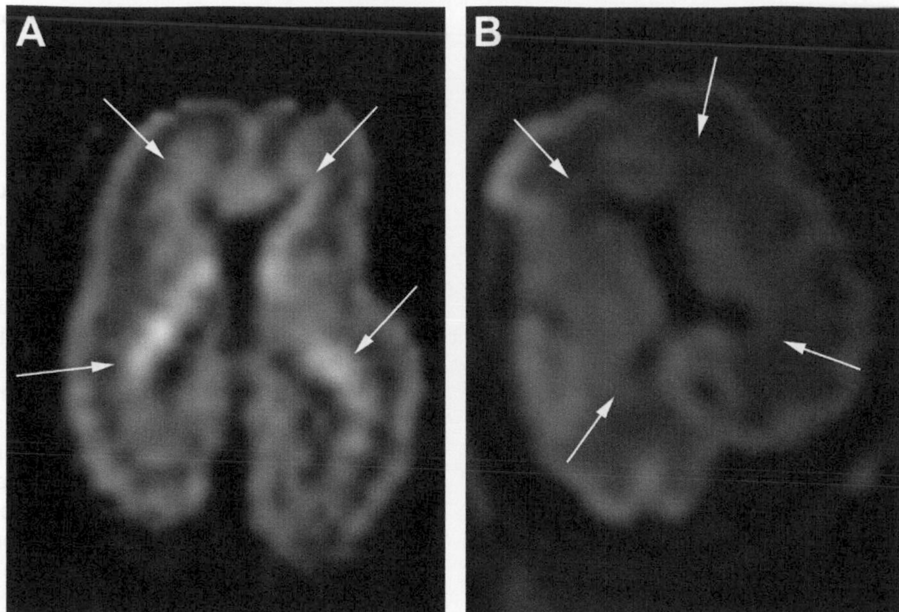

Fig. 3. DWI sequence in 2 different fetuses showing 3 parenchymal layers during the entire second and third trimesters. (*A*) A 21-week-old fetus showing expected thick band of high signal intensity in the periventricular region (*white arrows*). (*B*) A 30-week-old fetus demonstrating a thinner band of high signal within the periventricular region (*white arrows*).

by the hippocampal sulcus (18–23 weeks), parieto-occipital sulcus (22–23 weeks), calcarine sulcus (22–25 weeks), cingulate (24–25 weeks), central (26 weeks), collateral (26 weeks), precentral (27 weeks), superior temporal (27 weeks), marginal (27 weeks), postcentral (28 weeks), intraparietal (28 weeks), superior frontal (29 weeks), inferior frontal (29 weeks), inferior temporal (33–34 weeks), and occipitotemporal sulci (33–34 weeks)[2] (see **Fig. 7** B–D). By 35 weeks' gestation, all primary and most of the secondary sulci are present.[1,13,23]

It is imperative to know the fetal gestational age for accurate interpretation of the sulcation pattern and exclusion of malformations. Additional clinical history is important to exclude conditions known to delay fetal sulcation such as cardiac disease, congenital diaphragmatic hernia, intrauterine growth restriction, and chromosomal abnormalities. There may be a discrepancy of 2 weeks

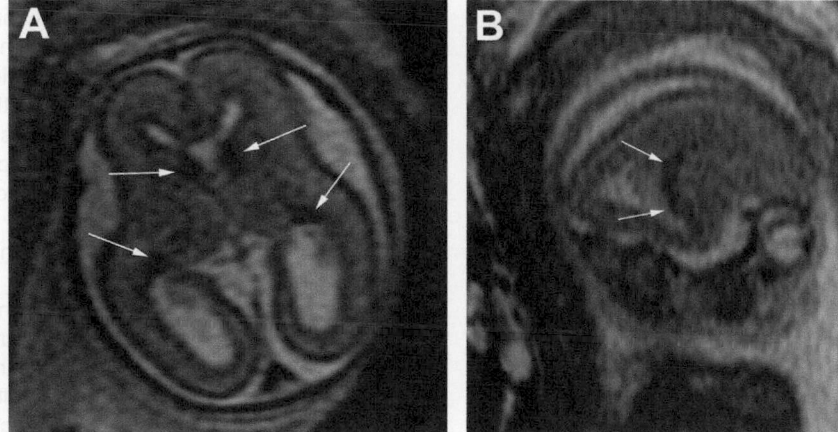

Figs. 4. (*A*) Axial ssFSE sequence of a 22-week-old fetus showing the normal T2 hypointense signal of the bilateral ganglionic eminences (*white arrows*). (*B*) Periventricular ganglionic eminences again seen on sagittal ssFSE of the same fetus (*white arrows*).

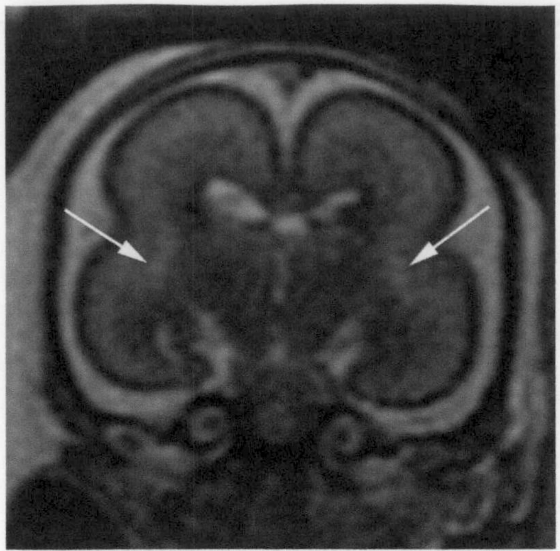

Fig. 5. Bilateral periventricular crossroads demonstrated on coronal ssFSE of a 22-week-old fetus (*white arrows*).

between sulcus identification on MRI and gestational age.[2,13] Mild asymmetry of cortical sulcation can be seen between the 2 cerebral hemispheres. For example, the right superior temporal gyrus may appear before the left,[2,24] and the calcarine

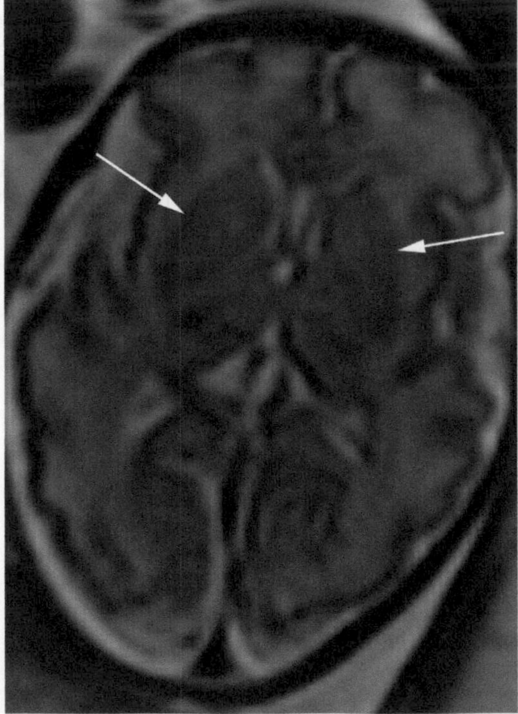

Fig. 6. 33-week-old fetus showing the normal T2 hypointense signal of the basal ganglia seen after 27 weeks of gestation.

fissures can show asymmetric development.[24,25] These variations should not be misinterpreted as malformations of cortical development.

MYELINATION

Although some brain myelination occurs in the fetus, most of the brain myelination occurs postnatally. Normal myelination demonstrates high T1 and low T2 signal and generally occurs from central to peripheral, inferior to superior and posterior to anterior. Myelination is first identified in the dorsal brainstem at about 21 to 22 weeks, progressing from the medulla, through the pons, to the midbrain.[1,2] At 28 to 29 weeks, the inferior and superior cerebellar peduncle are myelinated.[2,26] Supratentorial myelination is not apparent on MRI until late third trimester. After 32 weeks, myelination can be seen in the putamen, ventrolateral thalamus, and posterior aspect of the posterior limb of the internal capsule[2] (**Fig. 8**).

VENTRICULAR SYSTEM

There are 2 methods to measure the size of the lateral ventricles on fetal MRI. On the axial plane, it mirrors the traditional US measurement in the transventricular plane. The transventricular plane is an axial view of the brain at the level of the septum pellucidum, thalamus, and parietal-occipital sulcus. Measurements are made at the level of the parieto-occipital sulcus and glomus of the choroid plexus, with the calipers placed in the largest part of the atrium inside the ventricular wall[2,27] (**Fig. 9**A). The atrial diameter of the lateral ventricles is relatively constant during gestation, with normal values being less than 10 mm.[2,27] A 1 to 2 mm discrepancy with US measurements is within normal limits.[2,28] It is also important to know that lateral ventricular asymmetry of 2.4 mm without dilatation is considered normal.[2,29] Another way to measure the lateral ventricles is using the coronal plane at the level of the atrium where the glomus of the choroid plexus is visualized (see **Fig. 9**B). Measurements made by this method are highly concordant with those made by US.[2,30]

The third ventricle can be measured in the coronal plane at its largest transverse diameter (**Fig. 10**). A measurement of more than 4 mm is considered enlarged.[31] The third ventricular recesses and the aqueduct of Sylvius can be seen on a high-quality, well-positioned sagittal views of the fetal brain (**Fig. 11**). These structures can be difficult to fully delineate in young fetuses if motion degraded or off-midline images were obtained. They are better visualized in the third

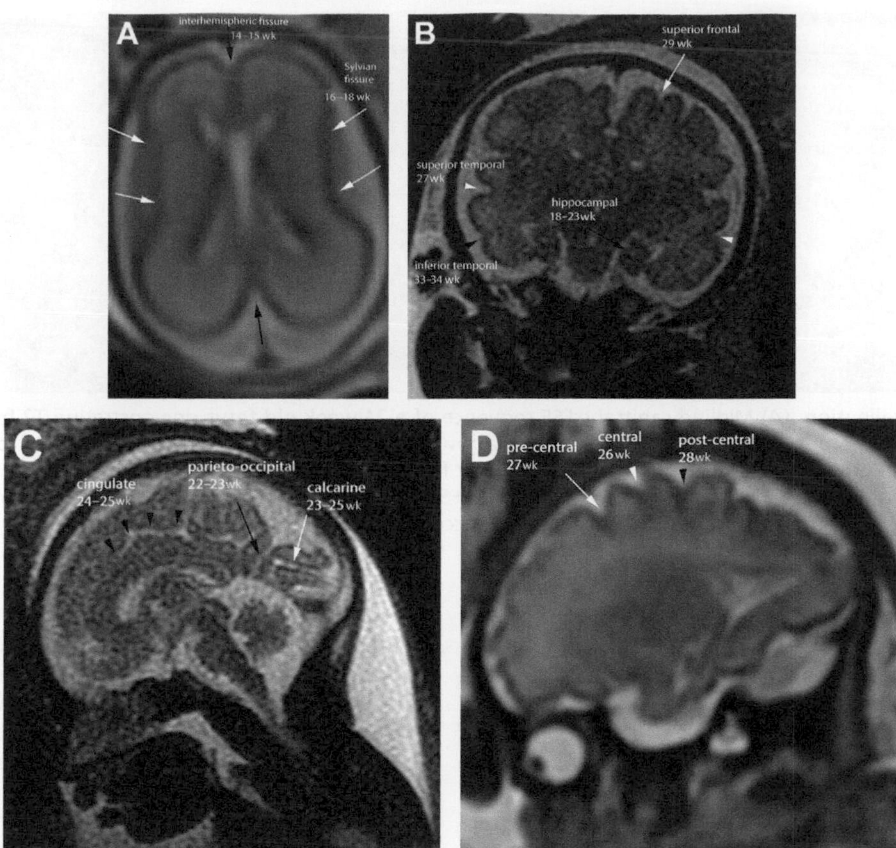

Fig. 7. Cerebral gyri demonstrated in different gestational ages. (*A*) Axial ssFSE sequence of a 20-week-old fetus demonstrating the presence of the interhemispheric fissure (*black arrow*), which appears at 14 to 15 weeks, and the Sylvian fissure (*white arrows*), which appears at 16 to 18 weeks. (*B*) Coronal ssFSE of a 33-week-old fetus demonstrating the hippocampal sulcus (*black arrow*), which appears at 18 to 23 weeks; the superior temporal sulcus (*white arrowheads*), which appears at 27 weeks; the superior frontal sulcus (*white arrow*), which appears at 29 weeks; and the inferior temporal sulcus (*black arrowhead*), which appears at 33 to 34 weeks. (*C*) Sagittal ssFSE of a 33-week-old fetus demonstrating gyri seen at the midline including the parieto-occipital gyrus (*black arrow*), which appears at 22 to 23 weeks; the calcarine fissure (*white arrow*), which appears at 23 to 25 weeks; and the cingulate gyrus and overlying cingulate sulcus (*black arrowheads*), which appears at 24 to 25 weeks. (*D*) Sagittal off-midline ssFSE of a 33-week-old fetus showing the central sulcus (*white arrowhead*), which appears at 26 weeks; the precentral sulcus (*white arrow*), which appears at 27 weeks; and the postcentral sulcus (*black arrowhead*), which appears at 28 weeks.

trimester or when abnormally dilated, such as in cases of aqueduct stenosis. In aqueduct stenosis, dilated third ventricular recesses and aqueduct funneling are typically present.[32]

The fourth ventricle can be measured on the midline sagittal image from the dorsal pons to the fastigial point (Fig. 12). A measurement of more than 7 mm is considered abnormal.[2,33]

Early in gestation (16–20 weeks), the ventricles and extra-axial spaces seem prominent relative to the thin cerebral parenchyma[13] (see Fig. 1A). This normal prominence should not be misdiagnosed as ventriculomegaly. With growth of the surrounding cerebral parenchyma, the lateral ventricles narrow and achieve their normal mature configuration.[1] The walls of the ventricle should be smooth without nodularity.[2]

CAVUM SEPTUM PELLUCIDUM AND CORPUS CALLOSUM

The cavum septum pellucidum is a transient space between the frontal horns of the lateral ventricles and is bordered by the septum pellucidum leaflets (Fig. 13). Its development is closely associated with the development of the forebrain commissures and the forniceal columns at the level of the lamina reuniens.[34] The cavum septum pellucidum can be visualized as early as 15 weeks, and it should be present by 18 weeks of gestation.[2,35] Its

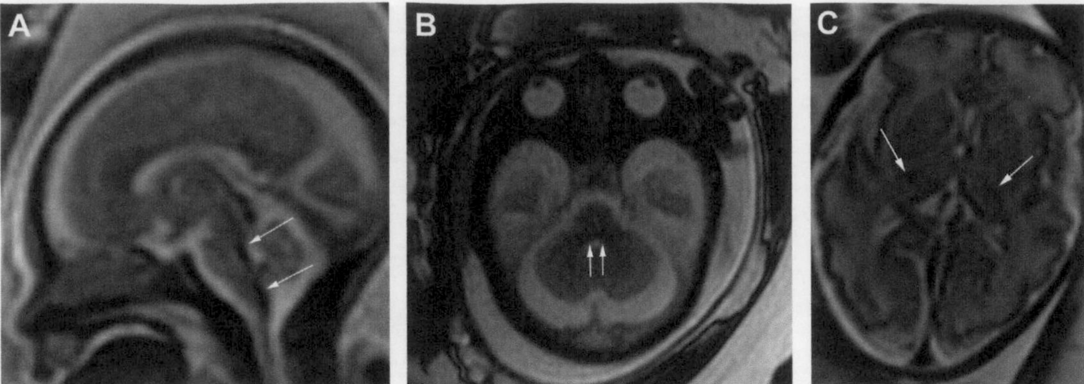

Figs. 8. Myelination. (*A*) Midline sagittal ssFSE sequence of a 24-week-old fetus demonstrating T2 hypointense signal along the dorsal pons and medulla (*white arrows*) corresponding to myelination after 21 to 22 weeks of gestation. (*B*) Axial ssFSE at the level of the posterior fossa in a 34-week-old fetus again demonstrating myelination along the dorsal pons (*white arrows*). (*C*) Axial ssFSE sequence of a 34-week-old fetus showing myelination within the ventrolateral thalami (*white arrows*) that occurs after 32 weeks of gestation.

normal diameter ranges between 2 and 10 mm.[2,34] The leaflets of the septum pellucidum begin to close from back to front during the third trimester of pregnancy. It may be closed as early as 37 weeks of gestation and will be closed in most infants by 3 to 6 months of age. Persistence until adulthood may occur as a normal variant.[2,31] Absent visualization of the septum pellucidum on US suggests a midline abnormality and is a common indication for fetal MRI.

The corpus callosum is the largest cerebral commissure connecting the 2 cerebral hemispheres. It is composed by the rostrum, genu, body, and splenium. It forms during 8 to 20 weeks of gestation, starting at the anterior body (ventral part of the lamina reuniens) and then develops anteriorly and posteriorly.[2] The corpus callosum is seen as a T2 hypointense crescentic linear structure on a midline sagittal image superior to the lateral ventricles (Fig. 14A). It may be difficult to visualize in its entirety in young fetuses or on motion-degraded examinations. In such cases, its presence can be confirmed by using images obtained in the coronal and axial planes (see Figs. 14B and C). Before 20 weeks of gestation, the delineation of its rostrum and splenium may be especially difficult, as the corpus callosum is still developing; this should not be interpreted as an abnormality.

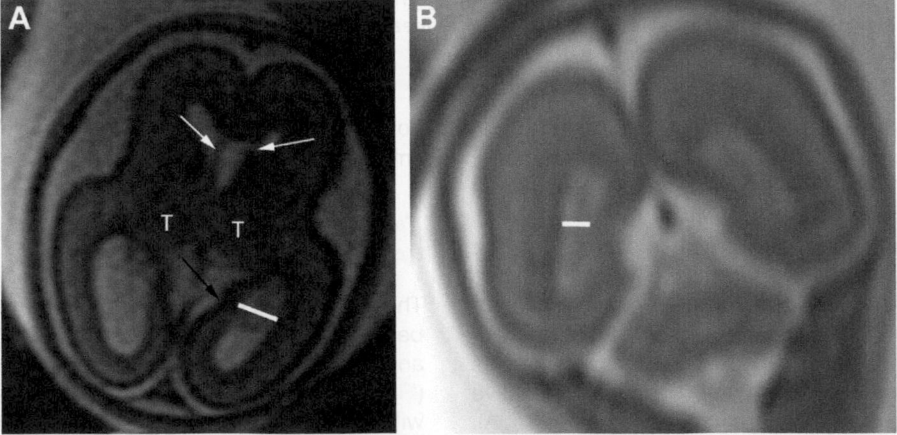

Fig. 9. Measurement of the lateral ventricles (*white lines*). (*A*) Axial plane measurement is performed similar to US transventricular plane—at the level of the septum pellucidum (*white arrows*), thalamus (T), and parietal-occipital sulcus (*black arrow*). (*B*) Coronal measurement is made at the level of the lateral ventricular atrium, where the glomus of the choroid plexus is seen.

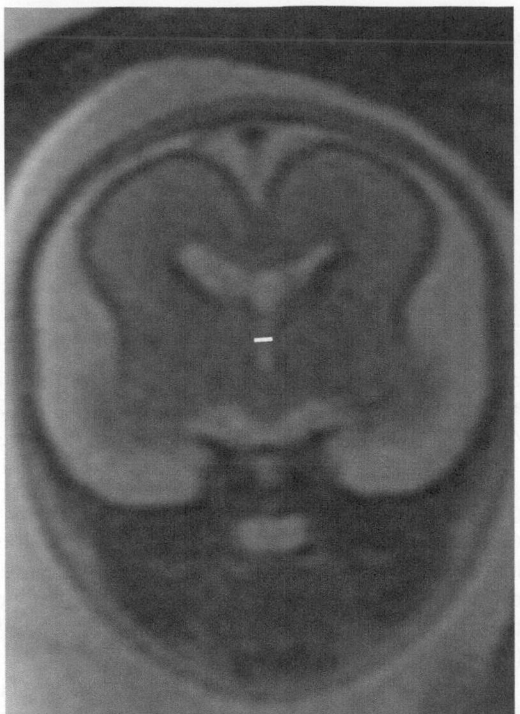

Fig. 10. Measurement of the third ventricle, performed on the coronal plane at its largest transverse diameter (*white line*).

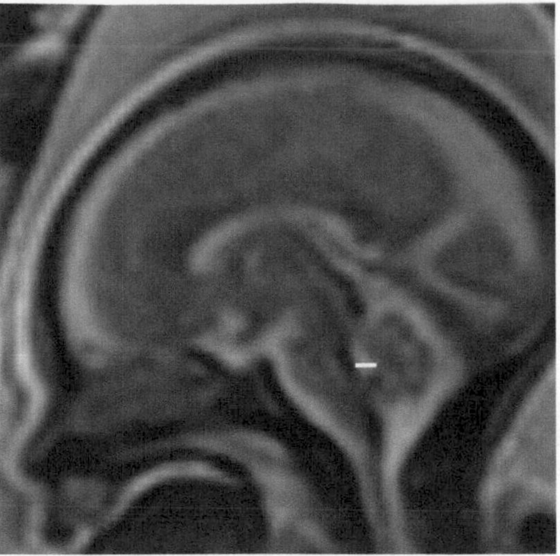

Fig. 12. Measurement of the fetal fourth ventricle, performed at the midline sagittal plane from the dorsal surface of the brainstem to the fourth ventricular fastigial point (*white line*).

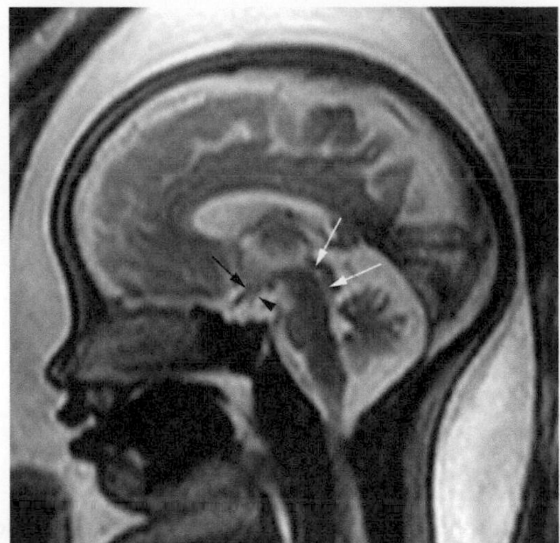

Fig. 11. Midline sagittal ssFSE sequence of a 33-week-old fetus demonstrating a patent cerebral aqueduct (*white arrows*) and normal morphology of the inferior third ventricular recesses (supraoptic recess—*black arrow* and infundibular recess—*black arrowhead*).

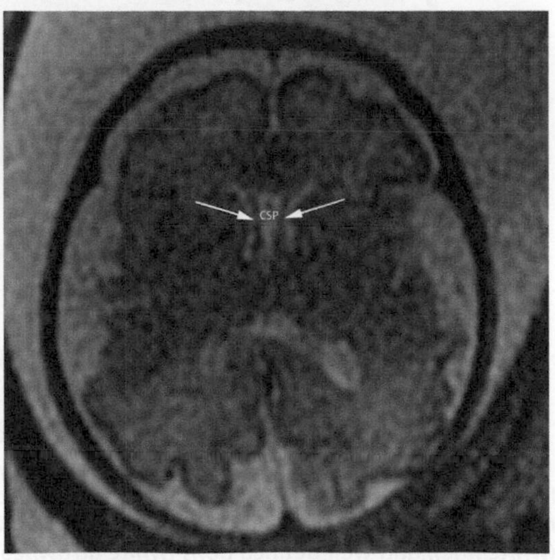

Fig. 13. Cavum septum pellucidum (CSP) seen on the axial plane, laterally demarcated by the septum pellucidum leaflets (*white arrows*).

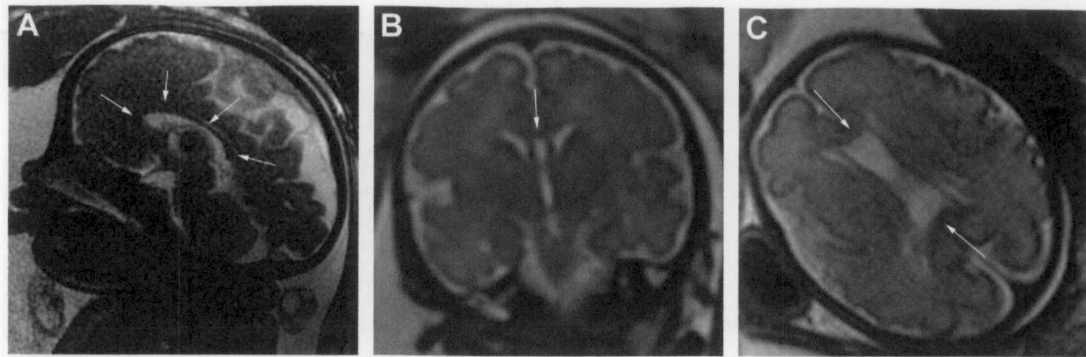

Fig. 14. Visualization of the corpus callosum. (*A*) Midline sagittal fast steady-state free precession sequence in a 33-week-old fetus showing the entire extension of the fetal corpus callosum (*white arrows*). (*B*) Coronal and (*C*) axial images can help confirm its presence when difficult visualization on the sagittal plane (*white arrows*).

POSTERIOR FOSSA DEVELOPMENT

The infratentorial brain develops from the mesencephalon and rhombencephalon. The midbrain derives from the mesencephalon. The cerebellum and pons mainly derive from the metencephalon portion of the rhombencephalon[36] with influences from the isthmic organizer at the midbrain-hindbrain boundary.[13] The medulla develops from the myelencephalon portion of the rhombencephalon.[13,36] At about 6 weeks of gestation, the cerebellum and the brainstem begin to form.[13,37] The brainstem undergoes a segmentation process that leads to patterning along the anteroposterior and dorsoventral neuraxis.[38] During the second and third trimesters of pregnancy, there is greater growth of the cerebellar and pontine areas compared with the midbrain and medulla; this leads to a change of the midbrain to pons to medulla area ratio from 2:1:1 in the early second trimester to 2:3:2 at the end of pregnancy[38] (**Fig. 15**A).

At 12 to 13 weeks of gestation the first cerebellar fissure, the posterolateral fissure located between the flocculonodular lobe and the remaining cerebellum, develops.[1] At 14 to 15 weeks of gestation, the primary fissure develops. The primary fissure is the deepest fissure in the vermis (see **Fig. 15**A) and an important anatomic landmark when evaluating the normal cerebellar anatomy.[1,2] At 15 to 16 weeks of gestation, the prepyramidal, preculminate, and precentral fissures develop. At

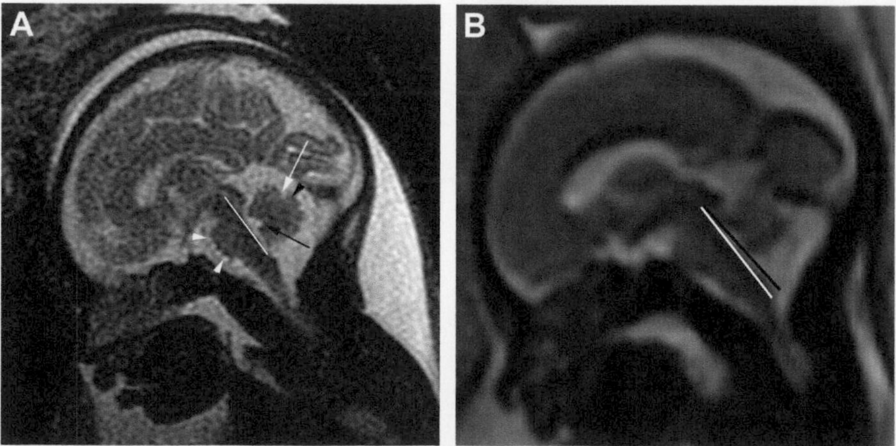

Fig. 15. (*A*) Midline sagittal ssFSE sequence of a 33-week-old fetus showing important posterior fossa anatomic landmarks on fetal MRI. These include the normal acute fourth ventricular fastigial point (*black arrow*), the primary fissure (*white arrow*), the cerebellar declive lobule (*black arrowhead*), a straight dorsal brainstem surface (*white line*), and well-defined pons (*white arrowheads*), which should be larger than the midbrain and medulla during the third trimester. (*B*) Midline sagittal ssFSE sequence of a 23-week-old fetus showing a normal tegmentovermian angle, which should be close to 0 after 20 weeks of gestation. The angle is measured between the lines drawn along the dorsal brainstem (*white line*) and the ventral vermis (*black line*).

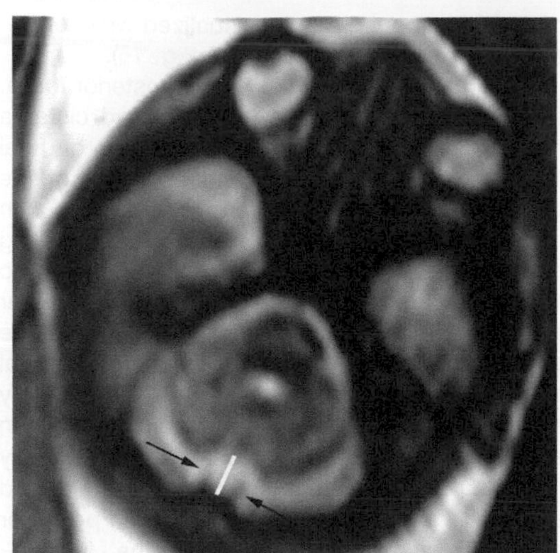

Fig. 16. Measurement of the cisterna magna on the axial plane from the cerebellar vermis to the calvarium (*white line*). Note the lateral walls of the Blake pouch (*black arrows*).

21 weeks of gestation, the horizontal fissure will be present.[1] The horizontal fissures are the deepest fissures in the cerebellar hemispheres.[2]

The cerebellar vermis develops in a craniocaudal fashion, with the inferior aspect of the vermis (known as the posterior vermian lobe) developing later than its superior aspect (known as anterior vermian lobe). The posterior vermian lobe will show its normal inferior contour, covering the inferior aspect of the fourth ventricle, at about 18 to 20 weeks of gestation.[2,13] Therefore, caution should be exercised while diagnosing vermian hypoplasia before 18 weeks of gestation. After 18 to 20 weeks of gestation, the posterior vermian lobe should be slightly larger than the anterior vermian lobe; this can be confirmed by drawing a line from the fastigial point to the declive (vermian lobulation just below the primary fissure). This line is referred to as the fastigial-declive line. The cerebellar tissue below this line should normally be larger than above, an important observation when evaluating a fetus with possible vermian hypoplasia.[39] Also, the tegmentovermian angle (angle between the dorsal brainstem and the ventral vermis) will be close to zero in most fetuses after 18 to 20 weeks[2,39,40] (see **Fig. 15**B).

The cerebellar parenchyma will show layers of low T2 signal on fetal MRI, at the deep cerebellar nuclei and cortex by 21 weeks of gestation and at the flocculonodular lobe by 30 to 31 weeks.[1] The tips of the cerebellar foliae are more hypointense on T2-weighted images than their deeper portions.[1]

The cisterna magna is an important posterior fossa structure, and its normal size should be documented on anatomic US. To accurately evaluate the cisterna magna, it is important to understand the Blake pouch. The Blake pouch represents an embryonic outpouching of the meninx primitiva that extends from the inferior forth ventricle into the retrocerebellar subarachnoid space. Blake pouch undergoes fenestration to form the foramina of Luschka and

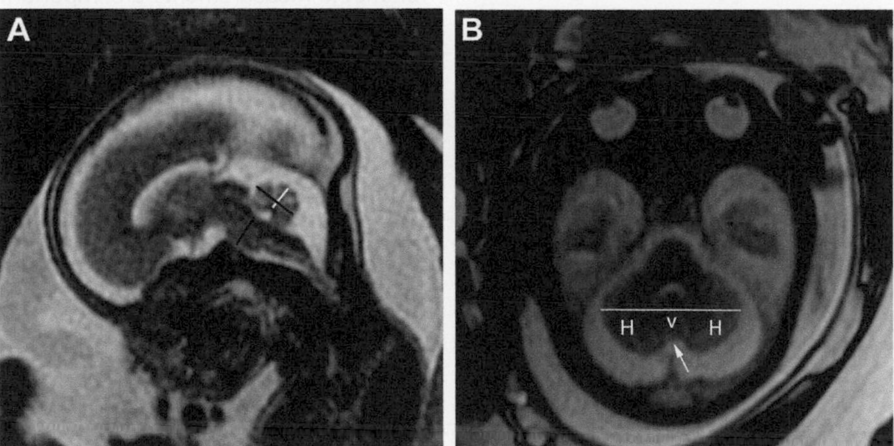

Figs. 17. Posterior fossa MRI biometric measurements. (*A*) The cerebellar vermis craniocaudal diameter (*black line*), the cerebellar vermis anteroposterior diameter (*white line*), and the pons anteroposterior diameter (*blue line*). (*B*) The transverse cerebellar diameter (*white line*). Also note the normal morphology of the cerebellum on the axial plane including the 2 symmetric cerebellar hemispheres (H) and the single midline cerebellar vermis (V). Note the presence of a focal concavity at the level of the cerebellar vermis (*white arrow*), an important landmark when evaluating the presence of the vermis.

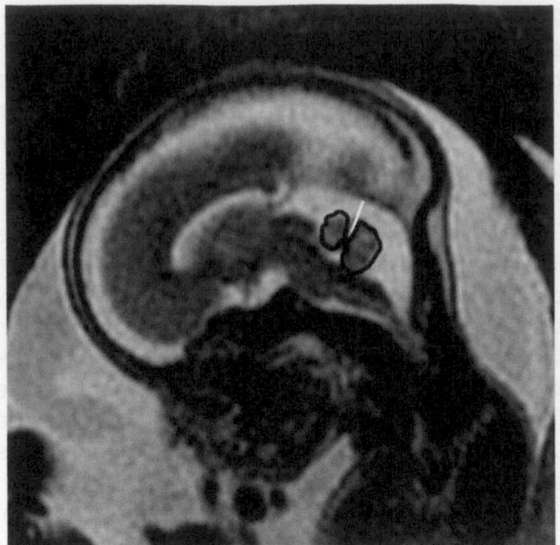

Fig. 18. Midline sagittal ssFSE sequence of a 22-week-old fetus demonstrating the relationship between the anterior vermian lobe (*blue*) and the posterior vermian lobe (*red*) after drawing a line from the fourth ventricular fastigial point to the cerebellar declive, known as the fastigial-declive line (*white line*). Note that the posterior vermian lobe (inferior vermis) is slightly larger than the anterior vermian lobe (superior vermis).

Magendie.[41,42] The cisterna magna represents the fenestrated Blake pouch and is seen as a focal cerebrospinal fluid space along the dorsal aspect of the posterior fossa. The normal cisterna magna should be measured from the vermis to the calvarium on axial transcerebellar images. Normal size should measure between 2 and 10 mm^2 (**Fig. 16**). Both on US and MRI, the lateral walls of the Blake pouch can be visualized while evaluating the cisterna magna[39] (see **Fig. 16**).

Suspected abnormalities of the posterior fossa, especially ones that cause an enlarged cisterna magna, is another common indication of fetal MRI. Fetal MRI allows the measurement of the posterior fossa structures and comparison with normative data for gestational age while providing detailed anatomic evaluation. Important biometric measurements include the transverse cerebellar diameter, the anteroposterior dimension of the pons, and the anteroposterior and craniocaudal dimensions of the cerebellar vermis (**Fig. 17**). Key anatomic landmarks include visualization of an acute fastigial point, the presence of the primary fissure, a near-zero tegmentovermian angle, and a normal ratio between the anterior and posterior cerebellar vermis after drawing the fastigial-declive line (see **Figs. 15**A–B and **Fig. 18**). On the axial plane, the dorsal contours of the cerebellum will show a focal concavity at the level of the cerebellar vermis, between the 2 cerebellar hemispheres; this is another important landmark when evaluating for the presence of the cerebellar vermis on fetal MRI (see **Fig. 17**). Also, it is important to note the normal anatomy of the brainstem, which includes a flat dorsal surface (without kinking or focal bulges) and a well-defined pons that are larger than the midbrain and medulla by the third trimester (see **Fig. 15**A).

SKULL, SCALP, AND ADDITIONAL INTRACRANIAL STRUCTURES

The overall shape of the fetal skull and normative biometric measurements are important additional information when evaluating a fetal MRI.

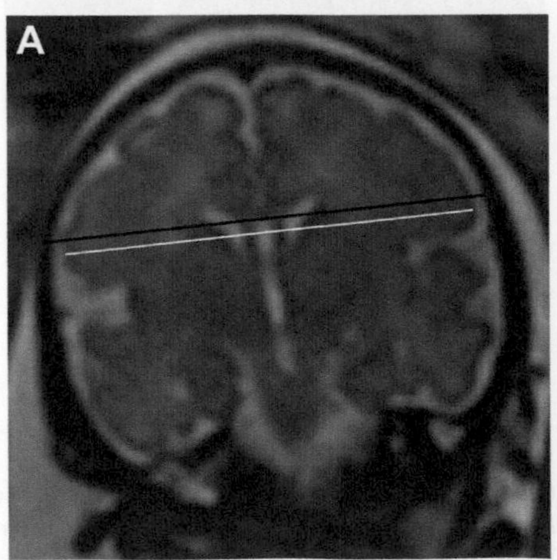

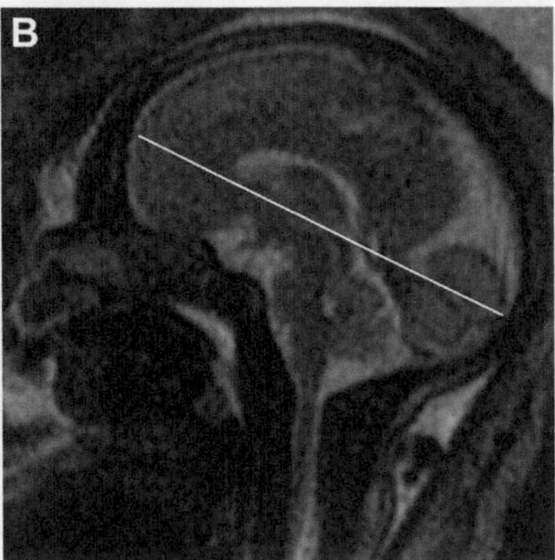

Fig. 19. Skull and cerebral MRI biometric measurements. (*A*) Bony biparietal diameter measured on the coronal plane from inner to outer skull table (*black line*) and cerebral biparietal diameter (*white line*). (*B*) Cerebral fronto-occipital diameter measured on the sagittal midline plane (*white line*).

Measurements include the biparietal diameters of the skull and brain, measured on the coronal plane, and fronto-occipital diameter, measured on the midline sagittal image (Figs. 19 A–B). The measurement of the brain biparietal diameter and fronto-occipital diameter on MRI estimates the actual brain size without the extra-axial spaces. These measurements are compared with established normative data for gestational age and help in the identification of skull abnormalities (such as dolichocephaly or brachycephaly seen with craniosynostosis, microcephaly, macrocephaly, and megalencephaly).[8] The integrity of the skull and scalp should be evaluated. Focal scalp masses should be ruled out.

Another intracranial structure visualized on fetal MRI is the pituitary stalk, which can be detected on coronal or sagittal images as early as 19 gestational weeks and in all fetuses after 25 weeks of gestation[13,43](Fig. 20).

The olfactory sulci and bulbs can be reliably detected in the coronal plane after 30 weeks of gestation[44] (Fig. 21).

HEAD AND NECK

Evaluation of the fetal facial profile is part of the routine fetal CNS evaluation, performed on T2 sagittal views of the fetal brain and face. Key facial structures seen on the sagittal plane include the frontal and nasal bones, hard palate, tongue, and mandible.[7] Patency of the upper airway can be also accessed (Fig. 22).

The nasal bones should be seen after 10 weeks of gestation. The nasal bones are best delineated on US but can also be seen on MRI as a linear T2 hypointense structure on the sagittal midline image (Fig. 23). When the nasal bone is absent, a flat fetal profile is noted. The absence or hypoplasia of the nasal bone is commonly associated with chromosomal abnormalities.[45]

In cases of suspected micrognathia, measurements of the inferior facial angle and jaw index can be performed (Fig.s. 24 A–B). The inferior facial angle is measured at the midline sagittal image by drawing a line along the glabella, perpendicular to the forehead, and a second line from the tip of the mentum to the anterior border of the upper lip[46](see Fig. 24A). The normal inferior facial angle should be greater than 50°. The jaw index is the ratio between the anterior–posterior diameter of the mandible (APD) and the bony biparietal diameter (BPD) calculated by the following formula: (APD/BPD) × 100. The anterior–posterior diameter of the mandible is measured on the axial plane from the mandibular symphysis to a line that connects the posterior borders of the masseter muscles[46,47](see Fig. 24 B). Normal jaw index should measure greater than 33.5.

The T2 axial plane demonstrates the nasal passages, choanae (Fig. 25), and ocular globes (Figs. 26 A–C). The orbits and ocular globes should be evaluated for presence, size, and morphology. Measurements of the interocular diameter (inner-to-inner margin between orbits) and binocular diameter (outer-to-outer margin of both orbits) can be performed and compared with normative data to identify the presence of hypo or hypertelorism[7,48] (Fig. 27). The transient fetal vasculature

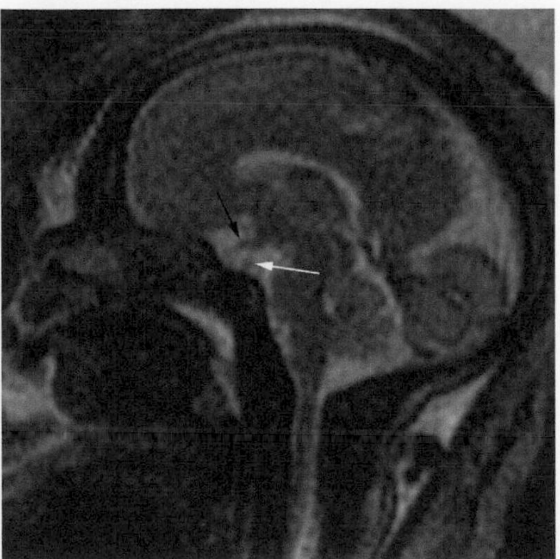

Fig. 20. Midline sagittal ssFSE sequence of a 28-week-old fetus demonstrating the normal pituitary stalk (*white arrow*). Also note the optic chiasm (*black arrow*) often seen at the same plane.

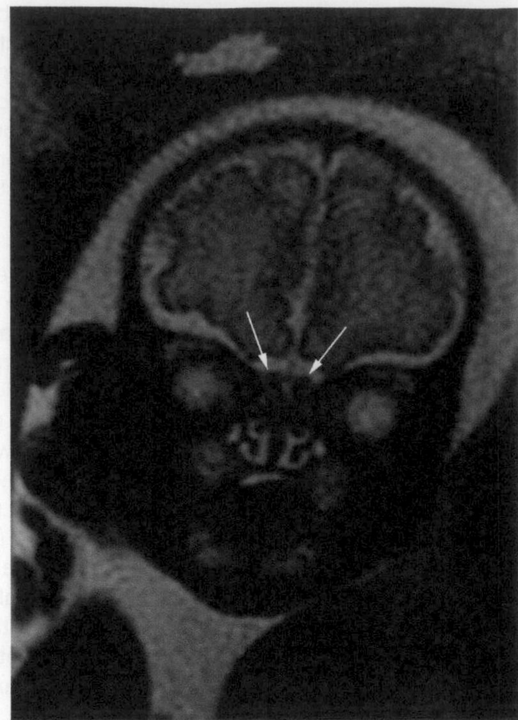

Fig. 21. The paired olfactory bulbs (*white arrows*) can be seen on the coronal T2-weighted sequence after 30 weeks of gestation.

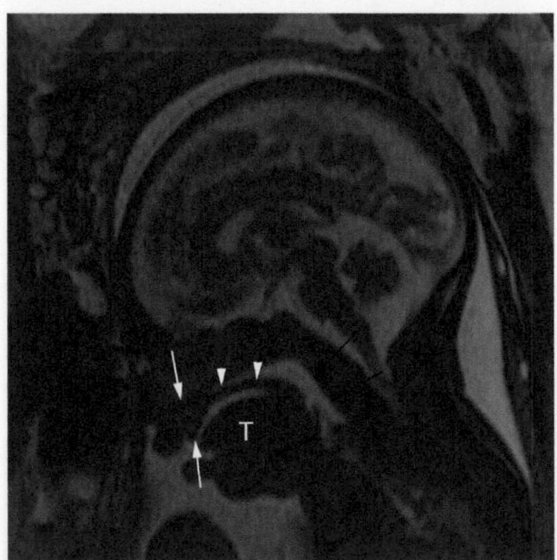

Fig. 22. Midline sagittal view of the brain and fetal profile demonstrating the normal primary palate (*white arrows*), secondary palate (*white arrowheads*), tongue (T) and the patent upper airway (*black arrows*).

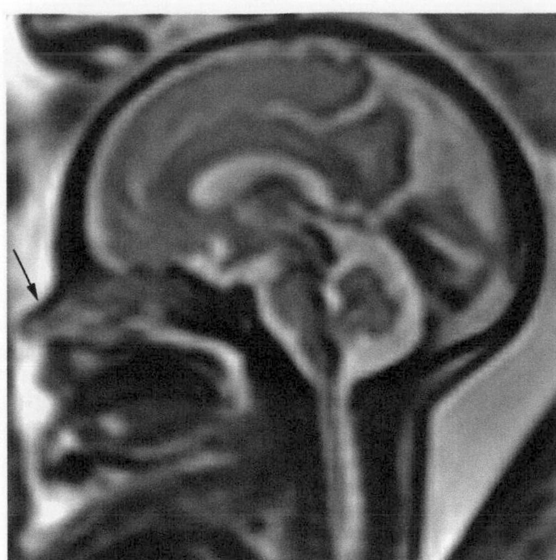

Fig. 23. The normal nasal bone (*black arrow*) seen as a linear band of hypointense T2 signal in the midline sagittal image.

(hyaloid artery) can be seen on fetal MRI as a linear band of hypointense T2 signal traversing the vitreous, from 17 to 24 weeks of gestation.[49] The morphology of the ocular globes changes during gestation. Before 29 weeks, the globes are flat along their posteromedial margins in the axial plane and conical in the sagittal plane (see Figs. 26A–B). After 29 weeks, the fetal ocular globes should assume their final rounded configuration[49] (see Fig. 26C).

The T2 coronal plane is helpful in the assessment of the fetal lip, palate, and ears (Fig. 28). Visualization of the pinna, middle ear cavity, and gross anatomy of the inner ear structures are possible in most pregnancies beyond 25 weeks of gestation. The external auditory canal patency is better seen after 29 weeks of gestation.[50]

The fetal thyroid gland is indistinct on T2-weighted sequences but identifiable on T1-weighted imaging as a small ill-defined hyperintense structure along the anterior neck[51] (Fig. 29); this is important when there is suspicion for fetal goiter or other neck masses.

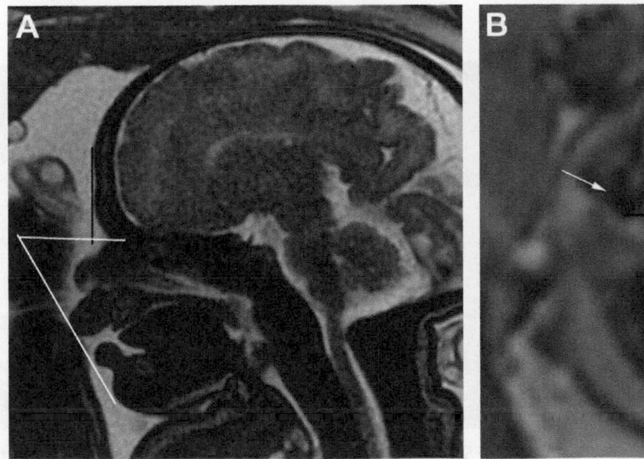

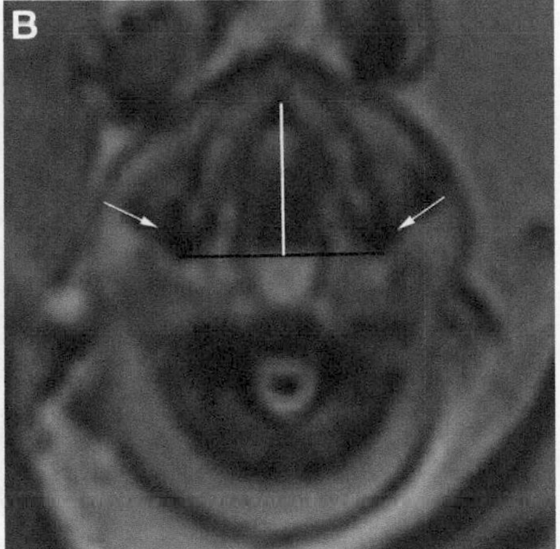

Figs. 24. Inferior facial angle and jaw index. (*A*) Measurement of the inferior facial angle on the sagittal midline plane. Normal angle should be greater than 50°. (*B*) Measurement of the anterior–posterior diameter of the mandible (APD—*white line*) on the axial plane from the mandibular symphysis to a line (*black line*) that connects the posterior borders of the masseter muscles (*white arrows*). The jaw index is calculated by the following formula: (APD/BPD) × 100. Normal jaw index should measure greater than 33.5.

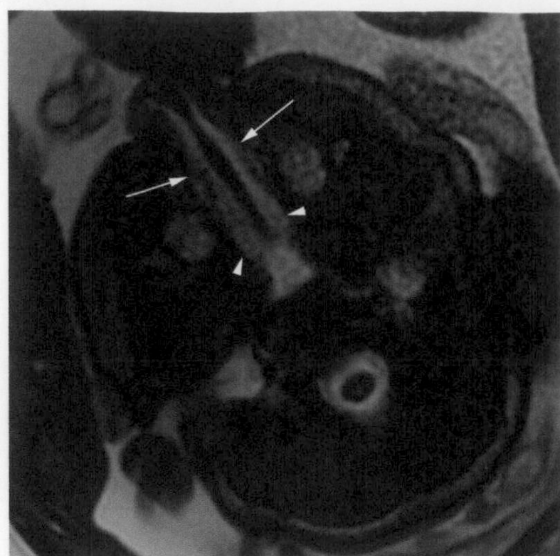

Fig. 25. Axial fast steady-state free precession sequence showing the normal patent bilateral nasal passages (*white arrows*) and choanae (*white arrowheads*).

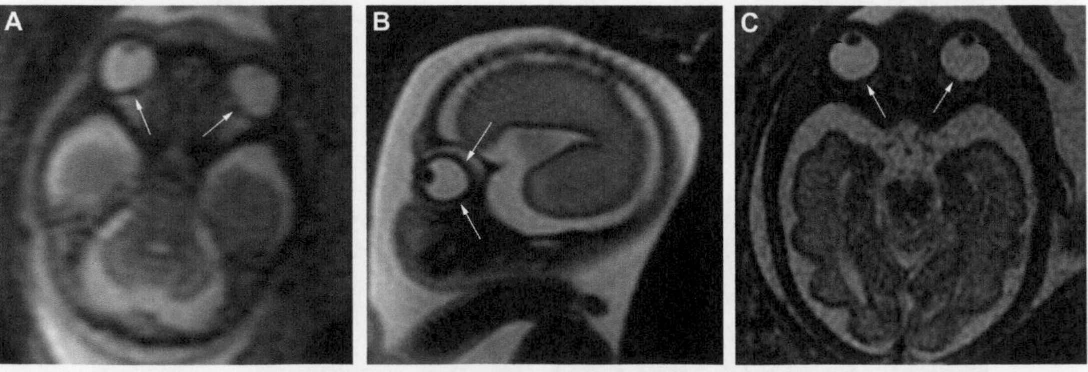

Figs. 26. Morphology of the ocular globes. (*A*) Axial ssFSE sequence of a 22-week-old fetus showing the normal morphology of the ocular globes before 29 weeks of gestation with flattening of its posteromedial contours (*white arrows*). (*B*) Sagittal ssFSE view of a 25-week-old fetus showing the conical shape of the posterior ocular globes before 29 weeks of gestation (*white arrows*). (*C*) Axial ssFSE sequence of the ocular globes in a 33-week-old fetus showing the normal rounded configuration of the ocular globes after 29 weeks of gestation (*white arrows*). Note also the normal T2 hypointense lens (*black arrows*).

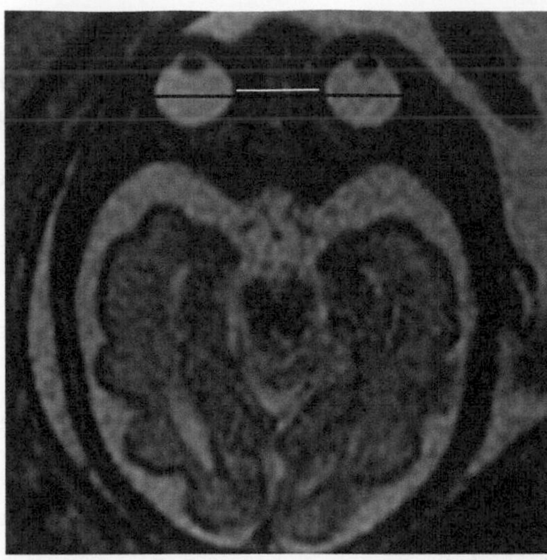

Fig. 27. Measurement of the interocular diameter from inner-to-inner margin of the ocular globes (*white line*) and binocular diameter from outer-to-outer margin of ocular globes (*black line*).

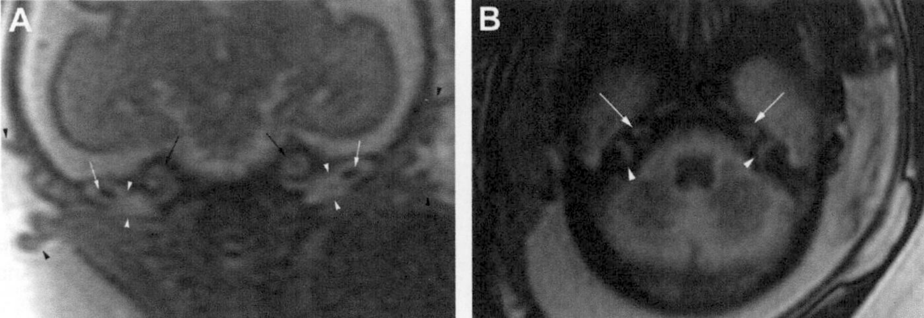

Figs. 28. Bilateral ears. (*A*) Coronal ssFSE sequence demonstrates the bilateral pinna (*black arrowheads*), fluid-filled middle ear cavities (*white arrowheads*), middle ear ossicles (*white arrows*), and the cochlea (*black arrows*). (*B*) Axial fast steady-state free precession sequence showing the cochlea (*white arrows*), vestibule, and portions of the lateral semicircular canal (*white arrowheads*).

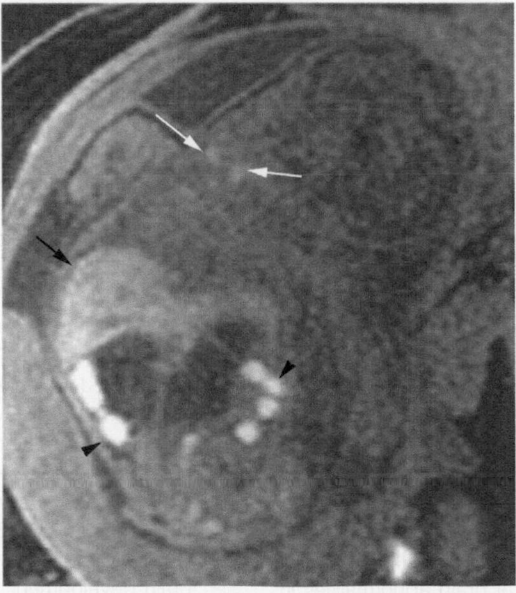

Fig. 29. Coronal T1-weighted sequence showing the normal small ill-defined T1 hyperintense thyroid gland (*white arrows*). Note also more prominent T1 hyperintense structures in the fetus, the liver (*black arrow*) and the meconium within the colon (*black arrowheads*).

SUMMARY

Accurate interpretation of fetal imaging is heavily based on knowledge of normal anatomy and developmental variants. The evaluation of the fetal CNS also depends on the knowledge of the extensive dynamic changes that occur normally during each stage of pregnancy. These changes have been temporally defined on both US and MRI, and normative data are available. MRI is performed when a CNS abnormality is seen or suspected on screening anatomic US. When interpreting a fetal MRI for CNS abnormalities, the radiologist should have knowledge of gestational age, prior US findings, maternal history, risk factors, and other fetal or pregnancy abnormalities. An understanding of normal fetal anatomy and the expected changes during gestation are also necessary to avoid misinterpretation.

CLINICS CARE POINTS

- **Between 20 to 28 weeks of gestation, MRI shows a 5-layer appearance of the fetal cerebral parenchyma on ssFSE corresponding to neuronal migration. After 28 weeks, only 3 layers should be visualized.**
- **The normal lateral ventricles should measure less than 10 mm at the level of the atrium.**
- **Important midline cerebellar vermis landmarks include an acute fastigial point and the presence of the primary fissure.**

DISCLOSURE

The authors have nothing to disclose.

REFERENCES

1. Prayer D, Kasprian G, Krampl E, et al. MRI of normal fetal brain development. Eur J Radiol 2006;57(2):199–216.
2. Kline-Fath BM. Ultrasound and MR Imaging of the Normal Fetal Brain. Neuroimaging Clin N Am 2019;29(3):339–56.
3. Griffiths PD, Bradburn M, Campbell MJ, et al. MRI in the diagnosis of fetal developmental brain abnormalities: the MERIDIAN diagnostic accuracy study. Health Technol Assess 2019;23(49):1–144.
4. Griffiths PD, Bradburn M, Campbell MJ, et al. Use of MRI in the diagnosis of fetal brain abnormalities in utero (MERIDIAN): a multicentre, prospective cohort study. Lancet 2017;389(10068):538–46.
5. Chartier AL, Bouvier MJ, McPherson DR, et al. The Safety of Maternal and Fetal MRI at 3 T. AJR Am J Roentgenol 2019;213(5):1170–3.
6. Safety ACRCoM, Greenberg TD, Hoff MN, et al. ACR guidance document on MR safe practices: Updates and critical information 2019. J Magn Reson Imaging 2020;51(2):331–8.
7. Mirsky DM, Shekdar KV, Bilaniuk LT. Fetal MRI: head and neck. Magn Reson Imaging Clin N Am 2012;20(3):605–18.
8. Saleem SN. Fetal magnetic resonance imaging (MRI): a tool for a better understanding of normal and abnormal brain development. J Child Neurol 2013;28(7):890–908.
9. Krishnamurthy U, Neelavalli J, Mody S, et al. MR imaging of the fetal brain at 1.5T and 3.0T field strengths: comparing specific absorption rate (SAR) and image quality. J Perinat Med 2015;43(2):209–20.
10. Tocchio S, Kline-Fath B, Kanal E, et al. MRI evaluation and safety in the developing brain. Semin Perinatol 2015;39(2):73–104.
11. Ray JG, Vermeulen MJ, Bharatha A, et al. Association Between MRI Exposure During Pregnancy and Fetal and Childhood Outcomes. JAMA 2016;316(9):952–61.
12. Committee Opinion No. 723: Guidelines for Diagnostic Imaging During Pregnancy and Lactation. Obstet Gynecol 2017;130(4):e210–6.
13. Glenn OA. Normal development of the fetal brain by MRI. Semin Perinatol 2009;33(4):208–19.
14. Kostovic I, Judas M, Rados M, et al. Laminar organization of the human fetal cerebrum revealed by histochemical markers and magnetic resonance imaging. Cereb Cortex 2002;12(5):536–44.
15. Maas LC, Mukherjee P, Carballido-Gamio J, et al. Early laminar organization of the human cerebrum demonstrated with diffusion tensor imaging in extremely premature infants. Neuroimage 2004;22(3):1134–40.
16. Brisse H, Fallet C, Sebag G, et al. Supratentorial parenchyma in the developing fetal brain: in vitro MR study with histologic comparison. AJNR Am J Neuroradiol 1997;18(8):1491–7.
17. Kinoshita Y, Okudera T, Tsuru E, et al. Volumetric analysis of the germinal matrix and lateral ventricles performed using MR images of postmortem fetuses. AJNR Am J Neuroradiol 2001;22(2):382–8.
18. Judas M, Rados M, Jovanov-Milosevic N, et al. Structural, immunocytochemical, and mr imaging properties of periventricular crossroads of growing cortical pathways in preterm infants. AJNR Am J Neuroradiol 2005;26(10):2671–84.
19. Lan LM, Yamashita Y, Tang Y, et al. Normal fetal brain development: MR imaging with a half-Fourier rapid acquisition with relaxation enhancement sequence. Radiology 2000;215(1):205–10.

20. Righini A, Bianchini E, Parazzini C, et al. Apparent diffusion coefficient determination in normal fetal brain: a prenatal MR imaging study. AJNR Am J Neuroradiol 2003;24(5):799–804.
21. Schneider JF, Confort-Gouny S, Le Fur Y, et al. Diffusion-weighted imaging in normal fetal brain maturation. Eur Radiol 2007;17(9):2422–9.
22. Garel C, Chantrel E, Elmaleh M, et al. Fetal MRI: normal gestational landmarks for cerebral biometry, gyration and myelination. Childs Nerv Syst 2003; 19(7–8):422–5.
23. Fogliarini C, Chaumoitre K, Chapon F, et al. Assessment of cortical maturation with prenatal MRI. Part I: Normal cortical maturation. Eur Radiol 2005;15(8): 1671–85.
24. Kasprian G, Langs G, Brugger PC, et al. The prenatal origin of hemispheric asymmetry: an in utero neuroimaging study. Cereb Cortex 2011;21(5):1076–83.
25. Habas PA, Scott JA, Roosta A, et al. Early folding patterns and asymmetries of the normal human brain detected from in utero MRI. Cereb Cortex 2012;22(1):13–25.
26. Adamsbaum C, Moutard ML, Andre C, et al. MRI of the fetal posterior fossa. Pediatr Radiol 2005;35(2): 124–40.
27. Society for Maternal-Fetal M, Norton ME, Fox NS, et al. Fetal Ventriculomegaly. Am J Obstet Gynecol 2020;223(6):B30–3.
28. Perlman S, Shashar D, Hoffmann C, et al. Prenatal diagnosis of fetal ventriculomegaly: Agreement between fetal brain ultrasonography and MR imaging. AJNR Am J Neuroradiol 2014;35(6):1214–8.
29. Guibaud L. Fetal cerebral ventricular measurement and ventriculomegaly: time for procedure standardization. Ultrasound Obstet Gynecol 2009;34(2):127–30.
30. Garel C, Alberti C. Coronal measurement of the fetal lateral ventricles: comparison between ultrasonography and magnetic resonance imaging. Ultrasound Obstet Gynecol 2006;27(1):23–7.
31. Sari A, Ahmetoglu A, Dinc H, et al. Fetal biometry: size and configuration of the third ventricle. Acta Radiol 2005;46(6):631–5.
32. Heaphy-Henault KJ, Guimaraes CV, Mehollin-Ray AR, et al. Congenital Aqueductal Stenosis: Findings at Fetal MRI That Accurately Predict a Postnatal Diagnosis. AJNR Am J Neuroradiol 2018;39(5): 942–8.
33. Garel C. Fetal cerebral biometry: normal parenchymal findings and ventricular size. Eur Radiol 2005;15(4):809–13.
34. Nagaraj UD, Calvo-Garcia MA, Kline-Fath BM. Abnormalities Associated With the Cavum Septi Pellucidi on Fetal MRI: What Radiologists Need to Know. AJR Am J Roentgenol 2018;210(5):989–97.
35. Jou HJ, Shyu MK, Wu SC, et al. Ultrasound measurement of the fetal cavum septi pellucidi. Ultrasound Obstet Gynecol 1998;12(6):419–21.
36. Ber R, Bar-Yosef O, Hoffmann C, et al. Normal fetal posterior fossa in MR imaging: new biometric data and possible clinical significance. AJNR Am J Neuroradiol 2015;36(4):795–802.
37. Tilea B, Alberti C, Adamsbaum C, et al. Cerebral biometry in fetal magnetic resonance imaging: new reference data. Ultrasound Obstet Gynecol 2009; 33(2):173–81.
38. Dovjak GO, Schmidbauer V, Brugger PC, et al. Normal human brainstem development in vivo: a quantitative fetal MRI study. Ultrasound Obstet Gynecol 2021;58(2):254–63.
39. Robinson AJ, Blaser S, Toi A, et al. The fetal cerebellar vermis: assessment for abnormal development by ultrasonography and magnetic resonance imaging. Ultrasound Q 2007;23(3):211–23.
40. Stazzone MM, Hubbard AM, Bilaniuk LT, et al. Ultrafast MR imaging of the normal posterior fossa in fetuses. AJR Am J Roentgenol 2000;175(3):835–9.
41. Robinson AJ, Goldstein R. The cisterna magna septa: vestigial remnants of Blake's pouch and a potential new marker for normal development of the rhombencephalon. J Ultrasound Med 2007;26(1): 83–95.
42. Kau T, Birnbacher R, Schwärzler P, et al. Delayed fenestration of Blake's pouch with or without vermian hypoplasia: fetal MRI at 3 tesla versus 1.5 tesla. Cerebellum Ataxias 2019;6(1):4.
43. Righini A, Parazzini C, Doneda C, et al. Prenatal MR imaging of the normal pituitary stalk. AJNR Am J Neuroradiol 2009;30(5):1014–6.
44. Azoulay R, Fallet-Bianco C, Garel C, et al. MRI of the olfactory bulbs and sulci in human fetuses. Pediatr Radiol 2006;36(2):97–107.
45. Kashikar SV, Lakhkar BN. Assessment of Fetal Nasal Bone Length and Nasofrontal Angle in the Second Trimester in Normal Indian Pregnancies. J Fetal Med 2014;1(3):137–41.
46. Nemec U, Nemec SF, Brugger PC, et al. Normal mandibular growth and diagnosis of micrognathia at prenatal MRI. Prenat Diagn 2015;35(2):108–16.
47. Paladini D, Morra T, Teodoro A, et al. Objective diagnosis of micrognathia in the fetus: the jaw index. Obstet Gynecol 1999;93(3):382–6.
48. Burns NS, Iyer RS, Robinson AJ, et al. Diagnostic imaging of fetal and pediatric orbital abnormalities. AJR Am J Roentgenol 2013;201(6):W797–808.
49. Whitehead MT, Vezina G. Normal Developmental Globe Morphology on Fetal MR Imaging. AJNR Am J Neuroradiol 2016;37(9):1733–7.
50. Moreira NC, Teixeira J, Raininko R, et al. The ear in fetal MRI: what can we really see? Neuroradiology 2011;53(12):1001–8.
51. Fujii S, Nagaishi J, Mukuda N, et al. Evaluation of Fetal Thyroid with 3D Gradient Echo T1-weighted MR Imaging. Magn Reson Med Sci 2017;16(3): 203–8.

Imaging of Normal Brain Aging

Yoshiaki Ota, MD, Gaurang Shah, MD, FACR, FASFNR*

KEYWORDS

• Structural MRI • DTI • fMRI • Aging mechanism • WMH • Lacunes • Microbleed • CAA

KEY POINTS

- Brain morphologic changes related to aging are characterized by cortical thinning, gray and white matter volume loss, sulcal widening, and ventriculomegaly.
- Structural MR imaging can help evaluate age-related brain morphologic and pathologic changes, and functional imaging can assess white matter fiber tract and brain connectivity.
- Gray matter changes are characterized by cortical thinning and gray matter volume loss driven by microstructural changes on the molecular, cellular, and tissue levels.
- White matter changes related to aging are characterized by atrophy, white matter tract disruption, demyelination, vascular impairment, and increased inflammation. Age-related ventricular change is characterized by ventriculomegaly owing to compromise of the ependymal wall, and vascular changes are characterized by lacunes/microhemorrhages owing to damages to small cerebral vessels, small arteries, arterioles, and venules.

INTRODUCTION

Brain aging is mainly characterized by physiologic changes that reduce cognitive abilities, by decreased physical fitness, and by increased mortality.[1] Functional decline, such as reduced physical fitness and cognitive abilities, typically accompanies aging.[1,2] Many diseases with high mortality, such as cardiovascular diseases and cancers, also increase with age, as does the rate of mortality, according to the Gompertz-Makeham law.[1] Structural brain MR imaging and advanced brain imaging techniques, such as diffusion tensor imaging (DTI) and functional MR imaging (fMR imaging), can help characterize morphologic changes of the aging brain and evaluate changes of white matter fiber tracts and connectivity.[3,4] Integration of these unique imaging techniques can enable a multiphysics approach to characterizing brain changes in aging and help uncover spatiotemporal progression patterns of aging mechanisms. Moreover, combining this longitudinal imaging and computational modeling of aging can deliver reliable biomarkers for the early diagnosis of abnormal aging patterns. The effects of the aging brain include global brain atrophy, gray and white matter changes, ventricular enlargement, and vascular changes, all of which involve various pathophysiological mechanisms.[2] This review summarizes the effect of aging on the brain, focusing on structural and functional imaging features and morphologic changes with aging.

IMAGING TECHNIQUES

Age-related changes are attributed to various structural and functional alterations without clinically significant impairment. Neuroimaging techniques play a crucial role in detecting age-related brain structural changes. In clinical settings, head computed tomography (CT) scan is often used for a quick survey of structural brain changes, with particular attention to eliminating acute

Division of Neuroradiology, Department of Radiology, University of Michigan, 1500 East Medical Center Drive, UH B2, Ann Arbor, MI 48109, USA
* Corresponding author. B2A209, Department of Radiology, 1500 East Medical Center Drive, UH B2, Ann Arbor, MI 48109, USA.
E-mail address: gvshah@med.umich.edu

Neuroimag Clin N Am 32 (2022) 683–698
https://doi.org/10.1016/j.nic.2022.04.010

pathologic conditions. Although CT can visualize gross atrophic changes, MR imaging is the most informative structural neuroimaging technique for age-associated neurodegenerative diseases.[5,6] The aging brain shows global and regional reduction in volume, and the ventricular system increases in size. Previous studies have shown that normal aging is mostly attributed to extensive changes in frontal and temporal cortical thickness, in subcortical volume, and in the putamen, thalamus, and nucleus accumbens.[5–7] However, use of structural MR imaging alone may be insufficient to describe the relative proportion of age-related alterations in different brain locations. Functional and molecular imaging also has an essential role in neuroimaging. DTI, fMR imaging, and fluorine-18-fluorodeoxyglucose (^{18}F-FDG) PET are the most commonly used imaging techniques for evaluating brain function and metabolism.

STRUCTURAL MR IMAGING

The most historically valuable and informative structural MR imaging sequences in the study of brain aging include T1-weighted images, which provide high-resolution structural details of brain anatomy. These images typically maximize the contrast difference between gray matter, white matter, and the cerebrospinal fluid (CSF) of the extra-axial spaces and ventricles. They are generally used to reveal the size of various cortical and subcortical structures and to reliably help evaluate volume changes in gray and white matter parenchyma, cortical thickness, degree of folding, and other features, including the ventricles.[2,8]

Other useful structural MR imaging sequences include T2-weighted and fluid-attenuated inversion recovery (FLAIR) MR. These images can depict perivascular spaces and abnormalities of cerebral white matter. In addition, hyperintensities of white matter are usually silent and often seen in the aging brain. T2*-weighted gradient recalled echo sequence (GRE T2*WI) also is often included in imaging protocols to detect microhemorrhages,[9] which can be seen in the aging brain. To collectively evaluate multiple common brain changes and their additional effects on brain function, the Brain Atrophy and Lesion Index (BALI) has been used and validated.[10–13] BALI is a semiquantitative rating scale (Table 1) used to assess global brain atrophy and white and gray matter lesions in the supratentorial and infratentorial compartments, including cortical infarcts, dilated perivascular spaces, lacunar infarcts, and white matter hyperintensities. All these can be evaluated using T1-weighted, T2-weighted, FLAIR, and GRE T2*WI structural MR imaging sequences (Fig. 1).

FUNCTIONAL AND METABOLIC NEUROIMAGING

Diffusion Tensor Imaging

DTI is a noninvasive imaging technique used for characterizing the structural integrity of anatomic connections in the brain. It also provides a quantitative assessment of brain white matter microstructure by detecting the quantity and direction of myelin water movement in extracellular and intracellular white matter spaces.[2,14] In extracellular spaces, fluid diffuses between fibers, whereas in intracellular spaces, fluid diffuses in the axoplasm.[14] DTI is sensitive to detecting white matter linear structures, composed principally of axons (Fig. 2A–D). Several patterns of white matter microstructural sparing have been identified. Those include the following: (1) lower fractional anisotropy (FA) and higher mean diffusivity (MD) in older than younger adults; (2) anterior and superior aspects of the brain are earlier and more severely affected than the posterior and inferior aspects of the brain; and (3) association fibers connecting cerebral cortex are more readily affected than projection fibers. Disruption of white matter microstructure detectable using DTI can reflect the breakdown of myelin, certain constituents of the cytoskeleton, and axon density.[14] This disruption can occur in a normal aging brain, along with a decline in the number and length of myelinated fibers.[15] FA, MD, axial diffusivity (AD), and radial diffusivity (RD) are commonly used to detect microscopic changes in white matter tissue integrity. Decreases in FA and AD and increases in MD and RD are interpreted as alterations in white matter microstructure integrity that can also be influenced by other factors, such as concussion injury, ischemia, or prolonged hypertension (see Fig. 2E–G). However, the structural connectivity investigated using DTI can be supplemented by functional connectivity investigated using fMR imaging.

Functional MR Imaging

Connectivity between different brain areas is crucial for effective cognitive functioning. Healthy aging significantly affects the organization and function of networks in the human brain. Functional connectivity is the phenomenon of connection between different brain regions that share the same functional properties. Many past fMR imaging studies have examined how functional connectivity during one task or at rest is affected by normal aging. However, resting-state fMR imaging is more suitable for investigating functional brain connectivity than task-based fMR imaging.

Table 1
Categorization and grading criteria of the Brain Atrophy and Lesion Index

Evaluation Categories	Rating Score
GM-SV: Gray matter lesions and subcortical dilated perivascular spaces	0 = absence; 1 = dotted abnormal signal intensity in gray matter or multiple dotted/liner abnormal signal intensity in subcortical areas; 2 = small patches of abnormal signal intensity in gray matter or diffuse and countless dotted/liner abnormal signal intensity in subcortical areas; 3 = patches of abnormal signal intensity in gray matter
DWM: Deep white matter lesions	0 = absence; 1 = dotted abnormal signal intensity; 2 = small patches of abnormal signal intensity; 3 = large patchy abnormal signal intensity; 4 = large patchy abnormal signal intensity involving all cerebral lobes; 5 = abnormal signal intensity involving complete deep white matter
PV: Periventricular white matter lesions	0 = absence; 1 = "cap" or pencil-thin lining; 2 = smooth "halo" with blurred margin; 3 = irregular periventricular abnormal signal intensities extending into the deep white matter
BG: Lesions in the basal ganglia and surrounding areas	0 = absence; 1 = 1 focal lesion; 2 = more than 1 focal lesion; 3 = patchy confluent lesions (regardless of dilated perivascular spaces)
IT: Lesions in the infratentorial compartment	0 = absence; 1 = 1 focal lesion; 2 = more than 1 focal lesion; 3 = patchy confluent lesions
GA: Global atrophy	0 = no obvious atrophy; 1 = mild atrophy; 2 = moderate atrophy; 3 = severe atrophy; 4 = most severe atrophy present especially in the medial temporal lobes; 5 = most severe atrophy present especially in the medial temporal lobes and cerebral cortex
MH: Microhemorrhage	0 = absence; 1 = 1 focal lesion; 2 = more than 1 focal lesion; 3 = diffuse lesions
Other findings: neoplasm, trauma, deformity, hydrocephalus	0 = no other kind of disease; 1 = any 1 kind of brain neoplasm, deformation or trauma; 2 = any 2 kinds of brain neoplasm, deformation, or trauma; 3 = simultaneous presence of brain neoplasm, deformation, and trauma

FMR imaging is based on the temporal correlations of spontaneous blood-oxygen level-dependent signal fluctuations between different brain areas. This connectivity method can allow evaluation of interactions between brain regions to be studied with or without a specific cognitive task and to investigate functional connectivity in aging. FMR imaging has different approaches and levels of complexity in functional connectivity, ranging from the study of connectivity between 2 regions (seed-to-seed–based analysis) to the research of whole-brain connectivity using complex network approaches, such as graph analysis. Connectivity and network integrity appear to decrease in healthy aging,[3] but this decline accelerates in neurodegenerative diseases, such as Alzheimer disease.

Discernible functional "communities" within the brain are called resting-state networks: these networks exhibit high-level functional coupling within the community. However, the connectivity between different communities is of lower or intermittent coupling. The most common 7 major resting-state networks are the default mode network, the executive control network, the dorsal attention network, the salience network, the auditory/limbic network, the visual network, and the somatomotor network (Fig. 3). Each of these networks is responsible for a particular task set (Fig. 4). Normal aging is associated with disruptions in the resting-state functional organization of the brain.

Functional connectivity is a relatively recent area of research, but it holds great promise in revealing how brain network dynamics change across the

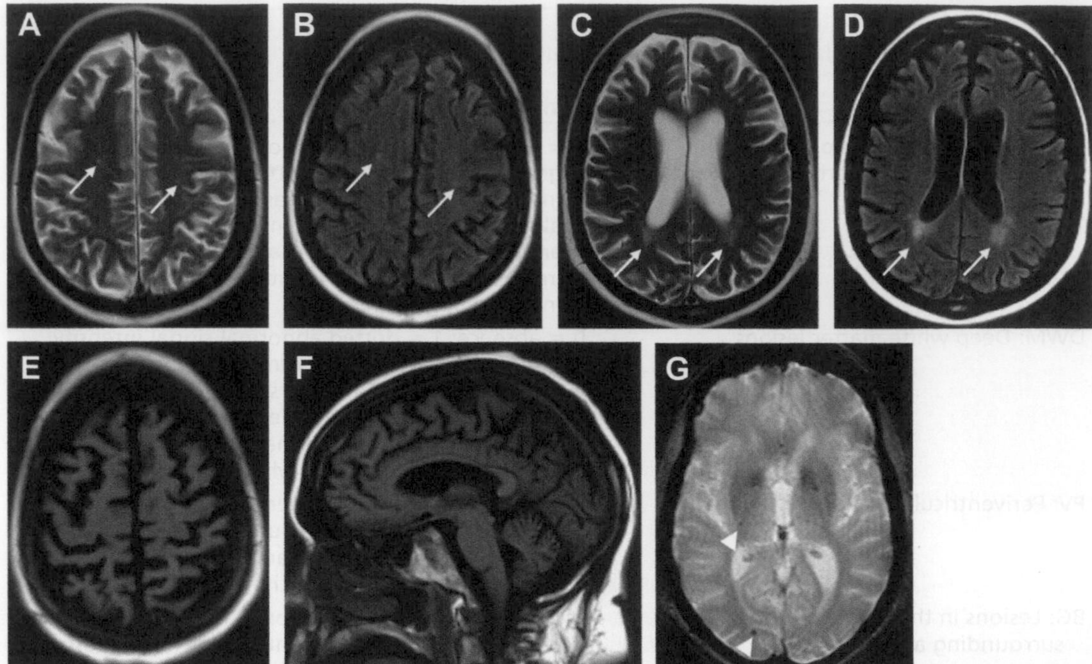

Fig. 1. Example of categorization and grading criteria of the BALI. A 76-year-old man with normal cognitive function presented with chronic headaches. (*A, B*) T2-weighted image and FLAIR show foci in deep and subcortical white matter (*arrows*) (GM-SV score = 1, DWM score = 1, respectively). (*C, D*) At the level of the lateral ventricles, there are periventricular white matter lesions with blurred margins, which extend into the deep white matter (*arrows*) (PV score = 3). (*E, F*) Axial and sagittal T1-weighted images show mild global atrophy (GA score = 1). (*G*) GRE T2*weighted image shows 2 punctate foci of susceptibility abnormality (*arrowheads*) (MH = 2). There is no lesion in the basal ganglia or infratentorial area (*not shown*).

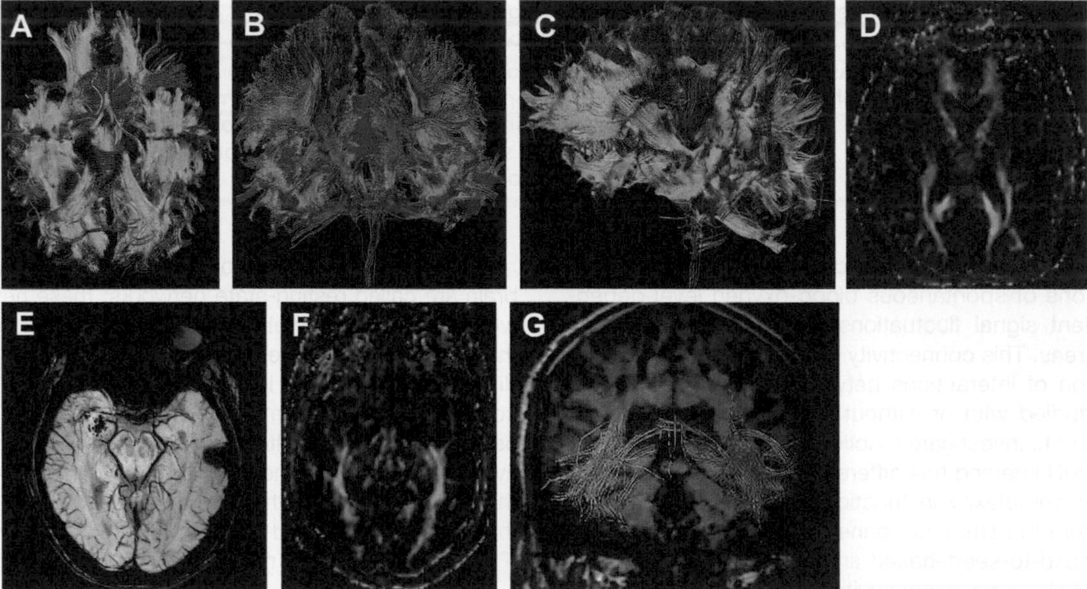

Fig. 2. DTI can complement structural brain MR imaging with information about brain white matter microstructure changes. The tractography mapping of the brain (*A–C*) and color-coded (x-axis: green; y-axis: red; z-axis: blue) brain mapping (*D*) exhibits the structural integrity of individual white matter tracts in the normal brain. In a patient with concussion and microhemorrhage in the right temporal lobe, seen on susceptibility-weighted imaging (SWI) (*E*), diminished fiber tracts and reduced FA values can be seen (*F, G*).

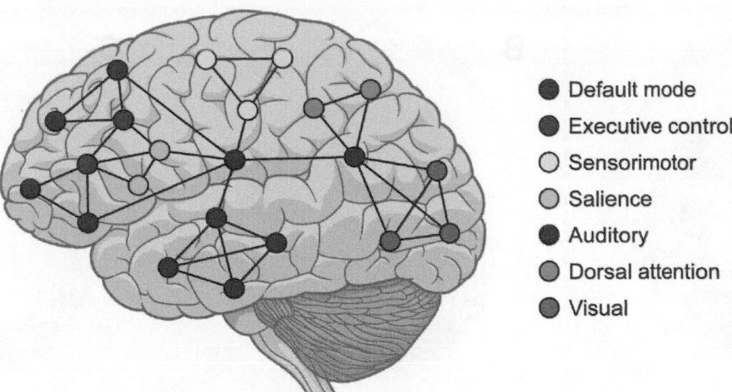

Fig. 3. fMR imaging: functional connectivity.

lifespan and in disease.[2,3] Structural imaging and functional neuroimaging can provide information about the anatomy and physiology of the brain, respectively. In addition, their combination enables a multiphysics approach to characterizing brain imaging changes in aging. It also helps to reveal spatiotemporal progression patterns of primary aging mechanisms. The combination of longitudinal imaging and computational modeling of aging will deliver reliable biomarkers for the early diagnosis of abnormal aging patterns.[2]

Positron Emission Tomography

^{18}F-FDG is the most commonly used radiotracer for assessing regional cerebral glucose metabolism as a biomarker of neural activity, synaptic density, and functioning.[16,17] ^{18}F-FDG-PET can

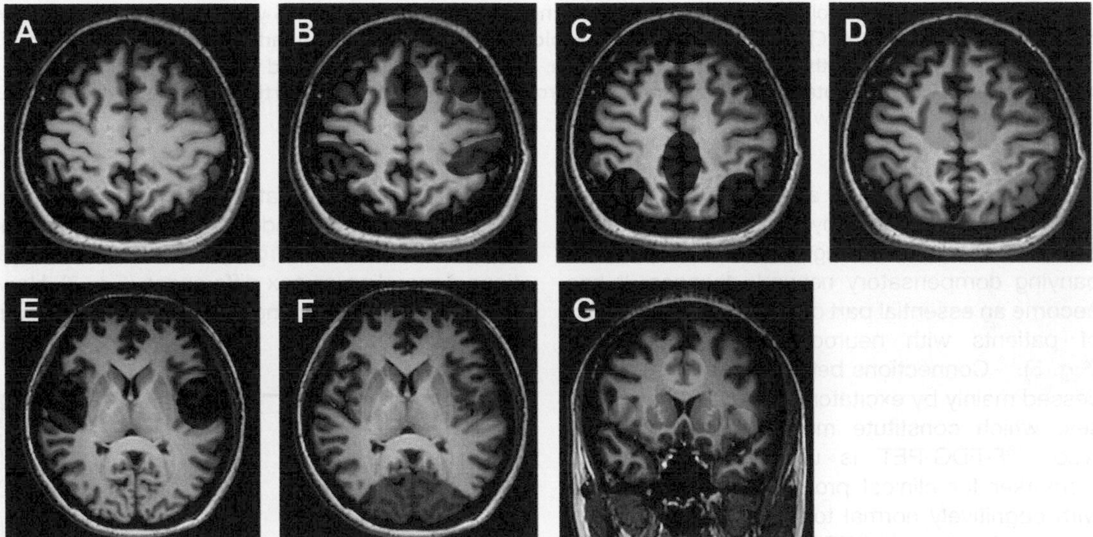

Fig. 4. fMR imaging: brain network and function. (*A*) Sensorimotor network: Primary sensorimotor cortex, supplementary motor area, and secondary somatosensory cortex. Function: Motor programming and execution and sensory integration. (*B*) Executive control network: Anterior cingulate, dorsolateral frontal areas, and parietal cortex. Functions: Working memory, sensorimotor learning, and attentive functions. (*C*) Default mode network: Ventromedial prefrontal cortex, precuneus and posterior cingulate, and bilateral inferior parietal areas. Functions: introspective ability and episodic memory, deactivation during the goal-based and attention-demanding task. (*D*) Dorsal attention network: Superior parietal and inferior parietal sulcus, superior frontal areas, and frontal eye fields. Functions: Attention and control demanding tasks. (*E*) Auditory network: Superior temporal gyrus, Herschel gyrus, and primary auditory and associated areas. Functions: primary and associative auditory processes. (*F*) Visual network: Striate cortex, occipital pole, and lateral visual areas. Functions: Primary and associative visual processes. (*G*) Salience network: Dorsal anterior cingulate and bilateral insulae. Function: Elaboration of salient inputs.

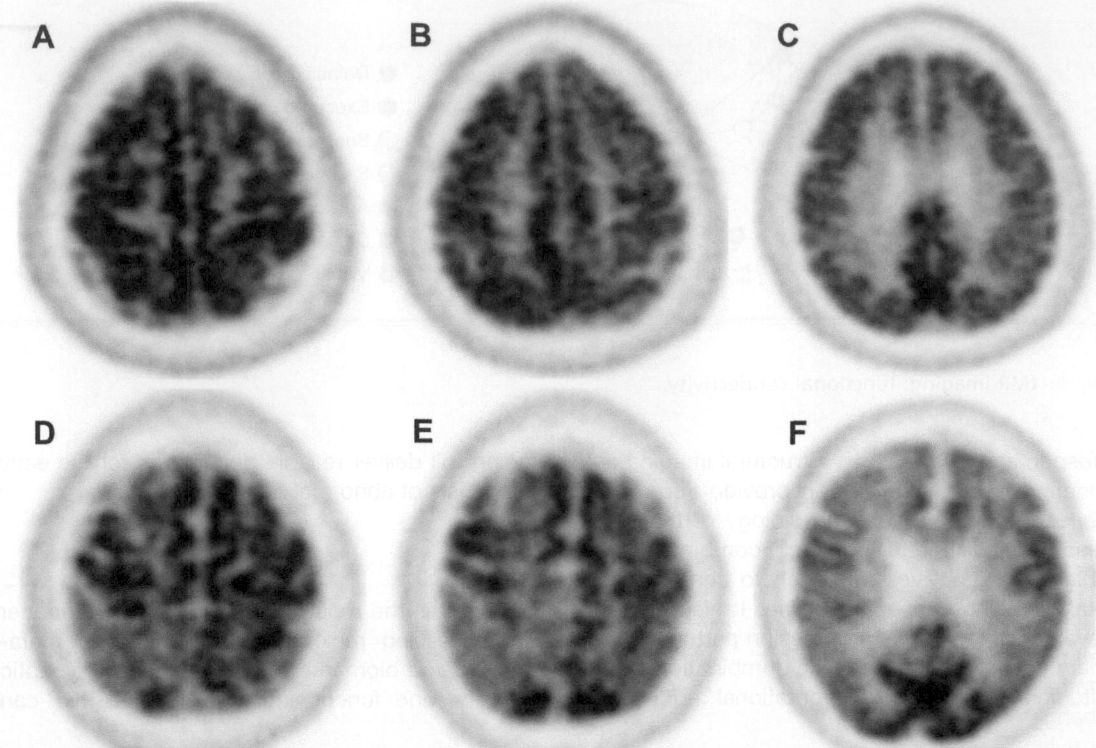

Fig. 5. PET-CT in a 69-year-old man with a history of lung cancer (*A, B, C*) and a 76-year-old man with cognitive dysfunction (*D, E, F*). (*A, B, C*) FDG-PET-CT of a 69-year-old man shows no reduced radiotracer uptake in the brain cortex. (*C, D, E*) On the other hand, FDG-PET-CT of a 76-year-old man presented with cognitive dysfunction showing low radiotracer uptakes in the bilateral temporoparietal and prefrontal cortices and the posterior cingulate precuneus, consistent with Alzheimer disease.

reveal disease-specific alterations of regional glucose metabolism by assessing synaptic dysfunction, neuronal degeneration, and accompanying compensatory network changes. It has become an essential part of the diagnostic workup of patients with neurodegenerative disorders (**Fig. 5**).[17] Connections between neurons are processed mainly by excitatory glutamatergic synapses, which constitute most cortical synapses. Also, ^{18}F-FDG-PET is used as a predictive biomarker for clinical progression from patients with cognitively normal to mild cognitive impairment or dementia.[18] PET is also used to quantify biomarker concentrations, such as tau and amyloid-beta, which are the 2 most prominent proteins in aging and neurodegenerative diseases, helping to reveal spatial and temporal brain changes and their impact on cognitive decline.[19]

BRAIN AGING MECHANISMS

The brain undergoes changes in morphology with aging. The most common hallmarks of age-related changes are thinning of the peripheral cortex,[20] both gray and white matter volume loss, widening of cerebral sulci,[21] and increased caliber of the ventricular system[22] (**Fig. 6**). There are also variations depending on sex differences (**Fig. 7**). However, the effect of aging on brain morphology is

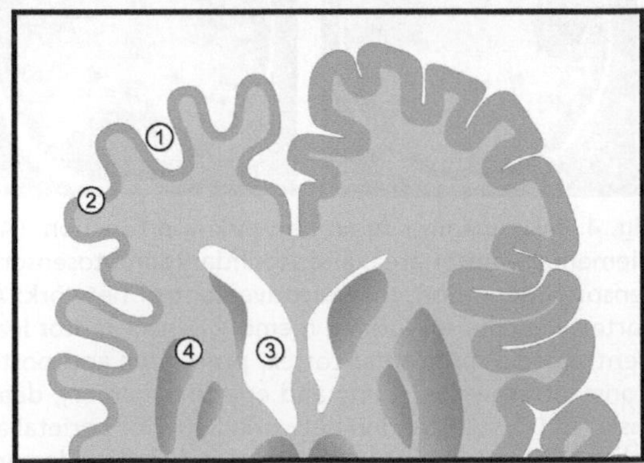

Fig. 6. Common feature of age-related morphologic brain changes. (1) Sulcal widening; (2) cortical thinning; (3) ventriculomegaly; (4) gray and white matter volume loss.

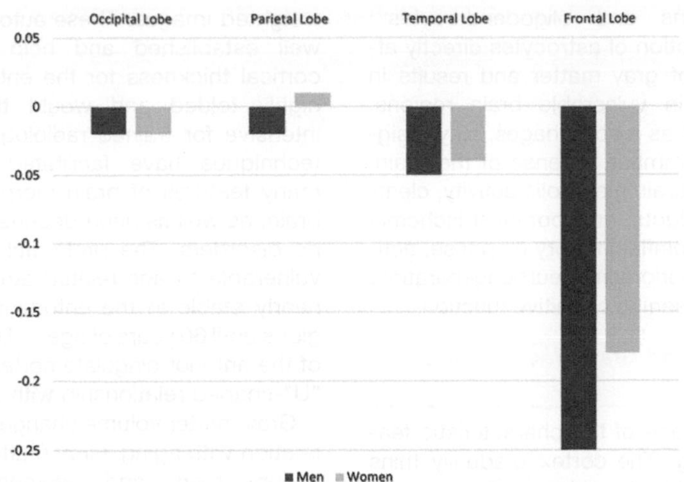

Fig. 7. Sex differences in yearly lobar brain volume change based on the Framingham Heart Study. The frontal and temporal lobe volumes are significantly different between men and women, whereas the volumes of the occipital and parietal lobes are not.

highly heterogeneous and exhibits spatial and temporal variations.[23] The authors discuss gray matter, white matter, ventricular, and vascular changes with aging, highlighting the observed quantitative changes, clinical features, sex differences, and imaging features.

Gray Matter Aging Mechanisms

Gray matter changes are driven by microstructural alterations on the molecular, cellular, and tissue levels, specific to the cortex. The gray matter layer comprises neuronal cell bodies and blood vessels, which account for 16% of the cortex. Axons and dendrites each consist of around 29%, and glial cells and extracellular space make up the rest of the gray matter layer. For several decades, neuronal cell death was considered the leading cause of cortical atrophy in healthy aging.[23] However, the total number of neurons is estimated to decrease by 2% to 4%, accounting for only up to 10% of overall gray matter volume loss.[24] Instead, it has been shown that a decrease in neuronal body size, degeneration of neuropil, degeneration of the dendritic network, and consequent loss of synapses are the driving forces behind cortical atrophy in the aging brain.[25]

Neurons with large cell bodies in particular, experience substantial volume loss owing to gradual loss of metabolic activity and mitochondrial dysfunction.[26] Dendritic arborization plays a central role in neuronal connectivity, because the dendritic spines are the principal sites of signal transmission between neurons.[27] Loss of spines or decay of the dendritic network affects synaptic events and leads to cognitive decline.[28] In the healthy brain, dendritic spines have excitatory synapses, the density of which varies across the brain and within the dendritic tree itself. Degeneration of dendrites, such as decreased dendritic length and spine density, is found in pyramidal neurons in prefrontal, precentral, and superior temporal cortical areas.[29]

Molecular Changes

Mitochondria play a significant role in cellular energy metabolism, Ca^{++} homeostasis, and apoptosis (programmed cell death) in healthy and pathologic conditions.[30] In the aging brain, enlargement or fragmentation of mitochondria and increased numbers of denatured mitochondria with depolarized membranes and impaired Ca^{++} handling have been observed.[31,32] Dysregulation of Ca^{++} in mitochondria in the hippocampus is commonly seen in neurodegenerative diseases, which leads to the generation of reactive oxygen species and activation of apoptosis. Accompanying oxidative stress in neurons causes typical energy metabolism impairment and disrupts protein function that controls subcellular calcium dynamics.[33]

Cellular Changes

Glial cells, such as astrocytes and microglia, play a central role in aging mechanisms. Astrocytes maintain a wide range of significant functions to support nutrient and ion transportation, mitigate neuroinflammation, and preserve the blood-brain barrier (BBB).[34,35] Astrocytes are unable to maintain their ability to carry out these functions in the aged brain and release a toxic factor that attacks neighboring neurons and oligodendrocytes[36] (Fig. 8). The dysfunction of astrocytes directly affects the integrity of gray matter and results in structural atrophy in vulnerable brain regions. Microglia, which act as macrophages, play a significant role in the immune defense of the brain. The gradual loss of brain metabolic activity, clearance of waste products, and potential ischemia contribute to a neuroinflammatory response, activating microglia, deteriorating neurodegeneration, and resulting in worsening cognitive function.[37]

Cortical Thinning and Gray Matter Volume Changes

Cortical thinning is one of the characteristic features of brain aging. The cortex gradually thins with aging across all brain regions[38,39] and correlates with cognitive decline and deterioration of memory function.[23] Therefore, cortical thinning may promise to provide a potential key biomarker for age-related cognitive decline. Cortical thickness is frequently calculated from brain MR images using software, such as NeuroQuant and FreeSurfer, on high-resolution 3-dimensional T1-weighted images. These automated methods are well established and help estimate accurate cortical thickness for the entire cortex, which is highly folded and would therefore be labor-intensive for trained radiologists to label. Those techniques have facilitated the evaluation of many features of brain morphology in the aging brain, as well as neurodegenerative and psychiatric disorders. The prefrontal cortex is the most vulnerable to age-related atrophy[40] and remains nearly stable in the entorhinal and temporal regions until 60 years of age.[41] The cortical thickness of the anterior cingulate cortex has an attenuated "U"-shaped relationship with age.[42]

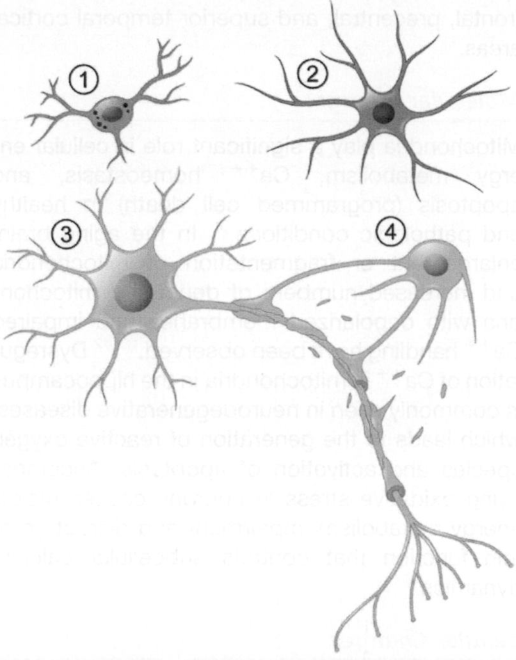

Fig. 8. Mechanism of gray matter change. (1) Astrocyte; (2) microglia; (3) neuron; and (4) oligodendrocyte. In the aging brain, the ability of astrocytes to support nutrient and ion transportation is decreased, and microglia cells lose their function of preserving brain immunity. This deterioration affects neurons and oligodendrocytes and decreases synaptic function, decreases myelination, and releases myelin debris.

Gray matter volume changes have a strong correlation with aging. Gray matter atrophy rates between men and women have been a controversial topic. One study reported no sex differences in volume changes affecting gray matter,[43] but another study reported significantly greater volume decline in men than in women.[44] One longitudinal study showed that annual gray matter atrophy rates were more significant in patients with Alzheimer disease than in healthy controls (2.76% ± 1.64% vs 0.49% ± 1.19%), proposing that gray matter atrophy rate can be used as a biomarker to differentiate between healthy aging and disease progression in Alzheimer disease.[45] The hippocampus has been extensively investigated with regard to assessing age-related changes in the brain because it has a crucial role in memory and learning. The hippocampus has been shown to be vulnerable to aging and neurodegeneration.[46] It has been shown that hippocampal atrophy progresses faster in patients with Alzheimer disease than in healthy adults.[47] The atrophy of the limbic system also progresses faster than that of the basal ganglia (0.4% per year for the hippocampus, 0.7% per year for the thalamus, and 0.2% per year for the caudate nucleus).[48]

White Matter Aging Mechanisms

White matter volume changes play a significant role in brain atrophy and loss of brain function. Age-related white matter volume changes are mainly characterized by atrophy, demyelination, disruption of white matter tracts, vascular impairment, and increased inflammation[49–53] (Fig. 9). Most of the white matter volume comprises myelinated axons (up to 60%). The extracellular spaces make up approximately 20%; blood vessels account for less than 3%, and the rest of the volume consists of glial cells.[54] Age-related white matter degeneration has been associated with behavioral changes and cognitive impairment.[55]

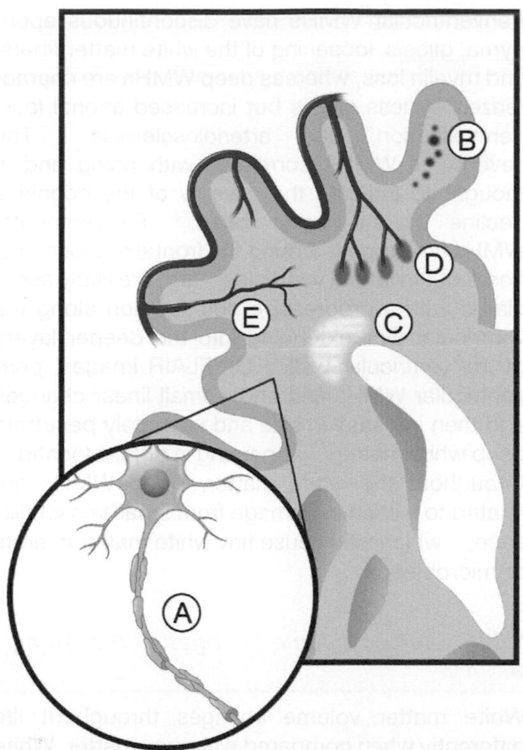

Fig. 9. White matter change in aging brain. Age-related white matter changes are characterized by (*A*) demyelination; (*B*) microbleeds; (*C*) white matter hyperintensities; (*D*) lacunar infarcts; and (*E*) vascular disruption.

White matter aging mechanisms related to axonal architecture, demyelination, and white matter hyperintense lesions (WMH) are reviewed in later discussion. Although structural imaging methods are used to quantify morphologic changes, DTI can increase sensitivity for detecting age-related white matter microstructural alternations.[56]

Axonal Architecture in Aging White Matter

The length of myelinated fibers reduces by almost 10% per decade between 20 and 80 years of age.[15] Axonal degeneration predominantly affects axons with small diameters and slender myelin sheaths compared with thicker axons.[57] DTI is the most promising imaging technique to quantify the degree of anisotropy in white matter tracts, mainly evaluated using 4 diffusion-based measurements, FA, MD, AD, and RD.[58] AD is associated with diffusion parallel to fiber tracts, and a decrease in AD can reflect damage to axons, reduced axonal diameters, or progressively less coherent axonal orientation.[14] RD is related to diffusion perpendicular to fiber tracts. An increase in RD can indicate the presence of axonal loss, loss of myelin, or low axonal packing density.[59] FA evaluates the degree of anisotropy concerning the axonal network based on the diffusivity of water molecules inside myelinated axons and the extracellular space. MD is calculated from RD and AD and can represent the overall magnitude of water diffusion.[58] An increase in MD reflects impaired white matter integrity owing to local axon and myelin degeneration.

In a cohort study with 282 subjects aged between 20 and 84 years of age, the annual FA percentage change decreased by a mean 0.3% globally, 0.5% in the frontal lobe, 0.2% in the parietal lobe, 0.2% in the occipital lobe, and increased by 0.1% in the temporal lobe.[60] Diffusion is highly anisotropic in myelin-rich axon tracts, although axonal diameter, fiber density, and myelin structure vary spatially. In the aging brains, multiple brain areas, especially in the midhippocampal and posterior thalamic areas, show increased AD and RD values with age resulting from progressive deterioration of axons and supporting myelin.[61] Additional factors associated with white matter changes in aging brains include corresponding changes in the supporting cell density, orientation, size, numbers, and volume of axonal fibers.[62] A decrease in axonal packing density owing to loss of myelin or axons in aging can increase extracellular water and the formation of white matter lesions.[62] The accumulation of extracellular fluid is thought to be associated with increased harmful substances, such as plasma proteins that originate from BBB breakdown and can be toxic to neighboring myelin and axons.[63] BBB dysfunction is associated with increased glial cell activation and results in age-related neuroinflammation and white matter lesions.[64,65] Another common feature related to white matter change is vessel wall stiffening.[66] A stiffened wall can change pressure gradients and molecular permeability in capillaries and increase free water in the interstitial space.

AGE-RELATED CHANGES IN THE BRAIN

Demyelination

Oligodendrocytes are the myelinating cells that extend their processes to neighboring axons to maintain myelin sheaths wrapped around axon segments.[67] Myelin accelerates signal transduction along axons, provides mechanical integrity, and increases white matter stiffness.[68] Demyelination of white matter axon bundles (see Fig. 9) is common in healthy brain aging.[69] Oligodendrocytes have a unique metabolic demand, including that required to produce and maintain myelin sheaths. Consequently, oligodendrocytes are susceptible to various insults, including chronic hypoperfusion and toxic products from activated microglia and excitotoxicity.[70] The loss of myelin in aging white matter may be caused by immune-mediated and ischemic pathways.[51] Immune-mediated myelin injury is driven by activated microglial cells or macrophages, which release toxic molecules and result in myelin sheath degeneration. Moreover, oligodendrocytes and glial cells are sensitive to ischemia-induced apoptosis.[71] Hypertensive vascular alterations may gradually obstruct blood flow to white matter areas and cause chronic ischemia, which results in progressive loss of myelin and oligodendrocytes.[51]

White Matter Hyperintensities

WMHs are a common feature in the aging brain and are found in more than 90% of people aged 60 to 64.[72] They are seen on FLAIR and T2-weighted images as bright white matter lesions (**Fig. 10**).[73] WMHs are thought to represent consequences of hypoperfusion caused by vascular obstruction, reactive gliosis, or infarcts.[73] The prevalence of WMHs increases with vascular risk factors, such as hypertension, diabetes, and smoking.[74] WMHs can be differentiated into periventricular and deep white matter lesions.[75] Both types of lesions are associated with small vessel disease, although having some differences with respect to microstructural properties and pathophysiology.[2,76]

DTI shows lower FA and increased MD, AD, and RD in periventricular than deep WMHs.[77] Periventricular WMHs have discontinuous ependyma, gliosis, loosening of the white matter fibers, and myelin loss, whereas deep WMHs are characterized by less gliosis but increased axonal loss, demyelination, and arteriolosclerosis.[77] The severity of WMHs correlates with aging and is thought to indicate the severity of the cognitive decline in the aging brain.[78] Periventricular WMHs first appear around the frontal and occipital horns of the lateral ventricles[79] and are likely associated with a progressive deterioration along the ventricular wall extending into the deeper layers of the ventricular wall.[80] On FLAIR images, periventricular WMHs first show small linear changes and then increase in size and ultimately penetrate deep white matter,[79] appearing in diffuse locations throughout the white matter. Deep WMHs are related to ischemic damage from small vessel disease,[77] which also cause tiny white matter infarcts or microbleeds.

White Matter Volume Changes in the Aging Brain

White matter volume changes throughout life differently when compared with gray matter. White matter volume increases and peaks at approximately 40 to 50 years of age.[81] Its volume then decreases in the later stages of life. It is thought that white matter volume loss typically starts later and rapidly progresses compared with gray matter.[82] It is estimated that white matter volume decrease at 70 years is approximately 6%, and at 80 years rapidly decreases to approximately 25%.[83] White

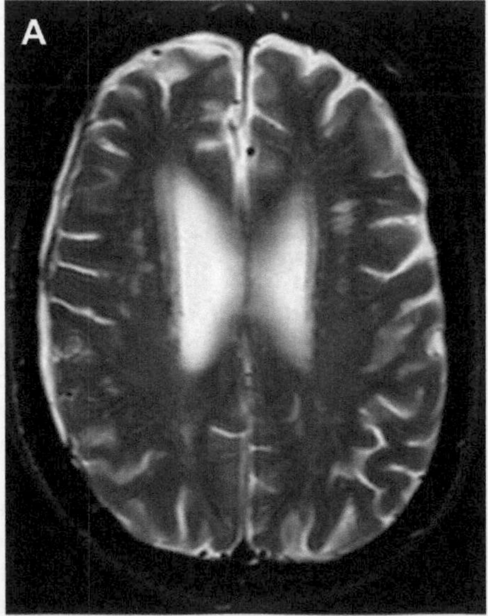

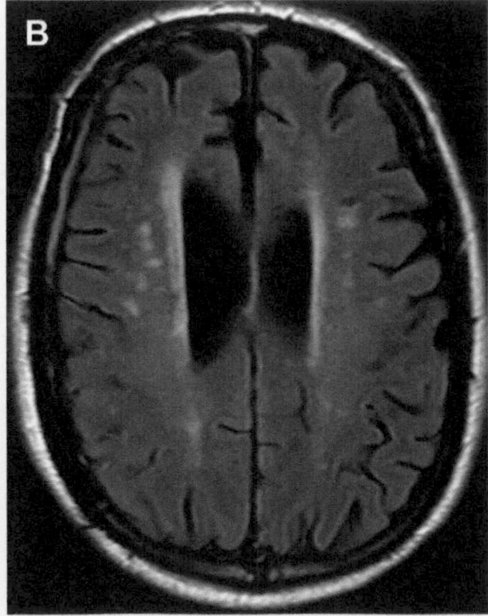

Fig. 10. A 75-year-old man presented with a headache. (*A*) T2-weighted image and (*B*) FLAIR show hyperintense lesions in the deep and subcortical white matter.

matter volume changes are most prominently seen in the frontal lobe.[84] In one study of subjects aged 59 to 85 years, the annual atrophy rate was 2.1% in the frontal lobe, 1.1% in the parietal lobe, 1.0% in the temporal lobe, and 0.8% in the occipital lobe.[85] The corpus callosum shows early development of age-related changes and degradation.[86]

Ventricular Aging Mechanisms

There is a possible link between venous drainage and ventricular enlargement in both normal and accelerated aging.[87] The brain contains 3 fluid systems: interstitial fluid, CSF, and vasculature. Although the interstitial fluid is secreted by endothelial cells, most CSF is produced by the choroid plexus, which is within the lateral, third, and fourth ventricles. The choroid plexus is a lobulated structure formed by a unique and continuous line of epithelial cells that originate from the ependymal wall of the ventricles. The ependymal cell layer lining the ventricular wall is connected by tight gaps and adherent junctions and contains the water channel protein aquaporin 4 (AQP4).[88] These junctions and AQP4 allow the ependymal lining to act as a bidirectional barrier and a fluid transport system for interstitial fluid and CSF, helping to transport toxic materials from the brain.[89] Biochemical changes to the ependymal cell layer can affect the function of its clearance mechanisms. Glial scarring owing to age-related ependymal wall failure can induce an increase in AQP4 water channels and inadvertently results in a disruption of interstitial solute clearance.[89] The 3 main factors that dictate the size of the ventricles are changes in brain tissue properties, CSF dynamics, and vascular parameters.[90] Throughout life, the hemodynamic loading of the ventricles causes ependymal cell stretching and leads to microtears in the ventricular membrane.[91] This compromise disrupts transependymal flow mechanisms.[76] Aging can lead to epithelial atrophy, thickening of the basement membranes, and decreased CSF production.[92]

Ventriculomegaly (Ventricular Enlargement)

The normal aging process can induce alterations in CSF circulation and affect neuronal performance.[93] Excessive CSF accumulation in the ventricular system in the elderly causes ventriculomegaly and consequent compression of the brain parenchymal blood vessels, which results in functional and neuropsychological abnormalities.[76,90] Also, vascular changes, the loss of neurons, the subsequent degeneration of axons, and the loss of cerebral white matter are linked directly to age-related ventricular enlargement.[94] Ventricular volume can be assessed using morphometry.[94] One study revealed that the CSF volume remains nearly constant until 50 years of age and gradually increases afterward.[95] The ventricular volume is significantly larger in men than in women, and gray matter and white matter are significantly smaller in men than in women.[96]

Vascular Changes

One of the main characteristics of vascular change with aging is vessel wall stiffness and damage to blood vessels.[97] Other changes include decreased capillary density and BBB breakdown.[98] Cerebral small vessels, including small arteries, arterioles, and venules, are commonly related to vascular change with aging.[99] Vessel walls become stiff

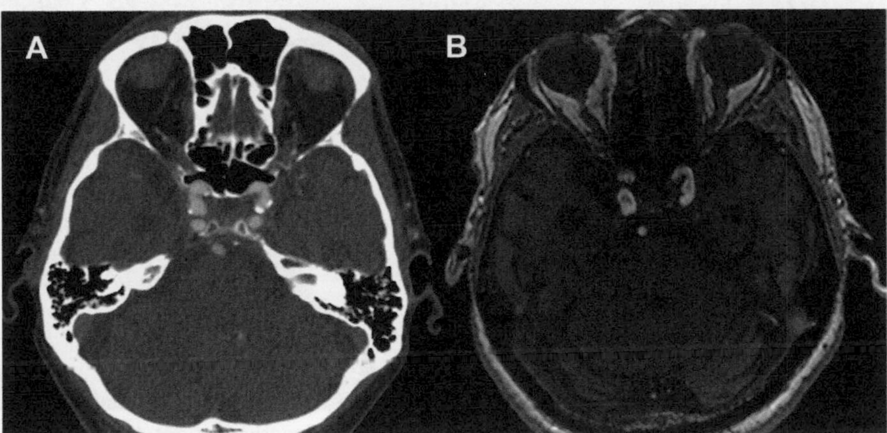

Fig. 11. CT and MR angiography of a 73-year-old man. (*A*) Head CT angiography shows atherosclerotic calcification in the bilateral internal carotid arteries. (*B*) Time-of-flight image of MR angiography shows a signal loss in the exact location.

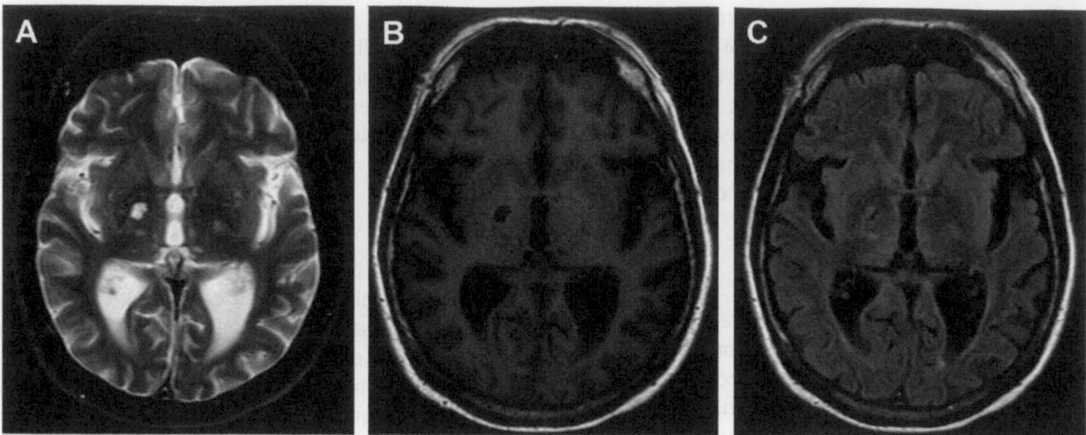

Fig. 12. Lacune in a 68-year-old man. (*A*) T2-weighted image and (*B*) T1-weighted image show a T2 hyperintense and T1 hypointense lesion in the right globus pallidus. (*C*) FLAIR shows a rim-hyperintense lesion in the corresponding region, compatible with a lacunar infarct.

and thicken, which result in a loss of elasticity with aging.[100] Excess collagen deposition in the walls of veins and venules constricts vessel lumina and causes decreased blood flow in white matter. This change also impairs the clearing of toxins through the bloodstream and the glymphatic system, which results in irreversible white matter damage.[99] Atherosclerotic plaque formation is often associated with the large arteries in the circle of Willis, which can be identified using MR angiography, although the gold standard of diagnosis remains catheter angiography (**Fig. 11**).[101] Cerebral amyloid angiopathy is one of the mechanisms of aging. This change can make the blood vessels susceptible to rupture. Cerebral amyloid angiopathy first involves the occipital cortex, followed by the frontal, temporal, and parietal lobes.[102] Cerebral amyloid angiopathy is also associated with stroke and intracerebral hemorrhage.[103]

Lacunes and Microbleeds

Lacunes are 3- to 15-mm fluid-filled cavities commonly seen in the basal ganglia and white matter.[104] Lacunes can be seen on FLAIR as hypointense lesions with peripheral hyperintense rims (**Fig. 12**). They appear following small infarcts in the vicinity of perforating arterioles.[99] Lacunes in the white matter can develop in perfusion-compromised regions, whereas lacunes in the basal ganglia are likely caused by arterial occlusions.[105]

Microbleeds are small circular lesions commonly seen in the basal ganglia, thalamus, and white

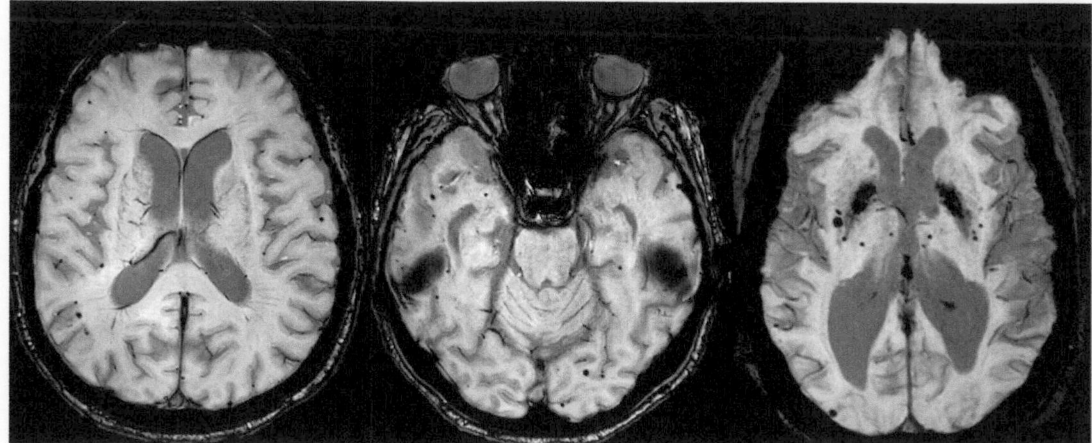

Fig. 13. SWI of a patient with cerebral amyloid angiopathy and a hypertensive patient. (*A, B*) SWI of a 72-year-old man shows punctate low signals in the lobar distribution, whereas (*C*) SWI of a 61-year-old hypertensive woman shows punctate low signals in the bilateral basal ganglia and thalami. Low signals in the globi pallidi represent mineral deposition.

matter, easily detected on susceptibility-weighted imaging (Fig. 13). They form upon rupture of blood vessels caused by vasculopathy or cerebral amyloid angiopathy.[106] Microbleeds in cerebral amyloid angiopathy are typically caused by vessel fragility and rupture and affect cortical and subcortical areas (so-called lobar locations) and the infratentorial regions. Microbleeds owing to hypertensive vasculopathy are caused by endothelial dysfunction and arterial remodeling, affecting the basal ganglia, pons, and cerebellar hemispheres.

SUMMARY

Normal brain aging is characterized by cortical thinning, gray and white matter volume loss, sulcal widening, and ventriculomegaly, which are tightly linked to age-related tissue-specific metabolic and microstructural changes. Structural, functional, and metabolic imaging enable qualitative and quantitative assessment of the aging brain. Age-related brain structural and functional changes are related to memory loss and cognitive decline. Integration of these imaging techniques enables a multiphysics approach to understanding aging mechanisms, early differentiation of normal aging from neurodegenerative diseases, and early treatment introduction.

CLINICS CARE POINTS

- Brain morphological changes related to aging are characterized by cortical thinning, gray and white matter volume loss, sulcal widening, and ventriculomegaly.
- Structural MRI can help evaluate age-related brain morphological and pathological changes.
- Functional and metabolic imaging can assess white matter fiber tract, brain connectivity, and neural activity.
- Aging mechanisms in gray matter, white matter, ventricular system, and vasculature are linked to tissue-specific metabolic and microstructural changes.

DISCLOSURE

The authors have nothing to disclose.

REFERENCES

1. MacDonald ME, Pike GB. MRI of healthy brain aging: a review. NMR Biomed 2021;34(9):e4564.
2. Blinkouskaya Y, Cacoilo A, Gollamudi T, et al. Brain aging mechanisms with mechanical manifestations. Mech Ageing Dev 2021;200:111575.
3. Dennis EL, Thompson PM. Functional brain connectivity using fMRI in aging and Alzheimer's disease. Neuropsychol Rev 2014;24(1):49–62.
4. Chen JJ. Functional MRI of brain physiology in aging and neurodegenerative diseases. Neuroimage 2019;187:209–25.
5. Lockhart SN, DeCarli C. Structural imaging measures of brain aging. Neuropsychol Rev 2014; 24(3):271–89.
6. Courchesne E, Chisum HJ, Townsend J, et al. Normal brain development and aging: quantitative analysis at in vivo MR imaging in healthy volunteers. Radiology 2000;216(3):672–82.
7. Pourhassan Shamchi S, Khosravi M, Taghvaei R, et al. Normal patterns of regional brain (18)F-FDG uptake in normal aging. Hell J Nucl Med 2018; 21(3):175–80.
8. Fischl B, Dale AM. Measuring the thickness of the human cerebral cortex from magnetic resonance images. Proc Natl Acad Sci U S A 2000;97(20): 11050–5.
9. Tang MY, Chen TW, Zhang XM, et al. GRE T2*-weighted MRI: principles and clinical applications. Biomed Res Int 2014;2014:312142.
10. Grajauskas LA, Guo H, D'Arcy RCN, et al. Toward MRI-based whole-brain health assessment: The brain atrophy and lesion index (BALI). Aging Med (Milton) 2018;1(1):55–63.
11. Guo H, Siu W, D'Arcy RC, et al. MRI assessment of whole-brain structural changes in aging. Clin Interv Aging 2017;12:1251–70.
12. Chen W, Song X, Zhang Y, et al. An MRI-based semi-quantitative index for the evaluation of brain atrophy and lesions in Alzheimer's disease, mild cognitive impairment and normal aging. Dement Geriatr Cogn Disord 2010;30(2): 121–30.
13. Guo H, Song X, Vandorpe R, et al. Evaluation of common structural brain changes in aging and Alzheimer disease with the use of an MRI-based brain atrophy and lesion index: a comparison between T1WI and T2WI at 1.5T and 3T. AJNR Am J Neuroradiol 2014;35(3):504–12.
14. Sullivan EV, Pfefferbaum A. Diffusion tensor imaging and aging. Neurosci Biobehav Rev 2006; 30(6):749–61.
15. Marner L, Nyengaard JR, Tang Y, et al. Marked loss of myelinated nerve fibers in the human brain with age. J Comp Neurol 2003;462(2):144–52.
16. Magistretti PJ. Cellular bases of functional brain imaging: insights from neuron-glia metabolic coupling. Published on the World Wide Web on 12 October 2000. Brain Res 2000;886(1–2): 108–12.

17. Meyer PT, Frings L, Rucker G, et al. 18)F-FDG PET in parkinsonism: differential diagnosis and evaluation of cognitive impairment. J Nucl Med 2017; 58(12):1888–98.
18. Ewers M, Brendel M, Rizk-Jackson A, et al. Reduced FDG-PET brain metabolism and executive function predict clinical progression in elderly healthy subjects. Neuroimage Clin 2014;4:45–52.
19. Lowe VJ, Wiste HJ, Senjem ML, et al. Widespread brain tau and its association with ageing, Braak stage and Alzheimer's dementia. Brain 2018; 141(1):271–87.
20. Madan CR, Kensinger EA. Cortical complexity as a measure of age-related brain atrophy. Neuroimage 2016;134:617–29.
21. Kochunov P, Mangin JF, Coyle T, et al. Age-related morphology trends of cortical sulci. Hum Brain Mapp 2005;26(3):210–20.
22. Coffey CE, Ratcliff G, Saxton JA, et al. Cognitive correlates of human brain aging: a quantitative magnetic resonance imaging investigation. J Neuropsychiatry Clin Neurosci 2001;13(4): 471–85.
23. Fjell AM, Walhovd KB. Structural brain changes in aging: courses, causes and cognitive consequences. Rev Neurosci 2010;21(3):187–221.
24. von Bartheld CS. Myths and truths about the cellular composition of the human brain: A review of influential concepts. J Chem Neuroanat 2018; 93:2–15.
25. Esiri MM. Ageing and the brain. J Pathol 2007; 211(2):181–7.
26. Castelli V, Benedetti E, Antonosante A, et al. Neuronal cells rearrangement during aging and neurodegenerative disease: metabolism, oxidative stress and organelles dynamic. Front Mol Neurosci 2019;12:132.
27. Dickstein DL, Weaver CM, Luebke JI, et al. Dendritic spine changes associated with normal aging. Neuroscience 2013;251:21–32.
28. Dickstein DL, Kabaso D, Rocher AB, et al. Changes in the structural complexity of the aged brain. Aging Cell 2007;6(3):275–84.
29. de Brabander JM, Kramers RJ, Uylings HB. Layer-specific dendritic regression of pyramidal cells with ageing in the human prefrontal cortex. Eur J Neurosci 1998;10(4):1261–9.
30. Mattson MP, Arumugam TV. Hallmarks of brain aging: adaptive and pathological modification by metabolic states. Cell Metab 2018;27(6):1176–99.
31. Grimm A, Eckert A. Brain aging and neurodegeneration: from a mitochondrial point of view. J Neurochem 2017;143(4):418–31.
32. Morozov YM, Datta D, Paspalas CD, et al. Ultrastructural evidence for impaired mitochondrial fission in the aged rhesus monkey dorsolateral prefrontal cortex. Neurobiol Aging 2017;51:9–18.
33. Camandola S, Mattson MP. Aberrant subcellular neuronal calcium regulation in aging and Alzheimer's disease. Biochim Biophys Acta 2011; 1813(5):965–73.
34. Ota Y, Capizzano AA, Moritani T, et al. Comprehensive review of Wernicke encephalopathy: pathophysiology, clinical symptoms and imaging findings. Jpn J Radiol 2020;38(9):809–20.
35. Liddelow SA, Guttenplan KA, Clarke LE, et al. Neurotoxic reactive astrocytes are induced by activated microglia. Nature 2017;541(7638): 481–7.
36. Clarke LE, Liddelow SA, Chakraborty C, et al. Normal aging induces A1-like astrocyte reactivity. Proc Natl Acad Sci U S A 2018;115(8):E1896–905.
37. Lull ME, Block ML. Microglial activation and chronic neurodegeneration. Neurotherapeutics 2010;7(4):354–65.
38. van Velsen EF, Vernooij MW, Vrooman HA, et al. Brain cortical thickness in the general elderly population: the Rotterdam Scan Study. Neurosci Lett 2013;550:189–94.
39. Fjell AM, Westlye LT, Grydeland H, et al. Accelerating cortical thinning: unique to dementia or universal in aging? Cereb Cortex 2014;24(4): 919–34.
40. Lemaitre H, Goldman AL, Sambataro F, et al. Normal age-related brain morphometric changes: nonuniformity across cortical thickness, surface area and gray matter volume? Neurobiol Aging 2012;33(3):617 e1-9.
41. Hasan KM, Mwangi B, Cao B, et al. Entorhinal Cortex Thickness across the Human Lifespan. J Neuroimaging 2016;26(3):278–82.
42. Sowell ER, Peterson BS, Kan E, et al. Sex differences in cortical thickness mapped in 176 healthy individuals between 7 and 87 years of age. Cereb Cortex 2007;17(7):1550–60.
43. Fotenos AF, Snyder AZ, Girton LE, et al. Normative estimates of cross-sectional and longitudinal brain volume decline in aging and AD. Neurology 2005; 64(6):1032–9.
44. Taki Y, Kinomura S, Sato K, et al. A longitudinal study of gray matter volume decline with age and modifying factors. Neurobiol Aging 2011;32(5): 907–15.
45. Anderson VM, Schott JM, Bartlett JW, et al. Gray matter atrophy rate as a marker of disease progression in AD. Neurobiol Aging 2012;33(7): 1194–202.
46. Geinisman Y, Detoledo-Morrell L, Morrell F, et al. Hippocampal markers of age-related memory dysfunction: behavioral, electrophysiological and morphological perspectives. Prog Neurobiol 1995;45(3):223–52.
47. Barnes J, Bartlett JW, van de Pol LA, et al. A meta-analysis of hippocampal atrophy rates in

Alzheimer's disease. Neurobiol Aging 2009;30(11):1711–23.

48. Narvacan K, Treit S, Camicioli R, et al. Evolution of deep gray matter volume across the human lifespan. Hum Brain Mapp 2017;38(8):3771–90.
49. Lemaitre H, Crivello F, Grassiot B, et al. Age- and sex-related effects on the neuroanatomy of healthy elderly. Neuroimage 2005;26(3):900–11.
50. Coelho A, Fernandes HM, Magalhaes R, et al. Signatures of white-matter microstructure degradation during aging and its association with cognitive status. Sci Rep 2021;11(1):4517.
51. Chen D, Huang Y, Shi Z, et al. Demyelinating processes in aging and stroke in the central nervous system and the prospect of treatment strategy. CNS Neurosci Ther 2020;26(12):1219–29.
52. Raj D, Yin Z, Breur M, et al. Increased White Matter Inflammation in Aging- and Alzheimer's Disease Brain. Front Mol Neurosci 2017;10:206.
53. Kalaria RN. Vascular basis for brain degeneration: faltering controls and risk factors for dementia. Nutr Rev 2010;68(Suppl 2):S74–87.
54. Duval T, Stikov N, Cohen-Adad J. Modeling white matter microstructure. Funct Neurol 2016;31(4):217–28.
55. Bennett IJ, Madden DJ. Disconnected aging: cerebral white matter integrity and age-related differences in cognition. Neuroscience 2014;276:187–205.
56. Maillard P, Fletcher E, Singh B, et al. Cerebral white matter free water: A sensitive biomarker of cognition and function. Neurology 2019;92(19):e2221–31.
57. Stahon KE, Bastian C, Griffith S, et al. Age-related changes in axonal and mitochondrial ultrastructure and function in white matter. J Neurosci 2016;36(39):9990–10001.
58. Basser PJ, Pierpaoli C. Microstructural and physiological features of tissues elucidated by quantitative-diffusion-tensor MRI. 1996. J Magn Reson 2011;213(2):560–70.
59. Solowij N, Zalesky A, Lorenzetti V, et al. Chronic Cannabis Use and Axonal Fiber Connectivity. Handbook Cannabis Relat Pathologies 2017;391–400.
60. Sexton CE, Walhovd KB, Storsve AB, et al. Accelerated changes in white matter microstructure during aging: a longitudinal diffusion tensor imaging study. J Neurosci 2014;34(46):15425–36.
61. Kumar R, Chavez AS, Macey PM, et al. Brain axial and radial diffusivity changes with age and gender in healthy adults. Brain Res 2013;1512:22–36.
62. Faizy TD, Thaler C, Broocks G, et al. The myelin water fraction serves as a marker for age-related myelin alterations in the cerebral white matter - a multiparametric MRI aging study. Front Neurosci 2020;14:136.
63. Yu X, Yin X, Hong H, et al. Increased extracellular fluid is associated with white matter fiber degeneration in CADASIL: in vivo evidence from diffusion magnetic resonance imaging. Fluids Barriers CNS 2021;18(1):29.
64. Norden DM, Godbout JP. Review: microglia of the aged brain: primed to be activated and resistant to regulation. Neuropathol Appl Neurobiol 2013;39(1):19–34.
65. Simpson JE, Wharton SB, Cooper J, et al. Alterations of the blood-brain barrier in cerebral white matter lesions in the ageing brain. Neurosci Lett 2010;486(3):246–51.
66. Maillard P, Mitchell GF, Himali JJ, et al. Aortic Stiffness, Increased White Matter Free Water, and Altered Microstructural Integrity: A Continuum of Injury. Stroke 2017;48(6):1567–73.
67. Salzer JL, Zalc B. Myelination. Curr Biol 2016;26(20):R971–5.
68. Weickenmeier J, de Rooij R, Budday S, et al. Brain stiffness increases with myelin content. Acta Biomater 2016;42:265–72.
69. Callaghan MF, Freund P, Draganski B, et al. Widespread age-related differences in the human brain microstructure revealed by quantitative magnetic resonance imaging. Neurobiol Aging 2014;35(8):1862–72.
70. Bartzokis G. Age-related myelin breakdown: a developmental model of cognitive decline and Alzheimer's disease. Neurobiol Aging 2004;25(1):5–18 [author reply: 49-62].
71. Lassmann H. Classification of demyelinating diseases at the interface between etiology and pathogenesis. Curr Opin Neurol 2001;14(3):253–8.
72. Wen W, Sachdev P. The topography of white matter hyperintensities on brain MRI in healthy 60- to 64-year-old individuals. Neuroimage 2004;22(1):144–54.
73. Wardlaw JM, Valdes Hernandez MC, Munoz-Maniega S. What are white matter hyperintensities made of? Relevance to vascular cognitive impairment. J Am Heart Assoc 2015;4(6):001140.
74. Wardlaw JM, Smith C, Dichgans M. Small vessel disease: mechanisms and clinical implications. Lancet Neurol 2019;18(7):684–96.
75. Chen J, Mikheev AV, Yu H, et al. Bilateral distance partition of periventricular and deep white matter hyperintensities: performance of the method in the aging brain. Acad Radiol 2021;28(12):1699–708.
76. Todd KL, Brighton T, Norton ES, et al. Ventricular and Periventricular Anomalies in the Aging and Cognitively Impaired Brain. Front Aging Neurosci 2017;9:445.
77. Griffanti L, Jenkinson M, Suri S, et al. Classification and characterization of periventricular and deep

white matter hyperintensities on MRI: a study in older adults. Neuroimage 2018;170:174–81.

78. Schmidt R, Ropele S, Enzinger C, et al. White matter lesion progression, brain atrophy, and cognitive decline: the Austrian stroke prevention study. Ann Neurol 2005;58(4):610–6.
79. Fazekas F, Chawluk JB, Alavi A, et al. MR signal abnormalities at 1.5 T in Alzheimer's dementia and normal aging. AJR Am J Roentgenol 1987; 149(2):351–6.
80. Jimenez AJ, Dominguez-Pinos MD, Guerra MM, et al. Structure and function of the ependymal barrier and diseases associated with ependyma disruption. Tissue Barriers 2014;2:e28426.
81. Liu H, Yang Y, Xia Y, et al. Aging of cerebral white matter. Ageing Res Rev 2017;34:64–76.
82. Gunning-Dixon FM, Brickman AM, Cheng JC, et al. Aging of cerebral white matter: a review of MRI findings. Int J Geriatr Psychiatry 2009;24(2): 109–17.
83. Allen JS, Bruss J, Brown CK, et al. Normal neuroanatomical variation due to age: the major lobes and a parcellation of the temporal region. Neurobiol Aging 2005;26(9):1245–60 [discussion: 1279-82].
84. Salat DH, Greve DN, Pacheco JL, et al. Regional white matter volume differences in nondemented aging and Alzheimer's disease. Neuroimage 2009;44(4):1247–58.
85. Resnick SM, Pham DL, Kraut MA, et al. Longitudinal magnetic resonance imaging studies of older adults: a shrinking brain. J Neurosci 2003;23(8): 3295–301.
86. Lebel C, Gee M, Camicioli R, et al. Diffusion tensor imaging of white matter tract evolution over the lifespan. Neuroimage 2012;60(1):340–52.
87. Aso T, Sugihara G, Murai T, et al. A venous mechanism of ventriculomegaly shared between traumatic brain injury and normal ageing. Brain 2020; 143(6):1843–56.
88. Ota Y, Srinivasan A, Capizzano AA, et al. Central nervous system systemic lupus erythematosus: pathophysiologic, clinical, and imaging features. Radiographics 2022;42(1):212–32.
89. Shook BA, Lennington JB, Acabchuk RL, et al. Ventriculomegaly associated with ependymal gliosis and declines in barrier integrity in the aging human and mouse brain. Aging Cell 2014;13(2):340–50.
90. Meunier A., Sawamoto K. and Spassky N., Rubenstein J, Rakic P, Chen B, Kwan KY, (Editors), Ependyma, Ependyma. Patterning and cell type Specification in the developing CNS and PNS, Second, 2020, Academic Press, 1021–1036.
91. Acabchuk RL, Sun Y, Wolferz R Jr, et al. 3D Modeling of the Lateral Ventricles and Histological Characterization of Periventricular Tissue in Humans and Mouse. J Vis Exp 2015;99:e52328.
92. Serot JM, Bene MC, Faure GC. Choroid plexus, aging of the brain, and Alzheimer's disease. Front Biosci 2003;8:s515–21.
93. Redzic ZB, Preston JE, Duncan JA, et al. The choroid plexus-cerebrospinal fluid system: from development to aging. Curr Top Dev Biol 2005; 71:1–52.
94. Breteler MM, van Amerongen NM, van Swieten JC, et al. Cognitive correlates of ventricular enlargement and cerebral white matter lesions on magnetic resonance imaging. Rotterdam Study *Stroke* 1994;25(6):1109–15.
95. Nagata K, Basugi N, Fukushima T, et al. A quantitative study of physiological cerebral atrophy with aging. A statistical analysis of the normal range. Neuroradiology 1987;29(4):327–32.
96. Resnick SM, Goldszal AF, Davatzikos C, et al. One-year age changes in MRI brain volumes in older adults. Cereb Cortex 2000;10(5):464–72.
97. Lin CH, Cheng HM, Chuang SY, et al. Vascular aging and cognitive dysfunction: silent midlife crisis in the brain. Pulse (Basel) 2018;5(1–4):127–32.
98. Watanabe C, Imaizumi T, Kawai H, et al. Aging of the vascular system and neural diseases. Front Aging Neurosci 2020;12:557384.
99. Ter Telgte A, van Leijsen EMC, Wiegertjes K, et al. Cerebral small vessel disease: from a focal to a global perspective. Nat Rev Neurol 2018;14(7): 387–98.
100. Shim YS, Yang DW, Roe CM, et al. Pathological correlates of white matter hyperintensities on magnetic resonance imaging. Dement Geriatr Cogn Disord 2015;39(1–2):92–104.
101. Qureshi AI, Feldmann E, Gomez CR, et al. Intracranial atherosclerotic disease: an update. Ann Neurol 2009;66(6):730–8.
102. Magaki S, Tang Z, Tung S, et al. The effects of cerebral amyloid angiopathy on integrity of the blood-brain barrier. Neurobiol Aging 2018;70:70–7.
103. Weller RO, Nicoll JA. Cerebral amyloid angiopathy: pathogenesis and effects on the aging and Alzheimer brain. Neurol Res 2003;25(6):611–6.
104. Benjamin P, Trippier S, Lawrence AJ, et al. Lacunar infarcts, but not perivascular spaces, are predictors of cognitive decline in cerebral small-vessel disease. Stroke 2018;49(3):586–93.
105. Gouw AA, van der Flier WM, Pantoni L, et al. On the etiology of incident brain lacunes: longitudinal observations from the LADIS study. Stroke 2008; 39(11):3083–5.
106. Martinez-Ramirez S, Greenberg SM, Viswanathan A. Cerebral microbleeds: overview and implications in cognitive impairment. Alzheimers Res Ther 2014;6(3):33.

Printed and bound by CPI Group (UK) Ltd, Croydon, CR0 4YY
03/10/2024
01040307-0003